国家中医药管理局中医药国际合作专项项目（项目编号：1601500000027-10）

——"一带一路"中医药国际教育培训基地教材丛书

A Special Project of International Cooperation on Traditional Chinese Medicine of the State Administration of Traditional Chinese Medicine（NO. 1601500000027-10）

——A Series of Textbook of the "B&R" TCM International Educational Training Center

名医大讲堂

——临床疑难杂病的中医药辨证论治

Lecture Room for Famous Doctors

TCM Differentiation of Clinical Rare and Miscellaneous Diseases

主编　应森林　主审　张伯礼

中国健康传媒集团

中国医药科技出版社

内 容 提 要

本书精选了慢性阻塞性肺疾病、慢性心力衰竭、类风湿关节炎等 12 种临床常见病及难治病进行了详细论述，既有西医病因诊断，也有中医辨证论治；既有常规治疗方法，也有名家验案分析，以中英双语的形式，旨在为海内外的中医药学者及临床从业人员提供可借鉴的中医药学习资源，对临床实践有所裨益。

图书在版编目（CIP）数据

名医大讲堂 . 临床疑难杂病的中医药辨证论治 / 应森林主编 . — 北京：中国医药科技出版社，2018.9
（"一带一路"中医药国际教育培训基地教材丛书）
ISBN 978-7-5214-0310-7

Ⅰ. ①名…　Ⅱ. ①应…　Ⅲ. ①疑难病—辨证论治—教材　Ⅳ. ① R2

中国版本图书馆 CIP 数据核字（2018）第 105565 号

美术编辑　陈君杞
版式设计　也　在

出版　**中国健康传媒集团** ｜ 中国医药科技出版社
地址　北京市海淀区文慧园北路甲 22 号
邮编　100082
电话　发行：010-62227427　　邮购：010-62236938
网址　www.cmstp.com
规格　$889 \times 1194mm\ ^{1}/_{16}$
印张　24¼
字数　561 千字
版次　2018 年 9 月第 1 版
印次　2018 年 9 月第 1 次印刷
印刷　三河市百盛印装有限公司
经销　全国各地新华书店
书号　ISBN 978-7-5214-0310-7
定价　**69.00 元**

国家中医药管理局中医药国际合作专项项目
——"一带一路"中医药国际教育培训基地教材丛书

A Special Project of International Cooperation on Traditional Chinese Medicine of the State
Administration of Traditional Chinese Medicine
—— A Series of Textbooks of the "B&R" TCM International Educational Training Center

主　审　张伯礼

Chief Proofreader: ZHANG Boli

总主编　李庆和　高秀梅

General Chief Editor: LI Qinghe ,GAO Xiumei

总编委（按姓氏笔画排序）

王丽莉　刘　刚　李　欣　李海南　应森林　张　杰
张　岩　张艳娜　金　军　郑　毅　聂静怡　徐　立
高　睿　储利荣　潘　淼

Chief Editorial Board Member (Names in strokes order)

WANG Lili, LIU Gang, LI Xin, LI Hainan, YING Senlin, ZHANG Jie,
ZHANG Yan, ZHANG Yanna, JIN Jun, ZHENG Yi, NIE Jingyi, XU Li,
GAO Rui, CHU Lirong, PAN Miao

名医大讲堂——临床疑难杂病的中医药辨证论治
Lecture Room for Famous Doctors
TCM Differentiation of Clinical Rare and Miscellaneous Diseases

主 编 应森林

Managing Editor: YING Senlin

副主编 储利荣 潘 淼

Associate Managing Editors: CHU Lirong, PAN Miao

编 委（按姓氏笔画排序）

于春泉 王 卫 孙中堂 邢淑丽 杜武勋 李桂兰

李新民 应森林 陆小左 罗美玉 孟静岩 徐 立

Chief Editorial Board Member (Names in strokes order)

YU Chunquan, WANG Wei, SUN Zhongtang, XING Shuli, DU Wuxun, LI Guilan,

LI Xinmin, YING Senlin, LU Xiaozuo, LUO Meiyu, MENG Jingyan, XU Li

校 译

刘 刚 李 鹏 郭 勖 张 颖

施 琪 李玲玲 陈彦竹 马娇阳

English Proofreaders

LIU Gang, LI Peng, Guo Xu, ZHANG Ying,

SHI Qi, LI Lingling, CHEN Yanzhu, MA Jiaoyang

序一

由天津中医药大学组织编写的《"一带一路"中医药国际教育培训基地教材丛书》即将出版，可喜可贺。

中医药自古以来就是古丝绸之路沿线国家交流合作的重要内容，并以不同形态成为沿线民众共享共建的卫生资源。随着健康观念和医学模式的转变，中医"治未病"的思想，天人合一、心身并重的整体观，以及在防治常见病、多发病、慢性病及重大传染性疾病中的确切作用日益得到国际社会的认可。屠呦呦研究员因发现青蒿素获得2015年诺贝尔生理学或医学奖、中医针灸列入联合国教科文组织"人类非物质文化遗产代表作名录"、《本草纲目》和《黄帝内经》入选"世界记忆名录"，无不体现了中医药在国际医学体系中的重要地位。目前中医药已传播到183个国家和地区，正为促进人类健康发挥着积极作用。

为推进中医药"一带一路"建设，加强与"一带一路"沿线国家在中医药领域的交流与合作，我局于2015年设立中医药国际合作专项项目，天津中医药大学作为首批建设单位积极承担了"'一带一路'中医药国际教育培训基地建设"项目，并勇于开拓，不断创新，在中医药国际教育诸多领域进行了有益尝试，组织了《世界中医教育核心教材》编写工作，开展了"一带一路"中医师资培训系统建设工作，在泰国、日本建立了中医孔子学院、孔子课堂，开展了中医药普及教学和中医体验工作，取得了较好效果。此套丛书也是成果之一，内容涉及中医药理论方法、医疗康复、中医养生、中医药膳、中医文化等诸多方面。内容深入浅出，通俗易懂，适合大众阅读；理论联系实际，可操作性强，具有实用性。

中医药凝聚着中华民族传统文化的精华，是中华文明与"一带一路"沿线国家人文交流的重要内容，希望丛书的出版，为沿线国家医疗、教育、文化的可持续发展提供借鉴参考，进一步促进与沿线国家的民心相通，为维护人类健康做出新的贡献。

国家中医药管理局

局长 于文明

2018 年 7 月 16 日

Prologue1

It is a congratulatory event The Series of Textbooks for "B&R" International Education and Training Base on TCM, compiled by Tianjin University of Traditional Chinese Medicine, is about to be published.

TCM has long been a significant content of communication and cooperation among the countries along the ancient Silk Road and has been the sharing of the co-construction of health resources for the peoples along the route in different forms. With the change of health concept and medical model, the TCM idea of preventive treatment of disease, the holistic view of integration of human and heaven and emphasis of both body and mind and its definite functions of prevention and cure of common, frequently-occurring, chronic and severe infectious diseases have been increasingly accepted. The discovery of artemisinin by Ms. TU Youyou won the Nobel Prize in Physiology or Medicine in 2015; TCM acupuncture and moxibustion have been enlisted in representative list of the intangible cultural heritage of humanity by UNESCO; and, Compendium of Materia Medica and The Inner Canon of Huangdi have been enlisted in the Memory of the World Register. All these have indicated invariably the significant position of TCM in the world medical system. At present, TCM has been spread to 183 countries and regions and is playing an active role in improving human's health.

In order to push forward the construction of "B&R" and enhance the communication and cooperation on TCM with the countries along B&R, our administration set up a special project of TCM international cooperation in 2015, in which Tianjin University of Traditional Chinese Medicine was assigned as the first institution undertaking "the Construction of TCM International Education and Training Center of 'B&R'" . Tianjin University of Traditional Chinese Medicine (TUTCM) has been endeavoring to explore and make innovations. The university has tried in many aspects of TCM international education, organized the compiled work of The Core Teaching Material of the World TCM, carried out the construction of "B&R" TCM Teacher Training System, set up a TCM Confucius Institute in Thailand and a Confucius classroom in Japan, and unfolded the TCM popularizing, training and experiencing. Their efforts have made achievements. The series of textbooks is one of the outcomes containing TCM theoretical method, medical recovery, regimen, medicated diet, TCM culture and etc. Explaining the profound in simple terms and easy-to-understand language, linking theory with applications, the books are suitable for common readers, operative and practical.

TCM, cohering the essence of traditional Chinese culture, has been an important content of communication between Chinese civilization and the countries along the "B&R". The publication of the series is hopefully to be reference for those countries to their sustainable development of medical treatment, education and culture and further more to make contribution in improving the friendship and maintaining human health in those countries.

YU Wenming

Director-General State Administration of Traditional Chinese Medicine of the PRC

July 16, 2018

序二

国粹医药，博大精深，仁医国术，唯我特有，佑我华夏，泽被他国，福祉大众，成就非凡。

《医学三字经》云："医之始，本岐黄，灵枢作，素问详，难经出，更洋洋，越汉季，有南阳，六经辨，圣道彰，伤寒着，金匮藏，垂方法，立津梁……"浩如烟海的中医古籍，敬畏已久的先贤圣医，效如桴鼓的临证医案，怎会不让人心驰神往？！

古往今来，名医辈出，先贤们以前无古人的勇气探索试验，以高尚的医德悬壶济世，以高超的医术救死扶伤，赢得了世人的尊敬和青睐，并把数千年之精髓流传至今，其医理之独特、疗效之神奇、方法之简便，深受各国患者喜爱，为世人争先习之。我大学积极响应国家"一带一路"倡议，携数十年中医药对外教育交流经验，以中医药在丝绸之路上发扬光大为己任，以国家中医药管理局国际合作项目为依托，成立了"一带一路中医药国际教育培训基地"，为更多的国家培养中医药人才提供高标准的教育和师资培训，让各国民众有机会享受真正中医药的魅力。

本书作为"一带一路中医药国际教育培训基地"配套系列教材之一，特别邀请了来自天津中医药大学及其附属医院的十二位中医名家担任编者，这些专家均活跃在国际中医药教育第一线，承担大学国际学生中医药教育，国外研修者培训，并赴国外讲授中医药，教学与临床经验俱丰。他们将各自擅长治疗病种的临床、教学经验和研究领域做一总结，实践心得与中外学者分享，同系中医缘，共筑中医梦。本书精选了中风、失眠、糖尿病等十二种临床常见病及难治病进行了详细论述，既有西医病因诊断，也有中医辨证论治；既有常规治疗方法，也有名家验案分析，以中英双语的形式，旨在通过"一带一路中医药国际教育培训"，为海内外的中医药学者及临床从业人员提供可借鉴的中医药学习经验，对临床实践有所裨益。此夙愿，如能实现，也不枉编者一番心血。

开卷有益。"问渠哪得清如许，为有源头活水来"，品读中医，需要一种溯本求源的执着；

掩卷冥思。"纸上得来终觉浅，绝知此事要躬行"，践行中医，需要一种不懈临证的坚持。

从温故知新到豁然开朗，中医的漫漫长路需要一代代海内外中医人的继往开来。

中医药源于中国，但终将福泽世界。乐为之序。

中国工程院院士

中国中医科学院院长　张伯礼

天津中医药大学校长

戊戌年初夏于津门

Prologue 2

Traditional Chinese Medicine (TCM) is of long standing history, extensive and profound intensions. It has been blessing and protecting the multiplication and growth of the Chinese people from generation to generation in the past, and been beneficial to the neighboring countries and has made extraordinary achievement.

In the Three-character Medical Verses, it says: "The medical skill started from Emperor Xuanyuan and his minister of Qibo when Lingshu and Suwen were compiled in details. The emergence of Classics on Medical Problems has greatly enriched TCM. In the late Eastern Han Dynasty, a doctor in Nanyang proposed the theory of Syndrome-Differentiation of the Six Meridians on the basis of theory of Internal Classic which made a further development in the theory of TCM in his two books-Febrile Diseases and Golden Chamber which were handed down to the present and have set up the standards for syndrome differentiation and treatment in diagnoses and treatment for doctors in later ages. It has become the only way which must be passed in studying medicine, just like ferry and bridge······" These Chinese medical books are as vast as the open sea, and those admirable sages and holy doctors, clinic guidelines and medical records with instant effects are just like beacon lights leaving endless dreams for those who are exploring in the medical field with fervent love.

The TCM doctors of all ages, with unprecedented courage to discover, experiment and practice in order to help the people with magnificent virtue, heal the wounded and rescue the dying with superb skills, have won respects and favors among common people, and have handed down the essence of medicine accumulated in the past thousands of years of to benefit the descendants. With unique medical thoughts, magnificent effects and easy means, it is loved by various foreign patients and trusted by more and more foreign students. Taking TCM generalization in the Silk Road as our own duty and in response of the state Belt & Road appeal, with decades of experience in TCM international education and duty of, our university has established the Belt and Road TCM International Educational Training Center under the State Administration of Traditional Chinese Medicine cooperative project to provide a high standard TCM education and training for more countries. So the common people in the respective countries may have the opportunity to experience the charm of real TCM.

The book has been appointed as one of the serial textbooks for the the Belt and Road TCM International Educational Training Center and the editor of this book invited 12 famous TCM doctors acting as editors from TUTCM and its affiliated hospitals. These experts have rich teaching and clinical experience and have been working actively on the front line of TCM international education, taking up the TCM education for international students of the university and training for scholars both domestic and overseas. They have summarized clinical and teaching experience in treating various diseases as well as their own specialized fields and shared that practical experience with readers worldwide. Bonded by TCM and a dream dreamt by all practitioners, this bilingual book has specially selected 12 common and rare diseases to discuss in details, integrating with etiological diagnosis of western medicine, TCM syndrome differentiation and treatment, conventional therapies and famous doctors with case analysis. It aims at providing advisable TCM study materials for TCM scholars and clinical practitioners in the world through the Training for Belt & Road TCM International Education. It is very helpful for clinical practice. If this long-cherished wish can be achieved, the efforts of the editors are not in vain.

Reading enriches the mind. "Why the pond is deep and clear, it is because it has water source providing constantly, so it never dries up." Studying TCM requires a kind of persistence to trace the source.

Thinking comes after a book. "Everything can only be done with profoundly understanding of the theories." Practicing TCM calls for indomitable persistence.

A suddenly enlightenment is followed by reviewing what have been learned. The course of TCM is a long journey and it is calling all the TCM practitioners of generations to carry forward the cause pioneered by our predecessors and forge ahead into the future.

TCM is derived from China but will benefit the world eventually.

ZHANG Boli

Academician of China Academy of Engineering

President of China Academy of Chinese Medical Science

President of Tianjin University of Traditional Chinese Medicine

Early summer of 2018, Tianjin

前言

　　中医药作为中国独特的卫生资源、潜力巨大的经济资源、具有原创优势的科技资源、优秀的文化资源和重要的生态资源，在经济社会发展的全局中有着重要意义，在世界卫生保健事业中起着重要作用。

　　天津中医药大学作为国家中医药管理局首批中医药国际合作专项建设单位，积极推进中医药在世界范围内的普及和发展。本丛书的出版，为落实国家"一带一路"重大发展倡议，以实现促进中医药的国际化发展，弘扬中华优秀文化，培育更多的中医药从业人员和爱好者，为应用中医药知识方法、预防保健、医疗康复服务，为实现人人享有基本医疗保健的宗旨贡献力量。丛书依托天津中医药大学中医药国际教育培训基地，组织中医药领域专家、学者共同编写，内容涉及中医药理论方法、医疗康复、中医养生、中医药膳、中医文化等诸多方面，内容深入浅出，通俗易懂。旨在为海内外中医药领域学者，以及教育、医疗、科研等相关人员和中医药爱好者提供学习参考。

　　我们衷心希望这套丛书能够成为世界各国中医药爱好者和从业人员了解中医药、学习中医药、使用中医药、传播中医药的工具和载体，弘扬中医药这一中国文化瑰宝，造福世界人民。

天津中医药大学
"一带一路"中医药国际教育培训教材丛书编委会
2018 年 3 月 18 日

Preface

Traditional Chinese medicine (TCM), as a featured health resource in China, it is of great economic potential, of inherent advantage of science and technology, of excellent culture and of ecologic importance, and it plays a significant role in the overall economic and social development as well as in world's hygiene and health care.

As one of the special construction units first approved by State Administration of Traditional Chinese Medicine (SATCM) for TCM international cooperation, Tianjin University of Traditional Chinese Medicine (TUTCM) has engaged herself in boosting worldwide popularization and development of TCM ever since. The publication of the series is a dedication in implementing the state initiative policy of "The Belt and Road (B&R)" to the promotion of the internationalization of TCM; to the development and expansion of the excellent Chinese culture; to the application of TCM in disease prevention, healthcare and rehabilitation; and to the realization of the objective of an overall basic healthcare. This set of books is compiled by experts and scholars in the field taking the advantage of the TCM International Education and Training Center of TUTCM and published particularly in compliance with the development strategy of "B&R" to reach the high-level goal of promoting TCM international development by education. This set of books covers the contents of TCM theories, medical rehabilitation, TCM health preservation, medicated diet, TCM culture and etc., which will be study and research reference for TCM scholars, amateurs and those who are concerning TCM education, treatment, research and etc. at home and abroad.

It is our sincere hope that this series of books can become the very tool and carrier by which TCM amateurs and practitioners worldwide could understand, study, use and generalize TCM, and carry forward the gem of Chinese culture – Traditional Chinese Medicine and bring benefits to people around the world.

Editorial Board of "B&R" Textbooks on TCM International Educational Training

Tianjin University of Traditional Chinese Medicine

March 18, 2018

目 录
Content

慢性阻塞性肺疾病

Chronic Obstructive Pulmonary Disease

一、概述

慢性阻塞性肺疾病（Chronic Obstructive Pulmonary Disease，COPD）是一种以持续气流受限为特征的可以预防和治疗的疾病。气流受限进行性发展，与气道和肺组织对烟草烟雾等有害气体或有害颗粒的慢性炎性反应增强有关，急性加重和并发症影响着疾病的严重程度和个体的预后。慢性炎性反应可以导致肺实质破坏（引起肺气肿），同时破坏正常的修复和防御机制（导致小气道纤维化）。COPD 的临床表现包括呼吸困难、慢性咳嗽、慢性咳痰、喘息和胸闷，上述症状可出现急性加重。COPD 多属于中医学的"咳嗽""喘病""肺胀"等范畴。

二、病因病机

（一）病因

1. 中医

（1）外邪侵袭：外感风寒，侵袭于肺，外阻皮毛，内遏于肺，肺气不宣，气机壅阻，发为咳喘；若素体肺热炽盛，或表邪未解，内已化热，则见外寒内热，热不得泄，肺失宣降，亦可发为咳喘；风热袭肺，肺气壅滞，升降失司，亦发为咳喘；热邪伤津液，聚而成痰，壅阻气机，发为喘咳。

（2）饮食不当：恣食生冷，寒饮内停，嗜食肥甘厚味，积痰生热，嗜酒无度或食海膻发物，导致脾失健运，痰湿内停，上犯于肺，阻遏肺气，气道失利，发为本病。

（3）久病体虚：长期呼吸困难、慢性咳嗽、慢性咳痰等病症，迁延不愈，久病体虚，肺虚卫外不固，外邪易袭，诱使本病发作，病情加重。金水相生，肺虚日久，不能下荫于肾，肾亦亏虚，肾不纳气而短气喘促，《景岳全书》说："五脏所伤，穷必及肾。"子病及母或素体脾虚，脾失健运，湿浊不化，聚而为痰，痰湿阻遏于肺，肺失宣降，诱发本病。

2. 西医

（1）吸烟：吸烟为重要的发病因素，吸烟者慢性支气管炎的患病率比不吸烟者高 2~8 倍，烟龄越长，吸烟量越大，COPD 患病率越高。烟草中含焦油、尼古丁和氢氰酸等化学物质，可损伤气道上皮细胞和纤毛运动，使气道净化能力下降；促使支气管黏液腺和杯状细胞增生肥大，黏液分泌增多；刺激副交感神经而使支气管平滑肌收缩，气道阻力增加；使氧自由基产生增多，诱导中性粒细胞释放蛋白酶，破坏肺弹力纤维，诱发肺气肿形成。

（2）职业性粉尘和化学物质：接触职业性粉尘及化学物质，如烟雾、变应原、工业废气及室内空气污染等，浓度过大或接触时间过长，均可能产生与吸烟无关的 COPD。

（3）空气污染：大气中的有害气体如二氧化硫、二氧化氮、氯气等可损伤气道黏膜上皮，使纤毛清除功能下降，黏液分泌增加，为细菌感染增加条件。

（4）感染：感染是 COPD 发生发展的重要因素之一。病毒、细菌和支原体是本病急性加重的重要因素。病毒主要为流感病毒、鼻病毒、腺病毒和呼吸道合胞病毒等；细菌感染常继发于病毒感染，常见病原体以肺炎链球菌、流感嗜血杆菌、卡他莫拉菌及葡萄球菌为多见。

（5）其他：免疫功能紊乱、气道高反应性、年龄增大等机体因素和气候等环境因素均与此病的发生和发展有关。如老年人肾上腺皮质功能减退，细胞免疫功能下降，溶菌酶活性降低，从而容易造成呼吸道的反复感染。寒冷空气可以刺激腺体增加黏液分泌，纤毛运动减弱，黏膜血管收缩，局部血循环障碍，可导致继发感染。

（二）病机

1. 中医

慢性阻塞性肺疾病是由于慢性肺系疾患病史多年，反复发作，迁延不愈，失治误治所引发，病变部位主要在肺，继则影响脾、肾功能。同样脾或肾功能失常，亦可引起肺失宣降，发为喘咳。

肺主气，司呼吸，开窍于鼻，在体合皮，其华在毛，与天气直接相通，故外邪从口鼻、皮毛入侵，大多首先犯肺。又因肺居高位，为其他脏腑之华盖，且为百脉所朝，故而其他脏腑之病变，易于上及于肺。无论外感还是内伤或者他脏病变，多易袭或者累及于肺，导致肺气宣降不利，上逆而为咳，升降失常则为喘，久则肺虚，主气功能失常。

肾为先天之本，主水，主纳气。因此，人体呼吸之气虽为肺所主，但其根在肾，故有"肺为气之主，肾为气之根"之说，肺与肾的关系称为金水相生，二者协调调节呼吸运动。如果肺气久虚，伤及肾气，而致肾不纳气，或者肾的精气不足，摄纳无权，气浮于上，均可出现喘咳、动则尤甚等症状。

脾为后天之本，气血生化之源，水谷之气的输布依赖于肺气宣降作用，久病肺虚，即子盗母气，导致脾失健运，出现肢倦乏力、食少便溏、形体消瘦、面色萎黄等症状。若脾失健运，水湿不化，凝聚而为痰饮，痰饮阻碍肺的气机，亦可出现咳喘等症状，因此有"脾为生痰之源，肺为贮痰之器"之说。

慢性阻塞性肺疾病的病理性质有虚实之分，实者主要在肺，外邪侵袭，或者痰浊壅阻，导致肺气宣降不利。虚者责之肺、脾、肾三脏，尤以气虚为主，脾失健运，肾失摄纳，均可引起肺失宣降。虚者复感外邪，或实者久病伤正，由肺及脾、肾，则病情表现虚实错杂。

慢性阻塞性肺疾病主要的病理产物为痰饮、瘀血。痰的产生，最初责之肺气的升降失常，气机不利，又肺为水之上源，肺通调水道功能失司，水液不行停聚为痰；肺病及脾，子耗母气，脾失健运，内湿由生，聚而为痰。慢性阻塞性肺疾病患者久病喘咳，肺气虚损，不能贯心而朝百脉，无力助血运行则血行瘀滞，出现瘀血。痰浊、瘀血相互夹杂，导致疾病更加缠绵难愈。

慢性阻塞性肺疾病是一种长期反复发作、时轻时重、缠绵难愈的疾病，尤其多见于中老年及久病体弱患者，由于素体正气不足，且脏腑功能渐衰，因此难以根治。若临床出现因虚引起的阴阳离决、孤阳浮越、冲气上逆，或者因实引起的邪气闭肺、胸闷如窒、呼吸窘迫等，均属于危重征象，必须及时救治。

2. 西医

（1）炎症机制：气道、肺实质及肺血管的慢性炎症是慢性阻塞性肺疾病的特征性改变，中性粒细胞、巨噬细胞、T淋巴细胞等炎症细胞均参与了慢性阻塞性肺疾病的发病过程。中性粒细胞的活化和聚集是慢性阻塞性肺疾病炎症过程的一个重要环节，通过释放中性粒细胞弹性蛋白酶等多种生物活性物质引起慢性黏液高分泌状态并破坏肺实质。

（2）蛋白酶－抗蛋白酶失衡机制：蛋白水解酶对组织有损伤、破坏作用；抗蛋白酶对弹性蛋白酶等多种蛋白酶具有抑制功能，其中 α_1-抗胰蛋白酶（α_1-AT）是活性最强的一种。蛋白酶和抗蛋白酶维持平衡是保证肺组织正常结构免受损伤和破坏的主要因素，蛋白酶增多或抗蛋白酶不足均可导致组织结构破坏，产生肺气肿。

（3）氧化应激机制：许多研究表明慢性阻塞性肺疾病患者的氧化应激增加。氧化物主要有超氧阴离子、次氯酸和一氧化氮等。氧化物可直接作用并破坏许多生化大分子如蛋白质、脂质和核酸等，导致细胞功能障碍或细胞死亡，还可以破坏细胞外基质；引起蛋白酶-抗蛋白酶失衡；促进炎症反应，如激活核因子 NF-κB，参与多种炎症介质的转录，如白细胞介素 8（IL-8）、肿瘤坏死因子 α（TNF-α）以及诱导型一氧化氮合酶（NOS）和环氧化物酶等的转录。

（4）其他机制：如自主神经功能失调、营养不良、气温变化等都有可能参与慢性阻塞性肺疾病的发生发展。

上述炎症机制、蛋白酶-抗蛋白酶失衡机制、氧化应激机制以及自主神经功能失调等共同作用，产生两种重要病变：①小气道病变，包括小气道炎症、小气道纤维组织形成、小气道管腔黏液栓等，使小气道阻力明显升高。②肺气肿病变，使肺泡对小气道的正常牵拉力减小，小气道较易塌陷；同时，肺气肿使肺泡弹性回缩力明显降低。这种小气道病变与肺气肿病变共同作用，造成慢性阻塞性肺疾病特征性的持续气流受限。

三、诊断要点与鉴别诊断

（一）诊断要点

（1）有慢性肺系疾患病史多年，反复发作，缠绵难愈，时轻时重。

（2）临床以呼吸困难、咳嗽、咳痰为主要表现。可见张口抬肩、鼻翼煽动、胸中满闷、喘息、动则加剧、咳嗽剧烈痰多等表现。

（3）常因外感而诱发，情志刺激或者劳倦过度也可诱发。

（4）肺功能检查见持续气流受限是慢性阻塞性肺疾病诊断的必备条件，吸入支气管扩张剂后 $FEV_1/FVC<0.70$ 为确定存在持续气流受限的界限。

（二）鉴别诊断

1. 慢性阻塞性肺疾病与咳嗽的鉴别

咳嗽仅仅以咳嗽为主要表现，不伴有呼吸困难；慢性阻塞性肺疾病往往咳、痰、喘并见，反复发作，时轻时重，常因久咳反复发作引起。

2. 慢性阻塞性肺疾病与哮病的鉴别

哮病亦可见呼吸困难、咳嗽、咳痰的症状，大多由慢性咳嗽经久不愈，逐渐加重而成咳喘，病情时轻时重，与慢性阻塞性肺疾病的区别在于：哮病间歇发作，突然起病，迅速缓解，喉中哮鸣有声，轻度咳嗽或不咳。

四、中医治疗

（一）辨证治疗

1. 风邪袭肺

主症： 咳嗽，喘息，痰白清稀，恶寒发热，无汗，鼻塞清涕，肢体酸痛，舌苔薄白，脉浮紧。

治法： 宣利肺气，疏风止咳。

方药： 止嗽散加减。桔梗、荆芥、紫菀、炙百部、白前、甘草、陈皮。

方解： 桔梗宣通肺气，泻火散寒；荆芥散风湿，清头目，利咽喉；紫菀补虚调中，消痰止咳；百部润肺止咳；白前下痰止嗽；陈皮调中，导滞消痰；炙甘草利咽止咳，调和诸药。

加减： 风寒重者加荆芥穗、防风、淡豆豉；风热加银花、前胡；咽痛加牛蒡子、生甘草、金灯；鼻塞加辛夷、苍耳子、鹅不食草；咽痒、过敏加蝉蜕、地肤子；咽干加桑叶、枇杷叶；内热加黄芩、黄连、生石膏；痰多色黄加鱼腥草、蒲公英。

2. 外寒内热

主症： 喘咳，甚则气急，鼻翼煽动，咳痰黏稠，咳吐不利，烦闷，有汗或无汗，身热不解，口渴，苔薄黄，脉滑数。

治法： 辛凉宣肺，清热平喘。

方药： 麻黄杏仁甘草石膏汤加减。麻黄、杏仁、炙甘草、石膏。

方解： 麻黄宣肺平喘；石膏甘寒，清泄肺热、生津；杏仁苦降肺气，止咳平喘；炙甘草顾护胃气，调和诸药。

加减： 表邪偏重，无汗而恶寒加荆芥、苏叶；肺热甚加重石膏用量，或加桑白皮、黄芩、知母、鱼腥草、蒲公英；痰多气急加葶苈子、枇杷叶；痰黄稠而胸闷加瓜蒌、贝母、黄芩、桔梗。

3. 外寒内饮

主症： 呼吸急促，喘憋气逆，胸膈满闷如塞，咳嗽，痰少咳吐不爽，色白而多泡沫，口不渴或渴喜热饮，形寒怕冷，天冷或受寒易发，面色青晦，舌苔白滑，脉弦紧或浮紧。

治法： 宣肺散寒，化痰平喘。

方药： 射干麻黄汤或小青龙汤加减。射干麻黄汤：射干、麻黄、生姜、细辛、紫菀、款冬花、大枣、半夏、五味子。小青龙汤：麻黄、芍药、细辛、干姜、炙甘草、桂枝、五味子、半夏。

方解： 射干麻黄汤：麻黄、射干宣肺平喘，化痰利咽；干姜、细辛、半夏温肺化饮降逆；紫菀、款冬化痰止咳；五味子收敛肺气；大枣、甘草和中。小青龙汤：麻黄、桂枝发汗解表，兼能宣肺平喘；芍药配桂枝以调和营卫；干姜、细辛内以温化水饮，外以发散风寒；半夏燥湿化痰，蠲饮降浊；五味子敛肺止咳；甘草缓和药性。

加减： 鼻塞清涕多加辛夷、苍耳子；有热象而烦躁者，加生石膏、黄芩；喉中痰鸣加杏仁；水肿加茯苓、猪苓。

4. 痰热壅肺

主症： 咳嗽气急，喘急面红，胸痛满闷，咳吐黄绿色浊痰、有腥味，口干咽燥，舌质红、舌苔黄腻，脉滑数。

治法： 清肺化痰，逐瘀排脓。

方药： 苇茎汤加减。苇茎、薏苡仁、瓜瓣、桃仁。

方解： 苇茎甘寒轻浮，清肺泻热；瓜瓣化痰排脓；桃仁活血祛瘀；薏苡仁清肺破毒肿。

加减： 热邪炽盛加银花、黄芩、黄连、生石膏、鱼腥草；胸闷加瓜蒌皮、郁金；痰多加半夏、杏仁、浙贝、天竺黄、胆南星、桔梗；腹胀加枳实、厚朴、莱菔子；胸痛加当归、川芎、乳香、没药；不能平卧加苏子、葶苈子、杏仁。

5. 肺气虚

主症： 咳喘无力，气短，动则加重，痰液清稀，声音低怯，神疲体倦，面色㿠白，畏风自汗，舌淡苔白，脉虚。

治法： 补肺益气，固表止咳。

方药： 玉屏风散加减。防风、黄芪、白术。

方解： 黄芪补脾肺之气，固表止汗；白术健脾益气，加强益气固表之功；防风走表散风，益气祛邪。

加减： 咳嗽较重加紫菀、前胡、白前；自汗较重加浮小麦、煅牡蛎、麻黄根；虚人易感加苏叶；咽干加桑叶、枇杷叶；内热加黄芩、黄连、生石膏。

6. 脾气虚

主症： 咳嗽，气短，喘息，肢倦乏力，食少便溏，形体消瘦，面色萎黄，舌体胖大、有齿痕，脉沉弱。

治法： 益气健脾，化痰止咳平喘。

方药： 参苓白术散加减。莲子肉、薏苡仁、缩砂仁、桔梗、白扁豆、白茯苓、人参、炙甘草、白术、山药。

方解： 人参、白术、茯苓益气健脾渗湿；山药、莲子肉健脾益气止泻；白扁豆、薏苡仁健脾渗湿；砂仁醒脾和胃，行气化滞；桔梗宣肺利气，通调水道，载药上行；炙甘草健脾和中，调和诸药。

加减： 痰多加半夏、杏仁；腹胀加枳实、厚朴、莱菔子；里寒而腹痛加干姜、肉桂。

7. 肾气虚

主症： 咳嗽，喘息，呼多吸少，气短，动则喘甚，腰膝酸软，耳鸣，夜尿多，咳而遗溺，面色淡白，神疲乏力，舌淡白，脉弱、沉缓。

治法： 补肾纳气平喘。

方药： 七味都气丸。五味子（制）、山茱萸（制）、茯苓、牡丹皮、熟地黄、山药、泽泻。

方解： 熟地黄滋补肾阴；山茱萸、山药补肝益脾，化生精血；泽泻、茯苓利水渗湿，防地黄之滋腻；丹皮清肝泄热；五味子补肾涩精止遗。

加减： 痰多加陈皮、半夏、苏子、白前；喘咳欲脱、汗出如珠加太子参；腰酸、气短较重加蛤蚧、冬虫夏草；不能平卧加苏子、葶苈子、杏仁。

（二）单方验方

（1）百部根捣取自然汁，和白蜜等份，熬膏，每日2次，每次一匙，适用于年久咳嗽。

（2）珍珠层粉60g、青黛少许，麻油调服，分8次服，每日2次，用于咳嗽之急。

（3）黄芩、瓜蒌皮、鱼腥草，水煎服，1日3次，适用于热痰咳嗽。

（4）川贝母、梨汁、冰糖，加水煎服，适用于阴虚咳嗽。

（5）千年矮（又名紫金牛）干枝25g、石膏15g、桔梗12g、干地龙9g、蜂蜜30g、猪苦胆1个、甘草5g，水煎服，用于实喘、热喘。

（6）红人参3g、五味子20粒（1次量），研末，1日2次，用于虚喘。

（7）人参6g、胡桃肉2枚（去壳不去皮）、生姜5片、大枣2枚，水煎服，用于虚喘。

（8）人参15g、蛤蚧（炙）1对、杏仁30g、川贝母30g、紫河车30g，研细末，每次服3g，1日2~3次，用于虚喘。

（三）中成药

1. 散寒止咳平喘

（1）通宣理肺丸：口服。大蜜丸1次2丸，1日2~3次。可解表散寒，宣肺止嗽。用于风寒袭肺引起的咳嗽咳痰等。

（2）止嗽青果丸：口服。1次2丸，1日2次。可宣肺化痰，止咳定喘。用于风寒束肺引起的咳嗽痰盛、胸膈满闷、气促作喘、口燥咽干等。

（3）冬菀止咳颗粒：温开水冲服。1次1袋，1日3次。可祛风散寒、宣肺止咳。用于风寒袭肺证，症见咳嗽、咯痰稀薄色白、咽痒、恶寒、发热等，急性支气管炎见上述证候者。

（4）小青龙合剂：口服。1次10~20ml，1日3次，用时摇匀。可解表化饮，止咳平喘。用于风寒水饮，恶寒发热，无汗，喘咳痰稀。

2. 清热止咳平喘

（1）清肺消炎丸：口服。1次60粒，1日3次。少儿6~12岁每次40粒；3~6岁每次30粒；1~3岁每次20粒；1岁以内每次10粒。可清肺化痰，止咳平喘。用于痰热阻肺，症见咳嗽气喘、胸肋胀痛、吐痰黄稠；上呼吸道感染、急性支气管炎、慢性支气管炎发作及肺部感染。

（2）止嗽定喘丸：口服。1次10粒，1日2~3次。可清肺热，平喘咳。用于发热口渴，咳嗽痰黄，喘促，胸闷。

（3）咳欣康片：口服。1次3~4片，1日3次。可降气平喘，清肺化痰。用于肺热咳嗽及气管炎咳嗽。

（4）哮喘宁颗粒：开水冲服。儿童5岁以下1次5g，5~10岁1次10g，10~14岁1次20g，成人可适量增加或遵医嘱，1日2次。可宣肺止咳，清热平喘。用于肺热哮喘。

（5）急支糖浆：口服。1次20~30ml，1日3~4次；儿童1岁以内1次5ml，1~3岁1次7ml，3~7岁1次10ml，7岁以上1次15ml，1日3~4次。可清热化痰，宣肺止咳。用于外感风热所致的咳嗽，症见发热、恶寒、胸膈满闷、咳嗽咽痛；急性支气管炎、慢性支气管炎急性发作见上述证候者。

（6）羚羊清肺丸：开水冲服。1次1丸，1日3次。可清肺利咽，清瘟止咳。用于肺胃热盛、感受时邪，症见身热头晕，四肢酸懒，咳嗽痰盛，咽喉肿痛，鼻衄咳血，口干舌燥。

（7）清金止嗽化痰丸：口服。1次6g，1日2~3次。可清肺，化痰，止嗽。用于肺热痰盛引起的咳嗽黄痰，胸膈不畅，喉痛音哑，大便干燥。

3. 化痰平喘

（1）安嗽化痰丸：口服。1次1丸，1日2次。可清肺化痰，润肺止嗽。用于阴虚肺热引起的咳嗽痰盛，气短喘促，咽干口渴，劳伤久嗽，痰中带血。

（2）百咳静糖浆：口服。1~2岁1次5ml；3~5岁1次10ml；成人1次20~25ml，1日3次。可清热化痰、平喘止咳。用于外感风热所致的咳嗽、咯痰；感冒，急、慢性支气管炎，百日咳见上述证候者。

（3）川贝止咳露：口服。1次15ml，1日3次。可止嗽祛痰。用于肺热咳嗽，痰多色黄。

（4）除痰止嗽丸：口服。1次2丸，1日2次。可清肺降火，除痰止嗽。用于肺热痰盛引起的咳嗽气逆，痰黄黏稠，咽喉疼痛，大便干燥。

（5）肺力咳胶囊：口服。1次3~4粒，1日3次；或遵医嘱。可止咳平喘，清热解毒，顺气祛痰。用于咳喘痰多，呼吸不畅，以及急、慢性支气管炎，肺气肿见上述症状者。

（6）泻白糖浆：口服。周岁以上每次10ml，周岁以下每次5ml，1日2次。可宣肺清热，化痰止咳。用于伤风咳嗽，痰多胸满，口渴舌干，鼻塞不通。

（7）哮喘丸：口服。1次10g，1日2次。可定喘，镇咳。用于年久咳嗽，年久痰喘。

（8）橘红痰咳液：口服。1次10~20ml，1日3次。可理气化痰，润肺止咳。用于痰浊阻肺所致的咳嗽，气喘，痰多；感冒、支气管炎、咽喉炎等见上述症状者。

4. 补肺平喘

（1）补肺丸：口服。1日1丸，1日2次。可补肺益气，止咳平喘。用于肺气不足，气短喘咳，咳声低弱，干咳痰黏等。

（2）参贝咳喘丸：口服。1次40丸，1日3次。可健脾化痰，补肺益肾，止咳平喘。用于慢性支气管炎属于虚寒型咳嗽，气喘者。

（3）人参保肺丸：口服。1次2丸，1日2~3次。可益气补肺，止嗽定喘。用于肺气虚弱，津液亏损引起的虚劳久嗽，气短喘促等症。

（4）玉屏风胶囊：口服。1次2粒，1日3次。可益气、固表、止汗。用于表虚不固，自汗恶风，面色㿠白，或体虚易感风邪者。

5. 纳气平喘

（1）喘泰颗粒：口服，温开水冲服。1日4次，1次3g。可宣肺定喘，益肾祛痰。用于支气管哮喘急性发作期表寒里热证。症见呼吸急促，喉中哮鸣，胸胁胀满，咳而不爽，吐痰黏稠，或见形寒，身热，烦闷，身痛，口渴等。

（2）泻肺定喘片：口服。1次5片，1日2次。可泻肺纳气，止咳定喘。用于肺气壅塞，肾不纳气所致的喘咳。

（3）固肾定喘丸：口服。1次1.5~2.0g，1日2~3次。可温肾纳气，健脾利水。可在有发病预兆前服用，也可预防久喘复发，一般15天为1个疗程。适用于脾肾虚型及肺肾气虚型的慢性支气管炎，肺气肿，支气管哮喘，老人虚喘。

（4）金水宝胶囊：口服。1次3粒，1日3次；用于慢性肾功能不全者，1次6粒，1日3次。可补益肺肾、秘精益气。用于肺肾两虚，精气不足，久咳虚喘，神疲乏力，不寐健忘，腰膝酸软，月经不调，阳痿早泄；慢性支气管炎、慢性肾功能不全、高脂血症、肝硬化见上述证候者。

（5）百令胶囊：口服。规格①1次5~15粒，规格②1次2~6粒，1日3次。慢性肾功能不全：1次10粒，1日3次，疗程8周。可补肺肾，益精气。用于肺肾两虚引起的咳嗽、气喘、咯血、腰背酸痛；慢性支气管炎的辅助治疗等。

6. 健脾化痰

（1）参苓白术散：口服。1次6g，1日3次。可健脾、益气。用于体倦乏力，食少便溏。

（2）陈夏六君丸：口服。水蜜丸1次6g，小蜜丸1次9g，大蜜丸1次1丸，1日2~3次。可补脾健胃，理气化痰。用于脾胃虚弱，食少不化，腹胀胸闷，气虚痰多。

（四）针灸治疗

1. 针刺

取穴： 主穴为肺俞（双）、大椎、风门（双）、定喘。咳甚者，配尺泽、太渊；体虚易感冒者，配合谷、足三里；痰多者，配足三里、中脘、丰隆、脾俞；痰壅气逆者，配天突、膻中；肾失摄纳者，配肾俞、关元、太溪；心悸者，配神门、内关、心俞。

操作： 针刺大椎、中脘、尺泽、关元，采用提插捻转相结合手法。针刺肺俞、风门、心俞、肾俞，采用提插捻转相结合手法。针刺合谷、太渊、内关、鱼际、太溪，以捻转为主，提插为辅进行。针刺天突穴，用小幅度提插捻转行针法，得气后不留针。针刺足三里，采用提插捻转相结合的行针手法。急性加重期每日针刺1次，稳定期每日或隔日针刺1次，每次留针30分钟，每隔10分钟行针1次。根据具体病情采取虚补实泻，即稳定期多为正虚，针用补法；急性加重期多为邪实，或虚实夹杂，故针用泻法或平补平泻法。10次为1个疗程，疗程间休息3~5天，继续治疗1个或2个疗程。

2. 灸法

取穴： 主穴为天突、肺俞、列缺、关元。实证、痰热证加定喘、尺泽、丰隆；虚证、寒证加肾俞、天突、膏肓、足三里。气虚、阳虚者，宜灸或针灸并用，取穴同上。

操作： 以艾条温和灸为主，在留针期间或起针之后进行，每穴灸 5~10 分钟，以局部潮红为度。每日 1 次，10 次为 1 个疗程。

3. 拔火罐

取穴： 感受风寒之邪选用肺俞、身柱、风门、外关；感受风热之邪选用大椎、风门、肺俞、曲池。

操作： 用较大火罐或广口玻璃瓶拔于穴位之上。如患者消瘦，可用小火罐。留罐 10 分钟左右。

4. 皮肤针

取穴： 颈背部督脉、膀胱经、喉两侧。

方法： 先用 75% 酒精消毒局部，然后用皮肤针轻或中度叩刺，每日 1 次，10 次为 1 个疗程。

（五）其他

1. 耳穴贴压

取穴： 主穴为肺、气管、肾上腺、大肠。喘重加平喘穴；痰多加脾穴。

操作： 先用 75% 酒精消毒一只耳，然后用 0.4cm×0.4cm 的胶布上放 1 粒王不留行籽，将其放到相应的穴位上，粘贴好，轻轻按压，使患者感耳廓发热、胀痛为止。并嘱其每日轻轻按压 3~5 次，两耳交替敷贴，4~5 天贴 1 次，5 次为 1 个疗程。

2. 穴位贴敷

取穴： 肺俞、肾俞、大椎、膏肓、定喘等穴。

药物： 麻黄、白芥子、延胡索各 20g，甘遂、细辛各 10g，将上述药物共研细末，加麝香 0.6g，用鲜姜汁调和均匀。

操作： 患者取坐位，穴位局部常规消毒后，将药物做成直径约为 1.5cm、厚约 0.5cm 的圆饼贴于上述穴位上，用 4cm×4cm 胶布固定，成人贴 4~6 小时，儿童贴 2~3 小时，治疗时间为三伏天、三九天，每 10 日敷 1 次，常配合服用中药。

五、名医专家经验方

（一）肺肾咳喘方（孟澍江）

适应证： 咳逆气喘。肺肾两虚、虚实夹杂的慢性支气管炎、肺气肿。

组方：麻黄 4g，杏仁 9g，甘草 3g，法半夏 9g，陈皮 6g，茯苓 10g，当归 9g，熟地 12g。

用法：水煎服。

功效：宣肺化痰，止咳平喘，补益肺肾。

按语：慢性支气管炎、肺气肿等病属中医咳喘病范围。本证的发生多由肺肾不足而痰湿内盛，并每为感受新邪而诱发，所以往往呈表里兼病、虚实夹杂之证。古人有平时治肾、发时治肺之说。对本病证的治疗，投用一般的止咳化痰平喘之剂，虽可取得一时之效，但效果总难令人满意。本方乃从张景岳金水六君煎化裁而来，方中用麻黄、杏仁宣肺化痰，且麻黄又有开肺疏表定喘之功；又用半夏、陈皮理气化痰，使气顺而痰降；所用茯苓可健脾化湿，以痰由脾虚而生，又为湿所化，所以用之既可健脾以杜生痰之源，又可祛湿以化痰，与半夏、陈皮相伍，即是二陈汤；配伍当归和血，熟地补肾纳气以治其本。本方用于屡治无效的慢性咳喘，往往能取得较好疗效。特别是在入冬之时病将发前坚持服用，每可使病情大为减轻。

（二）肺热咳喘方（麻瑞亭）

适应证：因表邪入里，内伤于肺，肺失清肃降敛，相火上炎，刑逼肺金，肺热气逆所致的肺热喘咳。

组方：生薏苡仁 12g，生甘草 6g，生杭芍 12g，粉丹皮 9g，干生地 12g，广橘红 9g，杏仁泥 9g，法半夏 9g，浙贝母 9g，柏子仁 9g，鲜芦根 25g，北沙参 12g。

用法：水煎服。

功效：平胆疏肝，清降肺胃，化痰止咳。

按语：肺热喘咳，包括急、慢性肺炎等肺家燥热型喘咳症。肺炎，属中医学之肺热喘咳或温热病范畴。本病一般起病较急，内外合邪，表里皆热，气火上冲，肺热郁隆，所以起即发热，咳嗽气喘，胸闷胸痛。部分患者起病急骤，变化迅速，病情危重，症见谵语妄言，昏昧撮空，寻衣摸床，烦躁不安，当配合西药以救急。若喘咳痰鸣，垂头闭目，声如浅锯者，为病势重危之象，命在旦夕，当以西药急救，以冀挽患者于冥途。肺为心之宅，心为神之舍，宅焚则神无所藏，必魂荡而神驰。心主血脉，君相火炎，热伤营血，必危及心君，故危重者见神昏谵语等心经症状。此即邪热内陷心包，叶天士谓之"温邪上受，首先犯肺，逆传心包"者是也。所以方中用柏子仁，意在养心强心以防脱；或加五味子、天门冬，清敛肺气，亦可防脱。

六、名医专家典型医案

（一）丁甘仁医案

朱左　新寒引动痰饮，渍之于肺，咳嗽气急又发，形寒怯冷，苔薄腻，脉弦滑。仿《金匮》痰饮之病，宜以温药和之。

川桂枝（八分），云苓（三钱），生白术（五钱），清炙草（五分），姜半夏（二钱），橘红（一钱），光杏仁（三钱），炙远志（一钱），炙白苏子（五钱），旋覆花（包，五钱），莱菔子（炒、研，二钱），鹅管石（一钱）。

暴寒外束，痰饮内聚，支塞于肺，肃降失司，气喘咳嗽大发，故日夜不能平卧，形寒怯冷，纳少泛恶，苔白腻，脉浮弦而滑。拟小青龙汤加减，疏解外邪、温化痰饮。

蜜炙麻黄（四分），川桂枝（八分），云苓（三钱），姜半夏（二钱），五味子（四分），淡干姜（四分），炙苏子（二钱），光杏仁（三钱），熟附片（一钱），鹅管石（一钱）。

哮吼，紫金丹（另吞，连服二天，两粒）。

二诊：服小青龙汤两剂，气喘咳嗽，日中大减，夜则依然，纳少泛恶，苔薄腻，脉弦滑。夜为阴盛之时，饮邪窃踞阳位，阻塞气机，肺胃下降之令失司，再以温化饮邪，肃降肺气。

川桂枝（八分），云苓（三钱），姜半夏（二钱），橘红（一钱），五味子（四分），淡干姜（四分），水炙远志（五分），光杏仁（三钱），炙苏子（五钱），旋覆花（包，五钱），熟附片（一钱），鹅管石（一钱）。

三诊：气喘咳嗽，夜亦轻减，泛恶亦止，惟痰饮根株已久，一时难以骤化。脾为生痰之源，肺为贮痰之器。今拟理脾肃肺，温化痰饮。

原方去旋覆花、远志二味，加生白术（五钱）、炒补骨脂（五钱）。

（二）吴佩衡医案

郑某某 女，25岁，已婚，云南省人。

初诊： 患慢性哮喘病已14年之久，现身孕4个月余，住昆明军区某医院，于1959年10月9日邀余会诊。询其病史，始因年幼体弱，感风寒而起病，药、食调理不当，风寒内伏，夹湿痰上逆于肺，经常喘咳，值天寒时令尤甚，迄今病已多年，转成慢性哮喘。症见咳嗽短气而喘，痰多色白，咽喉不利，时发喘息哮鸣。面色淡而少华，目眶、口唇含青乌色。胸中闷胀，少气懒言，咳声低弱，咳时则由胸部牵引小腹作痛。食少不思饮，溺短不清，夜间喘咳尤甚，难于平卧入寐。舌苔白滑厚腻，舌质含青色，脉现弦滑，沉取则弱而无力，此系风寒伏于肺胃，久咳肺肾气虚，阳不足以运行，寒湿痰饮阻遏而成是证。法当开提肺寒、补肾纳气、温化痰湿治之，方用小青龙汤加附片。

附片100g，杭芍10g，麻黄10g，北细辛6g，干姜30g，桂枝20g，五味子5g，半夏10g，甘草10g。

二诊： 服上方2剂后，咳吐大量清稀白痰，胸闷、气短及喘咳均已较减，能入睡四五小时，食思见增，唇舌转红，仍微带青色，厚腻白苔退去其半。上方虽见效，然阳气未充，寒湿痰饮尚未肃清，继以温化开提之剂治之。方用四逆、二陈合方加麻、辛、桂。

附片200g，干姜40g，茯苓30g，法夏15g，广陈皮10g，北细辛8g，麻黄（蜜炙）10g，上肉桂（研末，泡水兑入）10g，甘草10g。

服上方后喘咳皆有减少。治法不变，仍用此方，随症加减药味及分量，共服20余剂后，哮喘、咳嗽日渐平息。再服10余剂，病遂痊愈，身孕无恙，至足月顺产一子，娩后母子均健康。

按语： 昔有谓妇人身孕，乌、附、半夏皆所禁用，其实不然。盖乌、附、半夏，生者具有毒性，固不能服，只要炮制煎煮得法，去除毒性，因病施用，孕妇服之亦无妨碍。妇人怀孕，身为疾病所缠，易伤胎气而不固。因证立方用药，务使邪去而正安，此实为安胎、固胎之要义。《内经》云："妇人重身，毒之何如……有故无殒，亦无殒也。"此乃有是病而用是药，所谓有病则病当之，故孕妇无殒，胎亦无殒也。余临证数十年，思循经旨，多有所验，深感得益不少。

（三）赵绍琴医案

祁某 男，47岁。

初诊：喘咳10余年，遇寒即发，痰多清稀，甚则喘急不能平卧。近因感寒，喘咳又作，入夜尤甚。舌白苔腻水滑，脉象沉弦，按之紧数。寒饮相搏，气逆上冲，喘咳由是而作。温化寒饮，以定其喘。小青龙汤法。

麻黄6g，桂枝6g，半夏10g，细辛3g，白芍10g，干姜6g，炙甘草6g。7剂。

二诊：药后喘咳渐减，痰量亦少。脉仍沉弦，舌白且润。仍以前法进退。

麻黄3g，桂枝6g，半夏10g，细辛3g，干姜6g，白芍10g，炙草6g，杏仁10g，旋覆花10g。7剂。

三诊：两进小青龙汤，咳喘渐平，食少痰多，脉沉已起，舌白苔润。仍以宣肺化痰方法。

苏叶子各10g，杏仁10g，浙贝母10g，莱菔子10g，白芥子6g，炒枳壳6g，桔梗10g，焦三仙各10g，半夏10g，陈皮10g。7剂药后咳喘皆止，纳食增加，嘱其忌食寒凉饮食，运动锻炼以增强体质，预防感冒以防其复发。

按语：慢性喘息性支气管炎以反复发作的喘咳多痰为主要表现。常因感冒风冷而复发或加重。其病机为内饮外寒，即《内经》所说："形寒饮冷则伤肺，以其两寒相感，中外皆伤，故气逆而上行。"既为外寒内饮，当用仲景小青龙汤，外散表寒，内化寒饮。凡属此型者服之即效。切不可惑于炎症之名而用凉药。又须忌食寒凉饮食，如冷饮及生冷瓜果。病愈之后，须防复发。预防之法以防止感冒和忌食寒凉最为重要。患者本身应加强锻炼，增强体质，提高抗病能力。用药则以健脾胃助消化为主。脾胃健则痰湿不生，元气固则外邪难侵。故为根本之法。

七、预防与调护

1.注意季节气候，预防感冒

在寒冷季节或气候骤变时，要注意防寒保暖，积极防治感冒、慢性支气管炎、支气管哮喘等肺系疾病的反复发作，注意避免感受外邪，以防止诱发或加重肺气肿。坚持耐寒等适应性锻炼，可提高患者抵抗风寒的能力。

2.饮食宜清淡，忌辛辣刺激、生冷、油腻

饮食以高蛋白、高热量、高维生素、低盐、易消化的食物为宜，注意增加补益肺阴及健脾之品。痰浊阻肺者，忌生冷、肥腻厚味及甜食；肺气虚，忌寒凉之品，适当进食有温补肺气的食物，如羊

肉、猪肺等。肺热痰黄者应禁食辛辣、油腻等助火生痰之品。

3. 忌烟酒，避免刺激性气体、灰尘、花粉、动物

戒烟，避免烟尘，防止有害气体及不良因素对呼吸道的刺激，过敏性患者注意避开过敏原，例如刺激性气体、灰尘、花粉、动物等易致敏因素。

4. 避免过劳、饥饿和情志刺激

注意劳逸结合，起居有常，勿太过劳累。鼓励患者积极防治，配合治疗，树立战胜疾病的信心，保持心情舒畅，避免情绪激动。

5. 用药护理

遵医嘱正确使用药物，以避免擅自服用引起咳喘副作用的药物，服用补肺益肾中药时，宜早、晚空腹温服，咳嗽喘息时，少量多次服。出现失眠或烦躁时，非经医生许可，不能擅自使用药物。

（邢淑丽）

参考文献

［1］ Global strategy for the diagnosis, management and prevention of chronic obstructive pulmonary disease（updated2015）［EB/OL］.［2015-01］. http://www.goldcopd.org/guidelines-global-strategy-for-diagnosis-management.html.

［2］ 李建生，李素云，余学庆. 慢性阻塞性肺疾病中医诊疗指南（2011版）［J］. 中医杂志，2012，53（1）：80-84.

［3］ 孙丽萍，徐升，张念志. 慢性阻塞性肺疾病中医药研究进展［J］. 中医药临床杂志，2012，24（4）：368-370.

［4］ 刘淑珍，张玉珍，邢淑丽. 耳穴敷压法治疗"慢性阻塞性肺疾病"的临床观察［J］. 中国中医急症，1992，1（1）：40-41.

［5］ 杨进. 孟澍江——中国百年百名中医临床家丛书［M］. 北京：中国中医药出版社，2001.

［6］ 孙洽熙. 麻瑞亭治验集［M］. 北京：中国中医药出版社，2011.

［7］ 丁甘仁. 丁甘仁医案［M］. 上海：上海科学技术出版社，1960.

［8］ 吴生元. 吴佩衡医案［M］. 昆明：云南人民出版社，1979.

［9］ 彭建中，杨连柱. 赵绍琴临证验案精选［M］. 北京：学苑出版社，1996.

慢性心力衰竭

Chronic
Heart
Failure

一、概述

慢性心力衰竭是由于任何心脏结构或功能异常导致心室充盈或射血能力受损的复杂临床综合征，其主要临床表现为呼吸困难、乏力（活动耐量受限）以及液体潴留（肺淤血和外周水肿），相当于中医学"心悸""怔忡""喘证""水肿""痰饮""胸痹""积聚"等范畴。

心力衰竭为各种心脏疾病的严重和终末阶段，具有发病率高、死亡率高的特点，5年生存率与恶性肿瘤相近，严重者1年内病死率高达50%。据我国的流行病学调查显示，在过去40年中，由于老年化、心血管危险因素的增加，心衰引起的死亡增加了6倍，患病率约0.9%。我国部分地区42家医院，对10 714例心衰住院病例回顾性调查发现，其病因以冠心病居首，其次为高血压，而风湿性心脏瓣膜病比例则下降；各年龄段心衰病死率均高于同期其他心血管病，其主要死亡原因依次为左心功能衰竭（59%）、心律失常（13%）和猝死（13%）。据美国心脏病学会（AHA）2005年的统计报告显示，全美约有500万心衰患者，心衰的年增长数为55万。欧洲心脏病学会（ESC）近年来通过对51个国家的统计发现，在普通人群中，心衰的总患病率为2%~3%，而在70~80岁的老年人群中，则高达10%~20%。近年来心衰的发病率仍持续增长，正成为21世纪最重要的心血管疾病。

二、病因病机

（一）中医

慢性心力衰竭病因病机涉及脏腑亏损、阴阳失调及气血津液代谢紊乱等。其外因多为风、寒、湿、热等，内因多为饮食失宜、七情内伤、先天禀赋不足、年老体衰及久病等因素导致。当代基于病证结合的临床和研究对其病机的认识经历了长期的探索，文献分析及相关流行病学调查研究显示，当前对慢性心力衰竭的病机认识即本病多为本虚标实之证，本虚为气虚、阴虚、阳虚，标实为血瘀、水湿、痰饮，其病位在心，涉及肺、脾、肾、肝及三焦诸脏腑。

1. 气虚、阴虚、阳虚为本

《黄帝内经》中记载："手少阴气绝则脉不通，脉不通则血不流"，"若心气虚衰，可见喘息持续不已"。这些描述均与慢性心力衰竭的症状有关，其主要病机为心气亏虚。心主血脉，心气亏虚，鼓动无力，血行滞缓，血脉瘀阻，从而出现心力衰竭。而心气又有赖心阳的温煦激发，心阳不振，上不能助肺金，中不能温脾土，下不能暖肾水，则会出现胸闷、憋喘、腹胀、水肿等症状；心阳旺盛则心气充沛，心气充沛则血运正常。由于阴阳互根，久病阳损及阴，或原发病阴虚在先、治疗中利尿伤阴、饮食化源不足等，也可出现气阴匮乏、阴阳并损的情况。

2. 血瘀、水湿、痰浊为标

《血证论·吐血》载："气为血之帅，血随之而运行。"气虚则运血无力而致血瘀。气虚日久，损及阳气，阳气的温煦、推动作用减弱，出现气不行水、气不化水的病理状态，从而水聚成湿、凝聚为痰，甚则水泛为肿，出现咳嗽、咳痰、水肿等症。痰滞留脉中，血行不畅又可导致为瘀，张仲景在《金匮要略·水气病》中提出："血不利则为水。"水饮停聚，阻滞经络气血运行，血瘀、水湿又互相影响。血瘀、水湿、痰浊相互交织，可作为新的病理产物进一步致病。慢性心力衰竭，因虚致实，因实致虚，虚实夹杂，恶性循环。

3. 病位在心，涉及肺、脾、肾、肝及三焦诸脏腑

其病位在心，但不局限于心，五脏是一个有机的整体，在生理上既分工又合作，共同完成生理功能，在病理上相互影响，此脏发病可累及彼脏。一方面，"心为五脏六腑之大主也"，心阳亏虚，心血不行，血脉不畅，则五脏经脉失养，日久致肺、脾、肝、肾四脏俱损。另一方面，肺、脾、肝、肾、三焦失调，俱可伤及于心。肺主气，司呼吸，朝百脉，主宣降，通水道，肺气虚弱或肺失宣肃，则使心脉不畅，而见胸闷等症；脾为气血生化之源，津液运行之枢纽，脾虚则气血生化乏源，津液停滞而为水湿，助长心水的形成，而见腹胀、纳呆、呕恶等；肾为先天之本，寓元阴元阳，心本乎肾，心气心阳源于肾，赖肾气肾阳以温煦，心主火，肾主水，阴阳互根，水火既济，肾阳亏虚，气化不行，而为水肿，甚或凌心射肺，致喘促心悸；肝主藏血，主疏泄，若肝失疏泄，气机不畅，则

导致气滞血瘀，可有肝脏肿大、情志抑郁等。"三焦者，原气之别使也，主通行三气，经历五脏六腑"，"盖三焦者，水谷之道路，气之所终始也"，设三焦气塞，则水饮停滞，不得宣行，故腹胀气满，不得小便，溢为水胀。

（二）西医

1. 病因

（1）心肌舒缩功能障碍：心肌梗死、心肌炎、心肌病、心肌中毒、心肌纤维化等导致的心肌损害；维生素 B_1 缺乏、缺血、缺氧等导致的心肌代谢异常。

（2）心脏负荷过重：瓣膜关闭不全、动 - 静脉瘘、室间隔缺损、严重贫血、甲状腺功能亢进等导致的容量负荷过重；高血压、主动脉缩窄、主动脉瓣狭窄、肺动脉高压、肺动脉瓣狭窄等导致的压力负荷过重。

2. 诱因

据流行病学分析，约 60%~90% 心力衰竭的发生都有诱因的存在，常见的诱因有感染、心律失常、劳力过度、妊娠和分娩、肺栓塞、水和电解质代谢紊乱、酸碱平衡失调、治疗不当等。

三、诊断要点与鉴别诊断

（一）诊断要点

参考 2014 年中国心力衰竭诊断和治疗指南，慢性心力衰竭（CHF）的诊断需综合病史、症状、体征及辅助检查。依据左心室射血分数（LVEF），CHF 可分为 LVEF 降低的心力衰竭（HF-REF）和 LVEF 保留的心力衰竭（HF-PEF）。一般来说，HF-REF 指传统意义上的收缩性心力衰竭，而 HF-PEF 指舒张性心力衰竭，但部分心力衰竭患者两者并存。LVEF 是心力衰竭患者分类和预后判断的重要指标之一。

1. 慢性心力衰竭患者的临床评估

（1）病史、症状及体征：详细的病史采集及体格检查可提供线索。心衰患者多因下列 3 种原因之一就诊：运动耐量降低、液体潴留以及其他心源性或非心源性疾病，均会有相应症状和体征。接诊时要评估容量状态及生命体征，监测体质量，估测颈静脉压，了解有无水肿、夜间阵发性呼吸困难以及端坐呼吸。

（2）心力衰竭的常规检查：二维超声心动图及多普勒超声；心电图；实验室检查；生物学标志物：血浆利钠肽［B 型利钠肽（BNP）］或 N 末端 B 型利钠肽原（NT-proBNP）测定（BNP<35ng/L，NT-proBNP<125ng/L）不支持慢性心力衰竭诊断、心肌损伤标志物（cTn）、纤维化（可溶性 ST2、半乳糖凝集素 -3）、炎症、氧化应激、神经激素紊乱、心肌和基质重构的标记物；X 线胸片。

2. 慢性 HF-PEF 的诊断标准

（1）对本病的诊断应充分考虑下列两方面的情况。

① 主要临床表现：有典型心衰的症状和体征；LVEF 正常或轻度下降（≥45%），且左心室不大；有相关结构性心脏病存在的证据（如左心室肥厚、左心房扩大）和（或）舒张功能不全；超声心动图检查无心瓣膜病，并可排除心包疾病、肥厚型心肌病、限制型（浸润性）心肌病等。本病的 LVEF 标准尚未统一。LVEF 在 41%～49% 被称为临界 HF-PEF，其人群特征、治疗及预后均与 HF-REF 类似，这提示将 LVEF>50% 作为临床诊断标准可能更好。此外，有的患者既往出现过 LVEF 下降至 ≤40%，其临床预后与 LVEF 持续性保留的患者可能也不同。

② 其他需要考虑的因素：应符合本病的流行病学特征：大多为老年患者、女性，心衰的病因为高血压或既往有长期高血压病史，部分患者可伴糖尿病、肥胖、房颤等；BNP 和（或）NT-proBNP 测定有参考价值，但尚有争论。如测定值呈轻至中度升高，或至少在"灰区值"之间，有助于诊断。

（2）辅助检查：超声心动图参数诊断左心室舒张功能不全准确性不够、重复性较差，应结合所有相关的二维超声参数和多普勒参数，综合评估心脏结构和功能。二尖瓣环舒张早期心肌速度（e'）可用于评估心肌的松弛功能，E/e' 值则与左心室充盈压有关。左心室舒张功能不全的超声心动图证据可能包括 e' 减少（e' 平均 <9cm/s），E/e' 值增加（>15），E/A 异常（>2 或 <1），或这些参数的组合。至少 2 个指标异常和（或）存在房颤，增加左心室舒张功能不全诊断的可能性。

（二）鉴别诊断

（1）支气管哮喘应与左心衰竭相鉴别。左心衰竭夜间阵发性呼吸困难，常称之为"心源性哮喘"。前者多见于青少年有过敏史，后者多见于老年人有高血压或慢性心瓣膜病史；前者发作时双肺可闻及典型哮鸣音，咳出白色黏痰后呼吸困难常可缓解，后者发作时必须坐起，重症者肺部有干湿性啰音，甚至咳粉红色泡沫痰。测定血浆 BNP 水平对鉴别心源性哮喘和支气管哮喘有较重要的参考价值。

（2）心包积液、缩窄性心包炎时，由于腔静脉回流受阻同样可以引起颈静脉怒张、肝大、下肢水肿等表现，应根据病史、心脏及周围血管体征进行鉴别，超声心动图检查可得以确诊。

（3）肝硬化腹水伴下肢水肿应与慢性右心衰竭鉴别，除基础心脏病体征有助于鉴别外，非心源性肝硬化不会出现颈静脉怒张等上腔静脉回流受阻的体征。

（4）右心衰竭引起的水肿、腹水应与肾性水肿、心包疾患和肝硬化所引起者相鉴别。肾性水肿多出现于眼睑、颜面部组织较疏松的部位，且以晨起较明显，故不同于心力衰竭的重力性水肿。心包疾患和肝硬化的腹水征常较外周水肿为明显。

四、中医治疗

（一）辨证治疗

由于慢性心力衰竭是一个慢性进行性病变，一旦起始，即使没有新的心肌损害，临床亦处于稳定阶段，自身仍可不断发展。因此慢性心力衰竭是一个具有缓慢发展和急性加重特点的疾病，在其发展的过程中，自然表现为加重和缓解的反复交替出现，一旦存在诱发慢性心力衰竭加重的因素，如感染、心律失常、血压增高、电解质紊乱、输液过多过快、情绪激动等，患者就会进入加重期，临床表现为胸闷憋气、喘促、运动耐力减低、难以平卧、呼吸困难、咳嗽、双下肢水肿，甚至出现胸水、腹水，造成患者生活质量的下降。从中医学认识考虑，加重期临床主要为以血瘀、水湿、痰浊等标实证病机特点为主，其中以水肿为主，同时伴有气虚、阴虚、阳虚的本虚症状。而在缓解期，标实证血瘀、水湿、痰浊得到明显的缓解和好转，主要以气、阴、阳的亏损为主要病机特点。正是由于其缓慢发展和急性加重的疾病特点，加重期患者不得不进入医院住院治疗。由于目前临床医生"重住院治疗，轻院外治疗"，患者和家庭"重视加重期的治疗，轻视缓解期的治疗"，造成大量的患者处于加重住院、缓解出院、出院后缺乏系统合理的治疗，形成反复发作加重、反复住院的局面。因此，将慢性心力衰竭分加重期和缓解期，实际上是根据中医对慢性心力衰竭认识的"本虚标实证"为主要特点进行分类，体现了"急则治其标，缓则治其本"的中医药治疗疾病的原则。

1. 慢性心力衰竭加重期

慢性心力衰竭加重期分类方法，依据标实证作为疾病分类依据，在此期根据八纲辨证进行寒热分治，并结合气血津液辨证进行分类。根据机体寒热性质不同将慢性心力衰竭加重期分为寒瘀水结型和热瘀水结型两型。加重期，由于此期瘀水是不可分离的，血瘀、水湿、痰浊是其主要疾病病机特点，但是寒热性质的不同，中医药治疗的原则就不同，临床疾病不外寒热两端，寒热分类，充分体现了"寒者热之，热者寒之"的治疗原则。加重期治疗目的：迅速缓解慢性心力衰竭心衰症状，控制慢性心力衰竭发作。治疗原则：以利水消肿、泻肺平喘、清热祛痰、活血化瘀等治疗方法，体现出"急则治其标"的治疗原则，同时要根据"标本先后"的中医药治疗大法，兼顾患者为主要本虚症状，采用益气温阳、养阴生津等治疗方法，体现出"祛邪扶正"，做到祛邪不伤正。

（1）寒瘀水结

主症：喘咳倚息，不能平卧，咳吐泡沫状痰；下肢或全身水肿，按之凹陷，甚则阴肿；小便不利，心悸气短，动则尤甚；舌质淡胖、苔白滑，脉沉细无力或沉迟。

治法：温阳利水，泄浊活血。

方药：真武汤合苓桂术甘汤加减。黄芪、党参、制附子、桂枝、五加皮、泽泻、茯苓、白术、葶苈子、桑白皮、车前子、半边莲、泽兰、甘草。

方解：附子性热，补火助阳散寒；桂枝温经通脉、助阳化气；黄芪、党参补中益气，四者相配振奋阳气、温化水湿。葶苈子、桑白皮泻肺平喘、利水，祛除上焦水湿；茯苓健脾渗淡利湿，白术健脾燥湿，使中焦健运，水湿自除；五加皮温肾除湿，泽泻、车前子、半边莲渗湿利尿，泽兰利水，兼能活血，使下焦水道通利。炙甘草健脾补中，调和诸药，共奏温阳利水、泻浊活血之功。

加减：咳嗽痰多者，加半夏、竹茹以燥湿化痰；咳嗽喘息不得卧者，加前胡、白前、白果、桔梗宣肺理气；恶心呕吐者，加生姜、吴茱萸、半夏降逆温胃止呕，或砂仁、陈皮、佩兰化湿和胃；心下痞或腹中有水声者，可加枳实、生姜消痰散水；气滞腹胀者，加槟榔、大腹皮；肝脾肿大者加鳖甲、三棱、莪术等破血消积；少尿或无尿者，加猪苓、防己。

（2）热瘀水结

主症：喘咳倚息，不能平卧，咳嗽咳痰、咳痰黏稠或咳痰黄稠；下肢或全身水肿，按之凹陷，甚则阴肿；心悸气短，动则尤甚，胸闷憋气；腹胀纳呆，口干口渴，小便不利；舌质暗红或紫暗，苔黄厚或黄腻，脉滑数。

治法：清热活血，泻肺利水。

方药：己椒苈黄汤加减。汉防己、川椒目、葶苈子、大黄、桑白皮、枳壳、白花蛇舌草、半边莲、泽兰、泽泻、车前子、茯苓、白术、甘草。

方解：汉防己清热利水、泄下焦膀胱湿热，川椒目、白花蛇舌草、半边莲清热利湿、消除腹中水气，泽兰、泽泻、车前子共奏活血、泄热、利尿之功，葶苈子、桑白皮泻肺平喘、利水；茯苓、白术健脾渗湿，大黄清热泻下、逐瘀通经，枳壳行气宽中除胀，甘草调和诸药。全方清热活血，泻肺利水。

加减：肺热喘急者，加木防己、石膏清热利湿；痰涎壅盛者，加川贝母、胆南星、天竺黄、鱼腥草宣肺化痰；咯血者，加大小蓟、侧柏叶；呕吐者，加竹茹、生姜化痰止呕；腹肿满胀较重者，加川朴、莱菔子、槟榔、牵牛子；大便干结者，加制大黄、槟榔、柏子仁润肠通便；少尿或无尿者，加滑石、猪苓、冬瓜皮、冬瓜子通利小便，泄热于下。

2. 慢性心力衰竭缓解期

慢性心力衰竭缓解期，患者标实症状基本得到控制或减轻，此时脏腑功能亏虚导致的本虚症状成为主要临床表现。慢性心力衰竭缓解期分类方法，依据本虚证作为疾病分类依据，此期气、阴、阳亏虚为主要病机特点。在此期根据八纲辨证进行阴阳分治，并结合气血津液辨证。根据机体阴阳亏虚性质不同，慢性心力衰竭缓解期分为气阴两虚、瘀血内阻型和气阳两虚、瘀血内阻型两型。慢性心力衰竭缓解期血瘀是贯穿其发展全过程的病机特征，与加重期比较只是程度的不同。但是由于阴阳亏损的不同，临床疾病不外阴阳两端。阴阳分类，充分体现了"阴虚滋阴，阳虚补阳"治疗原则。缓解期的治疗应注重平衡阴阳气血，调理脏腑功能，在阴阳气血辨证基础上以心肺、脾胃、肝肾、三焦辨证病位进行加减治疗，目的在于增强患者抗病御邪能力，促进组织修复，改善生活能力，提高生活质量，减少心衰复发。一旦病情加重则进入加重期治疗。治疗原则应以益气温阳、养阴生津、平衡阴阳气血、调理脏腑功能为主，体现出"缓则治其本"。同时要根据"标本先后"的中医药治疗大法，兼顾患者血瘀、水湿、痰浊症状，活血化瘀、泻肺平喘、利水消肿等治疗方法，体现出"扶正祛邪"，做到扶正不忘祛邪。在缓解期充分发挥中医药"辨证论治、整体治疗、复杂干预、动态调整"的"既病防变"的防治特色，以期达到使患者不进入加重期，以恢复脏腑气化功能，提高慢性心力衰竭的整体疗效水平。

（1）气阴两虚，瘀血内阻

主症：喘促憋气，动则加剧；心悸心慌，疲乏懒动，动则汗出，心悸加重；失眠多梦，气短乏力，自汗或盗汗；五心烦热，口干口渴，面颧暗红，舌质红少苔，脉细数无力或结代。

治法：益气活血，滋阴纳气。

方药：生脉散加减。党参、麦冬、五味子、生地黄、黄芪、赤芍、当归、山茱萸、玉竹、葶苈子、茯苓、车前子。

方解：方中党参味甘，性平，补中益气、止渴、健脾益肺、养血生津；麦门冬甘寒养阴清热、润肺生津。党参、麦冬合用，益气养阴之功益彰。五味子酸温，敛肺止汗，生津止渴。三药合用，一补一润一敛，益气养阴，生津止渴，敛阴止汗，使气复津生，汗止阴存，气充脉复。生地黄、赤芍、当归、玉竹生津滋阴、养血、活血，黄芪增强补气之效，山茱萸酸敛生津，葶苈子泻肺平喘、利尿，茯苓健脾渗淡利湿，车前子入肾和膀胱经，渗湿利尿。全方益气活血，滋阴纳气。

加减：动则气喘明显者，加重党参、黄芪的量；心悸失眠甚，加珍珠母、生龙齿、酸枣仁安神定悸；皮肤蒸热，日晡尤甚，阴虚潮热者，加银柴胡、地骨皮、鳖甲滋阴退热；热伤阴津，烦热口渴者，加花粉、芦根清热生津；汗出明显者，加浮小麦敛汗；胃纳欠佳，可加砂仁、山药、焦三仙、炒鸡内金；腹泻者，可加芡实、炒山药、莲子；血瘀重者，加用当归、丹参、丹皮等；咯血者，加花蕊石、三七粉。

（2）气阳两虚，瘀血内阻

主症：喘促憋气，动则加剧，吐痰清稀；心悸心慌，疲乏懒动，动则汗出，喘息加重；失眠多梦，气短乏力，自汗或盗汗；神疲纳呆、胸满脘胀；颜面灰白，口唇青紫，四肢清冷，小便清少，舌质淡胖、苔白腻或水滑，脉细沉或结代。

治法：益气活血，温阳化瘀。

方药：保元汤加减。党参、黄芪、巴戟天、肉桂、茯苓、车前子、葶苈子、丹参、淫羊藿、菟丝子、甘草。

方解：党参、黄芪补中益气，巴戟天、淫羊藿、肉桂温补肾阳，菟丝子甘温，平补肝肾，茯苓健脾渗湿，车前子淡渗利湿，葶苈子泻肺平喘，丹参活血化瘀，甘草补气、调和诸药。全方益气活血，温阳化瘀。

加减：肾虚喘甚者，可选加紫河车、蛤蚧；痰多气急者，加半夏、苏子；阳虚畏寒肢冷明显者，加附子、菟丝子、仙茅、补骨脂等温补肾阳；阳脱者，加附子、干姜以回阳救逆；心悸心慌甚，加酸枣仁、炙远志；血瘀明显者，加川芎、桃仁、红花；大便秘结者，加肉苁蓉；脉结代，可选加炙甘草、生龙骨、生牡蛎等。

（二）专方治疗

中国中医科学院史大卓教授治疗慢性心力衰竭常用基础方为：人参10g，生黄芪30g，桂枝15g，丹参30g，泽兰30g，益母草30g，车前子30g，赤小豆30g。全方益气温阳、活血利水，治疗慢性心力衰竭常有较好疗效。

（三）单方验方

葶苈子 6~10g，煎服，1 日 1 剂；若用粉剂，1 次 1~2g，水冲服，1 日 3 次。可用于治疗心力衰竭。

（四）中成药

1. 芪苈强心胶囊

1 次 4 粒，1 日 3 次。可益气温阳，活血通络，利水消肿。用于冠心病、高血压病所致轻、中度慢性心力衰竭证属阳气虚乏、络瘀水停者。

2. 补益强心片

1 次 4 片，1 日 3 次。可益气养阴，活血利水。用于心慌，气短，乏力，胸闷、胸痛，面色苍白，汗出，口干，浮肿，口唇青紫等的气阴两虚兼血瘀水停型冠心病、高血压性心脏病所致的慢性心力衰竭（心功能分级 Ⅱ ~ Ⅲ 级）。

3. 参附强心片

1 次 2 丸，1 日 2~3 次。可益气助阳，强心利水。用于慢性心力衰竭而引起的心悸、气短、胸闷喘促、面肢浮肿等症，属于心肾阳衰者。

4. 芪参益气滴丸

1 次 1 袋，1 日 3 次。可益气通脉、活血止痛。用于气虚血瘀型胸痹，症见胸闷、胸痛，气短乏力、心悸、自汗、面色少华，舌体胖有齿痕、舌质暗或紫暗或有瘀斑，脉沉或沉弦。现代临床常用于无症状心力衰竭或梗死后心力衰竭恢复期的治疗。

（五）针灸治疗

1. 体针

主穴： 内关、间使、通里、少府、心俞、神门、足三里。

配穴： 水肿者，加水分、水道、阳陵泉、中枢透曲骨；或三阴交、水泉、飞扬、复溜、肾俞。两组穴位可交替使用。咳嗽痰多者，加尺泽、丰隆；嗳气腹胀者，加中脘；心悸不眠者，加曲池；喘不能卧者，加肺俞、合谷、膻中、天突。

2. 灸法

主穴： 心俞、百会、神阙、关元、人中、内关、足三里。

配穴： 喘憋者，加肺俞、肾俞；水肿者，加水道、三焦俞、阴陵泉。

操作： 每次选用 3~5 穴，艾条灸 15~20 分钟，灸至皮肤潮红为度，每日 1 次。

（六）推拿治疗

柔和的向心性按摩，对早期轻度心衰患者有一定疗效。

（七）其他

1. 耳针

取穴为心、肺、肾、神门、交感、定喘、内分泌，每次选取 3~4 穴，埋针或用王不留行籽贴压。

2. 穴位注射

有报道应用黄芪注射液足三里穴位注射、参附注射液内关穴位注射治疗慢性心力衰竭有显著疗效，能明显改善心功能。

3. 其他

取心俞、膻中、内关等穴位贴敷、穴位埋线；神阙穴中药超声导入疗法；中药沐足等。

五、名医专家经验方

（一）调心饮子（张琪）

适应证：心阳虚衰、血络瘀阻型心力衰竭。

组成：人参 15g，黄芪 25g，甘草 20g，小麦 50g，红枣 5 枚，附子（先煎）、桂枝、麦冬、五味子、红花各 15g，丹参 20g，鸡血藤 30g，赤芍 15g。

用法：水煎服，日 1 剂。

功效：益气温阳，活血通络。

（二）温阳益心饮（张琪）

适应证：心肾阳衰、水气凌心、血络瘀阻型心力衰竭。

组成：人参、附子各 15g，茯苓 20g，白术 15g，白芍 20g，桂枝、生姜各 15g，泽泻、丹参各 20g，红花 15g，葶苈子 20g，甘草 15g。

用法：水煎服，日 1 剂。

功效：益气温阳利水。

（三）温运阳气方（颜德馨）

适应证： 心气阳虚为主型心力衰竭。

组成： 熟附子 15g，炙麻黄 9g，细辛 4.5g，生蒲黄（包煎）9g，丹参 15g，葛根 15g。

用法： 水煎服，日 1 剂。

功效： 温运阳气。

（四）行气活血方（颜德馨）

适应证： 心血瘀阻为主型心力衰竭。

组成： 桃仁 9g，红花 9g，赤芍 9g，当归 9g，川芎 9g，生地黄 12g，柴胡 4.5g，枳壳 6g，牛膝 9g，桔梗 6g，降香 2.4g，黄芪 15g。

用法： 水煎服，日 1 剂。

功效： 行气活血。

六、名医专家典型医案

（一）杜武勋医案——热瘀水结

郝某 女，78 岁，体型偏胖。

初诊： 2011 年 10 月 24 日。慢性咳嗽病史 8 年，每于季节交替时发作，喘憋劳累及平卧位加重。症见喘憋，大汗出，夜间不能平卧，口干口苦，咳嗽痰黏稠，喉中痰鸣，腹胀，纳呆，大便干，3~4 天 1 次，夜寐欠安。爪甲青紫，口唇发绀，双下肢水肿（++），舌暗红、苔黄厚，脉滑数。查体：面色晦暗，颈静脉怒张，心率 106 次／分，律齐，双肺底可闻及少量干、湿啰音，肝肋下 2cm，血压 130/100mmHg。

西医诊断： 慢性心力衰竭；肺源性心脏病。

中医诊断： 喘证。属热瘀水结证。

治法： 清热活血，泻肺利水。

方药： 己椒苈黄丸加减。

汉防己 15g，川椒目 9g，葶苈子 30g，大黄 12g，黄芩 12g，鱼腥草 30g，茯苓 30g，白术 15g，桑白皮 30g，车前子 30g，泽泻 15g，白花蛇舌草 30g，半边莲 15g。

1 日 1 剂，水煎 2 次取汁 300ml，分早晚 2 次服，服 7 剂。

二诊： 2011 年 11 月 1 日。喘憋减轻，偶有咳嗽，小便量少，大便干。黄厚苔未减，双下肢水肿（+）。血压 120/80mmHg。初诊方中大黄、黄芩增至 15g。继服 7 剂。

三诊： 2011 年 11 月 8 日。患者静息状态下无明显喘憋，偶有气短、乏力，唇甲发绀，双下肢水肿明显消退。二便尚可，舌暗红，苔薄黄。二诊方加丹参 30g、黄芪 30g，继服 6 剂。

此后，继服该方 10 余剂，以巩固治疗。

按语： 慢性心力衰竭急性期常表现为咳、喘、痰、瘀、肿、悸等症，临床表现为虚实夹杂，邪盛正虚，寒热互见，为难治性危急重症。痰、热、水、瘀互结是该病常见证候，遵守辨证论治原则，以清热化痰、利水行瘀为治疗法则，杜师选用己椒苈黄丸加减治疗。该患者素体偏胖，痰湿积聚，脾失健运，壅滞胃肠，阻遏气机，气血运行不畅，瘀血内停，瘀久化热而致本病。证属慢性心力衰竭急性期热瘀水结证，治疗以己椒苈黄丸加减。方中葶苈子辛苦寒，祛痰定喘，泻肺行水；汉防己苦辛寒，善走下行，利水消肿；川椒目苦辛寒，化气行水，引诸药下行；大黄利水泄浊，活血通脉。加桑白皮泻肺平喘，茯苓、白术、泽泻、车前子、半边莲利水消肿，白花蛇舌草、黄芩、鱼腥草清热解毒，活血利水。全方共奏活血利水、清热解毒、泻肺平喘之功。二诊时黄厚苔不退、大便干，热象未减，故于初诊方基础上增加大黄、黄芩剂量以加强其清热泻火之力。三诊偶有气短、乏力症状，唇甲仍发绀，故加丹参、黄芪活血化瘀、益气固本。该方切中慢性心力衰竭痰热水瘀互结之病机，加减诸药以增强其化痰平喘、行气活血、利水消肿之力，诸药合用，宣上和中渗下，诸脏宣通，标本兼顾，扶正而不留邪，祛邪而不伤正。阴阳调和，升降周流，则脏腑畅达，病易向愈。

（二）孙光荣医案——阳虚水泛，气虚血瘀

侯某 男，81 岁。

初诊： 2014 年 3 月 7 日。胸闷气喘、动则尤甚已 2 月有余，加重 1 周。由轮椅推入病房。2014 年元月感冒后，开始咳嗽气短，胸闷气喘，下肢浮肿，常心悸，1 周前症状加重，动则心悸，心下及胸胁胀满，咳嗽吐泡沫清稀痰，难以平卧，时头汗出，冷汗淋漓，双下肢凹陷性水肿，纳差，少尿。舌淡胖，苔水滑，脉沉无力。查体：端坐呼吸，面色白，口唇轻度紫绀，颈静脉怒张，心率 100 次 / 分，律齐，两肺满布细湿啰音，X 线 DR 片示：双胸腔积液（约 800ml）。经结核病防治所检查排除了结核性胸膜炎。既往有糖尿病史多年，冠心病、高血压病史。

西医诊断： 心力衰竭 Ⅱ 度、心源性胸腔积液。

中医诊断： 喘证。属阳虚水泛、气虚血瘀证。

治法： 益气活血，温阳利水。

方药： 真武汤合调气活血抑邪汤（自拟方，组成：黄芪、人参、丹参）加减。

制附片（先煎）20g，生姜 20g，白芍 20g，白术 15g，茯苓 30g，泽泻 30g，人参 20g，黄芪 60g，丹参 30g，葶苈子 30g，大枣 10g，生半夏 15g，全瓜蒌 20g，干姜 10g，五味子 10g，细辛 10g，甘草 10g。

3 剂，水煎 500ml，分早、中、晚 3 次温服，1 日 1 剂。

上方服 3 剂后，尿量显著增加，每日达 1500ml，患者胸闷气喘好转，已能平卧，纳食改善，无心悸汗出，下肢肿好转。脉稍转有力。原方继进 3 剂。煎服法同前。服第 6 剂后浮肿消失，心率减慢，能下床轻微活动，X 线 DR 片示：双胸腔积液约 400ml。考虑还有胸闷、咳痰、短气等症，上方加入厚朴 6g、陈皮 6g 以宽胸理气燥湿化痰，入苏子 9g 以降气止咳。再服 5 剂后咳止，活动量大后可见胸闷、气喘症状，余症皆好转。舌淡及苔均有好转，脉较前有力。X 线 DR 片示：双胸腔积液

完全吸收。方改为制附片（先煎）10g，生姜10g，白芍20g，白术15g，茯苓15g，泽泻15g，人参20g，黄芪60g，丹参30g，麦冬10g，五味子10g，菟丝子10g，仙茅10g，补骨脂10g。服药1周，诸症悉除，心率85次/分，食纳正常，二便自调。

按语： 依据患者胸闷气喘，难以平卧，动则尤甚，汗出，下肢浮肿，面色白，口唇紫绀，舌淡胖而暗，苔水滑，脉沉无力可诊为喘证之阳虚水泛、气虚血瘀证。心主君火，肾主命火，君火命火互根互用。心力衰竭的本源是阳气不足，君命火衰，阳不化阴则水肿，气不行血必血瘀。心衰无力推动血行，血瘀则水停，故而水肿明显；水饮凌心射肺故可见胸闷气喘，心悸；气虚固摄无力故见汗出；因此心衰的治疗大法为温阳利水，行气化瘀；真武汤之附子温补命火以壮君火，白术、茯苓、泽泻补益中州、利水消肿，生姜温散水气；人参、黄芪、丹参益气活血、行气化瘀通血脉；葶苈子、大枣利水泻肺强心；生半夏、全瓜蒌宽胸理气化痰；干姜、五味子、细辛温肺化饮敛气；白芍利水活血兼敛阴和阳；甘草调和诸药。全方温阳利水强心，益气活血，化瘀祛痰，颇合病机，故收良效。

七、预防与调护

随着近年来我国人口老龄化趋势越来越明显，慢性心力衰竭的发病率日益增高，因此加强患者的日常调护，延缓疾病进展及预防急性加重，对于延长患者存活期、提高患者生存质量是大有裨益的。

（一）控制危险因素

（1）高血压。根据弗莱明翰心脏研究，高血压导致39%的男性和59%的女性心力衰竭；而控制高血压可使新发心力衰竭的危险降低约50%。高血压患者应积极控制血压，使血压长期达标。

（2）糖尿病。临床观察表明，糖尿病合并心力衰竭的发病率和死亡率是非糖尿病患者的4~8倍。糖尿病除引起大血管、微血管病变以外，还会引起心肌结构和功能的改变，胰岛素抵抗及高胰岛素血症可加重心脏和血管壁增厚，从而加速心力衰竭进展，特别是造成单纯舒张功能减退。故糖尿病患者应积极治疗原发疾病和并发症，预防心力衰竭的发生。

（3）改变生活方式。养成良好生活习惯，起居有时、饮食有度、生活规律、适当运动、戒烟戒酒、防止肥胖和高血脂等，可以有效减少心力衰竭的发生。在机体活动时，心率加快、耗氧量增加，因此应适当安排休息与活动。活动时以不感到疲劳，不加重症状为限，切忌参加重体力及长时间工作和学习，应做到积极休息及保证充足的睡眠时间。缓解期，则遵循"动"的原则，适当活动，防止静脉血栓形成或肺栓塞。

（4）避免使用心脏毒性的药物。决定应用此类药物前及用药后要充分评估心脏毒性的风险和患者的器官功能，注意药物累积剂量、种类剂型和给药方式，加强心功能检测及早预防心脏毒性和心力衰竭的发生。

（二）防止慢性心力衰竭加重

（1）防止液体潴留。钠盐和水摄入量过多不但能引起体内水分潴留且能提高神经肌肉的兴奋性，加重心脏负担。故应摄入适量的盐和水，教育心力衰竭患者每天定时测体重。

（2）各种感染（尤其上呼吸道和肺部感染）、肺梗死、心律失常［尤其伴快速心室率的心房颤动（房颤）］、电解质紊乱和酸碱失衡、贫血、肾功能损害、过量摄盐、过度静脉补液以及应用损害心肌或心功能的药物等均可引起心衰恶化，应及时处理或纠正。

毒性或细菌性感染均可直接或间接损害心肌收缩力、降低心脏功能，其中以上呼吸道感染最常见，风湿活动为诱发风湿性心脏病心力衰竭的主要诱因，也往往与呼吸道感染有关。严重的心律失常，尤其是快速型心律失常，由于心率过快，心脏工作量加大及心室舒张末期短，排血量减少，血压降低，心肌缺血等，可促使心力衰竭及心源性休克的发生，甚至死亡。

（3）规律服药。不足或停药过早等均可诱发或加重心力衰竭。

（三）防止精神刺激

情绪激动时可导致自主神经功能紊乱，交感神经兴奋，儿茶酚胺分泌增加引起心率加快，血压升高，从而增加心肌耗氧量，加重心脏负担。故应对各种心脏病患者都应做好心理调节，消除其对本病的恐惧紧张心理及悲观情绪，必要时酌情应用抗焦虑或抗抑郁药物。

（杜武勋）

参考文献

［1］中华医学会心血管病学分会，中华心血管病杂志编辑委员会. 中国心力衰竭诊断和治疗指南 2014［J］. 中华心血管病杂志，2014，42（2）：98-122.

［2］中华医学会心血管病学分会. 中国部分地区1980、1990、2000年慢性心力衰竭住院病例回顾性调查［J］. 中华心血管病杂志，2002，30（8）：450-454.

［3］陆再英，钟南山. 内科学［M］. 7版. 北京：人民卫生出版社，2008：170.

［4］Dickstein K, Cohen-Solar A, Filippatos G, et al. ESC Guidelines for the diagnosis and treatment of acute and chronic heart failure 2008 The Task Force for the Diagnosis and Treatment of Acute and Chronic Heart Failure 2008 of the European Society of Cardiology. Developed in collaboration with the Heart Failure Association of the ESC（HFA）and endorsed by the European Society of Intensive Care Medicine（ESICM）［J］. Eur J Heart Fail, 2008, 10（10）: 933-989.

［5］崔小磊，毛静远，王贤良，等. 心力衰竭中医证候流行病学调查表的设计［J］. 北京中医药，2009，28（3）：179-181.

［6］蔡辉，毛静远，王强，等. 慢性心力衰竭中医辨证规律的文献分析［J］. 四川中医，2011，29

（7）：22-25.

[7] 崔小磊，毛静远，王贤良，等. 心力衰竭中医证候的专家调查分析 [J]. 上海中医药大学学报，2009，23（2）：31-33.

[8] 崔小磊，毛静远，王贤良，等. 中医药治疗心力衰竭用药专家调查分析 [J]. 中成药，2009，31（9）：1431-1433.

[9] Jessup M, Abraham WT, Casey DE, et al. 2009 focused Update: ACCF/AHA guidelines for the diagnosis and management of heart failure in adults: a report of the American College of Cardiology Foundation/American Hearl Association Task Force on Practice Guidelines: developed in collaboration with the International Society for Heart and Lung Transplantation[J]. Circulation, 2009, 119: 1977-2016.

[10] Arnold JM, Liu P, Demers C. et al. Canadian Cardiovascular Society consensus conference recommendations on heart failure 2006: diagnosis and management [J]. Can J cardiol, 2006, 22: 23-45.

[11] Paulus WJ, Tschope C, Sanderson JE, eI al. How to diagnose diastolic heart failure: a consensus statement on the diagnosis of heart failure with normal left ventricular ejection fraction by the Heart Failure and Echocardiography Associations of the European Society of Cardiology [J]. Eur Heart J, 2007, 28: 2539-2550.

[12] 张扣启，孙青. 史大卓教授治疗慢性心功能不全经验撷菁 [J]. 中医药学刊，2003，21（1）：29.

[13] 中华中医药学会. 中医内科常见病诊疗指南（西医疾病部分）心力衰竭 [J]. 中国中医药现代远程教育，2011，9（18）：147.

[14] 谢燕萍，陈凤萍，黄国明，等. 黄芪注射液足三里穴位注射治疗慢性心力衰竭的临床观察 [J]. 实用中西医结合临床，2014，14（4）：5-6.

[15] 方居正，夏艳斐，黄巧婵，等. 中药穴位注射对慢性心衰患者 ICAM-1 等指标影响的观察 [J]. 人民军医，2013，56（10）：1192-1193.

[16] 孙元莹，吴深涛，姜德友，等. 张琪治疗充血性心衰经验介绍 [J]. 辽宁中医杂志，2006，33（11）：1394-1395.

[17] 严夏，周文斌，杨志敏，等. 颜德馨教授治疗心衰经验撷拾 [J]. 实用中医内科杂志，2003，17（6）：447.

[18] 刘辉. 运用国医大师孙光荣调气活血抑邪汤治疗疑难杂证的点滴体会 [J]. 光明中医，2015，30（4）：695-696.

中风

Stroke

一、概述

脑中风是以脑部缺血及出血性损伤症状为主要临床表现的疾病，又称脑卒中或脑血管意外，主要分为出血性脑中风（脑出血或蛛网膜下腔出血）和缺血性脑中风（脑梗死、脑血栓形成）两大类，临床上以脑梗死最为常见。本病发病率和死亡率较高，常留有后遗症，发病年龄也趋向年轻化，是世界上最重要的致死性疾病之一。

中医认为中风病是由于正气亏虚，饮食、情志、劳倦内伤等引起气血逆乱，产生风、火、痰、瘀，导致脑脉痹阻或血溢脑脉之外，此为基本病机，以突然晕倒，不省人事，伴口角㖞斜，言语謇涩或不语，半身不遂，或仅以口㖞、半身不遂为主要临床表现的病证。因其具有起病急、变化快、症见多端的特点，与风之善行数变特点相似，故名中风、卒中，有中经络、中脏腑之分。本病多见于中老年人。四季皆可发病，但以冬春两季最为多见。在本病的预防、治疗和康复方面，中医药具有较为显著的疗效和优势。不论是出血性还是缺血性脑血管病均可参考本节辨证论治。

二、病因病机

头为"诸阳之会"，五脏之精血，六腑之清气，皆上注于脑。中风之发生，其病位在心、脑，与肝、肾密切相关，乃上实下虚、阴阳互不维系的危重证候。

（一）病因

中风病因较多，其发生是多种因素所导致的复杂的病理过程，风、火、痰、瘀是其主要的病因。患者素体气血亏虚，心、肝、肾三脏功能失调，加之内伤积损，或饮食不节，或情志所伤，或外邪侵袭等诱因诱发。中风之病机复杂，但病因归纳起来不外虚（阴虚、血虚）、火（肝火、心火）、风（肝风、外风）、痰（风痰、湿痰）、气（气逆、气滞）、血（血瘀）六端。基本病机为阴阳失调、气血逆乱，病理性质多属本虚标实。肝肾阴虚、气血衰少为致病之本，风、火、痰、气、瘀为致病之标，两者可互为因果。

（二）病机

中风有中经络和中脏腑之别。若肝风夹痰，横窜经络，血脉瘀阻，气血不能濡养机体，则见中经络之轻证，症见半身不遂，口眼㖞斜，不伴神志障碍；若风阳痰火蒙蔽神窍，气血逆乱，上冲于脑，络损血溢，瘀阻脑络，则见中脏腑之重证，症见猝然昏倒，不省人事。

发病之初，邪气暴张，风阳痰火亢盛，气血上菀，故以标实为主；如病情剧变，在病邪的猛烈攻击下，正气急速溃败，可以正虚为主，甚则出现正气虚脱。后期因正气未复而邪气独留，可留后遗症。

1. 情志郁怒，化火生风

五志过极，心火暴盛，可引动内风。平素忧郁恼怒，情志不畅，肝气不舒，气郁化火，暴怒则肝阳暴亢，引动心火，气火俱浮，气血上涌于脑，神窍闭阻，遂致卒倒，昏不知人；或长期劳伤过度，阴精暗耗，虚火内燔，水不涵木，日久导致肝肾阴虚，复因情志所伤，肝阳暴亢，气血上逆，心神昏冒而发为中风。若青壮之年，素体阳盛，心肝火旺，亦有暴怒而致阳亢化风，突发本病者。

2. 饮食不节，痰浊内生

过食肥甘醇酒，辛香煎炸、烤炙之品。或饥饱无常，或饮酒过度，脾失健运，湿邪内停，聚而成痰，痰郁体内，阻滞经络，蒙蔽清窍。或痰湿生热，风火痰热内盛，引动肝风，窜犯经络，夹痰上扰，上阻头窍，猝然昏仆，半身不遂。

3.劳欲过度，内伤积损

操持过度，形神失养，阴亏血虚，虚阳化风，风火易炽。或纵欲伤精，引动心火，耗伤肾水，水不制火。或年老体衰，肝肾阴虚，肝阳偏亢，阳化风动，而致气血冲逆，上蒙神窍，突发本病。

4.气血不足，外风入中

年老久病，可致气血不足，脉络空虚，气候突变之际，风邪乘虚入中经络，气血痹阻，肌肉筋脉失于濡养。或痰湿素盛，形盛气衰，外风引动内风，痰湿闭阻经络，而致喝僻不遂。

5.血液瘀滞

气滞血行不畅，或气虚运血无力，或因暴怒血蕴于上，或因感寒收引凝滞，或因热伤阴液等均可造成血行滞涩而成血瘀。本病的病机多以暴怒血蕴或气虚血瘀最为常见。

三、诊断要点与鉴别诊断

（一）诊断要点

1.诱发因素

发病多与情志失调、饮食不当或劳累等诱因有关。

2.发病年龄

好发于 40 岁以上。

3.先兆症状

发病之前多有头晕、头痛、肢体一侧麻木等先兆症状。

4.临床表现

多发病较急，具有突然昏仆，不省人事，半身不遂，偏身麻木，口眼喝斜，言语不利等特点的临床表现。轻证仅见眩晕，偏身麻木，口眼喝斜，半身不遂等。

5.临床检查

中风类似于西医急性脑血管病，临床可根据具体情况作脑脊液、眼底及 CT、MRI 等检查。

（二）鉴别诊断

1.面瘫

面瘫可发于不同年龄阶段，常伴耳后疼痛，临床无半身不遂或神志障碍，以单侧面部肌肉瘫痪、口眼㖞斜、口角流涎，或伴言语不清等为主要表现，多因经络气血痹阻不通所致。

2. 眩晕

重证眩晕之仆倒与中风昏仆相似，但没有半身不遂、不省人事、口舌㖞斜等症。眩晕在临床上应注意与中风先兆的表现加以鉴别。

3. 厥证

厥证神昏时间短暂，常伴四肢逆冷的表现，大多可以自行苏醒，而无半身不遂、口舌㖞斜、言语不利等表现。

4. 痫证

痫病重证亦可有突然仆倒、不省人事之症，其苏醒后一如常人，无半身不遂、口眼㖞斜等症。

5. 痉证

痉证的发病可伴神昏，多于长时间抽搐之后出现，以四肢抽搐、颈背强直、角弓反张为主症，但临床上无半身不遂、口眼㖞斜等表现。

6. 痿证

痿证起病多缓慢，以双下肢瘫痪或四肢瘫痪为特征，或见肌肉萎缩、筋惕肉瞤为多，无神昏之症。

四、中医治疗

（一）辨证治疗

根据病情轻重和病位的深浅，中风临床分为中经络和中脏腑。中经络的治疗应以平肝息风、化痰祛瘀通络为主。中脏腑的治疗，其闭证当息风清火、豁痰开窍、通腑泄热；脱证应救阴回阳固脱；对于内闭外脱之证，应醒神开窍与扶正固脱之法兼用。恢复期及后遗症期，大多为虚实夹杂之证，应扶正祛邪、标本兼顾，当以平肝息风、化痰祛瘀与滋养肝肾、益气养血之法并用。

1. 中经络

以半身不遂、舌强语謇、口角㖞斜等为主症，一般无神志改变，临床可分为肝阳暴亢、风火上扰证；风痰瘀血、痹阻脉络证；痰热腑实、风痰上扰证；气虚血瘀证；阴虚风动证五种证型。

（1）肝阳暴亢、风火上扰

主症： 半身不遂，口舌㖞斜，舌强语謇或不语。面红目赤，眩晕头痛，偏身麻木，烦躁易怒，口苦咽干，大便秘结，小便黄赤，舌红或绛，苔黄或燥，脉弦滑有力。

治法： 镇肝息风，滋阴潜阳。

方药： 镇肝息风汤加减。怀牛膝、代赭石、龙骨、牡蛎、白芍、玄参、龟甲、天冬、茵陈、川楝子、生麦芽、甘草。

加减： 肝阳上亢甚者加天麻、钩藤以增强平肝息风之力；心烦甚者加栀子、黄芩以清热除烦；头痛较重者加羚羊角、石决明、夏枯草以清息风阳；痰热较重者，加胆星、竹沥、川贝母以清化痰热；若肝肾阴虚，脉弦细，舌质红等，加生地、何首乌、女贞子、枸杞子、旱莲草等滋养肝肾之药；若见口苦面红，便秘，小便赤，苔黄，脉弦数，可加郁金、龙胆草、夏枯草等以清肝泻火。

（2）风痰瘀血、痹阻脉络

主症： 半身不遂，口舌喎斜，舌强语謇或不语。肢体麻木或手足拘急，头晕目眩，舌质暗淡，苔白腻或黄腻，脉弦滑。

治法： 祛风，养血活血，化痰通络。

方药： 大秦艽汤加减。秦艽、羌活、独活、防风、当归、白芍、熟地、川芎、白术、茯苓、黄芩、石膏、生地。

加减： 年老体衰者，加黄芪以益气扶正；呕逆痰盛、苔腻脉滑甚者，去地黄，加半夏、南星、白附子、全蝎等祛风痰，通经络；无内热者可去石膏、黄芩。若痰浊郁久化热，可去白术加竹茹、枳实等行气清热燥湿；伴血瘀征象者可加桃仁、红花、川芎等活血祛瘀之品。

（3）痰热腑实、风痰上扰

主症： 半身不遂，口舌喎斜，舌强语謇或不语。头晕目眩，偏身麻木，口黏痰多，腹部胀满，便干便秘，舌质暗红或暗淡，苔黄腻或灰黑，脉弦滑而大。

治法： 清热化痰，理气通腑。

方药： 大承气汤（《伤寒论》）。大黄、枳实、厚朴、芒硝。

加减： 如药后大便通畅，则腑气通，痰热减，病情有一定程度好转。本方使用硝黄剂量应视病情及体质而定，一般控制在 10~15g 左右，以大便通泻、涤除痰热积滞为度，不可过量，以免伤正。腑气通后应予清化痰热、活血通络药，如胆南星、全瓜蒌、丹参、赤芍、鸡血藤。如头晕重，可加钩藤、菊花、珍珠母。若舌质红而口干咽燥，烦躁不安，彻夜不眠者，属痰热内蕴而兼津液大伤，可选加鲜生地、沙参、麦冬、玄参、茯苓、夜交藤等滋阴生津安神之品，但不宜过多，否则有碍涤除痰热。

（4）气虚血瘀

主症： 半身不遂，口舌喎斜，舌强语謇或不语。肢体软弱，偏身麻木，手足肿胀，心悸自汗，气短乏力，便溏，面色淡白，舌质暗淡，舌苔薄白或白腻，脉沉细，或细缓、细弦、细涩。

治法： 益气活血。

方药： 补阳还五汤加减。生黄芪、当归尾、川芎、赤芍、桃仁、红花、地龙。

加减： 如半身不遂较重加桑枝、穿山甲、水蛭等药加重活血通络、祛瘀生新作用；若肢体软弱，可加桑寄生、牛膝等补肝肾；言语不利甚者加菖蒲、远志以化痰开窍；手足肿胀明显者加茯苓、泽泻、薏仁、防己等淡渗利湿；大便溏甚者去桃仁加炒白术、山药以健脾。

（5）阴虚风动

主症： 半身不遂，口舌喎斜，舌强语謇或不语。肢体麻木、拘挛或蠕动，心烦失眠，眩晕耳鸣，手足心热，舌质红少苔或无苔，脉细弦或细数。

治法：滋阴息风。

方药：大定风珠加减。鸡子黄、阿胶、地黄、麦冬、白芍、龟甲、鳖甲、五味子、炙甘草。

加减：如偏瘫较重者可加牛膝、木瓜、地龙、蜈蚣、桑枝等通经活络之品；若心中烦热者，可加栀子、黄芩以清热除烦；如舌质暗红、脉涩等有血瘀证时加丹参、鸡血藤、桃仁、䗪虫等以活血祛瘀；语言不利甚者加菖蒲、郁金、远志开音利窍。

2. 中脏腑

以神志恍惚，迷蒙，嗜睡或昏睡，甚者昏迷，半身不遂为主症，分为闭证和脱证两类。

（1）闭证

主症：神昏恍惚，嗜睡或昏睡，甚者昏迷，半身不遂。兼见牙关紧闭，口噤不开，肢体强痉，呼吸急促，喉中痰鸣，二便不通，舌黄腻，脉洪大而数。

① 痰火瘀闭

兼症：面赤身热，气粗口臭，躁扰不宁，苔黄腻，脉弦滑而数。风火痰热之邪内闭经络，故见面赤身热，口噤，手握，气粗，口臭，便秘，苔黄腻，脉弦滑数。

治法：息风清火，豁痰开窍。

方药：羚羊钩藤汤（《通俗伤寒论》）。羚羊角、钩藤、桑叶、川贝母、鲜竹茹、生地黄、菊花、白芍、茯神木、生甘草。

加减：若痰热阻于气道，喉间痰鸣，可服竹沥水，以豁痰镇惊；肝火旺盛，面红目赤，脉弦有力，宜酌加龙胆草、山栀、夏枯草、代赭石、磁石等清肝镇摄之品；腑实热结，腹胀便秘，苔黄厚，宜加生大黄、元明粉、枳实；痰热伤津，舌质干红，苔黄燥者，宜加沙参、麦冬、石斛、生地。

② 痰浊瘀闭

兼症：面白唇暗，静卧不烦，四肢不温，痰涎壅盛，苔白腻，脉沉滑缓。

治法：化痰息风，宣郁开窍。

方药：涤痰汤（《济生方》）。茯苓、人参、甘草、橘红、胆星、半夏、竹茹、枳实、菖蒲。

加减：若兼有风动者，加天麻、钩藤平息内风；有化热之象者，加黄芩、黄连；见戴阳证者，属病情恶化，宜急进参附汤、白通加猪胆汁汤救治。

（2）脱证

主症：神志恍惚，迷蒙，嗜睡，或昏睡，甚者昏迷，半身不遂。气息微弱，呼吸短促，面色苍白，瞳神散大，目合口开，肢体软瘫，多汗肢冷，二便失禁，舌苔滑腻，脉散或微。

治法：补气回阳，救阴固脱。

方药：参附汤（《妇人良方》）合生脉散（《备急千金要方》）。人参、附子、青黛、麦冬、五味子。

加减：若阴不敛阳，阳浮于外，津液不能内守，汗出过多者，可加龙骨、牡蛎敛汗回阳；阴精耗伤，舌干，脉微者，加玉竹、黄精救护阴津。

3. 后遗症

（1）半身不遂

①气虚血滞，脉络瘀阻

主症：半身不遂，肢软无力外，并伴有患侧手足浮肿，语言謇涩，口眼㖞斜，面色萎黄，或暗淡无华，苔薄白，舌淡紫，或舌体不正，脉细涩无力等。

治法：补气活血，通经活络。

方药：补阳还五汤加味。

②肝阳上亢，脉络瘀阻

主症：患侧僵硬拘挛，兼见头痛头晕，面赤耳鸣，舌红绛，苔薄黄，脉弦硬有力。

治法：平肝潜阳，息风通络。

方药：镇肝息风汤或天麻钩藤饮加减。

（2）语言不利

①风痰阻络

主症：风痰上阻，经络失和，故舌强语謇，肢体麻木，脉弦滑。

治法：祛风除痰，宣窍通络。

方药：解语丹。方中天麻、全蝎、胆南星、白附子等以平肝息风祛痰；远志、菖蒲、木香等以宣窍行气通络；羌活祛风。

②肾虚精亏

主症：肾虚精气不能上承，故音喑失语，心悸、气短及腰膝酸软。

治法：滋阴补肾利窍。

方药：地黄饮子去肉桂、附子，加杏仁、桔梗、木蝴蝶开音利窍。

③肝阳上亢，痰邪阻窍

方药：可予天麻钩藤饮或镇肝息风汤加石菖蒲、远志、胆南星、天竺黄、全蝎以平肝潜阳、化痰开窍。

（3）口眼㖞斜：多由风痰阻于络道所致，治宜祛风、除痰、通络，方用牵正散。

（二）针灸治疗

1. 基本治疗

（1）中经络

治法：醒脑开窍，滋补肝肾，疏通经络。以手厥阴、督脉、足太阴经穴为主。

主穴：内关、水沟、三阴交、极泉、尺泽、委中。

配穴：肝阳暴亢加太冲、太溪；风痰阻络加丰隆、合谷；痰热腑实加曲池、内庭、丰隆；气虚血瘀加足三里、气海；阴虚风动加太溪、风池；口角㖞斜加颊车、地仓；上肢不遂加肩髃、手三里、合谷；下肢不遂加环跳、阳陵泉、阴陵泉、风市；头晕加风池、完骨、天柱；足内翻加丘墟透照海；便秘加水道、归来、丰隆、支沟；复视加风池、天柱、睛明、球后；尿失禁、尿潴留加中极、曲骨、关元。

操作：内关用泻法；水沟用雀啄法，以眼球湿润为佳；刺三阴交时，沿胫骨内侧缘与皮肤成45度角，使针尖刺到三阴交穴，用补法；刺极泉时，在原穴位置下2寸心经上取穴，避开腋毛，直刺进针，用提插泻法，以患者上肢有麻胀和抽动感为度；尺泽、委中直刺，使肢体有抽动感。

方义：心主血脉，内关为心包经络穴，可调理心气，疏通气血。脑为元神之府，督脉入络脑，水沟为督脉穴，可醒脑开窍，调神导气。三阴交为足三阴经交会穴，可滋补肝肾。极泉、尺泽、委中，疏通肢体经络。

（2）中脏腑

治法：醒脑开窍，启闭固脱。以手厥阴及督脉穴为主。

主穴：内关、水沟。

配穴：闭证加十二井穴、太冲、合谷；脱证加关元、气海、神阙。

操作：内关、水沟同前。十二井穴用三棱针点刺出血；太冲、合谷用泻法，强刺激。关元、气海用大艾炷灸法，神阙用隔盐灸法，直至四肢转温为止。

方义：内关调心神，水沟醒脑开窍。十二井穴点刺出血，可接通十二经气，调和阴阳。配太冲、合谷，平肝息风。关元为任脉与足三阴经交会穴，灸之可扶助元阳。神阙为生命之根蒂，真气所系，配合气海可益气固本，回阳固脱。

2. 其他治疗

（1）头针法：选顶颞前斜线、顶旁1线及顶旁2线，或颞三针，毫针平刺入头皮下，快速捻转2~3分钟，每次留针30分钟，留针期间反复捻转2~3次。行针后鼓励患者活动肢体。不寐或烦躁者，取额中线。

（2）眼针法：双上焦区、双下焦区为主穴，留针5~15分钟。

（3）电针法：在患侧肢体选取相应两个穴位组合，针刺得气后接通电针仪，以患者肌肉微颤为度，每次通电20分钟。

（4）皮肤针法：在患侧肢体选取以阳明经为主的相应经脉，用梅花针循经叩刺，取轻度叩刺法以刺激部位皮肤潮红为度。

五、名医专家典型医案

（一）张伯臾医案——肝阳上亢

黄某 女，54岁。

初诊：1976年10月14日。素有高血压病史，旬日前突然卒中，经中西医结合抢救好转。刻下：神志时清时昧，右半身不遂，言语謇涩，便秘，脉弦小，舌质红少津。

辨证：肾阴不足，水不涵木，风阳陡动，夹痰热内阻，上蒙心窍。

处方：仿地黄饮子之意。

大生地 18g，北沙参 18g，麦冬 15g，川石斛（先煎）18g，甜苁蓉 12g，朱远志 6g，丹参 12g，炒槐花 12g，天竺黄 9g，广郁金 9g，细石菖蒲 9g。6 剂。

二诊：1976 年 10 月 20 日。神志已清，右半身稍能活动，略能进食，但言语尚謇涩，舌红脉细。风阳渐平，肾阴损伤未复，痰热已有化机，再守原意增损。前方去广郁金，天竺黄，加大地龙 6g。12 剂。

三诊：1976 年 11 月 6 日。右半身活动日见好转，言语謇涩亦渐清楚，纳增，二便正常，舌红已润，脉细。肾阴损伤渐复，风阳痰热亦得平化，续予调补心肾。

大生地 12g，北沙参 18g，麦冬 15g，川石斛（先煎）18g，甜苁蓉 12g，制何首乌 15g，朱茯苓 9g，朱远志 6g，丹参 12g，炒枣仁 9g，淮小麦 30g，怀牛膝 9g。14 剂。

四诊：1976 年 11 月 27 日。言语已清，右半肢体已能活动且可扶杖行走，舌红润脉细小。类中在恢复之中，仍应前法调理以善后。原方续进 7 剂。

（二）王启才医案——中经络

赵某 女，72 岁。

初诊：1990 年 10 月 2 日。有高血压病史 20 余年。清晨上厕所时，感心痛，头昏，左侧肢体麻木，酸软无力，随即瘫倒于厕，但无意识障碍、失语和恶心呕吐，即送医院急救。查：左侧上下肢肌力 Ⅱ～Ⅲ级，伴口角㖞斜，脑 CT 示：右侧丘脑部位有一 1.31cm×1.31cm 高密度区。经急诊室观察处理后转针灸病房治疗。首次针灸双侧合谷、左侧地仓透颊车、曲池、足三里、阳陵泉、丰隆、太冲，中强刺激，加以语言暗示，动留针 30 分钟。起针后，即能在家属搀扶下行走数十米。

5 次治疗后，便能独自依杖而行，左侧上下肢肌力 Ⅳ级，仅存左侧口角及指、趾端麻木。3 周后痊愈出院。

（三）石学敏医案——中经络

张某某 男，67 岁，退休工人。

初诊：1980 年 9 月 23 日，住院号：9456。

主诉：左半身不遂伴语言欠流利 13 天。

病史：患者于 9 月 11 日夜间感受风寒，翌日晨出现左半身不遂。神清，肢麻言謇，主不能行，遂送某医院观察室观察。腰穿报告：脑脊液无色透明，糖五管（＋），诊为"脑意外"。予脉通、抗感染治疗。12 天后病情稳定，当时神清，口㖞，患肢无自主运动，语言欠流畅，无头痛、头晕，二便可控。既往否认高血压病史。9 月 23 日收住我科治疗。

查体：血压 240/120 毫米汞柱，脉率 60 次／分，神清体瘦，左侧中枢性面瘫，语言欠流利，双侧颈内动脉搏动对称；心音低钝，A2＞P2，律齐，左肺呼吸音粗；腹软，肠鸣音低；左上、下肢弛缓性瘫，生理反射均（＋），右掌颌反射（＋），左巴彬斯基氏征（＋）；舌质红，苔黄腻而干，脉弦细。

中医诊断：中风（中经络）。

西医诊断：高血压，动脉硬化，脑血栓形成。

辨证：患者年过八八，正气不足，肝肾已虚，肝阳偏亢，值感风寒，引动内风，上扰清窍，窍闭神匿，神不导气，故见口喎不遂。风邪引动痰湿，流窜舌络，则舌强语涩。

治则：醒脑开窍，滋补肝肾，疏通经络。

选穴：内关、人中、三阴交、极泉、尺泽、委中、风池、上星透百会。

操作：先针双侧内关，进针 1 寸，施捻转提插复式泻法，施术 1 分钟；继刺人中，进针 5 分，采用雀啄泻法，以眼球湿润或流泪为度；三阴交沿胫骨后缘与皮肤呈 45 度角，进针 1~1.5 寸，用提插之补法，使下肢抽动 3 次为度；极泉直刺 1~1.5 寸，用提插泻法，使上肢抽动 3 次为宜；尺泽操作及量学要求同极泉；委中穴采取仰卧位直腿抬高取穴，进针 1 寸，用提插泻法，使下肢抽动 3 次即可；风池针向结喉，针 2~2.5 寸，采用小幅度高频率捻转补法，施手法 1 分钟；上星透百会沿头皮向百会方向透刺，用捻转补法，以局部酸胀为度。

治疗经过：治疗一周后，左下肢直腿抬高 40 度，左上肢能屈肘，上举平胸，语音清。两周后搀扶行走，继之独立行走，左上肢抬举过头，唯左手握力稍差。四周左右四肢功能如常，语音清楚，痊愈出院。

六、预防与调护

（一）预防

（1）降低可能中风的危险因素：可能引起中风的疾病，如动脉硬化、糖尿病、冠心病、高血脂病、高黏血症、肥胖病、颈椎病等应及早治疗。

（2）注意中风的先兆征象：一部分患者在中风发作前常有血压升高、波动，头晕、头痛、昏沉嗜睡、性格反常、手脚麻木无力等先兆，发现后要尽早采取措施加以控制。

（3）有效地控制短暂性脑缺血发作：当患者有短暂性脑缺血发作先兆时，应让其安静休息，并及时到医院诊治，防止其发展为脑血栓形成。

（4）注意气象因素的影响：季节与气候变化会使高血压患者情绪不稳，血压波动，诱发中风，在这种时候更要防备中风的发生。应逐步适应环境温度，室内外温差不宜过大（特别是老年人）。此外，日常生活起床、低头系鞋带等动作要缓慢；洗澡时间不宜过长等。

（二）调护

（1）中医药对于中风的治疗效果较佳，早期介入针灸疗法效果更好，尤其对肢体运动、语言、吞咽等功能的恢复有较好的促进作用。

（2）中风急性期，出现高热、神昏、心衰、颅内压增高、上消化道出血等情况时，应采取综合治疗措施。

（3）中风卧床患者要定时翻身，保持皮肤干燥和血运良好，以避免褥疮的发生，同时注意保持呼吸道通畅。

（4）在治疗和恢复期间，功能锻炼对于促进瘫痪肢体运动功能的恢复大有益处。

（5）多食清淡饮食，避免或少食肥甘辛辣之品，可以防止蕴热生风，聚湿生痰。

（6）平时保持轻松愉悦，避免恼怒、抑郁、多虑和悲伤等不良情绪的影响。

（7）本病应注重预防，年过40岁，常有头晕头痛、肢体麻木、偶有发作性语言不利、肢体痿软无力等症状出现，应警惕中风先兆，应加强防治。

（徐　立）

参考文献

［1］天津中医学院第一附属医院针灸科．石学敏针灸临证集验［M］．天津：天津科技出版社，1990．

［2］王启才．针医心悟［M］．北京：中医古籍出版社，2001．

［3］严世芸，郑平东，何立人．张伯臾医案［M］．上海：上海科学技术出版社，2003．

［4］周仲瑛．中医内科学［M］．北京：中国中医药出版社，2003．

［5］石学敏，戴锡孟，王健．中医内科学［M］．北京：中国中医药出版社，2009．

［6］张伯礼．中医内科学［M］．北京：人民卫生出版社，2012．

［7］石学敏．针灸学（双语教材）［M］．北京：高等教育出版社，2005．

［8］高树中．针灸治疗学［M］．上海：上海科学技术出版社，2009．

［9］王启才．针灸治疗学［M］．北京：中国中医药出版社，2004．

失眠

Insomnia

一、概述

失眠在中医亦称"不寐""不得眠"，是指经常不能获得正常睡眠为特征的一种病证，在《内经》中又称为"不得卧""目不瞑"。病位在心，与肾、肝、脾、胃、胆密切相关。主要由心神不宁所致，临床表现为睡眠时间、深度的不足，轻者入睡困难，或寐而不酣，时寐时醒，或醒后不能再寐，重则彻夜不寐，常影响人们的正常工作、学习、生活和健康。为了提高人们对睡眠重要性的认识，国际精神卫生和神经科学基金学会发起了一项全球睡眠和健康计划，将每年 3 月 21 日定为"世界睡眠日"，可见失眠已逐步成为全球性的健康问题。

西医学中的神经官能症、更年期综合征、慢性消化不良、抑郁症、焦虑症、动脉粥样硬化症等以失眠为主要临床表现者，可参考本病内容辨证论治。

二、病因病机

（一）中医

失眠的发生主要与饮食不节、情志失调、劳逸失调、病后体虚及年迈衰弱等因素有关。正常睡眠依赖人体的气血充足、脏腑调和、阴平阳秘，以保证心神安定，入睡安稳。若思虑过度，内伤心脾，气血不足，心失濡养而心神不宁；若久病体虚，阴血不足，阴虚火旺，虚火上扰而心神不安；若暴受惊恐，心胆气虚，心神失养，神不守舍而心神难安；若情志不舒，气郁化火，肝火上炎，心火炽盛，扰乱神明而心烦不得眠；若饮食伤脾，宿食停滞，久化痰热，扰动胃腑而不得安眠。

1. 病因

《内经》认为失眠是邪气客于脏腑，卫气行于阳，不能入阴所得。《素问·逆调论》有"胃不和则卧不安"的记载。汉代张仲景的《伤寒论》将其病因分为外感和内伤两类，提出"虚劳虚烦不得眠"的观点。李中梓对不寐的病因提出了卓有见识的论述："不寐之故，大约有五：一曰气虚；一曰阴虚；一曰痰滞；一曰水停；一曰胃不和。"明代戴元礼《证治要诀·虚损门》提出"年高人阳衰不寐"之论。清代《冯氏锦囊·卷十二》提出"壮年人肾阴强盛，则睡沉熟而长，年老人阴气衰弱，则睡轻微易知。"说明失眠的病因亦与肾的阴阳虚衰有关。

（1）饮食不节：暴饮暴食，宿食内停，脾胃损伤，痰湿内生，壅遏于中，日久化热，痰热上扰，胃气失和，而不得安寐。《张氏医通·不得卧》阐述失眠原因曰："脉滑数有力不得卧者，中有宿滞痰火，此为胃不和则卧不安也。"

（2）情志失调：七情过极可导致脏腑功能失调而发生失眠病证。平日心情不舒或情志不遂，郁怒伤肝，肝气郁结，气郁化火，火扰神明，神不安而夜不寐；或因五志过极，心火内炽，扰动心神而不寐；或因喜笑无度，心神被扰，神魂不安而不寐；或因暴受惊恐，心胆虚怯，神魂不安而夜不能寐。《沈氏尊生书·不寐》记载："心胆俱怯，触事易惊，梦多不祥，虚烦不眠"。或因过度忧思，伤及心脾，营血不足，不能上荣于心而神不安夜难寐。《类证治裁·不寐》记载："思虑伤脾，脾血亏虚，经年不寐"。

（3）劳逸过度：劳倦过度伤脾，过逸少动亦伤脾。脾虚气弱，运化不健，气血生化之源不足，不能上养于心，以致心神失养而失眠。《景岳全书·不寐》记载："劳倦、思虑太过者，必致血液耗亡，神魂无主，所以不眠。"可见脾失健运，气血不生造成血虚，神明失养导致失眠。

（4）病后体虚：久病阴血不足，年迈体虚，导致心血不足，心失所养，心神不安不得寐，正如《景岳全书·不寐》所说："无邪而不寐者，必营气不足也，营主血，血虚则无以养心，心虚则神不守舍。"亦可因年迈体虚，阴阳亏虚而致不寐。若素体阴虚，兼因房劳过度，肾阴耗伤，阴衰于下，不能上奉于心，水火不济，心火独亢，火盛神动，心肾失交而神志不宁。如《景岳全书·不寐》记载："真阴精血不足，阴阳不交，而神有不安其室耳。"

2.病机

失眠的病因很多，但其基本病机是心神不宁，总归于阳盛阴衰，阴阳失交。即一为阴虚不能纳阳，一为阳盛不得入于阴。其病位主要在心，与肝、脾、胃、肾、胆密切相关。心主神明，神安则寐，神不安则不寐。因阴阳气血之来源，为水谷之精微所化生，上奉于心，则心神得养；受藏于肝，则肝体柔和；受养于胆，则胆气盛神气安；统摄于脾，则生化无穷；调节有度，化而为精，内藏于肾，肾精上承于心，心气下交于肾，则阴精内守，神志安宁。

失眠的病理性质有虚、实两种。若肝郁化火，或痰热内扰，或心火炽盛，心神不安者以实证为主。心脾两虚，气血不足，或由心胆气虚，或由心肾不交，水火不济，心神失养，神不安宁，多属虚证。若日久病长，可表现为虚实夹杂，亦可为瘀血所致。

失眠的预后一般较好，若失治误治可发生病机转化。如肝郁化火者，误治使病情加重，火热伤阴耗气，则由实转虚；心脾两虚者，饮食不节，进一步损伤脾胃，食积内停，而见虚实兼夹。往往因病情不一，预后亦各异。病程短，病情单纯者，治疗收效较快；病程较长，病情复杂者，治疗难以速效。因失治误治，病程延长，易产生情志病变，使病情更加复杂，治疗难度亦增加。

（二）西医

失眠按病因可划分为原发性和继发性两类。

1.原发性失眠

通常缺少明确病因，或在排除可能引起失眠的病因后仍遗留失眠症状，主要包括心理生理性失眠、特发性失眠和主观性失眠3种类型。原发性失眠的诊断缺乏特异性指标，主要是一种排除性诊断。当可能引起失眠的病因被排除或治愈以后，仍遗留失眠症状时即可考虑为原发性失眠。心理生理性失眠在临床上发现其病因都可以溯源为某一个或几个长期事件对患者大脑边缘系统功能稳定性的影响，边缘系统功能的稳定性失衡最终导致了大脑睡眠功能的紊乱，出现失眠。

2.继发性失眠

常由于躯体疾病、精神障碍、药物滥用等引起，与睡眠呼吸紊乱、睡眠运动障碍等相关。

失眠常与其他疾病同时发生，有时很难确定这些疾病与失眠之间的因果关系，故近年来提出共病性失眠（comorbid insomnia）的概念，用以描述那些同时伴随其他疾病的失眠。

三、诊断要点与鉴别诊断

（一）诊断要点

1.中医

（1）失眠，轻者入睡困难，或寐而易醒，或醒后不寐，或时寐时醒，或寐而不酣，连续3周以上，严重者彻夜难眠。

（2）可伴有头昏、头痛、心悸、健忘、神疲乏力、心神不宁、多梦等。

（3）常有饮食不节，情志失常，劳倦、思虑过度，病后、体虚等病史。

（4）经全面的系统及实验室检查，未发现有妨碍睡眠的其他器质性病变。

2.西医

（1）有失眠的典型症状：以睡眠障碍为几乎唯一的症状，其他症状均继发于失眠，包括入睡困难，易醒，多梦，晨醒过早，醒后不能再睡，醒后不适、疲乏或白天困倦。

（2）上述睡眠障碍每周至少发生3次，并持续1个月以上。

（3）失眠引起显著的苦恼，或精神活动效率下降，或妨碍社会功能。

（4）不是任何一种躯体疾病或精神障碍症状的一部分。

（二）鉴别诊断

失眠应与一时性不寐、生理性少寐、他病痛苦引起的不寐相区别。失眠是指单纯以不寐为主症，表现为持续的、严重的睡眠困难。若因一时的情志影响或生活环境改变引起的暂时性不寐不属病态。至于老年人少寐早醒，亦多属生理状态。若因其他疾病痛苦引起的不寐者，则应以治疗有关病因为主。

1.精神因素所致的失眠

精神紧张、焦虑、恐惧、兴奋等可引起短暂性失眠，临床主要为入眠困难及易惊醒，当精神因素解除后，失眠即可缓解。

2.躯体因素引起的失眠

各种躯体疾病引起的疼痛、瘙痒、鼻塞、呼吸困难、气喘、咳嗽、尿频、恶心、呕吐、腹胀、腹泻、心悸等均可引起入眠困难或睡眠不深，当躯体疾病解除后，失眠即可改善。

3.生理因素

由于生活工作环境的改变、初到异乡、不习惯的环境、饮浓茶咖啡等可引起失眠，当脱离不适环境或短期适应后，失眠即可缓解。

4.大脑弥散性病变

慢性中毒、内分泌疾病、营养代谢障碍、脑动脉硬化等各种因素引起的大脑弥散性病变，失眠常为早期症状，表现为睡眠时间减少、间断易醒、深睡期消失，当病情缓解时，失眠即可缓解；当病情加重时失眠加重，病情过于严重时可出现嗜睡或意识障碍。

四、中医治疗

（一）辨证治疗

1. 肝火扰心

主症： 难以入睡，不寐多梦，甚则彻夜不眠，烦躁易怒，伴头晕头胀，目赤耳鸣，口干而苦，不思饮食，便秘溲赤，舌红苔黄，脉弦而数。

治法： 疏肝泻火，镇心安神。

方药： 龙胆泻肝汤加减。龙胆草、栀子、柴胡、黄芩、生地、泽泻、当归、木通、车前子、生甘草、生龙骨、生牡蛎、磁石。

方解： 本方有清泻肝胆实火之功效，主要适用于肝郁化火上炎所致的失眠多梦，头晕头胀，目赤耳鸣之症。龙胆草、黄芩、栀子清肝泻火；泽泻、车前子清湿热解郁火；当归、生地滋阴养血以防泻火伤阴；柴胡疏肝解郁；甘草和中；生龙骨、生牡蛎、磁石镇心安神。

加减： 兼有胸闷胁胀，善太息者，加香附、郁金、佛手以增强疏肝解郁之功；兼有不思饮食，嗳腐吞酸者，重用黄连、吴茱萸以增强清泻肝火，降逆和胃之功；兼有彻夜不眠，头昏目眩，头痛欲裂，心烦易怒，大便秘结者，可改用当归龙荟丸。

2. 痰热扰心

主症： 心烦不寐，胸闷脘痞，泛恶嗳气，伴口苦口臭，头昏头重，目眩，舌红苔黄腻，脉滑数。

治法： 清化痰热，健中安神。

方药： 黄连温胆汤加减。黄连、竹茹、枳实、半夏、陈皮、甘草、生姜、茯苓、龙齿、珍珠母、磁石。

方解： 本方有清心降火。化痰安中之功效，主要适用于痰热上扰心神所致的心烦不寐，头昏多梦之症。半夏、陈皮、茯苓、枳实健脾化痰，理气和胃；黄连、竹茹清心降火化痰；龙齿、珍珠母、磁石镇惊安神。

加减： 兼有胸闷嗳气，脘腹胀满，大便不爽，苔腻脉滑者，加用半夏秫米汤健脾和胃降气；兼有饮食停滞，胃中不和，嗳腐吞酸，脘腹胀痛者，加用神曲、焦山楂、莱菔子以消导和中；兼有痰热壅盛，痰火上扰心神，彻夜不眠，大便秘结者，加用礞石滚痰丸以泻火逐痰。

3. 心火炽盛

主症： 心烦不寐，躁扰不宁，口干舌燥，小便短赤，口舌生疮，舌尖红，苔薄黄，脉数有力或细数。

治法： 清心泻火，安神宁心。

方药： 朱砂安神丸加减。朱砂、黄连、当归、生地、甘草、黄芩、栀子、莲子心。

方解：本方有清热泻火，除烦安神之功效，主要适用于心火亢盛所致的心烦不寐，躁扰不宁之症。朱砂重镇安神，黄连苦寒泻火，清心除烦，两药配伍，共奏泻火清热除烦、重镇以安神志之功；当归养血，生地滋阴，补充被炽盛之火耗伤之阴血；甘草调和诸药。可加黄芩、栀子、莲子心，加强本方清心泻火之功。

加减：兼有胸中懊恼，胸闷泛恶者，加豆豉、竹茹，以宣通胸中郁火；兼有便秘尿赤者，加大黄、淡竹叶、琥珀，引火下行，以安心神。

4. 胃失和降

主症：烦躁不寐，脘腹胀满，嗳腐吞酸，恶心呕吐，大便不爽，或大便恶臭，或便秘腹痛，舌红，苔黄腻，或黄糙，脉弦滑或滑数。

治法：和胃化滞，宁心安神。

方药：保和丸加减。山楂、神曲、莱菔子、陈皮、半夏、茯苓、连翘、远志、柏子仁、夜交藤。

方解：本方有消食，导滞，和胃安神之功效，主要适用于食积停滞，胃失和降所导致的胸脘痞满，腹胀时痛，烦躁不寐之症。山楂善消油腻肉滞；神曲能消酒食陈腐之积；莱菔子消面食痰浊之滞；陈皮、半夏、茯苓理气和胃，燥湿化痰；连翘散结清热，诸药共奏消食和胃之功；可加远志、柏子仁、夜交藤以宁心安神。

加减：兼有胸闷嗳气，脘腹胀满重者，加用枳实、枳壳行气消积；兼有胃中不和，恶心呕吐者，加用白术、厚朴、香附健脾利湿，宽中止呕；兼有气郁停滞，倒饱嘈杂，胸腹胀痛者，可改用越鞠保和丸以疏肝解郁，开胃消食。

5. 血脉瘀阻

主症：失眠多梦，烦躁不安，健忘，记忆力减退，口干口苦，头晕头痛，倦怠乏力，大便干结，小便黄赤，舌质暗红，舌边有瘀斑，舌苔黄腻或薄黄，脉弦细。

治法：活血化瘀，宁心安神。

方药：血府逐瘀汤合酸枣仁汤加减。当归、川芎、赤芍、桃仁、红花、牛膝、柴胡、桔梗、枳壳、生地、当归、酸枣仁、知母、茯苓、甘草。

方解：本方具有祛瘀通脉，养血安神之功效，主要适用于瘀血阻滞，清阳不升所致的心脾两虚所致的心悸、健忘、失眠之症。当归、川芎、赤芍、桃仁、红花活血化瘀；牛膝祛瘀滞而通血脉，引瘀血下行；柴胡疏肝解郁，升达清阳；桔梗开宣肺气，载药上行，与枳壳一升一降，开胸行气，使气行则血行；生地、当归合用养阴润燥，使祛瘀而不伤阴血；酸枣仁、知母、茯苓养血安神；甘草调和诸药。诸药合用既行血分瘀滞，又解气分郁结，活血而不耗血，祛瘀又能生新，故瘀血除，心神安。

加减：兼有入睡困难者，加用夜交藤、合欢皮、柏子仁养心安神；兼有不寐较重，心悸怔忡者，加用生龙骨、生牡蛎、珍珠母镇静安神。

6. 心脾两虚

主症：不易入睡，多梦易醒，心悸健忘，神疲食少，头晕目眩，四肢倦怠，腹胀便溏，面色少华，舌淡苔薄，脉细无力。

治法：健脾益心，养血安神。

方药：归脾汤加减。人参、白术、甘草、当归、黄芪、远志、酸枣仁、茯神、龙眼肉、木香。

方解：本方有健脾养心，益气补血之功效，主要适用于心脾两虚所致的不寐健忘，心悸怔忡，面黄食少之症。人参、白术、甘草健脾益气；当归、黄芪补气生血；远志、酸枣仁、茯神、龙眼肉补益心脾安神；木香行气疏脾。

加减：兼有心血不足较甚，心悸健忘者，加用熟地、芍药、阿胶以养心血；兼有难以入睡者，加用五味子、夜交藤、合欢皮、柏子仁养心安神；兼有不寐较重，心悸怔忡者，加用生龙骨、生牡蛎、琥珀粉镇静安神；兼有脘闷纳呆，苔腻者，重用白术，加用苍术、半夏、陈皮、茯苓、厚朴健脾燥湿，理气化痰。若老人夜寐早醒而无虚烦者，多属气血不足，重用当归、黄芪补益气血。

7. 心肾不交

主症：心烦不寐，入睡困难，心悸多梦，伴头晕耳鸣，腰膝酸软，潮热盗汗，咽干少津，男子遗精，女子月经不调，舌红少苔，脉细数。

治法：滋阴降火，交通心肾。

方药：六味地黄丸合交泰丸加减。熟地黄、山萸肉、山药、泽泻、茯苓、丹皮、黄连、肉桂。

方解：六味地黄丸以滋补肾阴为主，主要用于头晕耳鸣，腰膝酸软，潮热盗汗等肾阴不足之证；交泰丸以清心降火，引火归原，主要用于心烦不寐，梦遗失精等心火偏亢证。熟地黄滋阴补肾，填精益髓；山萸肉补养肝肾，并能涩精；山药补益脾阴，亦能固肾；三药合用以达滋补肾肝脾之功。泽泻利湿而泄肾浊，以减熟地之滋腻；茯苓淡渗脾湿，助山药之健运；丹皮清泻虚热，制约山茱萸之温涩；黄连清心降火；肉桂引火归原。

加减：兼有心阴不足者，加用天王补心丹滋阴养血，补心安神；兼有心烦不寐，彻夜不眠者，加用朱砂、磁石、龙骨、龙齿重镇安神；兼有阴血亏虚，心火亢盛者，加用朱砂安神丸。

8. 心胆气虚

主症：失眠多梦，易于惊醒，胆怯心悸，触事易惊，终日惕惕，伴气短懒言，易惊易恐，自汗出，倦怠乏力，舌淡苔白，脉弦细无力。

治法：益气镇惊，安神定志

方药：安神定志丸合酸枣仁汤加减。酸枣仁、人参、茯苓、甘草、茯神、远志、龙齿、石菖蒲、川芎、知母。

方解：安神定志丸以镇惊安神为主，主要用于心烦不寐，气短自汗，倦怠乏力之症；酸枣仁汤偏于养血清热除烦，用于虚烦不寐，终日惕惕，触事易惊之症。人参、茯苓、甘草补益心胆之气；茯神、远志、龙齿、石菖蒲化痰宁心，镇惊安神；川芎调血养心；知母清热除烦。

加减：兼有惊悸汗出，证属心肝血虚者，重用人参，加用白芍、当归、黄芪补养肝血；兼有肝木乘脾土，胸闷，善太息，纳呆腹胀者，加用柴胡、陈皮、山药、白术以疏肝健脾；兼有心悸甚，惊惕不安者，加用龙骨、生牡蛎、朱砂以重镇安神。

（二）单方验方

（1）夜交藤、生地各 10g，麦冬 6g。水煎服，于午休与晚上临睡前各服 1 次。用于阴虚火旺所致的失眠。

（2）莲子心 2g，生甘草 3g。开水冲泡，代茶饮，每日数次。用于心火内炽所致的烦躁失眠。

（三）中成药

1. 肝火扰心

中成药：龙胆泻肝丸。每次 3~5g，每日 2~3 次。

方义：方用龙胆草、黄芩、栀子清肝泻火；泽泻、木通、车前子利小便而清热；柴胡疏肝解郁；当归、生地养血滋阴柔肝；甘草和中。

若肝胆火旺，心烦不宁，头晕目眩，耳鸣耳聋，胁肋疼痛，可加用泻肝安神丸。若头痛欲裂，不寐欲狂，脘腹胀痛，大便秘结者，可用当归龙荟丸泻火通便。若情绪紧张，烦躁易怒者，可选用加味逍遥丸疏肝解郁，改善睡眠。

2. 痰热扰心

中成药：礞石滚痰丸。每次 6~12g，每日 1 次。

方义：方用礞石治实热顽痰；酒蒸大黄以豁痰通便；黄芩以清其热；沉香以行其滞。四味药合用为善治热痰之良方。

若痰热上蒙心神，惊惕不安，可加用清心滚痰丸以镇惊定志，逐痰安神；若宿食积，嗳腐吞酸，脘腹胀痛，可加用枳实导滞丸以消导和中安神。若痰热蒙蔽清窍，头昏头重，彻夜不眠，可选用牛黄清心丸以泻火豁痰，开窍安神。

3. 心火炽盛

中成药：朱砂安神丸。每次 6g，每日 2 次。

方义：方用黄连苦寒泻火，清心除烦，朱砂重镇安神，两药配伍共奏清泻心火，重镇安神之功；当归、生地滋阴养血；甘草调和诸药。

若心火亢盛，躁扰不宁，可加用牛黄上清丸清热除烦，镇惊安神；若心悸、坐立不安，可加用安神定志丸以安心神。若心火炽盛，消耗心血，不仅失眠，健忘，心悸、心慌，且手脚心热，口干舌燥，口舌生疮，可选用天王补心丹清热滋阴重镇安神。

4. 胃失和降

中成药：保和丸。每次 6g，每日 2 次。

方义：方用山楂消油腻厚味之滞；神曲消酒食陈腐之积；莱菔子消面食痰浊之滞；陈皮、半夏、茯苓健脾燥湿，宽胸理气，和胃降逆；连翘清热散结，诸药共奏消食和胃理气降逆之功。

若脘腹胀满，食欲不振，可加用同仁疏肝和胃丸以疏肝解郁，和胃止痛；若气郁停滞，两胁胀满，嗳腐吞酸，打嗝呕吐，胃脘疼痛，大便失调，可改用越鞠保和丸以疏肝解郁，开胃消食。

5. 血脉瘀阻

中成药：血府逐瘀胶囊。每次 2.4g，每日 2 次。

方义：方用桃仁、红花活血化瘀；当归、川芎、赤芍增强活血祛瘀之功；牛膝祛瘀血，通血脉，引瘀血下行；柴胡疏肝解郁，升达清阳；桔梗、枳壳一升一降，开胸行气，使气行则血行；生地凉血清热，合当归又能养阴润燥，使瘀血祛而不伤阴；甘草解毒，调和诸药。诸药合用既行血分瘀滞，又解气分郁结，活血而不耗血，祛瘀又能生新，故瘀血除心神安。

若失眠多梦，烦躁不安，健忘，记忆力减退，可加用安神定志丸以活血化瘀，宁心安神。

6. 心脾两虚

中成药：人参归脾丸。每次 1 丸，每日 2 次。

方义：方用人参大补元气，复脉固脱，补脾益肺，生津，安神；白术补脾，益胃，燥湿，和中；茯苓渗湿利水，健脾和胃，宁心安神；炙黄芪益气补中；当归、龙眼肉补益心脾，养血安神；酸枣仁养肝，宁心，安神；远志安神益智；木香理气调中；炙甘草益气滋阴，通阳复脉。

若心悸怔忡，健忘失眠，多梦易惊，可加用安神补心丸以养心益阴，安神定志；若面色萎黄，食少体倦，可选用养血安神丸。

7. 心肾不交

中成药：六味地黄丸合交泰丸。每次各 1 丸，每日 2 次。

方义：方用熟地黄、山萸肉、山药三药合用以达滋补肾肝脾之功；泽泻利湿泄浊，以减熟地之滋腻；茯苓淡渗脾湿，以助山药之健运；丹皮清泻虚热，以制山萸肉之温涩；肉桂引火归原，与黄连共用交通心肾，水火相济，心神可安。

若心烦心悸，梦遗失精者，可加用安神补心胶囊滋阴养心安神；若失眠，健忘，头晕者，可选用枣仁安神液养心、安神、益智。

8. 心胆气虚

中成药：安神定志丸。每次 1 丸，每日 2 次。

方义：方用人参补益心胆之气；茯苓、茯神、远志宁心安神；龙齿、石菖蒲镇惊开窍宁神。

若失眠健忘，易惊易恐，可加用同仁柏子养心丸以养心益气；若老年体虚，失眠多梦，心悸乏力，口干津少，可选用安神健脑液以益气养神，安神生津。

（四）针灸治疗

1. 肝火扰心

主穴：安眠、行间、足窍阴、风池、神门。

配穴：胁痛甚者加期门。

方义：安眠为治疗失眠的经验穴，对于各种失眠均有良好效果；行间为肝经之荥穴，平肝降火；

足窍阴为胆经之井穴，降胆火以除烦；风池疏调肝胆而止头痛头晕；神门宁心安神，神安则能寐；期门疏肝降火安神。

刺法：毫针刺，施泻法。

2. 痰热扰心

主穴：安眠、丰隆、内庭、公孙、神门。

配穴：头晕甚者加百会、印堂。

方义：安眠为治疗失眠的经验穴；丰隆清化痰浊，配内庭清泻脾胃蕴热；公孙健脾运湿；神门为心经之原穴，宁心安神；百会、印堂清热开窍。

刺法：毫针刺，施泻法。

3. 心火炽盛

主穴：安眠、神门、少府、劳宫。

配穴：口舌生疮加少冲、少泽。

方义：安眠为治疗失眠的经验穴；神门为心经之原穴，能镇静安神；少府、劳宫用泻法可清泻心火；少冲为心经之井穴，少泽为小肠经之井穴，点刺放血可清泻心火，使之不致上炎。

刺法：毫针刺，施泻法，少冲、少泽点刺放血。

4. 胃失和降

主穴：安眠、中脘、足三里、神门。

配穴：胁胀胃痛加太冲；脘腹胀满，嗳腐吞酸，恶心呕吐加内关、公孙；大便不爽加天枢。

方义：安眠为治疗失眠的经验穴；中脘、足三里健脾和胃，降气和中；神门为心经之原穴，能镇静安神；太冲疏肝理气，和胃降逆；内关、公孙宽胸和胃止呕；天枢调理胃肠，消食通便。

刺法：毫针刺，施泻法，或补泻兼施。

5. 血脉瘀阻

主穴：安眠、膈俞、血海、百会、神庭、神门。

配穴：健忘，记忆力减退加四神聪；头晕头痛加上星。

方义：安眠为治疗失眠的经验穴；膈俞、血海活血通络祛瘀；百会疏通脑络；神庭、神门镇静安神；四神聪健脑益智；上星通络止痛。

刺法：毫针刺，施泻法，或补泻兼施。

6. 心脾两虚

主穴：安眠、心俞、神门、足三里、三阴交、脾俞。

配穴：脘闷纳呆者加中脘。

方义：安眠为治疗失眠的经验穴；心俞、神门为俞原配穴法，能补益心之气血，养心安神；足三里、三阴交为健脾益气养血之要穴，配脾俞更能扶助后天之本，以资气血生化之源；中脘健脾和胃。

刺法: 毫针刺,行补法,并可加灸。

7. 心肾不交

主穴: 安眠、太溪、神门、心俞、大陵、照海、申脉。

配穴: 腰酸无力加肾俞。

方义: 安眠为治疗失眠的经验穴;太溪为肾经之原穴,功擅滋补肾阴,水盛则心火不亢;神门为心经之原穴,大陵为心包经之原穴,心俞为心之背俞穴,三穴合用,可清降心火,宁心安神;肾俞强腰壮脊;照海、申脉为八脉交会穴,分别与阴跷脉、阳跷脉相通,阴、阳跷脉主睡眠,若阳跷脉功能亢盛则失眠,故补阴泻阳使阴、阳跷脉功能协调,不眠自愈。

刺法: 太溪、心俞、肾俞、照海施补法,申脉施泻法,余用平补平泻法。

8. 心胆气虚

主穴: 安眠、心俞、神门、大陵、胆俞、丘墟、照海、申脉。

配穴: 食少无力者加足三里。

方义: 安眠为治疗失眠的经验穴;心俞、大陵、神门温养心气,使神不外逸,安居于内;胆俞、丘墟补益胆气,使中清之腑不虚,则惊悸不生;足三里健运脾胃,以资气血生化之源;照海、申脉为八脉交会穴,分别与阴跷脉、阳跷脉相通,阴、阳跷脉主睡眠,若阳跷脉功能亢盛则失眠,故补阴泻阳使阴、阳跷脉功能协调,不眠自愈。

刺法: 毫针刺,申脉用泻法,余穴施补法。

(五)推拿治疗

1. 头部按摩

①双手用拿法施于头部两侧 10 遍左右。②按揉印堂 1 分钟,再由印堂以两拇指交替直推至神庭 5~10 遍,拇指由神庭沿头正中线(督脉)点按至百会穴,指振百会穴约 1 分钟。③双手拇指分推前额、眉弓至太阳 3~5 遍。指振太阳穴约 1 分钟。④侧击头部,掌振两颞、头顶,约 2 分钟。上述操作以患者有深沉力透感和轻松舒适感为宜。每日治疗 1 次,连续 15 天为 1 个疗程。

2. 腹部按摩

①掌摩腹部约 6 分钟,逆时针方向操作,顺时针方向移动。②按揉或一指禅推法施于中脘、神阙、气海、关元各 1 分钟,指振各穴。手法宜轻柔。③双掌自肋下至耻骨联合,从中间向两边平推 3~5 次。④掌振腹部约 1 分钟。每日治疗 1 次,连续 15 天为 1 个疗程。

3. 背部按摩

①提拿两肩井约 1 分钟。使患者有轻松舒适感为宜。②直推背部督脉及两侧太阳经 10 次左右,手法要深沉有力,速度均匀和缓。③按揉背部太阳经,重点按揉心俞、脾俞、胃俞、肾俞,以局部酸沉为度。④双掌交替轻轻叩击背部两侧太阳经。每日治疗 1 次,连续 15 天为 1 个疗程。

（六）其他

1. 耳针疗法

取穴： 皮质下、交感、神门、心、肝、脾、肾、垂前、耳背心。

方法： 每次取 3~4 穴，毫针刺，留针 30 分钟，每日 1 次；或揿针埋藏，每周 2 次；或王不留行籽贴压，每周 2~3 次。

2. 皮肤针法

取穴： 自项至腰部督脉和足太阳膀胱经第一侧线。

方法： 用皮肤针自上而下叩刺，叩至皮肤潮红为度，每日 1 次。

3. 拔罐法

取穴： 自项至腰部足太阳膀胱经背部第一、二侧线。

方法： 走罐，沿背部自上而下走罐，至皮肤潮红或皮下瘀紫为度，每周 1~2 次。

4. 电针法

取穴： 四神聪、太阳。

方法： 用较低频率，每次刺激 30 分钟。

五、名医专家经验方

（一）经验方（李培生）

组成： 五味子 50g，茯神 50g，合欢花 15g，法半夏 15g。

用法： 水煎服，日 1 剂。

功效： 滋阴和阳，健脾宁神。

（二）潜阳宁神汤（张琪）

组成： 夜交藤 30g，熟枣仁 20g，远志 15g，柏子仁 20g，茯苓 15g，生地黄 20g，玄参 20g，生牡蛎 25g，生赭石（研）30g，川连 10g，生龙骨 20g。

用法： 水煎服，日 1 剂。

功效： 滋阴潜阳，清热宁心，益智安神。

（三）枸杞枣仁汤（彭静山）

组成： 枸杞 30g，炒枣仁 40g，五味子 10g。

用法： 每日用药 1 份，置于茶杯中，开水浸泡，当茶频频饮之。或日饮 3 次，每次至少 50ml。

功效： 滋补肝肾，养血安神。

六、名医专家典型医案

（一）李桂兰医案——肝郁化火，火扰心神

李某 女，61 岁。

初诊： 2009 年 10 月 5 日。患者于 2 年前由于工作劳累加之情志不畅而出现夜寐欠安，表现为入睡困难，多梦易醒，时伴心慌乏力。一月前患者自觉失眠明显，每日睡眠二、三小时，心烦乏力，纳少，因害怕西药副作用，欲寻求中医药治疗，遂前来就诊。现症：患者神清，精神欠佳，心烦，左侧头胀不适，右胁肋胀满不舒，夜寐不安，入睡困难，口干，纳少，恶心，二便调。

辨证： 肝郁化火，火扰心神。

治法： 疏肝解郁，调心安神。

方药： 柴胡 12g，半夏 12g，黄芩 15g，夏枯草 30g，酸枣仁 30g，合欢皮 15g，珍珠母 15g，夜交藤 15g，生姜 3 片，大枣 5 枚，甘草 10g。水煎服，每日 1 剂。

针灸处方： 主穴：百会、四神聪、神庭、神门、风池、太冲、三阴交、安眠。配穴：行间、内关。操作：百会、四神聪、神庭、内关用平补平泻手法；三阴交、安眠用捻转补法；风池、太冲、行间用捻转泻法留针 30 分钟，隔日 1 次。

二诊： 2009 年 11 月 13 日。坚持治疗一月后各种症状均较前改善。患者神清，精神可，未诉心烦，未发头胀及右胁肋胀满不适，食量增多，入睡较快，睡眠时间延长，二便调，舌质红，苔薄白，脉弦。为进一步巩固疗效，继续予以针灸及中药治疗一周后，诸症消失，随诊未见复发。

按语： 脑为奇恒之府，主思维、情绪、决断，一切精神、意识、思维、情感、记忆等活动均为脑所支配。《本草纲目·辛夷条》记载："脑为元神之府。"《景岳全书·不寐》曰："盖寐本乎阴，神其主也，神安则寐，神不安则不寐。"是故脑的功能失调，易致失眠。

李教授认为脑失所养，肝失条达，气郁日久化火，上扰心神而发不寐。治疗上针药并用，以安神调心、疏肝解郁为基本治疗原则。针刺治疗取四神聪、百会、神庭、风池、太冲、内关、三阴交、安眠，严格按手法量学标准施术，依法在各穴进行针刺治疗。百会、四神聪为脑部局部取穴，重在宣上导下，调节周身气血，舒畅脑部气机。内关为八脉交会穴、手厥阴心包经络穴，直通阴维脉，联络三焦经，能宁心安神，收敛浮越之阳，使心有所主。神庭为督脉穴，针之有镇脑安神之效。三阴交为肝、脾、肾三经交会穴，能益肾肝，补阴血，和胃降浊，引火归原，促进阴阳气血平衡。风池为足少阳胆经穴，又为少阳经、阳维脉、阳跷脉的交会穴，足少阳经别贯心，阳维脉维系诸阳经，

故有宁心安神之效。太冲为肝经原穴，具泻肝火平肝阳、疏肝解郁的作用。安眠奇穴，有镇静安神之效，针之，可调节颅内外血管和神经功能。同时配合中药汤剂治以安神定志、清心除烦之法。

（二）李桂兰医案——肝胃不和

杨某 男，46岁。

初诊： 2010年2月28日。患者由于长期工作劳累而出现夜寐欠安，表现为入睡困难，睡后易醒，醒后难于入睡，每日睡眠仅3~4小时。1个月前因工作压力大，用脑过度而失眠复发，开始用安眠药有效，后来效果不佳，多梦心烦，每夜仅能睡2~3小时，且出现胃肠不适症状，因害怕西药的耐药性及副作用，遂前来寻求中医治疗。现症：患者神清，精神欠佳，夜寐不安，入睡困难，头晕，胸中烦闷不安，嗳气吞酸，咽干口干，纳差，二便调。

辨证： 肝气郁结，横逆犯胃，胃失和降。

治法： 安神解郁，健脾和胃。

方药： 柴胡15g，白芍20g，当归20g，茯苓20g，生栀子20g，郁金15g，川楝子20g，丹参30g，川芎15g，酸枣仁40g，合欢花20g，石菖蒲20g，首乌藤20g，白术20g，砂仁12g，北沙参20g，莱菔子15g，神曲30g，五味子15g，甘草10g。水煎服，每日1剂。

针灸处方： 主穴：百会、四神聪、神庭、神门、风池、太冲、三阴交、安眠。配穴：行间、内关、足三里、中脘。操作：百会、四神聪、神庭、神门、内关用平补平泻手法；三阴交、足三里、中脘、安眠用捻转补法；风池、太冲、行间用捻转泻法。留针30分钟，隔日1次。

二诊： 2010年3月6日。诉夜寐状况较前稍好，但仍入睡困难，时心烦，纳少吞酸，无恶心，口已不干，二便可，舌质红，苔薄黄，脉弦细。针灸处方如前，中药处方为前方加远志15g。

三诊： 2010年4月2日。患者睡眠已恢复正常，无不适症状，达到治愈标准。

按语： 《普济本事方·卷一》曰："平人肝不受邪，故卧则魂归于肝。神静而得寐。今肝有邪，魂不得归，是以卧则魂扬若离体也。"李教授认为肝主疏泄，可调畅气机，疏泄正常，则气之升降出入有序，血之运行输布如常，气血调和，使人精力充沛，心境平和，神魂安宁。若脑神失养不能统摄肝神，致肝失条达，肝气郁久，则易化火，正如朱丹溪所言"气有余便是火"，火气上扰于心，则神不守舍，神不安则不寐。同时，因劳倦太过，思虑过度损伤脾胃，脾伤则食少，纳呆，加之土失木疏，气壅而滞，胃失和降，肝胃不和则见嗳气吞酸，纳少，《内经》中曰"胃不和则卧不安"，故亦可致不寐。舌质红，咽干口干，苔薄黄，脉弦细，乃肝郁化火耗阴之象。治疗上针药并用，以安神调心、疏肝解郁、健脾和胃为基本治疗原则。

七、预防与调护

（1）注重精神调摄，避免不良的精神刺激，《内经》曰："恬淡虚无，真气从之，精神内守，病安从来"，积极进行心理情志调整，做到喜怒有节，保持精神舒畅。

（2）生活起居要有规律，避免过于安逸，不要过度劳累，养成良好的睡眠习惯。

（3）创造良好的睡眠环境，床铺要舒适，卧室光线要柔和，并努力减少噪音，去除各种可能影响睡眠的外在因素。

（4）晚餐不宜过饥或过饱，宜进清淡、易消化的食物。

（5）睡前避免饮用浓茶、可口可乐、咖啡及引起过度兴奋刺激的饮料。

（6）为提高睡眠质量，睡前可采取温热水泡足20分钟，或饮用一杯热牛奶。

（7）由其他疾病引起失眠者，应同时治疗其原发病。

（8）针灸治疗在下午或晚上效果更好。

（9）避免长期服用镇静催眠药物所产生的依赖性、成瘾性等副作用。

（10）从事适当的体力活动或体育锻炼，劳逸结合，逐渐增强体质。

（李桂兰）

参考文献

［1］石学敏.针灸学"十一五"国家级规划教材［M］.北京：中国中医药出版社，2010：227.

［2］王华.针灸学"十二五"国家级规划教材［M］.北京：高等教育出版社，2013：228.

［3］高树中.针灸治疗学"十二五"国家级规划教材［M］.北京：中国中医药出版社，2014：64.

［4］吴勉华.中医内科学"十二五"国家级规划教材［M］.北京：中国中医药出版社，2014：149.

［5］王娜娜.李桂兰教授健脑调肝针药并施治疗失眠症验案2则［J］.现代中医药，2012，32（4）：1-2.

慢性萎缩性胃炎

Chronic Atrophic Gastritis

一、概述

慢性萎缩性胃炎（Chronic Atrophic Gastritis，CAG）是慢性胃炎的一种类型，是一种以胃黏膜上皮和固有腺体萎缩、黏膜变薄，或伴有肠上皮化生、异型增生为病理特点的临床常见消化系统疾病。慢性萎缩性胃炎是消化系统一种常见病、多发病、难治病，1978年世界卫生组织将其列为胃癌的癌前疾病或癌前状态。其发展模式：慢性胃炎→慢性萎缩性胃炎→肠化生→不典型增生→胃癌。随着对该病认识的加深，我们认识到了本病与胃癌间的密切联系。因此，治疗和逆转慢性萎缩性胃炎在控制消化道肿瘤中占据十分重要的地位。目前，西医对慢性萎缩性胃炎尚缺乏有效的治疗方法，对症处理和定期复查成为西医治疗该病的主要方法。大量临床报道显示，中医药在减轻症状、促进胃黏膜修复以及抑制肠上皮化生等方面有显著疗效。根据临床症状，慢性萎缩性胃炎的中医病名归属为"胃痞""痞满""虚痞"等范畴。

二、病因病机

（一）中医

中医认为慢性萎缩性胃炎的病因主要与饮食不节，情志失调，劳倦过度，感受外来毒邪、素体虚弱等因素有关。病位在胃，发病与脾、胃、肝（胆）关系最为密切，以脾胃虚弱、升降失常为本，热毒侵袭、肝胃郁热为标，久病入里、气血瘀滞为变。脾胃虚弱又以脾气虚、胃阴亏为多，而气滞血瘀则贯穿病程始终。脾胃为气血生化之本，中气旺盛，则化生气血，充养五脏六腑，脾胃小得自养；若脾胃功能衰减，则纳运失常、生化乏源，在临床上必会导致气机不得舒展畅运，郁而化热，湿热内阻，瘀毒蕴结，久则胃之脉络自痹，气血运行受阻，胃黏膜不得荣养，继而萎缩。近代医家也认为慢性萎缩性胃炎之病机以脾胃虚弱为本，瘀血阻络为标，气虚、血瘀互为因果。其病机特点为本虚标实、虚实夹杂。

（二）西医

西医学认为慢性萎缩性胃炎的发病主要与幽门螺杆菌（HP）感染、胆汁反流、血管活性因子及细胞因子改变、免疫因素等多种因素有关。萎缩性胃炎是西医从病理的角度分型的一种胃病，是胃黏膜的萎缩变化。常见胃黏膜萎缩变薄，腺体减少或消失，有的伴有肠上皮细胞不同程度的病变。有的学者认为萎缩性胃炎是胃癌的前期病变与息肉并存时，发生胃癌的可能性更大。由此提示人们要重视对萎缩性胃炎的治疗。

三、诊断要点与鉴别诊断

（一）诊断要点

1.临床表现

上腹部不适，痞满，时发疼痛，纳呆便溏，后期厌食，消瘦乏力，贫血，舌淡苔白，脉弦细。

2.相关检查

诊断慢性萎缩性胃炎主要依靠胃镜和病理诊断。

（1）胃镜诊断：胃镜可见黏膜颜色改变，呈灰白、灰色或灰黄色，黏膜萎缩可呈局限性也可为弥漫性，境界常不清晰。黏膜变薄，黏膜皱襞变平或变细小。萎缩初期可见黏膜内小血管，后期可见黏膜下大血管。腺体萎缩后腺窝增生延长或伴肠上皮化生表现，黏膜表面多粗糙，有颗粒感或结节样改变。

（2）病理诊断：根据悉尼系统要求取标本行常规活检，有如下病理表现即可诊断：①淋巴滤泡形成。②固有腺体萎缩，主要为腺体上皮细胞体积缩小，细胞量减少。腺体间纤维组织增生，间质病变。③固有膜炎症。④黏膜肌层增厚。⑤肠上皮化生或假幽门腺化生。

（二）鉴别诊断

1. 胃癌

慢性胃炎的症状如食欲不振、上腹不适、贫血等少数胃窦胃炎的 X 线征与胃癌的症状相似，需特别注意鉴别。绝大多数患者胃镜检查及活检有助于鉴别。

2. 消化性溃疡

两者均有慢性上腹痛，但消化性溃疡以上腹部规律性、周期性疼痛为主，而慢性胃炎疼痛很少有规律性并以消化不良为主。鉴别诊断依靠 X 线钡餐透视及胃镜检查。

3. 慢性胆管疾病

慢性胆囊炎、胆石症常有慢性右上腹腹胀、嗳气等消化不良的症状，易误诊为慢性胃炎。但该病胃肠检查无异常发现，胆囊造影及 B 超异常可最后确诊。

4. 其他

如肝炎、肝癌及胰腺疾病亦可因出现食欲不振、消化不良等症状而延误诊治，全面细微的查体及有关检查可防止误诊。

四、中医治疗

（一）辨证治疗

1. 肝胃不和

主症：胃脘胀痛，攻撑胸胁，嗳气吞酸，口干口苦，食欲不振，大便不畅，且发病多与情志因素相关，舌质红，苔薄白或薄黄，脉弦或弦数。

治法：疏肝和胃，行气消胀。

方药：柴胡疏肝散加减。柴胡、枳壳、香附、当归、白芍、木香、元胡、佛手、川楝子、佛手、蒲公英、丹参。

加减：若肝胃气郁化火或肝热犯胃，症见胃脘灼痛、泛酸、烧心、口苦、嘈杂、心烦易怒者，可用左金丸合金铃子散或丹栀逍遥散加减。胃纳不振明显者，加六神曲、炒谷芽、炒麦芽、焦山楂等。兼见恶心呕吐者，则可加竹茹、半夏、陈皮等。

2. 脾胃湿热

主症： 胃脘痞闷不适或灼痛不已，嘈杂嗳气，口苦口黏，渴不欲饮，或有腹胀便溏，舌质红，苔黄厚或腻，脉弦数或滑数。

治法： 清热化湿，健脾和胃。

方药： 三仁汤加减。白蔻仁、杏仁、薏苡仁、厚朴、半夏、通草、滑石、竹叶、黄连、茵陈、丹参。

加减： 兼有表湿者，加香薷、藿香以解表化湿。恶心呕吐者，加竹茹、生姜以和胃降逆。食欲不振明显者加鸡内金、神曲、麦芽以消食导滞。此型亦可用黄连平胃散加味治疗。

3. 脾胃虚弱

主症： 胃脘隐痛，喜得温按，脘腹痞满，食后加重，纳差少食，肠鸣便溏，或伴倦怠乏力，少气懒言，四肢酸软，舌质淡红，苔薄白或白或有齿痕，脉沉细。

治法： 益气和中，健脾养胃。

方药： 香砂六君子汤或参苓白术散加减。党参、炒白术、薏苡仁、茯苓、木香、砂仁、陈皮、半夏、麦芽、当归、白芍、桂枝、蒲公英、丹参、黄芪。

加减： 腹痛便溏，四肢不温，苔白，脉紧，虚寒偏重者，治以温补脾胃，方用黄芪建中汤合良附丸加减。食后脘腹胀甚者，可加鸡内金、莱菔子、佛手等。见呕吐大量清水者，可重用陈皮、半夏、茯苓；上泛酸水明显者，可配用左金丸。脾虚便溏甚者，可加山药、莲子肉、生扁豆等健脾化湿之品。见便黑者，加干姜炭、伏龙肝、白及、地榆炭。中阳虚者合理中汤加乌梅、白芍等。

4. 胃阴不足

主症： 胃脘隐痛或灼痛，嘈杂似饥，口干舌燥，便干，舌红少津有裂纹，少苔、无苔或花剥苔，脉细数。

治法： 清热生津，养阴益胃。

方药： 沙参麦冬汤或益胃汤加减。沙参、麦冬、石斛、天花粉、乌梅、白芍、山楂、甘草、党参、山药、茯苓、蒲公英、丹参。

加减： 兼见烦渴、干呕、齿衄，证属胃阴亏损，虚火内灼者，方选玉女煎加减。兼见胸胁腹痛，口干口苦，脉弦数，证属肝胃阴虚，血燥气郁者，方选一贯煎加减。兼见脘痞气滞，宜用行气药中润剂如佛手、绿萼梅、厚朴花、枳壳等。大便干结甚者，可合用增液汤。阴虚热盛者，可酌加生石膏、知母，以增强清热生津之功。夹湿者，可用薏苡仁、白蔻仁、茵陈清热化湿。兼有瘀滞者，加丹参、当归、桃仁，以活血化瘀。此型亦可用一贯煎加减。

5. 胃络瘀血

主症： 胃脘疼痛日久不愈，或痛有定处，拒按，痛如锥刺，或兼见吐血、黑便，舌质紫暗或暗红或有瘀斑，脉沉。

治法： 活血化瘀，通络止痛。

方药：桃红四物汤合失笑散加减。桃仁、红花、当归、川芎、赤芍、五灵脂、生蒲黄、元胡、丹参、泽兰、降香。

加减：气虚者，可加黄芪、党参、白术、黄精以益气；气滞明显者，可酌加枳壳、青皮、木香、砂仁以行气。兼见吐血、黑便者，若出血鲜红，舌红苔黄，脉弦数，可用泻心汤以清热凉血止血；若出血暗红，面色萎黄，四肢不温，舌淡脉弱，系脾不统血，可用黄土汤以温脾益气摄血。有息肉者可加丹参、当归、红花、三棱、莪术、九香虫。

6. 寒热错杂

主症：胃脘胀满疼痛、喜温喜按、恶心欲吐、嗳气泛酸、口渴善饥、便秘溲赤、舌质淡胖、舌苔黄白相间、脉弦细数。

治法：辛开苦降，寒热并调。

方药：半夏泻心汤加减。法半夏、黄芩、黄连、党参、干姜、茯苓、佛手、甘草、白术。

加减：胃酸不足者加乌梅、木瓜；纳差配以谷芽、鸡内金。肠上皮化生者，均应加刺猬皮、炮山甲以软坚散结，消息肉、化瘀滞，或加白花蛇舌草、土茯苓。有部分慢性萎缩性胃炎系自身免疫所致，对此应重用活血化瘀药。

（二）专方治疗

1. 肝胃不和类

（1）舒胃汤

组成：柴胡、郁金、香附、半夏、枳壳、砂仁各10g，白芍15g，薏苡仁30g，甘草5g。

主治：慢性萎缩性胃炎证属肝胃不和型。

（2）四逆散加味

组成：柴胡、白芍、枳实、佛手、麦芽、蒲公英各10g，甘草5g，黄连、吴茱萸各3g。

主治：慢性萎缩性胃炎证属肝脾不和型。

（3）疏肝健脾汤

组成：柴胡、枳壳、白芍、郁金、陈皮、白术各10g，太子参、茯苓各15g，甘草6g。

主治：慢性萎缩性胃炎属肝郁脾虚证。

2. 脾胃湿热类

（1）益气活血养胃汤

组成：黄芩、党参、莪术、乌梅各15g，丹参、蒲公英、白花蛇舌草各25g，干姜、三七粉（冲服）、川黄连各8g，枳实10g。

主治：慢性萎缩性胃炎属气虚热郁证。

（2）加味黄连温胆汤

组成：黄连2g，陈皮6g，半夏10g，茯苓12g，甘草3g，枳实、竹茹各6g。

主治：慢性萎缩性胃炎证属痰热中阻、胃失和降者。

（3）建中活血汤

组成： 白花蛇舌草、丹参各 30g，赤芍、白芍、黄芩、柴胡各 10g，太子参、白术各 15g，甘草 6g。

主治： 慢性萎缩性胃炎属肝胃郁热夹瘀证。

3. 脾胃虚弱或兼血瘀类

（1）治萎合剂

组成： 黄芪、党参、龙葵、菝葜各 30g，白术、当归、白芍、茯苓、石斛、丹参各 15g，甘草 9g，红枣 10g。

主治： 萎缩性胃炎属脾胃虚弱证。

（2）温润建中汤

组成： 黄芩、丹参各 20g，党参、仙草、百合各 15g，莪术、蒲公英各 12g，淫羊藿、炒白术、白芍各 10g，乌药 5g，炙甘草 6g。

主治： 萎缩性胃炎属热郁气虚血瘀证。

（3）健脾抗萎汤

组成： 党参 15g，白术、黄芪、丹参各 30g，枳壳、香附、莪术各 10g，黄连、连翘各 12g，甘草 6g。

主治： 慢性萎缩性胃炎属气虚血瘀证。

4. 胃阴不足类

（1）养阴护胃汤

组成： 沙参、麦冬、玄参、石斛、玉竹、白芍、甘草、乌梅、木瓜。

主治： 慢性萎缩性胃炎证属胃阴不足型。

（2）楂梅益胃汤

组成： 沙参 30g，麦冬 10g，玉竹 10g，生地 10g，木瓜 10g，山楂 15g，山药 15g，石斛 12g，乌梅 12g，白芍 12g，甘草 6g。

主治： 慢性萎缩性胃炎证属脾阴不足、胃土燥热者。

（3）董建华方

组成： 沙参、麦冬、石斛、元参、川楝子、香附各 10g，天花粉、生地各 12g，乌梅、甘草、元胡各 5g。

主治： 慢性萎缩性胃炎证属胃阴不足型。

（4）阴虚肝郁萎胃方

组成： 白芍、乌梅、木瓜、太子参各 12g，蒲公英、白花蛇舌草各 15g，佛手、绿梅花、薏苡仁各 10g，甘草 5g。

主治： 萎缩性胃炎证属阴虚肝郁型。

5. 胃络瘀血类

（1）益气活血汤

组成： 黄芪 30g，丹参、蒲公英各 20g，党参、白术、当归、五灵脂、延胡索各 15g，甘草、三七粉各 5g。

主治： 慢性萎缩性胃炎属气虚血瘀证。

（2）健脾活血汤

组成： 黄芪 30g，白术、党参、白芍各 20g，丹参 15g，元胡、莪术、枳壳各 10g，三七粉、甘草各 6g。

主治： 慢性萎缩性胃炎属气虚血瘀证。

6. 寒热错杂类

（1）萎胃方

组成： 黄芪、白芍各 15g，生地、乌梅各 12g，白术、木香、山楂各 10g，川连、甘草各 5g，吴茱萸 3g。

主治： 慢性萎缩性胃炎证属寒热错杂型。

（2）和中消痞汤

组成： 党参 12g，半夏 10g，干姜、川连各 6g，白芍 12g，甘草 5g，丹参、蒲公英各 15g。

主治： 慢性萎缩性胃炎，胆汁反流性胃炎等证属寒热错杂型。

（三）单方验方

1. 单方治疗

（1）枸杞子

组成： 宁夏枸杞子。

主治： 肝肾阴虚型慢性萎缩性胃炎。

用法： 将枸杞子洗净，烘干打碎分装，每日 20g，分 2 次于空腹时嚼服，2 个月为 1 个疗程。

（2）扁豆饮

组成： 炒扁豆、党参、玉竹、山楂、乌梅各等份。

主治： 各型胃炎，尤其是慢性萎缩性胃炎。

用法： 水煎至豆熟透时，加白糖适量饮用。

2. 验方治疗

（1）胃萎汤

组成： 太子参 15g，茯苓 15g，生白术 15g，生白芍 15g，铁树叶 20g，蒲公英 20g，丹参 20g，柴胡 9g，莪术 9g，枳壳 9g，佛手 9g，炙甘草 6g。

功效： 健脾疏肝，益气活血，清热解毒。

主治：慢性萎缩性胃炎，上腹饱胀或钝痛，恶心嗳气，食欲减退，舌淡红或偏红，苔薄白或腻，甚至消瘦贫血。

加减：脾胃阴亏者，加麦冬 10g、石斛 10g、乌梅 9g；脾肾阳虚者，加干姜 6g、吴茱萸 3g、补骨脂 15g；胃浊上泛、恶心、嗳气者，加法半夏 10g、陈皮 6g、苏梗 10g；胃湿苔腻者，加厚朴 6g、藿香 9g；Hp 感染，加黄芩 9g、川连 3g；肠腺上皮化生及不典型增生严重者，还可加平地木 20g、半枝莲 20g。

用法：每日煎服 1 剂，每日 3 次。

（2）玉竹黄精饮

组成：玉竹 30g，黄精 30g，石斛 30g，当归 15g，白芍 15g，川芎 15g，白梅花 15g，玫瑰花 15g，乌梅 15g，五味子 15g，炙甘草 6g。

功效：滋阴养胃，活血通络。

主治：慢性萎缩性胃炎，上腹隐痛，饥饿嘈杂，饥不欲食，口干咽燥不欲饮，大便干燥，舌质红或紫暗，苔薄或少苔，脉弦数或细弱等。

加减：气虚者，加生黄芪、怀山药各 15g；兼湿热者，加黄芩 15g、川连 6g、生甘草 6g；肝郁气滞者，加柴胡、郁金各 10g。

用法：水煎服，每日 1 剂，每日 3 次。

（3）抑肝扶脾方

组成：柴胡、枳壳、白芍、白术、陈皮、薏苡仁、山楂、丹参、莪术、三七、川黄连、甘草。

功效：抑肝扶脾，活血化瘀。

主治：慢性萎缩性胃炎，上腹部胀满、隐痛，伴有恶心、嗳气、纳呆、便溏或便秘不畅，还可见面色无华、神疲乏力及体重减轻。

加减：脾胃虚弱者，加党参、茯苓；肾阳虚衰者，加肉豆蔻、附子；胃阴不足者，加沙参、麦冬；湿热下注者加白头翁、车前子。

用法：每日 1 剂，每剂煎 3 次，分 2 次于饭前半小时服。

（四）中成药

1. 温胃舒胶囊

组成：党参、白术、附子、肉桂、山药、乌梅、砂仁、陈皮、补骨脂、山楂、黄芪、肉苁蓉等。

功效：扶正固本，温胃养胃，行气止痛，助阳暖中。

主治：慢性萎缩性胃炎、慢性胃炎症见胃脘冷痛、胀气、嗳气、纳差、畏寒、无力等。

用法：每日 3 次，每次 2~4 粒，饭前半小时服。

2. 养胃舒胶囊（颗粒）

组成：黄精（蒸）、党参、白术（炒）、山药、菟丝子、北沙参、玄参、乌梅、陈皮、山楂、干姜。

功效： 益气养阴，健脾和胃，行气导滞。

主治： 脾胃气阴两虚所致的胃痛，症见胃脘灼热疼痛、痞胀不适、口干口苦、纳少消瘦、手足心热；慢性胃炎见上述证候者。

用法： 每日 3 次，每次 2~4 粒，饭前半小时服。

3. 三九胃泰

组成： 三桠苦、九里香、白芍、生地、木香。

功效： 消炎止痛，理气健胃。

主治： 浅表性胃炎、糜烂性胃炎、萎缩性胃炎等各类型慢性胃炎。

用法： 每日 3 次，每次 1 袋，饭前半小时服。

4. 猴菇菌片

组成： 猴头菌。

功效： 消炎止痛，扶助正气。

主治： 慢性萎缩性胃炎、消化性溃疡、胃癌、食管癌等。

用法： 每日 3 次，每次 2~4 片，饭前半小时服。

5. 气滞胃痛颗粒

组成： 柴胡、香附（炙）、白芍、延胡索（炙）、枳壳、炙甘草。

功效： 疏肝理气，和胃止痛。

主治： 肝郁气滞，胸痞胀满，胃脘疼痛；慢性胃炎见上述证候者。

用法： 每日 3 次，每次 1 袋，饭前半小时服。

6. 胃苏颗粒

组成： 紫苏梗、香附、陈皮、枳壳、槟榔、佛手、香橼、鸡内金（制）。

功效： 理气消胀，和胃止痛。

主治： 气滞型胃脘痛，症见胃脘胀痛，窜及两胁，得嗳气或矢气则舒，情绪郁怒则加重，胸闷食少，排便不畅、舌苔薄白、脉弦；慢性胃炎及消化性溃疡见上述证候者。

用法： 每日 3 次，每次 1 袋，饭前半小时服。

（五）针灸治疗

1. 脾胃虚弱、气滞血瘀型

处方： 脾俞、胃俞、膈俞、中脘、章门、气海、内关、足三里、血海。

方义： 脾俞、胃俞、中脘三穴相配，可健脾和胃，温补中州；足三里为胃经之下合穴，可补中益气，升清降浊，有调理脾胃功能，为治疗脾胃虚弱之要穴；内关善治胸胃疼痛；章门为脾经募穴，八会穴之脏会，可以治疗腹痛、腹胀等消化系统疾病；膈俞、血海二穴同治血病；气海具有补元气、行气散滞功能。

操作：脾俞、胃俞、膈俞、章门用补法，气海、内关、足三里用平补平泻法，中脘、血海用补法加灸，留针30~40分钟，温针灸或艾条灸15~20分钟。

2. 肝胃不和、郁火燥热型

处方： 太冲、内关、中脘、足三里。

方义： 太冲为肝经之原穴，能疏肝理气，降逆和胃；内关善治胸胃之疼痛；中脘配足三里，健脾培土以抑肝木。

加减： 胃火盛配内庭穴，肝火盛配行间穴，大便秘结配天枢穴。

操作： 内关、中脘、足三里穴用平补平泻法，余穴均用泻法，留针30分钟，每10分钟行针1次。

3. 胃阴不足、血瘀络脉型

处方： 胃俞、中脘、内关、足三里、三阴交、血海。

方义： 胃俞、中脘穴为俞募配穴法，具有健脾和胃、补益中州之功；内关善治胸胃之疼痛；足三里为胃之下合穴，三阴交为脾经穴，二穴相配有健脾益阴之效；血海具有运化脾血的功效。

加减： 便秘加天枢。

操作： 胃俞、血海、中脘穴用补法，内关、三阴交、足三里穴用平补平泻法，天枢穴用泻法，留针30~40分钟，每10分钟行针1次。

4. 脾虚肝郁、气失和降型

处方： 中脘、内关、足三里、太冲、公孙。

方义： 中脘配足三里穴，健脾培土以抑肝木。内关、公孙穴为八脉交会穴相配，宽胸解郁，善治胸胃之疼痛。太冲为肝经之原穴，能疏肝理气，降逆和胃。

操作： 均用平补平泻法，偏虚证者中脘穴加隔姜灸3~5壮，留针30分钟，每隔10分钟行针1次。

（六）食疗方

1. 牛乳粥

组成： 鲜牛乳250g，粳米60g，白糖20g。

功效： 补虚损，益五脏。

适应证： 胃酸过少，体虚，便秘患者食用尤佳。

制作： 将粳米淘洗干净，放入锅内，加水适量，置武火上烧沸，再用文火煮成粥；再在锅内放入白糖、牛奶，烧沸即成。

2. 山楂煮瘦肉

组成： 山楂、芡实粉各20g，瘦猪肉250g，生姜、葱各10g，食盐6g，素油20 g。

功效： 化积食，增胃酸。

适应证： 胃酸缺乏。

制作：将山楂切片，瘦肉切薄片，姜切丝，葱切段；将猪肉用芡实粉上浆，把炒锅置武火上烧热，再加入素油，烧六成热时，加入姜、葱爆锅，加入清水适量，下山楂，烧沸，再下入挂好芡实粉的瘦肉，煮熟，加入盐即成。

3. 羊芪糯枣温胃粥

组成：新鲜羊肉200g，黄芪10g，糯米100g，大枣10枚，生姜5g。

功效：补养脾胃，常服可温阳补气健脾。

适应证：胃溃疡、胃神经官能症、慢性胃炎等伴有胃寒、四肢怯冷、胃痛时有发作者。

制作：将新鲜羊肉（煮烂切细）200g，加入黄芪10g，糯米100g，大枣10枚，生姜5g煮粥，待煮熟后加入适量细盐、味精、胡椒粉。

（七）其他疗法

1. 护胃袋

组成：姜半夏30g，白术30g，白芍30g，佛手花30g。

功效：健脾和胃，行气止痛。

主治：各种慢性胃炎伴有胃脘胀满疼痛诸症。

制作：用手帕做成小袋，将药物全部纳入袋中，放入冷水浸湿，然后放在炉上隔水蒸10分钟取出，先用一块毛巾盖于药袋外部，防太热烫伤皮肤，稍冷却即可将药袋放置肚脐部（神阙穴）。令患者静卧，1次半小时，敷2次，1日换药袋1个，3个月为1个疗程。

2. 益胃散护胃袋

组成：白芥子4g，砂仁1g，丁香0.4g，吴茱萸0.4g，白蔻仁0.4g，乌药2g，细辛1g，红花0.4g，冰片0.5g等。

功效：温胃止痛，行气降逆。

主治：畏寒型胃脘痛。

制作：上药干燥、粉碎、过80目筛。以棉纸分装10g为1小袋，外敷神阙穴，每日换药1次，30天为1个疗程。

3. 耳穴贴压

取穴：交感、神门、胃、脾、肝、皮质下。

功效：健脾益气，通经活血。

主治：各种慢性胃炎的胃脘部不适等症。

操作：将耳廓常规消毒，再以王不留行籽贴压。两耳交替使用，每周交替1次，10次为1个疗程，并嘱患者每日按压耳穴3~5次，每次以自感耳廓充血、发热、发胀为度。

4. 腹部按摩

（1）推、拉法：是做腹部按摩的首用和常用手法，应根据痞块状态及深度和患者腹壁的厚薄来确定力度，一般 10~30kg。要点是让患者不感到太痛为宜（痞块多在触摸时伴有压痛）。

（2）归挤法：是指医者用双手从腹部两侧向脐中部同时用力的手法，此法对深部痞块的治疗起主要作用。但较难掌握，医者需要较好的体能方可做到。

（3）托提法：医者用单手或双手自脐下以"之"字型向上慢慢托提的手法，本法主要用于下腹部痞块。

（4）揉按法：医者以脐为中心，双手稍用力揉按，逆时针揉按的直径要小些，顺时针揉按的直径要大一些。本法多为治疗结束前的手法。

以上手法可穿插运用，1 次治疗应分两三段进行。主治各种慢性胃炎伴有胃脘、腹部胀满症。

本套手法是根据腹腔的平滑肌特点而设，并结合痞块的位置和硬度、深浅来确定。患者治疗体位同腹诊一样，但还需让患者配合做深呼吸，最好是腹式呼吸。因为只有在呼气时运用手法才是最佳时刻。腹部按摩结束后最好配合背部按摩或踩跷术以提高疗效。治疗以 15~30 次为 1 个疗程，隔日 1 次或隔两日作 1 次为宜。

五、名医专家经验方

（一）益胃平萎汤（周信有）

组成： 党参 20g，炒白术 9g，黄芪 20g，陈皮 9g，姜半夏 9g，香附 9g，砂仁 9g，鸡内金 9g，炒白芍 20g，莪术 20g，蒲公英 15g，甘草 6g。

功效： 益气和胃，祛瘀止痛，生肌平萎。

主治： 萎缩性胃炎，临床以胃脘胀痛，嗳气，纳差，疲乏无力，胃酸减少为特点。

用法： 水煎服，每日 1 剂，每日 2 次。

（二）清中消痞汤（李寿山）

组成： 太子参 15g，麦冬 15g，制半夏 7.5g，柴胡 6g，生白芍 10g，炒栀子 7.5g，牡丹皮 7.5g，青皮 10g，丹参 15g，甘草 6g。

功效： 养阴益胃，清中消痞。

主治： 浅表性胃炎、反流性胃炎、萎缩性胃炎等，症见胃脘痞塞，灼热似痛，似饥不欲食，口干不欲饮，五心烦热，纳呆食少，大便燥秘，舌红少津或舌苔光剥龟裂，脉细或数等。

用法： 先将药物用冷水浸泡 20 分钟，浸透后煎煮。首煎沸后文火煎 30 分钟，二煎沸后文火 20 分钟。煎好后两煎混匀，总量以 200ml 为宜，每日服 1 剂，早晚分服，饭前或饭后 2 小时温服。视病情连服 3 剂或 6 剂停药 1 天。候病情稳定或治愈后停药，服药过程中，停服其他中西药物。慢性萎缩性胃炎一般需坚持治疗 3 个月为 1 个疗程。

（三）萎胃安汤（张镜人）

组成： 太子参 9g，炒白术 9g，丹参 9g，柴胡 6g，赤白芍各 9g，炙甘草 3g，徐长卿 15g，白花蛇舌草 30g，炒黄芩 9g。

功效： 调气活血。

主治： 慢性萎缩性胃炎。

用法： 水煎服，每日 1 剂，早晚分服。

（四）萎胃宁汤（于己百）

组成： 半夏 10g，黄芩 10g，黄连 6g，党参 12g，炙甘草 10g，干姜 10g，代赭石 20g，莱菔子 15g，枳实 10g，芍药 15g。

功效： 辛开苦降，健脾和胃。

主治： 慢性萎缩性胃炎。

加减： 胃脘疼痛较甚者加木香 10g、白芷 12g，行气消滞，和血散瘀，解痉止痛。肠鸣泄泻，大便溏薄者，以炮姜 10g 易干姜，加焦山楂 15g，温中散寒，健胃止泻。纳呆、食少加陈皮 10g、砂仁 6g，或焦山楂 15g、炒麦芽 15g，以醒脾开胃，消食导滞。夜卧不安、失眠加酸枣仁 30g、川芎 12g，以养心安神。寒偏盛者加细辛 10g、川椒 10g，温中散寒；热偏胜者去干姜，加槟榔 10g、蒲公英 20g，清解胃热；阴虚者去干姜，加沙参 10g、麦冬 12g、石斛 10g，养阴生津；瘀重者去干姜，加丹参 20g、生山楂 15g，活血祛瘀。慢性萎缩性胃炎伴有肠化或不典型增生者，加三棱 10g、莪术 10g，消瘀散结，抑制肠化；加黄药子 30g，或半枝莲 30g、山慈菇 12g，以抗癌防癌。

按语： 于己百教授强调慢性胃炎矛盾的主要方面在于胃气失于和降，治疗时重点采取和胃降气之法，该病宜缓图，取效贵在一个"守"字。于教授师仲景之本意，以半夏泻心汤为主，旋覆代赭汤为辅，又随证增损之。综观全方，寒热并用，苦辛并进，补泻兼施，标本兼治，服后可使寒热平调，阴阳和谐，升降复常，中气振作。

六、名医专家典型医案

（一）单兆伟医案——脾胃气虚

周某 男，45 岁。

初诊： 2011 年 11 月 29 日。诉 2 月前无明显诱因出现胃脘部隐痛，2011 年 10 月 24 日查胃镜示：①慢性胃炎；②疣状胃炎 APC 术后。病理：（窦小）轻度萎缩性胃炎，伴肠上皮化生，灶性区腺上皮轻度不典型增生。Hp（-）。刻下：胃脘部隐痛，空腹嘈杂，口有异味，苔薄黄，舌暗红，脉细弦。

辨证： 脾胃气虚。

治则： 益气和胃。

处方： 二参三草汤加减。太子参10g，黄芪10g，炒白术10g，炒薏苡仁15g，仙鹤草15g，白花蛇舌草15g，紫丹参15g，炙甘草5g，佛手5g。14剂，水煎服，每日1剂，每剂2服。

二诊： 药后胃脘隐痛时作，食后为甚，嘈杂，口有异味，胃纳不香，口干苦，舌暗红，苔薄黄，脉细弦。治再前方出入。前方去炙甘草，加炒谷芽、炒麦芽各15g，消食导滞。14剂，水煎服，每日1剂，每剂2服。

三诊： 药后胃脘隐痛减轻，脘胀，时有嘈杂，口有异味，胃纳转香，胃寒，喜热食，舌质暗，苔薄黄，脉细弦。治再前方出入。前方去炒谷芽、炒麦芽，加干姜2g胃中散寒。14剂，水煎服，每日1剂，每剂2服。

四诊： 药后胃脘隐痛不著，嘈杂不显，口中异味减轻，血压偏高，证仍属脾胃气虚，治再前法出入。前方去干姜，加钩藤15g、天麻10g潜降肝阳。14剂，水煎服，每日1剂，每剂2服。

五诊： 于2012年3月31日复查胃镜示：慢性胃炎，病理示:（窦小）重度浅表性胃炎。Hp（-）。诸症缓解，治再前法巩固疗效。太子参10g，黄芪10g，炒白术10g，炒薏苡仁15g，仙鹤草15g，白花蛇舌草15g，紫丹参15g，佛手5g，百合15g，夜交藤15g。14剂，水煎服，每日1剂。

按语： 二参三草汤是单兆伟教授根据慢性萎缩性胃炎久病脾胃气虚夹有血瘀的病机特点所拟，是单兆伟教授治疗慢性萎缩性胃炎的常用方之一。方中太子参、黄芪二药，益气健脾，补气为主，扶正固本。白术、薏苡仁，可补中健胃，运脾燥湿。仙鹤草一味，为单兆伟教授治疗脾胃病必备之品，能健胃补虚，清热止血。《百草镜》谓其可"下气活血，理百病，散痞满"；《本草纲目拾遗》云其能"消宿食，散中满，下气，疗吐血各病，翻胃噎膈"。白花蛇舌草清热解毒，现代药理研究，白花蛇舌草可抑制肠上皮化生，防止萎缩性胃炎发生肠上皮化生，发展为肿瘤，正所谓"防患于未然"；白花蛇舌草还可抑制肿瘤细胞的增殖、浸润，又体现了"既病防变"思想。丹参一味，活血补血为要，《妇人名理论》赞其"一味丹参，功同四物"，既可活血通络，又可养血生血；丹参与黄芪、党参相配，意在气为血之帅，使气充则血行，血行则瘀祛；血为气之母，使"阳得阴助而生化无穷"，共奏益气生血，养血活络之功；佛手疏肝理气，和胃止痛；甘草缓中，兼以调和诸药。

（二）徐景藩医案——中虚夹有温热

撒某　男，60岁，工人。

初诊： 1992年12月2日。患者素患胃脘痛已10余年，本次因解黑便而住院。查纤维胃镜示：慢性萎缩性胃炎伴肠上皮化生，浅表性十二指肠炎。血Hp抗体阳性。大便隐血（++）。入院后经冲服三七粉、白及粉及汤药芩连平胃散加减以清化湿热、和胃止血等治疗，黑便消失，大便隐血转阴。但入院40余天胃脘痛未除，并见苔黑似酱。症见胃脘隐痛，纳少乏味，口干欲饮，两便尚调。舌质红、苔黑黄黏腻、如罩霉酱，脉弦数。

辨证： 中虚夹有湿热。

治则： 清化湿热、理气和中。

处方： 冬瓜子30g，佩兰10g，黄连3g，薏苡仁20g，地榆10g，陈皮10g，法半夏10g，炙鸡内金10g，佛手6g，白术10g，怀山药15g，生甘草3g。每日1剂。

二诊:1992年12月16日,患者药后脘痛不显,胃纳渐振,口中已和,黑黄腻苔渐退。治守原方,略事增减,共服20余剂,诸症缓解而出院。

按语:《舌鉴辨证》谓"霉酱色者,有黄赤兼黑之状,乃脏腑本热,而加有宿食也"。说明霉酱苔主病湿热久郁。本案虚实夹杂,中虚为本,湿热为标。湿热蕴蒸,上泛于舌则化生黑黄腻苔,状似霉酱。徐老从标为主而治之,着重以清化和中为法,俾中焦湿热去而脾运得健,则垢苔自消。冬瓜子习用作清肺化痰排脓之药,而徐老独具慧眼,认为冬瓜子能清胃肠湿热、泄肠腑热毒,并能开胃,常用其治疗湿热中阻证的慢性胃炎。方中冬瓜子合黄连、地榆清热燥湿解毒;取佩兰、薏苡仁、半夏化湿浊;陈皮、佛手理气和中;鸡内金、白术、山药健脾养胃,并防苦寒伤中;甘草缓中,兼以调和诸药。

七、预防与调护

(一)预防

(1)定期检查,必要时作胃镜检查。

(2)遇有症状加重、消瘦、厌食、黑粪等情况时应及时到医院检查。

(3)节制饮酒,不吸烟,以避免尼古丁对胃黏膜的损害;避免长期服用消炎止痛药。

(4)所食食品要新鲜并富于营养,保证有足够的蛋白质、维生素及铁质摄入。按时进食,不暴饮暴食,不吃过冷或过热的食物,不用或少用刺激性调味品,如鲜辣椒粉等。

(二)调护

(1)饮食治疗原则:养成良好的饮食习惯和生活习惯。吃饭时要细嚼慢咽,使食物与消化液充分混合。饮食宜清淡、少刺激性,晚餐勿过饱,待食物消化后再入睡。否则,会增加胃部不适感。细嚼慢咽,使食物在口腔内的"机械加工"和部分"化学加工"进行得充分。牙齿松动、脱落不全者应及时修补,这样可大大减轻胃的负担。

(2)保持乐观开朗的情绪:胃肠道有十分丰富的神经分布,其总量仅次于大脑与脊柱,精神情绪通过它们或影响消化道(包括胃)的运动,或干扰消化腺的分泌,结果使胃炎症状加重。

(3)加强身体锻炼,力求生活规律。

(4)应戒烟、戒酒:长期大量饮酒伤胃,尽人皆知,但人们对吸烟伤胃则不以为然,殊不知烟草中有多种化学成分可毒害胃黏膜,甚至引起溃疡病。

八、结语

总之，中医药治疗慢性萎缩性胃炎具有显著优势，能够消除或改善临床症状、促进胃黏膜萎缩性病变恢复、阻断病情发展、减少复发，无明显毒、副作用。但是目前中医治疗也存在一定的不足：缺乏统一的辨证分型标准，多以个人经验为依据用药；疗效评估没有统一的参考依据；临床辨病多于辨证治疗，个案报道、经验总结样本量少；诊疗后随访不足。因此，我们应加强对中医药方剂的药理研究，制定统一的、规范的慢性萎缩性胃炎辨证分型标准、疗效评价标准，为推广中医药治疗慢性萎缩性胃炎提供更确切的理论依据。

（孟静岩）

参考文献

［1］陈佳，李守英，徐红．慢性萎缩性胃炎的研究进展［J］．中国老年学杂志，2013，33（14）：3540-3542．

［2］王水琴，王岩花，王菲．慢性萎缩性胃炎的中医辨证论治［J］．中国药业，2015，24（12）：125-127．

［3］杨维维，周晓虹．中医药治疗慢性萎缩性胃炎的研究进展［J］．世界科学技术－中医药现代化，2014，16（10）：2166-2169．

［4］高东五，刘小卫，陈万军．慢性萎缩性胃炎的诊断及中西医结合治疗［J］．临床和实验医学杂志，2012，11（10）：748-749．

［5］沈开金．常见胃肠病中医药诊治［M］．合肥：安徽科学技术出版社，2006．

［6］李建中，周吕，柳力公，等．针灸治疗慢性萎缩性胃炎36例临床观察［J］．针刺研究，2002，27（4）：280-285．

［7］张栋．名老中医屡试屡效方［M］．北京：人民军医出版社，2009．

［8］陈光顺，李金田，邓沂，等．于己百教授验方证治［J］．中医研究，2007，20（7）：50-53．

［9］顾诚，单兆伟．单兆伟运用自拟二参三草汤治疗慢性萎缩性胃炎验案［J］．长春中医药大学学报，2013，29（2）：222-223．

［10］徐青．徐景藩胃病医案2则［J］．中医杂志，1993，34（12）：722．

肾病综合征

Nephrotic
Syndrome

一、概述

肾病综合征（Nephrotic Syndrome，NS）是由多种病因引发，其临床表现为4大特点：大量蛋白尿；低蛋白血症，主要表现为血浆白蛋白降低，常低于30g/L；高脂血症，以胆固醇升高为主；不同程度的水肿，严重的患者可出现胸水、腹水。肾病综合征可分为原发性及继发性两大类。原发性肾病综合征的病理类型主要包括：微小病变肾病、系膜增生性肾小球肾炎、膜增生性肾小球肾炎、膜性肾病以及局灶性节段性肾小球硬化等，发病人群以儿童和青少年为多见。继发性肾病综合征病因明确，可由免疫性疾病（如系统性红斑狼疮，过敏性紫癜）、糖尿病以及继发感染（如细菌、乙肝病毒等）、循环系统疾病、药物中毒等多种途径引起。

中医学中并无"肾病综合征"这一病名，根据临床症状属于"水肿""腰痛""虚劳""尿浊"之范畴。水肿多为本病病变早期的主要表现，最早叙述见于《灵枢·水胀》："水始起也，目窠上微肿，如新卧起之状，其颈脉动，时咳，阴股间寒，足胫肿，腹乃大，其水已成矣；以手按其腹，随手而起，如裹水之状，此其候也"。

二、病因病机

肾病综合征虽然是一种常见的肾脏疾病，但是这方面的流行病学数据相当缺乏。研究者很少直接统计肾病综合征的发病率，而常常分析临床表现为肾病综合征的各种原发疾病的发病率。Llach 报道成人肾病综合征的年发病率在十万分之三。大部分肾病综合征由原发性肾小球疾病所致，但没有确切的数据显示肾病综合征中原发性和继发性各占多少，可供参考的是肾小球疾病中原发性占 60%。

肾病综合征的疾病谱有很大的地区差异，多数研究认为最常见的是局灶节段性肾小球硬化症，随后是膜性肾病和微小病变肾病。Kitiyakara 等报道膜性肾病和局灶节段性肾小球硬化症各占原发性肾病综合征的 1/3，微小病变肾病和 IgA 肾病约占 1/4，膜增殖性肾炎比较少见。来自东亚的研究数据则有很大差异，如日本报道 IgA 肾病占 1/3 以上，局灶节段性肾小球硬化症仅占 10%。北京的一项研究显示原发性肾病综合征中按所占比例由高到低依次为膜性肾病（29.5%）、微小病变肾病（25.3%）、IgA 肾病（20.0%）、系膜增生性肾小球肾炎（12.7%）、局灶节段性肾小球硬化症（6.0%）、膜增生性肾小球肾炎（1.5%）等。施素华等收集了 1993–2010 年南京军区福州总医院病理科肾穿活检病例 36 379 例，其中包含了全国各地近 200 家医院肾穿刺活检远程邮寄标本。发现总体肾脏疾病患者男女比例接近，男性略高（51.0%），肾脏疾病的高发年龄段为 18~37 岁。在病理类型分布中，发病率最高的为肾小球疾病（96.2%），其中原发性肾小球疾病所占比例较大（72.5%），狼疮性肾炎是继发性肾小球疾病的最常见病理类型（41.8%），原发性肾小球疾病表现为肾病综合征的患者其病理类型以系膜增生性肾小球肾炎最为常见。这些差异可能和种族、环境及肾活检指征等因素相关。

中医认为肾病综合征是由先天禀赋不足，或后期烦劳过度，损伤正气，或因久病失治、误治，引起脏腑气血、阴阳不调，甚至脾肾亏虚。脾虚则致精微物质和气血生化无源，加之肾虚外泄，则可造成机体精气亏损，故而出现低蛋白血症；肾虚则失封藏，肾气不固，精气外泄，下注膀胱则出现大量蛋白尿。脾虚水湿运化失司，肾虚气化不利，水湿内停，泛溢于肌肤则为水肿；脾肾俱虚，损及肝脏，而使肝阴亦虚，肝阴虚则肝阳上亢。在疾病发展过程中，肝、脾、肾三脏功能紊乱，导致气血阴阳不调，为本病之本，水湿、湿热、瘀血壅滞为本病之标，最终表现为虚中夹实之复杂的病理过程。因正气虚弱，易复感外邪而加重病情，形成恶性循环，正气愈虚，邪气愈盛，湿浊诸邪更甚，致病情迁延难愈。

三、诊断要点与鉴别诊断

（一）诊断要点

肾病综合征的分类根据病因分为原发性和继发性。如考虑为继发性应积极寻找病因，在排除继发性肾病综合征，如过敏性紫癜肾炎、糖尿病肾病、乙肝相关性肾炎、狼疮肾炎、肾淀粉样变等之后才能诊断为原发性肾病综合征。诊断标准如下：

（1）大量蛋白尿：尿蛋白 ≥ 3.5g/d，是肾病综合征最主要的诊断依据。

（2）低白蛋白血症：血清白蛋白 ≤ 30g/L。

（3）水肿：多较明显，严重者可出现胸腔、腹腔及心包积液。

（4）高脂血症：血浆中几乎各种脂蛋白成分均增加。

前两项是诊断肾病综合征的必要条件，后两项为次要条件。临床上只要满足上述两项必要条件，肾病综合征的诊断即可成立。实际上"大量蛋白尿"是肾病综合征的特征性表现和始动因素，后三者是其引起的结果，因此有学者认为用肾病范围（nephrotic range）蛋白尿来描述更为准确。关于大量蛋白尿的量曾有许多不同的标准，目前一般认为成人尿蛋白量 ≥ 3.5g/（1.73m·d）或 3.5g/d 为大量蛋白尿；在儿童则要根据体重计算，为尿蛋白 ≥ 50mg/（kg·d）。也可以用随时尿的尿蛋白与肌酐比值作为标准，尿蛋白/肌酐 ≥ 2mg/mg（0.25mg/mmol）即为大量蛋白尿。

（二）鉴别诊断

1. 慢性肾小球肾炎

本病可发生于任何年龄，但以中青年为主，主要临床表现为蛋白尿、血尿、水肿、高血压，可有不同程度肾功能减退，尿蛋白常在 1~3g/d，结合实验室检查，一般不难明确诊断。

2. 系统性红斑狼疮肾炎

本病发病率女性高于男性，常见于 20~40 岁女性，临床特征主要有：①患者多有发热；②多发性关节痛；③皮疹；④血液系统受累等。血清抗核抗体、抗双链 DNA（ds-DNA）、抗（SM）抗体阳性，血清补体水平下降，肾活检光镜下除系膜增生外，病变有多样性特征。

3. 慢性肾盂肾炎

多有反复发作的泌尿系感染病史，可能有腰痛、低热的症状，尿沉渣中常有白细胞，尿细菌学检查阳性即可鉴别。

4. 糖尿病肾病

本病发生率男性高于女性，多发生于糖尿病病史 10 年以上的患者。早期可表现为尿微量白蛋白排出增加，以后逐渐发展成大量蛋白尿。糖尿病病史及糖尿病视网膜病变有助于鉴别诊断。

5. 过敏性紫癜性肾炎

除有血尿、蛋白尿、水肿、高血压等肾炎的特点外，还伴有皮肤紫癜、关节痛、腹痛及消化道出血等特征表现。若紫癜特征表现不典型，易误诊为原发性肾病综合征。血抗核抗体为阴性。肾活检常见病理改变为弥漫系膜细胞增生，免疫病理主要沉积物为 IgA 及 C3，故不难鉴别。

四、中医治疗

水肿治疗，《素问·汤液醪醴论》指出："开鬼门，洁净府，去宛陈莝。"《金匮要略·水气病脉证并治》谓："诸有水者，腰以下肿，当利小便；腰以上肿，当发汗乃愈"。还可根据《丹溪心法·水肿》中阴水、阳水的不同病因病机进行治疗方法的选择，阴水为里、虚、寒证，应扶正为主，行温肾健脾疗法；阳水为表、实、热证，应祛邪为主，行发汗、利小便、攻逐等法。通常认为，发病始以外邪为主，可根据症状不同行发汗、利小便、攻逐、化瘀以祛邪，并辅以健脾温肾，使标本得以兼顾。而至病程后期，此时患者正气渐衰，治疗原则当属扶正固本，可着重温肾健脾，视其标实证的程度运用扶正祛邪法。

（一）辨证治疗

水肿在《内经》称"水""肾风""风水""水胀"等。《金匮要略》将水肿分为风水、皮水、正水、石水，并提出治法和方药。后世医家在此基础上不断发展，形成了中医治疗水肿比较完善的一套辨证论治体系，现将临床分型介绍如下。

1. 风水泛滥

主症： 先见眼睑及颜面浮肿，然后迅速波及全身，肢节酸重，小便不利，其中有兼见恶风寒、鼻塞、咳嗽、苔薄白、脉浮紧的风寒证和兼咽部红肿疼痛、舌红苔黄、脉浮数的风热证。

治法： 祛风散寒，利水渗湿；或祛风清热，利水渗湿。

方药： ①风寒为主者用麻杏五皮饮加减。生麻黄、杏仁、茯苓皮、陈皮、大腹皮、桑白皮、车前草、生姜皮。②风热为主者用越婢汤合麻黄连翘赤小豆汤加减。生麻黄、生石膏、连翘、白茅根、黄芩、赤小豆、鲜芦根、鱼腥草、桔梗。

加减： 若表邪解，可去麻黄、杏仁或石膏；尿检仍有蛋白或红细胞者，可加入雷公藤多苷片，每次 20mg，每日 3 次。

2. 湿热蕴结

主症： 遍身浮肿，皮色润泽光亮，胸腹痞闷，烦热口渴，大便干结，小便短赤，或皮肤有疮疡疖肿，舌红，苔黄腻，脉滑数。

治法：分利湿热。

方药：疏凿饮子加减。商陆、泽泻、赤小豆、川椒目、槟榔、大腹皮、茯苓皮、生大黄、苍术、厚朴、羌活。

加减：药后仍大便不通，湿热郁闭而病势急迫者，可仿己椒苈黄丸及巴黄丸意，倍大黄，加汉防己、葶苈子。另暂用生巴豆研末装入胶囊内吞服。有皮肤疮疡热肿者，可加金银花、连翘，或蒲公英、紫花地丁等清热解毒。

3. 瘀阻肾络

主症：面浮肢肿，迁延日久，皮肤甲错，或出现红丝、赤缕，瘀点瘀斑，或腰痛尿赤，舌淡或红，舌边有瘀点，舌下筋脉瘀紫，舌薄黄或腻，脉细涩。

治法：益肾行瘀。

方药：桃红四物汤加减。桃仁、红花、当归、川芎、赤芍、益母草、水蛭、泽兰。

加减：瘀阻甚者，加大上述用量并加䗪虫、蜈蚣；兼肾气虚者，加党参、黄芪、淫羊藿；肝肾阴虚者，加地黄、鳖甲；脾肾阳虚者，加白术、附子；有热邪者，加金银花、紫花地丁；血尿明显者加蒲黄、三七。

4. 肾气亏虚

主症：晨起面浮，傍晚跗肿或肿不甚，但感腰酸身重，形体困倦，甚则疲行于行立、不耐久坐，舌淡红，苔薄，脉偏沉细。

治法：补益肾气。

方药：济生肾气丸加减。附子、桂枝、熟地黄、山茱萸、山药、茯苓、泽泻、牡丹皮、淫羊藿、川牛膝、车前子、黄芪。

5. 脾肾阳虚

主症：面色㿠白，形寒肢冷，遍身悉肿，按之没指，甚者可伴胸腹水，胸闷气急，小便短赤，大便溏薄，舌淡体胖，脉沉细。

治法：温补脾肾，通阳利水。

方药：真武汤合实脾饮加减。附子、桂枝、白术、生白芍、干姜、赤猪苓、茯苓、泽泻、槟榔、葫芦壳。

加减：若兼恶寒无汗、发热头痛、咳嗽鼻塞等风寒外感者，去干姜、白术，加麻黄、细辛。阳虚水泛，喘促不能平卧，症情急迫者，合己椒苈黄丸攻逐水湿，以助阳气伸展。

6. 肝肾阴虚

主症：浮肿不甚，口干，咽喉干痛，头目昏眩，性情急躁，腰酸尿赤，盗汗，烦热，舌红，脉细弦数。

治法：滋补肝肾，兼化水湿。

方药：二至丸合杞菊地黄丸加减。女贞子、旱莲草、干地黄、菊花、枸杞子、牡丹皮、泽泻、茯苓、山药、益母草。

加减：水肿较甚者，加车前草、半边莲、半枝莲；尿赤不已者，加生茜草、生地榆。

7. 正气衰惫，浊毒内留

主症：面色萎黄，眼睑虚肿，神疲乏力，语音低怯，胸腹痞闷，呕吐厌食，口中有尿臭，或小便短少，或夜尿多，甚至昏愦、抽搐、皮肤瘙痒，黑粪，舌淡无华，苔腻或腐，脉细或滑，按之无力。

治法：温脾益肾，通阳泄浊。

方药：内服用温脾汤加减。人参、制附子、丹参、吴茱萸、黄连、晚蚕沙、六月雪、玉枢丹、制大黄、法半夏。外用灌肠方灌肠。生大黄、生牡蛎、附子、地榆。

加减：若呕吐不已者，加藿香、苏叶；黑便者，加三七或云南白药；昏愦者，加郁金、石菖蒲；抽搐者，加牡蛎、鳖甲、龟甲；水犯高原，湿浊凌心，致气急不得卧者，加葶苈子，增大黄用量；便溏者，用制大黄。灌肠方一般药液量为 150~200ml，温度 37℃~40℃左右。高位保留灌肠，药液灌入后，要抬高臀位，慢慢拔出肛管，嘱患者平卧休息半小时。尽量保持较长时间。

（二）专方治疗

戴陆庆认为真武汤益气温阳利水、健脾益肾的作用，能够改善肾脏微循环，纠正体内高凝状态，减少肾小球毛细血管病变，从而降低肾小球内压而减少蛋白尿的漏出。郝开花将 90 例本病患者随机分为两组，45 例患者给予常规治疗加用加味真武汤为治疗组，45 例患者只给予常规治疗为对照组，进行临床疗效观察。结果：治疗组治愈率为 40.00%，总有效率达 87.67%；对照组治愈率为 24.44%，总有效率为 66.67%（$P < 0.05$）。

夏建华将 100 例肾病综合征患者随机分为两组，治疗组采用小柴胡汤加味（药物组成：柴胡、黄芩、法半夏、党参、炒白术、茯苓、猪苓、白花蛇舌草、炙水蛭、生黄芪、白茅根、炙甘草、茜草、益母草）治疗，对照组采用激素加双嘧达莫治疗。结果显示：治疗组 24h 尿蛋白定量明显减少、血浆白蛋白升高、总胆固醇降低（$P < 0.01$）。小柴胡汤加味对本病消除患者蛋白尿、降血脂等有较好的治疗作用。

研究发现许多古方如十枣汤或控涎丹、血府逐瘀汤、柴苓汤、柴苓汤合桃红四物汤等，亦具有消除蛋白尿、水肿，提高血浆蛋白，改善高脂血症的作用，对治疗本病均取得了较好的疗效。

（三）中成药

1. 肾炎康复片

肾炎康复片主要包括：西洋参、人参、地黄、杜仲、山药、白花蛇舌草、黑豆、土茯苓、益母草、丹参、泽泻、白茅根、桔梗，具有补肾健脾之功效。主治慢性肾小球肾炎证属于气阴两虚、脾肾不足、毒热未清者，表现为神疲乏力、腰膝酸软、面浮、双下肢浮肿、头晕耳鸣、蛋白尿、血尿等症。主要药理作用有：①修复受损肾小球足细胞，减少蛋白丢失；②降低高血压，抗炎、利水、消肿，改善肾脏功能；③拮抗糖皮质激素的副作用。肾病综合征在水肿期，证属脾肾两虚，治疗宜攻补兼施,在温肾健脾的基础上利尿消肿。殷士涛等发现肾炎康复片联合激素治疗原发性肾病综合征,不仅试验组总有效率高于对照组,而且在24h尿蛋白定量、血肌酐、血清白蛋白、总胆固醇及甘油三酯等指标均有所改善。说明肾炎康复片在抑制尿蛋白的丢失、纠正低蛋白血症、降脂方面发挥了作用。

2. 黄葵胶囊

黄葵胶囊为黄蜀葵花经提取制成的胶囊剂,主要功能有清热利湿、解毒消肿,常用于慢性肾炎之湿热证,临床表现为浮肿、腰痛、蛋白尿、血尿、舌苔黄腻等症。现代药理研究表明黄葵胶囊具有抗肾小球免疫炎症反应、清除循环系统免疫复合物、抗血小板聚集、降低尿蛋白、保护肾功能等作用。有动物试验表明,黄葵胶囊能有效地清除氧自由基,降低尿蛋白,提高血清蛋白水平。孙毅等发现黄葵胶囊联合雷公藤多苷片治疗原发性肾病综合征,两者可以减少蛋白尿,延缓肾功能的进一步衰竭,同时能够调节免疫,减轻激素的毒副作用。

3. 金水宝胶囊、百令胶囊

金水宝胶囊和百令胶囊是经过现代工艺发酵冬虫夏草菌粉制成的中成药。富含氨基酸、多糖、有机酸、多种微量元素及甾醇类等多种化学成分,具有保护肝肾功能、抗炎及调节免疫作用等。郝丽通过冬虫夏草及雷公藤多苷对糖尿病肾病大鼠足细胞影响的实验研究发现,冬虫夏草联合雷公藤多苷,具有降低蛋白尿的功效,同时可以减轻雷公藤多苷的不良反应。

4. 雷公藤多苷片

雷公藤为卫矛科雷公藤属植物,其根、茎、花均有毒性,药用部分为去两层皮的根木质部,是迄今为止免疫抑制作用最可靠的中药之一。在肾病治疗中的作用机制主要包括:①抗炎及免疫抑制作用;②保护和修复足细胞损伤;③保护肾小管上皮细胞;④抑制系膜细胞增殖。目前有关雷公藤治疗原发性肾病综合征的研究报道均为小型、单中心研究,大都与糖皮质激素(简称激素)联合使用,报道有效率在73.1%~96.9%。有学者提出,雷公藤多苷的疗效与病理类型有关,病理类型为微小病变肾病及系膜增殖性肾炎疗效较佳,有效率可达到90%以上,对于病变较重,尤其是小管间质损害较重者会影响本药的疗效。过去基于对雷公藤毒性的考虑,提出的雷公藤常规使用剂量为1mg/($kg \cdot d$)。近年来的研究证实,作为诱导治疗,使用双倍剂量[2mg/($kg \cdot d$)]更为合适。南京军区总院的多项研究证实,双倍剂量雷公藤多苷治疗肾病综合征具有显著的疗效,4周的疗效总缓解率达83.3%。而且对于激素治疗无效的病例,双倍剂量的雷公藤总苷同样有效。双倍剂量雷公藤多苷治疗的时间以8~12周为宜,在减量的过程中,为避免复发,应像激素一样逐渐减量,即先减量至1.5mg/($kg \cdot d$),1个月后再减至1mg/($kg \cdot d$)维持。肾病综合征患者均能很好耐受双倍剂量的雷公藤多苷治疗,不良反应发生率并无明显增加。

（四）其他

1. 灸法

又称艾灸，是指将艾绒点燃后直接或间接熏灼体表穴位的方法，具有升阳举陷、振奋阳气的作用。临床分为艾条灸、艾炷灸、温针灸和温灸器灸等多种形式。张伟石运用温针灸治疗肾病综合征，同时加用中药，穴位主要为关元、气海、水分，治疗患者 51 例，其中 31 例完全缓解，8 例基本缓解，9 例部分缓解，3 例无效，有效率为 94%。庄克生运用艾炷隔姜灸法，穴位选取为关元、中极、气海、水分、足三里，治疗肾病综合征型紫癜性肾炎，疗程 4 周，结果显示：尿蛋白定量、血白蛋白、血胆固醇、尿沉渣红细胞数均有改善。

2. 穴位贴敷法

指将贴敷药物放在体表穴位上，通过对穴位的刺激发挥治疗作用，是一种融合经络、穴位、药物为一体的复合性疗法。张振中运用自制肾康敷剂（丁香、黄芪、肉桂、黄精、大黄、甘遂、山甲、䗪虫），用姜汁、大蒜调制，外敷于肾俞、涌泉及神阙穴。结果表明：实验组优于对照组，该疗法能够改善临床症状，降低蛋白尿，同时可减轻激素的副作用，降低复发率。王君运用中药贴敷（甘遂、大戟、芫花、制附子、小茴香、车前子、冰片）治疗原发性肾病综合征，贴敷穴位为神阙、肾俞、水分、水道、三焦俞、委阳、阴陵泉。结果显示：试验组患者水肿减轻、尿量增加、尿蛋白减少，疗效优于单纯应用西药基础治疗组。

3. 穴位注射法

又称"水针"，是选用中西药物注入特定穴位以治疗疾病的方法，具有提高机体免疫力、预防疾病的作用。曹阳运用穴位注射配合泼尼松治疗肾病综合征，穴位采用肾俞、足三里，注射药物为鱼腥草注射液，其中肾俞注射 1.5ml，足三里注射 2ml，连续治疗 2 个月。实验组总有效率 96.4%，对照组总有效率 63.2%，两组差异具有统计学意义（$P < 0.05$）。结论为穴位注射药物配合泼尼松能有效提高患者免疫能力。尹保奇运用黄芪注射液足三里、肾俞穴位注射辅助治疗原发性肾病综合征，随访 2 月，24 小时尿蛋白定量、血浆白蛋白、血胆固醇分别与治疗前相比较，指标均有所改善，差异有统计学意义（$P < 0.05$）。

4. 中药灌肠法

指将中药药液或者掺入散剂灌肠，利用直肠黏膜的吸收功能，从而达到治疗目的。赵卫运用中药合剂保留灌肠（生黄芪、炒白术、山药、黄芩、丹参、芡实、陈皮、金樱子、乌梅、甘草，制成 250ml 的煎剂，每天 2 次），治疗小儿原发性肾病综合征，实验组总有效率 93.33%，对照组 80.00%，治疗前后差异有统计学意义（$P < 0.01$），临床疗效较好。黄玲丽用中药保留灌肠（黄芪 30g、山药 15g、党参 20g、茯苓 15g、川芎 15g、益母草 20g、锁阳 15g、泽兰 15g、芡实 15g、防风 10g、白茅根 30g、黄柏 15g，制成煎液 200~300ml 灌肠量）治疗小儿难治性肾病综合征，3 岁以下的患儿每次 50~80ml，3 岁以上的患儿每次 80~120ml。结果显示：与单纯用西药组比较，症状、血脂、尿蛋白定量

均有所改善，差异有统计学意义（$P < 0.05$）。运用自拟肾析春灌肠液（生黄芪 30g、生牡蛎 30g、红花 15g、大黄 15g、蒲公英 30g、地丁 30g）治疗肾病综合征及肾衰患者。嘱患者将肾析春灌肠液温度控制在 37~40℃，每次 250ml；采取右侧躺姿，并将左腿自然弓起，将灌肠管轻轻放进肛门约 15 厘米深，打开止水阀约 1/3。速度视各人情况调整，如果忍不住便意可放慢速度，或是先关掉止水阀，忍住 30 秒到 1 分钟，等便意减低再继续；滴完后躺正，进行身体按摩左侧腹部约 3~5 分钟，以保证药物在体内充分吸收。此疗法在改善患者蛋白尿、降低肌酐指标有良好的效应。

五、名医专家经验方

辨证论治又称辨证施治。是中医学认识和处理疾病的过程，是运用中医学理论辨析有关疾病的资料、症状、体征，通过分析、综合以确立证候，论证其治则治法方药并付诸实施的思维和实践过程。现将名医专家的经验介绍如下。

（一）以"通"为用治肿（张琪）

张琪教授在治疗难治性肾病综合征水肿时，认为水液的运化与诸脏相关，最终是因"三焦停滞，经络壅塞"不"通"而形成水肿，在水肿病中，张老强调以"通"为用，认为调畅肺、脾、肾、三焦气化为治肿之先。将治疗法归纳为以下几类。

（1）提壶揭盖法：为朱丹溪创制，是"以升为降"之意。张老认为难治性肾病综合征患者由于长期反复服用激素及免疫抑制剂，导致太阴、少阴阳气不足，出现"内不得入于脏腑，外不得越于皮肤，客于玄府，行于皮里，传为胕肿"之风水。临床常用加味越婢汤（麻黄 15g、生石膏 50g、生姜 15g、红枣 3 个、甘草 7g、杏仁 10g、苍术 10g、西瓜皮 50g、红小豆 50g、车前子 25g）以宣肺通卫而利水。

（2）清利三焦水热法：此法针对水邪夹热弥散三焦，水热互结之证，用于慢性肾炎、肾病综合征，症见全身浮肿，腹部膨大，小便不利，尿黄量少，大便秘结，口舌干燥而渴，舌苔厚腻，脉沉滑或沉数有力。方用增味疏凿饮子（槟榔 20g、大腹皮 15g、茯苓皮 15g、川椒目 15g、商陆 15g、红小豆 50g、秦艽 15g、羌活 15g、木通 15g、姜皮 15g、车前子 15g、萹蓄 20g、海藻 30g、二丑 20g）。

（3）益气养阴，清利湿热法：此法用于气阴两虚、湿热留恋之证，症见四肢倦怠、少气懒言、口舌干燥、食少纳呆、五心烦热、轻微浮肿或无浮肿，舌尖红，苔白微腻，脉细数或滑。处以清心莲子饮加减（石莲子 15g、党参 20g、地骨皮 15g、茯苓 15g、柴胡 15g、麦冬 15g、车前子 15g、黄芩 15g、生黄芪 30g、白花蛇舌草 30g、益母草 30g、甘草 10g）。

（4）补肾填精法：本法针对肾气不固，精气外泄之病机而设。症见腰膝酸软，头晕耳鸣，遗精滑泄，舌体偏胖，舌质淡红，脉沉或无力。方用八味肾气丸化裁（附子 7g、肉桂 7g、熟地黄 20g、山茱萸 15g、山药 20g、茯苓 20g、丹皮 15g、泽泻 15g、菟丝子 20g、枸杞 20g、桑螵蛸 15g、金樱子 20g）。

（二）分期专治儿童肾病综合征（李少川）

（1）初期：证属素体本虚，脾失运化功能，风邪外袭，肺气郁遏，水湿浸渍，横逆泛滥所致。常用越婢加术汤、银翘四苓汤（银翘散合四苓汤）、杏苏散、疏风通气汤化裁治疗。常用药物有麻黄、杏仁、苏梗、苏叶、白术、茯苓、知母、泽泻、金银花、连翘等。

（2）迁延期：①脾虚湿困证，治以健脾利湿为主，佐以行气之味，方以胃苓汤加减。常用药物有苏梗、茯苓、厚朴、泽泻、麦门冬、陈皮、太子参、神曲等。②湿郁化热证，治以芳香化浊，清热利湿，选用甘露消毒丹，目的在于清热而不致碍湿，渗湿而不致伤阴，湿热兼治，加以调畅气机。常用药物有藿香、连翘、白蔻仁、厚朴、茯苓、泽泻、苏梗、滑石、知母、黄柏等。③阴虚火旺证，治以滋补肝肾为主，佐以健脾和胃，方用玉女煎、镇肝息风汤、知柏地黄汤，三方合胃苓汤化裁。常用药物有熟地黄、山茱萸、知母、黄柏、麦冬、山药、苍术、茯苓、厚朴、苏梗、泽泻、补骨脂、生地等。

（3）缓解期：此期的特点为水肿逐渐消退，尿蛋白转阴，饮食增加，面色少华，倦怠懒言，自汗易感，舌淡红苔白，脉数。肺脾气虚是肾病后期常见证型，易感复发是此期的关键，患儿无论是感冒或者腹泻，均可导致病情的复发。缓解期的主要治法是健脾益气，每以参苓白术散、天宝采薇汤、肥儿丸加减治疗。常用药物有太子参、茯苓、白术、山药、葛根、羌活、独活、柴胡、陈皮、厚朴、知母等。李老在治疗肾病上重视健脾利湿的思想，将健脾渗湿与滋阴润燥相互为用，防其燥利伤阴。

（三）辨证治疗肾病综合征水肿（黄文政）

（1）脾肾阳虚证：治以温阳利水，方药以真武汤合五苓散、济生肾气汤、肾水散（经验方）化裁。附子 12g，白术 12g，茯苓 30g，生姜 10g，泽泻 15g，肉桂 10g，猪苓 15g，胡芦巴 10g，仙茅 10g。

（2）脾虚湿困证：治以益气健脾，燥湿利水，方药以防己茯苓汤合参苓白术散、胃苓汤加减。防己 15g，桂枝 10g，生黄芪 30g，茯苓 30g，党参 12g，白术 12g，薏苡仁 15g，扁豆 10g，山药 15g，甘草 6g。

（3）风邪犯肺证：治以疏风宣肺利水，方药以越婢加术汤合五虎饮、麻黄连翘赤小豆汤。炙麻黄 10g，生石膏 30g，甘草 10g，生姜 3 片，大枣 4 枚，白术 12g，桑白皮 10g，茯苓皮 30g，陈皮 15g，大腹皮 10g。

（4）气滞水停证：治以行气利水，方药以大橘皮汤、木香流气饮加减。橘皮 10g，滑石 12g，赤茯苓 15g，猪苓 15g，泽泻 15g，肉桂 5g，生姜 2 片，木香 6g，槟榔 10g，乌药 12g，威灵仙 10g，木瓜 6g。

（5）瘀水交阻证：治以活血化瘀利水，方药以当归芍药散加减。当归 12g，赤芍 15g，川芎 10g，茯苓 15g，白术 12g，泽泻 15g，丹参 30g，桃仁 10g，红花 10g，益母草 30g，车前子 15g。

（6）湿热蕴结证：治以清热祛湿散结，方药以萆薢分清饮、五味消毒饮，阴虚挟湿热者可用猪苓汤加减。萆薢 15g，石菖蒲 10g，白术 10g，丹参 15g，莲子心 6g，茯苓 15g，黄柏 10g，车前子 10g，金银花 30g，连翘 10g，蒲公英 10g，紫花地丁 10g。

（四）结合临床特点辨证治疗（赵玉庸）

（1）水肿属阴水证多用健脾益气、消肿利水的方法，常采用五皮饮合五苓散加减：茯苓15g，猪苓10g，白术10g，泽泻10g，大腹皮10g，桂枝6g，桑白皮10g，陈皮6g，益母草20g，白茅根20g。复感风邪，也可以表现为阳水，治疗风寒为主者以麻杏五皮饮加减：生麻黄6g，杏仁9g，茯苓皮15g，陈皮6g，大腹皮9g，桑白皮12g，生姜皮3g，车前子15g。表邪解者去麻黄、杏仁，加玉米须30g，白茅根30g。若风热为主者以越婢汤合麻黄连翘赤小豆汤加减：生麻黄6g，生石膏30g，连翘9g，黄芩12g，赤小豆30g，鱼腥草15g，桔梗3g，鲜茅根15g，鲜芦根30g。

（2）低蛋白血症属脾肾亏虚证，治疗上常用健脾益气的六君子汤等，另外黄芪在改善低蛋白血症方面有较好的疗效，常用剂量10~40g。黄芪益气固表、利水消肿，是治疗肾脏病的常用药。多用生黄芪，同时配合理气、活血药物治疗。

（3）针对肾络瘀阻型患者，赵玉庸教授常采用益肾通络、活血化瘀法，用桃红四物汤加减：当归12g，生地黄15g，赤芍12g，桃仁9g，红花9g，川芎9g，益母草12g，淫羊藿12g，丹参12g，炙山甲片6g，瘀血严重者加水蛭3g。对于顽固性蛋白尿而无明显瘀血症状体征者，也可加入虫类药，如乌梢蛇、地龙、僵蚕、蝉蜕、全蝎、蜈蚣等，此类药物具有降低蛋白尿的作用。一些患者也可加入雷公藤、青风藤等药物，这类药物具有调节免疫的作用。雷公藤在使用中，一要去皮，二应久煎，以减少其毒副作用。

六、名医专家典型医案

（一）邹云翔医案——气血痰湿郁滞

孙某 男，16岁，1972年6月26日初诊。

1972年2月因浮肿就医，尿检：蛋白（+++），脓细胞（+），红细胞1~3，找到颗粒管型及透明管型。3月份查胆固醇23.34mmol/L，血浆白蛋白27g/L，球蛋白24g/L。某医院诊断为"肾病综合征"，于4月20日收住院治疗。用激素治疗2个月，因激素副作用已较明显，而于6月20日出院，26日至邹老处转服中药治疗。

刻下：腰府胀痛，头痛不舒，脱发汗多，形体肥胖，周身浮肿，尿量减少，脉弦，苔腻。尿检：蛋白以（+++）为多，并见脓细胞、上皮细胞、红细胞，颗粒管型少许。

辨证：气血痰湿郁滞。

治法：疏泄法。

方药：制苍术6g，生苡仁12g，云茯苓9g，法半夏6g，陈广皮6g，合欢皮15g，糯根须15g，川续断6g，红花9g，白蒺藜9g，越鞠丸12g。水煎服，每日2剂。

气短加用太子参、黄芪、潞党参、大枣；贫血加当归、白芍、枸杞子、磁石、全鹿丸；口干加天花粉、川石斛、沙参、玄参、生地；纳少便稀加用炒山药、芡实；腰痛明显者加用辽功劳叶；尿检：红细胞（++）时加用白茅根、琥珀、墨旱莲、女贞子。

按上方加减治疗3个月，浮肿渐退，尿量每日1000ml左右，尿检：蛋白（+）~（++）。治疗5个月，尿蛋白微量。至1973年秋季，已无自觉症状，浮肿全消，精神恢复，尿检蛋白极微，尿比重1.012，血压110/68mmHg，追访至1977年夏季未曾反复。

按语： 邹老根据《内经》升降出入的理论尝指出："出入废则神机化灭，升降息则气立孤危。"《素问·五常政大论篇》载："升降出入，四者之有，而贵常守，反常则灾害至矣。""四者分之为升降，为出入，合之则一气字而已。夫百病皆生于气。"《丹溪心法》云："气血冲和，百病不生；一有怫郁，百病生焉。"郁则气滞，气滞则升降出入之机失度，当升者不升，当降者不降，当出者不出，当入者不入，清者化为浊，行者阻而不通，表失护卫而不和，里失营运而不顺。因激素引起的柯兴氏综合征，即表现为人体的升降出入功能紊乱，起初伤于气分，久则延至血分，气血精微转化为湿浊痰瘀，阻于脏腑络脉肌腠而成。《素问·六元正纪大论篇》说："木郁达之，火郁发之，土郁夺之，金郁泄之，水郁折之。"邹老根据《内经》之理论，对肾病综合征、药物性柯兴氏综合征的治疗，创造了疏郁泄浊法，方用苍术、苡米、香附、郁金、合欢皮、半夏、陈皮、当归、红花、川芎、桃仁、神曲、茯苓、芦根等疏之泄之，疏其气血，泄其湿浊痰瘀，使失常之升降出入功能得以恢复，取得了满意的疗效。

（二）祝谌予医案——脾肾两亏，水湿内停

杨某 男性，18岁。1978年4月5日初诊。

主诉： 全身水肿2年余。患者2年前水肿伴大量蛋白尿，后经医院确诊为肾病综合征，期间服用激素治疗，效不佳，故来诊。刻时口服泼尼松400mg/d，检查尿蛋白（3+~4+），24小时尿蛋白定量大于3g。

现症： 双下肢浮肿明显，按之凹陷不起，尿量不少。形体丰腴但弱不禁风，感冒后极易咽痛。腰膝酸软，周身乏力。舌体胖大，舌尖红，边有齿痕，脉沉细。

辨证： 脾肾两亏，水湿内停。

治法： 培补脾肾，利水消肿。

方药： 六味地黄汤、防己黄芪汤加减。生地黄10g，熟地黄10g，五味子10g，山药10g，丹皮10g，茯苓25g，泽泻10g，黄芪30g，防己10g，白术10g，炙甘草5g，石莲子15g，旱莲草15g，车前草30g，白花蛇舌草30g。水煎服，每日2剂。

前方加减服用30余剂，患者自觉体力增加，感冒次数减少，水肿减轻，化验24小时尿蛋白定量2.3~3.2g。守方再加菟丝子15g，续服45剂，患者水肿大减，体力基本恢复，查尿蛋白（-）。口服泼尼松减至30mg/d，前后服药共计90余剂。经治疗3个月，患者水肿消退，化验24小时尿蛋白微量，口服泼尼松减至20mg/d维持，乃将原方稍事加减，改配丸药，缓图收功。

按语： 前贤论治水肿，总不离乎肺、脾、肾三脏。如张景岳云："凡水肿等证，乃肺脾肾三脏相干之病。盖水为至阴，故其制在脾；水化于气，故其标在肺；水惟畏土，故其制在脾。"可知攻水与补虚乃治疗水肿两大法规。本案病程2年，肿势严重且正气已虚，治之较难。若径用攻逐利水之法，虽可取快一时，但复伤正气，绝非良策。

（三）张琪医案——湿热蕴结

邹某 男，35岁。1989年5月初诊。

西医诊断为"肾病综合征"。高度胀满（腹水），恶心呕吐，不欲食，口干舌燥，尿少（24小时约200~300ml），面红，苔黄腻，脉沉。尿蛋白（++++），尿素氮13.9mmol/L，肌酐176.8μmol/L，屡用中西药剂、利尿剂均罔效，故来求诊。

辨证：脾湿胃热，湿热中阻，清浊混淆，肾关不利。

治法：健脾除湿，苦寒清热分消。

方药：川连15g，云苓15g，半夏15g，砂仁15g，川朴15g，枳实15g，陈皮15g，知母15g，泽泻15g，姜黄15g，茯苓15g，猪苓15g，白术10g，党参15g，甘草10g。水煎服。

患者服药5剂，腹胀满大减，尿量增多，水肿明显减轻。以此方化裁连服30余剂，食欲增加，症状消失，舌苔已化，脉转和缓，尿蛋白（+），尿素氮6.35mmol/L，后连续治疗，尿蛋白转阴。

按语：张琪教授认为脾湿胃热、湿热中阻、肾关不利是本病的病机。此方原名中满分消丸，东垣用以治湿热胀满。方中芩、连苦寒泻热消痞，干姜、砂仁暖胃健脾除湿，姜黄、枳、朴行气散满，知母滋补肾阴，茯苓淡渗利湿，参、术、陈、草健脾益胃。此消补兼施，寒温并举，以使湿热分消，清升浊降、脾健胃和而肿胀自除。

（四）于春泉医案——脾肾两虚

王某 男，66岁。2015年1月21日初诊，主因双下肢浮肿就诊。

患者诉1月前出现双下肢肿胀，遂于天津某三甲医院肾病科门诊诊治。查：24h尿蛋白定量5.80g/24h，白蛋白32.0g/L，总胆固醇5.65mmol/L，诊断为"肾病综合征"。治疗效果不佳，求助中医。现患者双下肢肿胀，平素血压160/100mmHg，腰痛，纳差，乏力，眠安，小便泡沫较多，大便量少，两日一行，偏干，舌质淡紫少苔，脉弦滑。

辨证：脾肾两虚。

治法：健脾益肾，活血利水。

方药：生黄芪30g，茯苓15g，猪苓15g，泽泻15g，白术15g，桂枝15g，当归15g，防己15g，熟地黄10g，山茱萸10g，山药10g，地龙10g，僵蚕8g，乌梢蛇8g，焦麦芽30g，酸枣仁15g，首乌藤15g。水煎服，日2剂。

此方化裁连续治疗3个月，尿蛋白恢复正常，双下肢未见浮肿，平素继续服用降压药（苯磺酸氨氯地平片），建议患者生活规律，加以调摄。

按语：运用五苓散和防己黄芪汤治以温阳化气，利湿行水，重用黄芪至30g，黄芪有利尿的作用已被现代科学证实，而且有补气之功，气足湿退，水肿得消。又佐以当归、地龙、乌梢蛇、僵蚕，其中乌梢蛇搜风通络；地龙、僵蚕化瘀通络；当归养血活血、化瘀。肾病综合征符合病久入络、肾络瘀阻的病机，使用乌梢蛇、地龙、僵蚕等虫蚁辛咸之品，能深达络脉以搜剔息风解痉通络。大量临床实践证明，在治疗慢性肾小球疾病中加入活血化瘀药物，能够控制免疫复合物的形成、防止延缓肾硬化。

七、预防与调护

在肾病综合征患者中，感染者有着较高患病率。在肾病综合征合并感染的患者中，常见感染部位为呼吸道、泌尿系、腹膜及皮肤软组织等。此类的患者肺组织间隙、胸膜腔容易水钠潴留，为细菌的生长提供了便利的条件。由于呼吸道与外界相通，致病菌容易经呼吸道进入人体，故肾病综合征患者合并感染时的最常见部位为呼吸道。因此，笔者特别重视中医"上工不治已病治未病"的思想，每每嘱咐患者加强自我调理，特别是预防呼吸道疾病，平时忌生冷油腻、辛辣之品以及海鲜牛羊肉之食。有研究表明高蛋白饮食可以增加肾小球的高灌注和高滤过，使肾脏肥大，同时增加肾单位的工作负荷，损坏肾脏结构；而高滤过的程度可以通过食用低蛋白饮食来减轻，同时能够减缓肾小球滤过滤下降的速度，延缓肾脏功能的恶化。关于饮食蛋白种类的选择，红肉（猪肉、牛肉、羊肉）白肉（鸡肉、鱼肉）比对肾脏血液动力学的影响较大。在预防慢性肾脏疾病患者肾功能进展的治疗措施中，低蛋白饮食近年来被认为是有效的措施之一。

（于春泉）

参考文献

［1］叶任高，陈裕盛，方敬爱，等. 肾脏病诊断与治疗及疗效标准专题讨论纪要［J］. 中国中西医结合肾病杂志，2003，4（6）：355-357.

［2］Llach F. Thromboembolic complications in the nephrotic syndrome. Coagulation abnormalities, renal vein thrombosis and other conditions［J］. Postgrad Med, 1984, 76（6）：111-114, 116-118, 121-123.

［3］Nachman PH, Jennette JC, Falk RJ. Primary Glomerular Disease. In：Brenner BM eds. Brenner and Rector's The Kidney［M］. 8th ed. Philadelphia：WB Saunders, 2007：987-1066.

［4］Kitiyakara C, Kopp JB, Eggers P. Trends in the epidemiology of focal segmental glomerulosclerosis［J］. Semin Nephrol, 2003, 23：172-182.

［5］Research Group on Progressive Chronic Renal Disease. Nation-wide and long term survey of glomerulonephritis in Japan as observed in 1850 biopsied cases［J］. Nephron, 1999, 82：205-213.

［6］Zhou FD, Zhao MH, Zou WZ, et al. The changing spectrum of primary glomerular disease within 15 years：a survey of 3331 patients in a single Chinese centre［J］. Nephrol Dial Transplant, 2009, 24：870-876.

［7］施素华. 中国36379例肾小球疾病病理分型及流行病学分析［D］. 福州：福建医科大学，2012.

［8］Orth SR, Ritz E. The nephrotic syndrome［J］. N Engl J Med, 1998, 338：1202-1211.

［9］Eddy AA, Symons JM. Nephrotic syndrome in childhood［M］. Lancet, 2003, 362：629-639.

［10］戴陆庆. 真武汤加减治疗肾病综合征12例［J］. 赣南医学院学报, 2005, 25（6）：834.

［11］郝开花, 张永奎. 真武汤治疗肾病综合征90例［J］. 光明中医, 2015, 30（6）：1231-1232.

［12］夏建华. 小柴胡汤加味治疗原发性肾病综合征60例［J］. 山东中医杂志, 2010, 29（3）：159-160.

［13］江尔逊. 对肾病综合征用十枣汤控涎丹利尿消肿的经验［J］. 河南中医, 1981, 1（6）：32-33.

［14］田文敬, 邹杰. 血府逐瘀汤治疗肾病综合征机理研究概况［J］. 实用中西医结合临床, 2005, 5（5）：90-91.

［15］藤田康介, 陈以平. 日本汉方治疗小儿肾病综合征进展［J］. 中国中西医结合肾病杂志, 2008, 9（1）：81-82.

［16］徐达良, 刘晨曦. 柴苓汤合桃红四物汤治疗肾病综合征高脂血症的研究［J］. 现代中西医结合杂志, 2004, 13（6）：722-723.

［17］谢红, 黄智勇, 刘玉, 等. 肾炎康复片治疗肾小球肾炎的作用机理及疗效观察［J］. 河南中医学院学报, 2005, 20（5）：22-23.

［18］殷士涛, 彭月萍. 肾炎康复片联合坎地沙坦治疗原发性肾病综合征临床观察［J］. 北京中医药, 2012, 31（7）：539-541.

［19］尹莲芳, 刘璐, 弓玉祥, 等. 黄蜀葵花对肾病综合征模型大鼠肾小管损伤保护作用的研究［J］. 首都医科大学学报, 2000, 21（3）：209-211.

［20］孙毅, 付滨. 黄葵胶囊联合雷公藤多苷片治疗原发性肾病综合征临床观察［J］. 吉林中医药, 2012, 32（6）：596-597.

［21］郝丽, 潘梦舒, 郑云, 等. 冬虫夏草及雷公藤多苷对糖尿病肾病大鼠足细胞影响的实验研究［J］. 中国中西医结合杂志, 2012, 32（2）：261-265.

［22］路艳青. 雷公藤总苷联合泼尼松治疗原发性肾病综合征26例［J］. 中国民间疗法, 2004, 12（12）：46.

［23］翟雪松. 雷公藤总苷与泼尼松合用治疗肾病综合征32例疗效分析［J］. 现代医药卫生, 2004, 20（21）：2246-2247.

［24］朱小利. 双倍剂量雷公藤总苷加泼尼松治疗原发性肾病综合征的临床研究［J］. 浙江医学, 2007, 9（2）：764-765.

［25］陈彦, 黄建萍, 丁洁, 等. 对雷公藤治疗原发性肾病综合征不同方案的评价［J］. 中国医刊, 2006, 41（2）：41-44.

［26］李学旺. 中药雷公藤在慢性肾脏疾病治疗中的应用［J］. 肾脏病与透析肾移植杂志, 2003, 12（3）：251-252.

［27］胡伟新, 唐政, 姚小丹, 等. 双倍剂量雷公藤多苷治疗原发性肾病综合征的近期疗效［J］. 肾脏病与透析肾移植杂志, 1997, 6（3）：210-213.

［28］戎殳, 胡伟新, 刘志红, 等. 系膜增殖性肾小球肾炎的新疗法——雷公藤多苷新治疗方案的疗

效观察［J］.肾脏病与透析肾移植杂志，1998，7（5）：409-413.

［29］刘志红，李世军，吴燕，等.雷公藤多苷联合小剂量激素治疗特发性膜性肾病前瞻性对照研究［J］.肾脏病与透析肾移植杂志，2009，18（4）：303-309.

［30］黎磊石，刘志红.中国肾脏病学［M］.北京：人民军医出版社，2008.

［31］张伟石.温针灸治疗肾病综合征50例临床观察［J］.中外医疗，2009，28（30）：96.

［32］庄克生，李连朝，李英琛，等.培元灸法辅助治疗肾病综合征型紫癜性肾炎近期疗效观察［J］.中国中医急症，2015，23（10）：1803-1805.

［33］张振中，岳军，李建国，等.肾康敷剂治疗原发性肾病综合征40例［J］.中医外治杂志，2000，9（2）：12.

［34］王君，土贺男.中药穴位贴敷治疗原发性肾病综合征水肿临床观察［J］.山西中医，2015，31（2）：30-31.

［35］曹阳，张燕敏.穴位注射配合泼尼松治疗肾病综合征临床疗效观察及对免疫功能的影响［J］.中国针灸，2005，25（12）：857-859.

［36］尹保奇，宋鹏娟.足三里、肾俞穴位注射辅助治疗成人原发性肾病综合征疗效观察［J］.新中医，2013，45（1）：109-111.

［37］赵卫，陈春红.中药合剂保留灌肠治疗小儿原发性肾病综合征的临床应用［J］.中国医药导报，2010，7（12）：118-119.

［38］黄玲丽.中药保留灌肠治疗护理小儿难治性肾病综合征［J］.湖北中医杂志，2014，36（10）：8-9.

［39］高燕翔，张佩青，张琪，等.张琪教授以"通"为用治疗难治性肾病综合征水肿经验［J］.中国中西医结合肾病杂志，2014，15（8）：663-664.

［40］马融.健脾利湿除肾病——李少川教授治疗儿童肾病综合征的学术思想［J］.天津中医，2002，19（3）：7-9.

［41］黄文政.中西医结合治疗肾病综合征的经验体会［J］.天津中医药大学学报，2006，25（3）：142-145.

［42］Soeiro E M, Koch V H, Fujimura M D, et al. Influence of nephrotic state on the infectious profile in childhood idiopathic nephrotic syndrotne［J］. Rev Hosp Clin Fac Med Sao Paulo, 2004, 59（5）：273-278.

［43］张吉吉，池芝盛.饮食蛋白对糖尿病肾病的影响［J］.国外医学：内分泌学分册，1998，18（4）：26-29.

［44］Teplan V, Schuck O, Votruba M, et al. Metabolic effects of keto acid--amino acid supplementation in patients with chronic renal insufficiency receiving a low-protein diet and recombinant human erythropoietin—a randomized controlled trial［J］. Wien Klin Wochenschr, 2001, 113（17-18）：661-669.

糖尿病

Diabetes

一、概述

糖尿病是一组以高血糖为特征的全身性、代谢性疾病。而高血糖的原因则是由于胰腺的胰岛素分泌不足或缺陷，或其生理作用不能正常发挥，或上述原因兼而有之所引起。糖尿病患病之后长期存在的高血糖，将可能导致身体多种组织，特别是眼、肾、心脏、血管、神经的慢性损害及功能障碍，进而形成多种并发症。

此病相当于中医所说的消渴病，但实际上中医所说消渴病的临床范围要大于糖尿病，比如西医学的"尿崩症"也可以按照中医的"消渴"来辨证论治，只是"尿崩症"的临床发病率要比"糖尿病"低得多。"消"有消耗、消瘦、乏力的意思；"渴"就是口渴、饮水多。消渴作为中医病名，它的基本临床特点就是多饮、多尿、多食，且身体乏力、消瘦。

中医认为，消渴病的基本病理变化是阴虚内热，主要涉及肺、胃、肾三个脏腑。病理变化侧重在肺的称为"上消"，症状表现以口渴多饮较为显著；侧重在胃的称为"中消"，症状表现以多食、易饥较为显著；侧重在肾的称为"下消"，症状表现以多尿、生殖系统功能异常和大便异常较为显著。所以"消渴"又称为"三消"。

二、病因病机

（一）中医

1. 饮食不节

饮食过量，尤其是多食肥甘厚味，多食油腻、辛辣、煎炸食物，积生内热。

2. 劳逸失度

多坐少动，活动量不足，久坐容易伤脾，导致气血运行不畅，气机壅滞，日久化热。

3. 情志失调

用心用脑思虑过度，或因所欲不遂而焦虑急躁，日久耗伤阴血，阴虚而生内热。

4. 酒色过度

过量饮酒，过于频繁的性生活，都容易导致消渴病的发生。因为酒性湿热，可以销铄、消耗津液营血；而饮酒又容易使人色欲过度，耗伤肾精，二者均可导致精、血、津液不足而生内热。

5. 先天因素

本病具有遗传倾向，若父母、（外）祖父母等上辈亲属中有罹患此病者，则子辈亲人相对高发。

（二）西医

胰腺的胰岛损伤，胰岛素分泌不足，胰岛素功能障碍，造成血糖升高，是其基本的病理变化。而其原因则有生活方式因素、家族遗传因素、感染因素等多个方面。

三、诊断要点与鉴别诊断

（一）诊断要点

1. 中医

（1）临床上出现口干、口渴、多饮，多食，易饥饿，尿量增多，乏力，易疲劳，或有身体消瘦。

（2）具有上述病因病机方面的 4 种生活方式及家族遗传史。

2. 西医

空腹血糖大于或等于 7.0mmol/L，和 / 或餐后 2 小时血糖 ≥ 11.1mmol/L 即可确诊。

（1）1 型糖尿病：发病年龄较轻，多小于 30 岁，起病突然，多饮、多尿、多食、消瘦症状明显，血糖水平高，较多患者以酮症酸中毒为首发症状，血清胰岛素和 C 肽水平低下，ICA、IAA 或 GAD 抗体可呈阳性。单用口服降糖药疗效差，一般需用胰岛素治疗。

（2）2 型糖尿病：常见于中老年人，肥胖者发病率高，常可伴有高血压、血脂异常、动脉硬化等疾病。起病较慢或隐袭发病，早期无明显症状，或仅有轻度乏力、口渴，血糖增高不明显者需做糖耐量试验才能确诊。血清胰岛素水平早期正常或增高，晚期低下。

（二）鉴别诊断

（1）一般的热证如胃肠热证、肝胆热证等也可出现口干、口渴、多饮等症状，但尿量不多或少尿，也少见乏力、易疲劳的症状，应该注意与消渴病的鉴别。

（2）甲状腺功能亢进、慢性肾功能不全、肝硬化等疾病，以及外伤等应激状态下也会出现血糖升高，应该注意鉴别。

四、中医治疗

（一）辨证治疗

前已述及，中医认为消渴病的基本病理变化是阴虚内热，主要涉及肺、胃、肾三个脏腑。从临床患者的具体情况来说，病变侧重在肺的"上消"大多同时与心的功能异常相关联，侧重在胃的"中消"大多同时与脾的功能异常相关联，侧重在肾的"下消"大多同时与肝的功能异常相关联，所以中医认为，消渴一病与人体上、中、下三焦多个脏腑的功能失调都有关系，是一种全身性疾病，只是在不同的患者身上其病理变化和临床表现可以有所侧重，因而表现为不同的证候类型。

1. 肺阴虚、心火旺

主症： 口干、口渴，饮水后仍不解渴，易急躁，可能失眠，舌苔干燥少津，舌尖红或全舌红，脉数或浮数、细数。

治法： 养阴清热，生津止渴。

方药： 玉泉散加减。天花粉、生地、麦冬、知母、葛根、桔梗、淡竹叶、生甘草、五味子。

方解： 天花粉、知母、桔梗、葛根清泻肺热，生津止渴；生地、麦冬、五味子滋阴生津；淡竹叶、生甘草清泻上焦心肺之热。综合配伍，达到养阴清热、生津止渴的作用。

2. 心肺气阴两虚

主症： 口干、口渴，饮水后仍不解渴，体力疲乏，精神倦怠，舌干少津，脉虚数或细数。

治法： 养阴益气，生津止渴。

方药： 沙参麦门冬汤加减。沙参、麦冬、玉竹、桑叶、天花粉、白扁豆、生黄芪、地骨皮、生甘草、葛根。

方解： 沙参、麦冬、玉竹、生黄芪养阴益气生津；桑叶、天花粉、地骨皮、葛根清热泻火生津；白扁豆、生甘草健脾化湿益气。综合配伍，达到养阴益气，生津止渴的作用。

3. 肺胃津伤、阴虚火旺

主症： 口干、口渴，易饥多食，食欲亢进，大便秘结，或黏腻不爽，舌质红、少苔，或舌苔干黄，脉细数或虚数。

治法： 养阴清热，益胃生津。

方药： 玉女煎加减。生地、麦冬、知母、生石膏、黄连、胡黄连、天花粉、茯苓、葛根、芦根。

方解： 生地、麦冬生津养阴清热；石膏、知母、黄连、胡黄连、天花粉、葛根清热泻火，生津止渴；茯苓、芦根健脾化湿，利尿泻热。

4. 脾胃气阴两虚

主症： 口干、口渴，易饥多食，或饥不欲食，面色萎黄不华，神倦力乏，便秘或便溏，脉细数或虚数或沉细。

治法： 健脾益气，养阴生津。

方药： 参苓白术散加减。人参、白茯苓、山药、白扁豆、黄精、葛根、桔梗、莲子肉、薏苡仁。

方解： 人参、山药、黄精、莲子肉健脾益气养阴；茯苓、白术、扁豆、薏苡仁健脾益气化湿；葛根、桔梗生津止渴。

5. 脾胃湿热

主症： 口干、口渴，多食易饥，或饥不欲食，大便秘结，或黏腻难解，舌质红，舌苔黄腻或白腻，脉濡数或沉数或沉弦。

治法： 健脾和胃，化湿清热。

方药： 平胃散合连朴饮加减。苍术、陈皮、厚朴、砂仁、佩兰、黄连、黄芩、苏梗、滑石、芦根。

方解： 苍术、陈皮、厚朴、砂仁、佩兰、苏梗健脾和胃化湿；黄芩、黄连清中焦湿热；滑石、芦根利尿泻热，生津止渴。

6. 肝肾阴虚

主症： 口干、口渴，腰膝酸软，急躁易怒，疲乏无力，头晕耳鸣，大便秘结，尿黄，或有盗汗，失眠，舌质红，少苔，脉细数或虚数。

治法： 滋补肝肾，清热养阴。

方药： 增液汤合六味地黄丸加减。生地、玄参、麦冬、山萸肉、五味子、菊花、地骨皮、山药、茯苓、丹皮、泽泻、怀牛膝。

方解： 生地、玄参、麦冬滋阴生津清热；山萸肉、五味子、怀牛膝滋补肝肾阴精；山药、茯苓、泽泻健脾化湿；菊花、丹皮、地骨皮清解肝肾虚火。全方合用，达到滋补肝肾阴精，清泻虚火的目的。

7. 肾精虚损

主症： 口干、口渴，腰膝酸软，头晕，耳鸣、耳聋，视物不清，神倦力乏，记忆力下降，多尿，可有尿液混浊，便秘或便溏，舌干少津，脉沉细或细数。

治法： 补肾，益气，填精。

方药： 六味地黄丸加减。生地、山萸肉、五味子、菟丝子、枸杞子、山药、怀牛膝、桑寄生、生黄芪、白术、茯苓、泽泻。

方解： 生地、山萸肉、五味子、菟丝子、枸杞子、怀牛膝、桑寄生滋补肝肾阴精；黄芪、白术、山药益气健脾，脾肾双补；茯苓、泽泻化湿利尿，使全方补而不滞。

8. 肝脾肾阴阳两虚

主症： 口干、口渴，腰膝酸软，头晕，耳鸣、耳聋，视物不清，记忆力下降，神倦力乏，肢端麻木，面色黧黑，尿频量多，男人可见阳痿，女人可见月经失调，大便溏泄，舌淡而干燥少津，苔剥或少苔，脉沉细。

治法： 补肝肾，益脾胃，助阳气。

方药： 八味肾气丸合四君子汤加减。生地、山萸肉、五味子、菟丝子、枸杞子、山药、怀牛膝、生黄芪、党参、白术、制附子、桂枝、淫羊藿、茯苓、泽泻。

方解： 生地、山萸肉、五味子、菟丝子、枸杞子、怀牛膝滋补肝肾；党参、黄芪、山药、白术补中益气；附子、桂枝、淫羊藿助脾肾之阳气；茯苓、泽泻化湿利尿，使补而不滞。

（二）专方治疗

鹤芝堂消渴万灵方，主治消渴病。白术 15g，苍术 15g，葛根 15g，天花粉 15g，蚕茧 30g，霜桑叶 30g，干玉米须 20g，生黄芪 15g，鸡内金 15g，枳壳 10g。水煎服，每日 1 剂，分两次空腹温服。

（三）单方验方

翻白草 30~50g，开水冲泡，代茶饮，对轻型糖尿病有效。

（四）中成药

（1）金匮肾气丸：适用于消渴病之肾阴、肾阳两虚证。

（2）六味地黄丸：适用于消渴病之肾阴虚证。

（3）参苓白术丸：适用于消渴病之脾气虚兼有湿气证。

（4）补中益气丸：适用于消渴病之中气不足，易受外感证。

（5）金芪降糖片：适用于消渴病之气虚兼热证。

（6）消渴丸：适用于消渴病之气阴两虚兼热证。

（五）针灸治疗

消渴病一般不提倡针刺疗法，因为针刺所造成的皮肤创伤有可能导致针眼局部感染，且感染后难以愈合，尤其是全身状况营养不良，且症情较为严重的患者不适宜做针刺治疗。灸法可选用足三里、肾俞、膈俞等穴位，需要长期坚持，方为有益。

（六）推拿治疗

推拿按摩方法，选用的穴位可以参照前述辨证用药的思路，从上中下三消入手，上焦选择肺经、心经的穴位，中焦选择脾胃经的穴位，下焦选择肝经、肾经、膀胱经的穴位。常用穴位如膏肓俞、肺俞、心俞、膈俞、肝俞、云门、命门、足三里、三阴交、然谷（骨）、涌泉等穴位。手法以较为轻柔的保健手法为主，手法可以由轻渐重，以穴位局部有轻度至中度酸胀、酸痛的感觉为度，取点压法或旋转式点压法。时间每次不少于15分钟，一般以30~60分钟为宜。按摩时间宜避开饱腹及空腹时。

六、名医专家典型医案

丁甘仁治消渴医案——肺胃津伤、阴虚阳亢、肝肾不足

尹某 诊脉左三部弦数，右三部滑数，太溪细弱，趺阳濡数。临床表现为消谷善饥，身体消瘦，饮食不充肌肤，神疲乏力，虚里穴动，自汗盗汗，头面烘热，汗后畏冷，头眩眼花。皆由阴液亏耗，不能涵木，肝阳上僭，心神不得安宁，虚阳逼津液而外泄则多汗，消灼胃阴则消谷。头面烘热，汗后畏冷，营虚失于内守，卫虚失于外护故也。脉数不减，颇虑延成消证。姑拟养肺阴以柔肝木，清胃阴而宁心神，俾得阴平阳秘，水升火降，方能渐入佳境。

辨证： 肺胃津伤，阴虚阳亢，肝肾不足。

治法： 滋阴潜阳，清热生津。

方药： 大生地12g，抱茯神9g，潼蒺藜9g，川贝母6g，浮小麦12g，生白芍6g，左牡蛎12g，熟女贞9g，天花粉9g，肥玉竹9g，花龙骨9g，冬虫夏草6g，五味子3g。

按语： 本案以肺胃肝肾俱阴液不足，阴虚阳亢，心肾不交为主要病机，属于较为典型的多个脏腑功能异常的消渴病。遣方用药则五脏兼顾，考虑周全，确实具有大家用药之风范。

七、预防与调护

（一）预防

（1）消渴病的形成与生活方式有较为密切的关系，尤其是有本病家族史的人群，青少年甚至童年时代即应引起注意。

（2）养成良好健康的生活方式，尽量少吃甜食，少吃煎炸类主食及菜肴，合理控制脂肪尤其是动物性脂肪的摄入量。

（3）根据不同年龄段，科学合理地并且最好是持之以恒地安排好体育锻炼或体力劳动，如50岁以前以及健康状态较好、体力较佳的人可以坚持每周不少于3次的中等强度的运动锻炼，50岁以后以及健康状况较差、体力较弱的人可以坚持每周不少于5次的低等强度的运动锻炼。

（4）上班族尤其是白领阶层的工作人员，一定要注意劳逸结合，避免久坐，避免超过一个小时的坐姿电脑办公。

（5）情绪方面注意避免大喜、大悲等过于剧烈的情感刺激，保持心态平和，开朗乐观。

（二）调护

（1）已经发现有此病的患者，首先需要引起重视的是，必须做到饮食有节，少吃甜食及饮用碳酸类饮料，酒类饮料要根据自己的身体实际状况酌情而定，但总的原则是以少饮为宜，控制高脂饮食尤其动物脂肪类饮食。适当吃些粗粮，不要只吃精米白面，适宜多吃些豆类食品及蔬菜。

（2）坚持有规律的运动锻炼，运动强度、锻炼方式及每次运动时间的长短可以根据自己的实际情况酌情而定，但不论哪一种锻炼方式都要持之以恒，运动强度及时间以身体微微出汗为宜，运动后注意补充水分。

（3）生活起居要有规律，睡眠、起床、进餐要有相对固定的时间，否则血糖就容易波动。

（4）保持心态乐观，情绪稳定，尽量避免过于剧烈的精神刺激。

（5）如果空腹血糖已经 > 9mmol/L 者，必须规范用药。

（孙中堂）

头痛

Headache

一、概述

头痛是以头部疼痛为主要症状的一种病症，是临床常见的一种自觉症状，可由多种疾病引起，也可单独出现。可见于多种急、慢性疾病中，凡外感六淫、内伤杂病引起以头痛为主症的病症均可称为头痛。如痛在一侧的名"偏头痛"；痛在头顶的名"颠顶痛"；痛在前额的名"额头痛"；痛在后脑的名"后头痛"；日久不愈者，名为"头风"；头脑尽痛，手足冷至节者，名为"真头痛"。本病属于中医"头风""脑风""偏头痛""厥头痛"等范畴。

在西医学看来，头痛的病因繁多，神经痛、颅内感染、颅内占位病变、脑血管疾病、颅外头面部疾病以及全身疾病如急性感染、中毒等均可导致头痛。不是所有头痛均可按本节所介绍的内容治疗，一般认为西医学中的高血压、颅内肿瘤、三叉神经痛、偏头痛、神经官能症等疾患若以头痛为主症者，可参考本病进行辨证论治。临床治疗是以神经性头痛为主，包括紧张性头痛、功能性头痛及血管神经性头痛等。

二、病因病机

（一）中医

头痛最早的记载见于《内经》，有"脑风""首风"之名，《素问》载有头痛35处，《灵枢》载有18处。在病因病机方面认为外邪入侵是头痛的主要原因，五脏疾病与头痛有关，六经皆有头痛，提出年龄不同部位有异，"年长者则求之于腑，年少者则求之于经，年壮者求之于脏。"《难经》提出"厥头痛"与"真头痛"，前者为气厥，后者为痰厥，病情凶险。《伤寒论》系统地提出头痛的病因病机及治法方药，共有记载14处，分布于太阳、阳明、少阳、厥阴四经。《东垣十书》将头痛分为内伤头痛和外感头痛。《丹溪心法》提出："头痛多主于痰，痛甚者火多。"《普济方·头痛附论》言："若人气血俱虚，风邪伤于阳经，入于脑中，则令人头痛也。"明代王肯堂言："天门真痛，上引泥丸，夕发旦死，旦发夕死。"

头乃人之首汇，头有"精明之府""诸阳之会""髓海所居处"之称，既有清窍与内外相通，又有经络与脏腑相连，故五脏六腑之气血津液，皆与头相关，汇聚于头部。《类证治裁》说："头为天象，诸阳经会焉，若六气外侵，精华内痹，郁于空窍，清阳不运，其痛乃作。"凡六淫之邪侵袭，上犯清窍，遏阻经脉；恼怒忧思，风阳上扰，气郁化火；饮食不节，脾伤湿聚，痰湿上聚；久病劳倦，气血不足，脑失所荣；先天不足，纵欲过度，精亏髓少；跌打损伤，瘀血内停，脑络受阻，皆可导致头痛。

1. 病因

一般认为，头痛之病因多端，但不外乎外感和内伤两大类。外感有风热、风寒、风湿之分，内伤有肝阳上亢、肾精亏虚、脾胃虚弱、痰湿阻滞、瘀血阻络之别。

（1）外感头痛：多因起居不慎，坐卧当风等感受六淫之邪，上犯颠顶，清阳之气受阻，气血凝滞，阻碍脉络而致头痛。然风为百病之长，"伤于风者，上先受之"，所以外感六淫所致之头痛仍以风邪为主，多挟时气而发病，尤以挟寒、热、湿邪为多见。

①风寒外侵：风寒多见于冬季，气候多寒，生活起居失宜，而致体虚气亏，卫外不固，寒邪侵袭，寒邪束表，卫阳被遏。寒邪入经，血脉凝滞，阻遏脉络，血瘀于内而致头痛。《素问·举痛论篇》说："寒气入经而稽迟，泣而不行，客于脉外则血少，客于脉中则气不通，故卒然而痛。"

②风热入侵：气温乍暖，将息失宜，或住室气流不畅，热气熏蒸，毛窍疏稀，温热之邪乘袭，风热相搏，肌腠疏泄不畅，火性炎上，清窍被扰，气血逆乱而致头痛。

③风湿入侵：久居潮湿之地，或冒雨涉水，或汗出入水，或雨湿之年，起居不慎，湿邪浸渍。且湿为阴邪，遏伤阳气，阻碍气机，其性氤氲黏腻，湿邪蒙蔽清窍，清阳不升而致头痛。《素问·生气通天论篇》说："因于湿，首如裹。"指的是头部有湿，头重痛而昏，似巾缠头，抠而发紧的感觉。

（2）内伤头痛："脑为髓之海"，主要依赖于肝肾之精的充养（肾藏精、主骨生髓，肝肾同源），以及脾胃运化的水谷之精的濡养，故内伤头痛的发生多与肝、脾、肾三脏相关。

①肝阳上亢：肝性喜条达而恶抑郁，又易升动，故有"肝为刚脏"之称。肝气的疏泄主要关系到人体气机的升降与调畅。只有在肝气疏泄正常的情况下，人才能气血和平，心情舒畅，而不为病伤。反之，若情志不和，郁怒伤肝，则肝失条达，肝气郁结，气郁化火。《临证指南医案·郁》云："郁则气滞，气滞久则必化热。"火性炎上，火邪上扰清空之窍而致头痛。如果气郁化火日久，就要耗伤津液，使肝阴不足，肝失濡养。或肾水不足，大多为房劳伤精所致，水不涵木，致肝肾阴亏，肝阳亢盛，再耗伤肝阴，下耗肾水，使肝肾阴液更加不足，形成"恶性循环"。"肝为风木之脏"，风火相煽，火随气窜，上扰颠顶，则发为头痛。

②肾精亏虚：多由于禀赋不足或房劳过度，使肾精久亏。《素问·逆调论篇》云："肾不生则髓不能满"，《灵枢·海论》说："脑为髓之海"。髓的生成来源于肾，肾主骨生髓，髓上通于脑，因此脑髓有赖于肾精的不断化生。如果肾精久亏，脑髓空虚就会发生头痛。如果肾阴久损，阴损及阳（阴阳互根）或久病体虚，都会导致肾阳虚弱，清阳不展而为头痛。

③脾胃虚弱：脾胃为后天之本，气血生化之源，全身四肢百骸，五脏六腑，无不赖于气血的濡养。饥饱劳倦或病后、产后体虚，脾胃虚弱，气血化源不足，致使营血亏虚，不能上荣于脑髓脉络而致头痛。

④痰湿阻滞：多由脾胃虚弱，化生痰浊，或因嗜酒肥甘，脾虚无力运化水湿而生痰，痰浊上扰清窍，阻遏清阳，清阳不升而致头痛。

⑤瘀血阻络：外伤或久病入络，均会导致气滞血瘀，"气为血之帅，血为气之母"，气行则血行，气滞则血凝，久病气虚，气不帅血，血流不畅。或头部外伤，气血瘀滞，瘀血阻于脑络，不通则痛，头痛随之而发。

2. 病机

头痛的病机是指不通则痛、不荣则痛、不平则痛。疼痛的发生，多与经脉不利有关。邪实阻滞，气血逆乱，脉道失于通利；脾胃虚弱，滋养乏源，气血失于濡养；或阴阳失衡，阳亢阴伤，气机逆乱，上扰于脑，头部脉络失利，皆可导致头痛症状的发生。

（1）不通则痛：《证治要诀》云："痛则不通，通则不痛。"不通为疼痛发生的重要原因之一。其病机关键主要在于邪实、痰浊、气滞、瘀血、食积等病理因素的聚积，脑络不通，引发头痛。若风寒之邪凝滞气血，阻遏脉络；或风热之邪上扰清窍，导致气血逆乱；或风湿之邪蒙蔽清窍，导致清阳不升；饮食不节，痰湿内生，阻遏清阳；气血不畅，络脉瘀阻；情志不和，肝气不舒，气郁化火，上扰清窍；久病入络，脑络不通等，皆可引起头痛。

（2）不荣则痛：《素问·举痛论篇》说："脉泣则血虚，血虚则痛。"《医宗金鉴》说："伤损之证，血虚作痛。"不荣则痛的病机关键在于精亏、气虚、血虚。先天禀赋不足，肾精不能上充于脑；或阴损及阳，肾阳衰微，清阳不升，脑府失养；劳倦过度，饮食不节，损伤脾胃，导致气血化源不足，脑失濡养；或久病耗损，气血两虚，脑窍失养，皆可引发头痛。

（3）不平则痛：气血通百病不生，物不平则鸣、人不平则病。平是指人体应当达到的阴平阳秘的状态。若这个平衡状态被破坏，那么疾病相应产生。除了不通而痛、不荣而痛，也存在不平则痛的情况。不平则痛的病机关键在于气逆、阳亢。阴阳不平，肝肾阴亏，火盛伤阴，肝阳上亢，上扰清窍；情志失调，气血逆乱，气逆上扰，皆可引发头痛。

（二）西医

头痛是由多种病因引起的综合性疾病，多种原因均可导致头痛。当头颈部的痛觉末梢感受器受到异常的神经冲动刺激后，往往会引发头痛。一般可分为4类：颅内病变所致头痛，如中风、脑动脉硬化、高血压脑病等；颅外头颈部病变引起的头痛，如偏头痛、丛集性头痛等；头颈部皮肤肌肉颅骨病变引起的头痛，如头皮急性感染、紧张性头痛等；五官及口腔病变引起的头痛，如青光眼、鼻窦炎等。常见的头痛病因如下所述。

1. 血管性头痛

多由颅内外动脉的扩张或破裂出血导致，如偏头痛、蛛网膜下腔出血等引起的头痛就常常与血管因素相关。

2. 牵引性头痛

多由颅内痛觉敏感组织被牵引或移位导致，当颅内发生水肿时，水肿部位对脑膜组织进行挤压，从而引发头痛。

3. 脑膜刺激性头痛

多由颅内外感觉敏感组织发生炎症导致，当颅内发生炎症性渗出时，渗出的炎性物质对脑膜神经及血管有一定的刺激，从而引发头痛。

4. 紧张性或肌肉收缩性头痛

多由颅内外的肌肉收缩导致，这种情况多因为精神因素导致，患者颅内往往没有病变，但有明显的精神症状。

5. 神经炎性头痛

多由传导痛觉的脑神经和颈神经直接受损或发生炎症导致，颅内的痛觉对第5对、第9对、第10对脑神经和第2~3对颈神经传导敏感，当上述神经发生炎症时，往往会产生头痛的感觉。

6. 牵涉性头痛

多由五官病变的疼痛扩散导致，面部三叉神经、颈神经等受到刺激时，可能会导致头部疼痛，此时颅内无病变。

7. 遗传性头痛

多由遗传因素导致，患者有明显的家族遗传病史。

三、诊断要点与鉴别诊断

（一）诊断要点

头痛的病因复杂，在病史采集中应重点询问头痛的起病方式、发作频率、发作时间、持续时间、头痛的部位、性质、疼痛程度，有无前驱症状，及有无明确的诱发因素、头痛加重和减轻的因素等。头痛的伴随症状繁多，应以头痛的部位、头痛性质、病程及舌脉象等作为诊断要点。

1. 中医

（1）以疼痛部位辨病位：头为诸阳之会，三阳经均循头面，厥阴经亦上会于颠顶。辨别头痛，可根据经脉加以判断。太阳头痛：多在头后部，下连于项；阳明头痛：多在前额及眉棱；少阳头痛：多在头之两侧，连及耳部；厥阴头痛：在颠顶部位，或连于目系；少阴头痛：在脑中，或牵及于齿。

（2）以疼痛性质辨病性：掣痛者多为筋脉阻痹引发；跳痛者多为肝阳上亢或血热引发；灼痛多为风热、火热或阴虚引发；胀痛者多为气滞或肝阳上亢、肝火上炎引发；重痛者多为风湿引发；隐痛者多为气血亏虚引发；空痛者多为肾精亏损引发；昏痛者多为体虚湿阻引发；刺痛（痛如锥刺，痛处固定不移）多为瘀血引发。

（3）以病程分外感内伤：新病之头痛，多因外邪所致，大多痛势较剧，多表现为掣痛、跳痛、灼痛、胀痛、重痛，痛无休止。久病之头痛，多因内伤所致，大多痛势较缓，多表现为隐痛、空痛、昏痛，痛势悠悠，遇劳则剧，时作时止。

（4）以舌象脉象明确诊断：舌苔薄白者多风寒头痛；舌苔薄黄者多风热头痛；舌苔白腻者多风湿或痰浊头痛；舌红苔黄者多肝阳上亢头痛；舌红苔少者多阴血亏虚头痛；舌瘦少苔者多肾虚头痛；舌质紫或有瘀斑、瘀点者为瘀血头痛。

脉浮紧者多风寒头痛；脉浮数者多风热头痛；脉濡者多风湿头痛；脉滑或弦滑者多痰浊头痛；脉弦者多肝阳上亢头痛；脉细数者多阴虚头痛；脉沉细者多肾虚头痛；脉细涩者多瘀血头痛。

2. 西医

突发性头痛伴有出汗、恶心、呕吐，吐出后头痛缓解者可见于偏头痛发作；头痛同时伴有剧烈的恶心、呕吐、颈项强直等脑内压增高及脑膜刺激征者，多见于脑内肿瘤、脑脊髓膜炎、蛛网膜下腔出血、脑出血等；头痛伴有明显的眩晕者，提示颅后窝病变；如果在头痛的同时出现精神症状，特别在早期出现欣快、幻觉、哭笑无常等表现可为颞叶肿瘤或病毒性脑炎；头痛时发生自主神经功能紊乱的症状如冷汗、面色潮红或苍白、血压波动、恶心、呕吐、乏力、心悸、腹泻等，则多为血管性头痛。

头痛发于头顶部者多为功能性或神经性头痛；发于后枕部者可能为蛛网膜下腔出血、脑脊髓膜炎、高血压性头痛、颈性头痛、颅后窝肿瘤、枕大神经痛；发为眼部或眼眶周围者多为颅内高压性头痛、青光眼、丛集性头痛、一氧化碳中毒性头痛、三叉神经痛；发于侧头的偏头痛多为血管性偏头痛、耳源性偏头痛、齿源性偏头痛；全头痛者多为脑肿瘤、紧张性头痛、颅内高压性头痛、感染性头痛者。

（二）鉴别诊断

1. 紧张性头痛

由于长期的精神紧张、焦虑、疲劳等致头颈部肌肉紧张，血管收缩，组织缺血，代谢异常，致痛物质释放所致。头痛的特点是发生于双侧额、枕、颞部，疼痛呈持续性钝痛，紧箍感、重压感，时轻时重，从无缓解。常伴有神经衰弱诸症。抗抑郁药、安定药能减轻头痛，麦角胺类药无效。

2. 颅内压增高

头痛是颅内压增高的主要症状，也是唯一的早期症状。头痛常呈持续性钝痛，可伴恶心呕吐，随着病情的发展，头痛也逐渐变得剧烈。头痛以清晨时明显，或可在夜间痛醒，任何可使颅内压增高的因素如咳嗽、喷嚏、大便用力等均可使头痛加重。临床上可根据病史、脑 CT、脑血管造影、磁共振成像（MRI）等进行鉴别。

3. 高血压性头痛

严重的高血压一般都有枕部及额部头痛，头部低俯或屏气用力时使头痛加剧。头痛与高血压之间有直接联系，控制高血压后可使头痛缓解。而偏头痛为发作性痛，一般为一侧搏动性痛。监测血压变化可鉴别。

4. 头痛性癫痫

头痛性癫痫发作起病急骤，常无先兆症状，头痛剧烈，可伴有意识障碍，头痛以颞部、额部多见，发作持续时间长短不一，发作可以自行停止。发作时脑电图多为阵发性高波幅：4~7 次 / 秒节律为主，或为棘波、尖波、棘慢波综合等。常两侧对称性同步出现，间隙期多为正常。

5. 神经症头痛

神经症患者常有头痛，主要是疼痛耐受性的阈值降低与肌肉紧张，非发作性痛，亦无先兆。通常伴有失眠、注意力不集中、记忆力减退、头昏、烦躁不安等症，症状的出现或加剧常与患者的精神状态有关。

6. 颞动脉炎

头痛为主要症状，常位于颞部与眼眶周围部，也可漫及额部与枕部。为一种强烈搏动性和持续性痛。并有一种其他血管性头痛中所没有的烧灼感。患者可在咀嚼时出现疼痛，并可以此为首发症状。常见症状有视觉障碍，有部分或完全视力丧失的可能。因约 1/3 颞动脉炎病例视网膜动脉也被侵及，眼底检查可见视网膜中央动脉血栓形成和缺血性神经炎。全身症状有发热，倦怠不适，食欲不振，肌肉疼痛，肢体无力，焦虑、忧郁以及血沉快，活检可确定诊断。激素治疗有显效。

7. 三叉神经痛

三叉神经痛无先兆期，其疼痛为急骤发作的阵发性、电击样或火烙样疼痛，部位限于三叉神经三支分布区域，疼痛持续数秒至数分钟。可因刺激皮肤触发点诱发。药用苯丙英钠有效。

四、中医治疗

（一）辨证治疗

辨证治疗要根据病机，以通、补、平为主。一般初病多实，治宜祛邪，以通为主，但又要根据不同病因施以不同治法，如风寒头痛则以疏风散寒为治，风热头痛则以疏风清热为治，风湿头痛则以祛风胜湿为治。久病多虚，治宜固元气，以补虚为主，但虚中挟实者，如瘀血、痰浊等当权衡主次，有补有通。肝阳头痛有虚有实，实者宜平肝潜阳，本虚标实者宜滋补肝肾之阴而平肝。如《景岳全书》中"暂病者应重邪气，久病者当顾元气"就是此意。头痛一证由于临床表现繁多复杂，各有不同，所以治疗应按不同的临床表现和不同阶段进行。急性发作期重在通，予以疏风、降火（潜阳）、化痰、祛瘀为主；缓解期应着重补，以健脾、养肝、补肾为治，以防复发。对于发作缓慢，痛势悠悠者，可以单纯用中医药进行综合治疗，但重度头痛者，起病较急，痛势急迫，难以忍受，应予以中西医结合治疗，待病情缓解之后再用中药进行调理以巩固疗效。

1. 外感头痛

（1）外感风寒

主症： 头痛时作，痛连项背，恶风寒，遇风尤剧，常喜裹头，得温则减，口不渴。舌淡红，苔薄白，脉浮。

治法： 疏风散寒。

方药： 川芎茶调散加减。川芎、羌活、白芷、细辛、薄荷、荆芥、防风、甘草、白芍。

加减： 若头痛剧，无汗，遇寒即甚，寒象明显可加熟附片、麻黄。若兼见咳嗽，痰稀色白，可在上方基础上加杏仁、前胡、苏叶增强宣肺止咳之力。

方解： 方中川芎主治少阳、厥阴经头痛，羌活主治太阳经头痛，白芷主治阳明经头疼，白芍缓挛急，止疼痛，均为主药；细辛、薄荷、荆芥、防风辛散上行，疏散上部风邪，协助上述各药，以增强疏风止痛之效，均为辅药；甘草调和诸药，又可以制约上药过于温燥，升散，使升中有降，为佐使。其中川芎可行血中之气，祛血中之风，上行头目，为临床治头痛之要药。诸药合用，共成疏散风邪，止头痛之功。原方本为外风头痛的主治方，而顽固性头痛又可以此方疏风、通络、止痛。研究表明川芎茶调散能促进血液循环，增强大脑供血，改善微循环，缓解头颈部肌肉疲劳，治疗神经性头痛也恰到好处。

（2）外感风热

主症：头胀而痛，甚则如裂，发热恶风，面红目赤，口渴欲饮，便秘溲黄。舌红，苔薄黄，脉浮数。

治法：疏风清热。

方药：芎芷石膏汤加减。川芎、白芷、菊花、石膏、丹皮、赤芍、薄荷、黄芩、栀子、连翘、芦根、桔梗、细辛、甘草。

加减：若症见高热、口渴、鼻干、心烦、舌红、少津等热甚伤津之证，可加葛根解肌，生石膏、知母、天花粉清热生津。若咳嗽不爽，痰稠而黄，口渴咽痛，可于前方加川贝母、瓜蒌仁、沙参等化痰生津。

方解：方中川芎、白芷、石膏、菊花疏风清热透表，共为君；丹皮、赤芍凉血活血，薄荷疏散风邪，黄芩、栀子、连翘清热透表，表证自解；芦根升清生津以养阴；配以甘草使风热之邪得去，又不伤阴伤正；桔梗开宣肺气，气机升降相宜，使风邪无以伤人。细辛止痛，诸药合用，共奏疏风解表、通络止痛之功。

（3）外感风湿

主症：头痛如裹，肢体困重，纳呆胸闷，大便溏泻，小便不利，舌淡红苔白腻，脉濡。

治法：疏风除湿。

方药：羌活胜湿汤加减。羌活、独活、防风、藁本、川芎、蔓荆子、白芍、牛膝、细辛、甘草。

加减：若伴见呕吐者，加姜半夏、姜竹茹以降逆止呕。若见烦闷，纳呆，口苦黏，小便黄，苔黄腻，脉濡数，此为湿郁化热所致，可加黄芩、黄连、黄柏、半夏以清热。如见胸闷腹胀，四肢困重，纳差，大便溏泻，可加苍术、厚朴、陈皮、枳壳等以祛湿和中。

方解：方中羌活、独活、防风、藁本都能祛风胜湿、散寒止痛，散在表之风寒，祛在表之湿邪；川芎活血行气，祛风止痛；白芍缓挛急，止疼痛，牛膝活血止痛，蔓荆子祛风止痛、清利头目，细辛止痛，与羌活、独活、防风等配伍，止头痛作用更为显著；因风能胜湿，所以多兼用风药；加以甘草制诸药之峻，矫味和中；共成发表散寒、祛湿止痛之功则头痛可愈。

2. 内伤头痛

（1）肝郁头痛

主症：受情志影响，或与妇女月经来潮有关，头痛偏于一侧，左右不一，或牵延至眉棱骨，多呈胀痛，其痛反复，胸闷不舒，喜太息，情志抑郁或心烦易怒，或兼胁痛，舌淡红，色暗，苔薄，脉弦。

治法：疏肝解郁。

方药：逍遥散加减。柴胡、香附、当归、白芍、白术、茯苓、甘草、煨姜、薄荷、细辛、牛膝、川芎。

加减：因风寒之邪入侵而诱发，加白芷、藁本祛风散寒；若因风热之邪而诱发，加葛根、白芷、菊花疏风清热；肝郁化火，口干苦，目赤者加丹皮、栀子、菊花、黄芩清肝泻火；头晕目眩者加天麻、钩藤平肝息风；恶心欲吐者，加半夏、竹茹和中止呕。

方解：方中柴胡疏肝解郁；当归、白芍补血养肝柔肝；白术、茯苓培土抑木，健脾祛湿，使运化有权；甘草益气和中，缓肝之急，生姜和中理气，薄荷增强疏散条达之功，加香附以调畅气机，川芎、牛膝行气活血，细辛止痛，诸药合用，共奏疏肝解郁、健脾和胃、理气止痛之效。

（2）肝火上炎

主症：头痛如裂，面红目赤，心烦易怒，口干口苦，失眠，尿黄便秘，舌红苔黄，脉弦数有力。

治法：清肝泄火。

方药：龙胆泻肝汤加减。龙胆草、黄芩、栀子、当归、生地、柴胡、车前子、泽泻、木通、生甘草。

加减：头晕目眩耳鸣者加菊花、天麻、磁石（先煎）平肝潜阳；烦热、口干口苦明显者，加丹皮、黄连清热泻火；恶心、呕吐黄水者，加竹茹、黄连、苏叶清心和胃；大便秘结者加生大黄通便泻热。

方解：方中龙胆草泻肝胆实火，清下焦湿热；黄芩、栀子清热泻火；泽泻、木通、车前子清热利湿；当归、生地养血柔肝；柴胡调达肝胆气机，引诸药入肝胆；生甘草泻火解毒，调和诸药。诸药合用，以达疏肝解郁、清肝泻火之功效。综观全方，泻中有补，利中有滋，以使火降热清，循经所发诸证可相应而愈。

（3）肝阳上亢

主症：头痛而眩，心烦易怒，睡眠不宁，面红目赤，口苦，舌红苔黄，脉弦数。

治法：平肝潜阳。

方药：天麻钩藤饮加减。天麻、钩藤、石决明、黄芩、栀子、牛膝、杜仲、寄生、夜交藤、茯神、细辛、赤芍、益母草。

加减：如日久不愈，头痛绵绵不已，腰痛腿酸、舌红脉细，证属肝病及肾。水亏火旺，可酌加生地、何首乌、女贞子、旱莲草、枸杞子、石斛等滋养肝肾之药。若头痛甚剧，面红目赤，口苦胁痛，便秘溲赤，苔黄脉弦数，此主要是肝火偏旺，宜清肝泻火，上方可加龙胆草、夏枯草。

方解：方中天麻甘平质润，性微寒，归肝经，功能息风止痉，平肝潜阳，祛风通络，止痛；钩藤、石决明均有平肝息风之效；山栀、黄芩清热泻火，使肝经之热不致偏亢；益母草活血利水；牛膝引血下行，配合杜仲、桑寄生补益肝肾；夜交藤、茯神安神定志。诸药合用使肝火清而风不作，脑络通而痛自止。

（4）痰浊上泛

主症：头痛昏蒙，胸脘满闷，呕恶痰涎，肢重体倦，纳呆，舌胖大有齿痕，苔白腻，脉沉弦或沉滑。

治法：化痰降逆。

方药：半夏白术天麻汤加减。半夏、白术、天麻、陈皮、茯苓、川芎、白芷、苍术、刺蒺藜、僵蚕、白芍、牛膝。

加减：头痛甚者，可加蔓荆子、川芎。伴气虚者，症见神疲乏力，面色萎黄不泽可加黄芪、人参之类以益气健脾。若伴见口苦，烦闷，胸闷腹胀，口渴不欲饮，尿赤，苔黄腻，脉濡数，此为痰湿郁久化热所致，可加黄芩、竹茹、枳实等以清热化痰。胸脘痞闷，纳呆呕恶者，加厚朴、藿香、佩兰以化湿宽胸降逆。兼气虚者，加党参、黄芪以益气健脾。呕吐甚者，加旋覆花（包煎）、代赭石以降逆止呕。痰郁化热，口苦苔黄腻者，去川芎、苍术，加黄芩、川连、天竺黄以清热化痰。

方解： 方中重用半夏、天麻，白芍、牛膝祛风化湿，活血行气止痛为其所长，西医学研究证明，半夏所含挥发油状生物碱物质对中枢神经系统有抑制作用，天麻有广泛的镇痛作用；白术、茯苓健脾、渗湿、化痰之功益佳；苍术燥湿健脾兼祛风，川芎、白芷行气散风，通络止痛，刺蒺藜下气行血，陈皮理气化痰，僵蚕祛风定惊、化痰散结；天麻、刺蒺藜平肝息风，为治头痛、眩晕之要药。诸药相伍，化痰降浊，理气止痛。

（5）瘀血头痛

主症： 头痛经久不愈，其痛如刺，固定不移，或头部有外伤史者，面色晦滞，唇色紫暗，舌紫或有瘀斑、瘀点，苔薄白，脉沉细或细涩。

治法： 活血化瘀。

方药： 通窍活血汤加减。川芎、白芷、细辛、白芍、甘草、柴胡、羌活、全蝎、藁本、白芥子、黄芩、牛膝、香附。

加减： 头痛甚者，加全蝎、蜈蚣、白芷、露蜂房镇痉止痛；兼寒象加桂枝、细辛温经散寒止痛；健忘失眠加菖蒲、远志、夜交藤安神定志；瘀久血虚者，加熟地、鸡血藤活血养血止痛；气虚加黄芪益气活血。

方解： 方用白芷、柴胡、羌活、藁本疏散风邪，为治疗头痛之要药；川芎、牛膝活血化瘀，利气止痛；细辛散寒止痛；白芍、甘草缓急止痛；全蝎、白芥子通络止痛。久痛气易滞，热易蕴，故加香附理气，黄芩清热。

（6）气血两虚

主症： 头痛痛势绵绵，时发时止，遇劳加剧，神疲体倦，口淡乏味，面色白，舌淡苔白，脉沉细而弱。

治法： 补益气血。

方药： 补中益气汤加减。当归、熟地黄、白芍、牛膝、川芎、党参、白术、黄芪、刺蒺藜、细辛、白芷、半夏、升麻、生甘草、阿胶（烊化）。

加减： 血虚重者，加何首乌养血；心悸失眠加炒枣仁、柏子仁养心安神；两目干涩加枸杞子、女贞子养肝明目；本证可因风寒入侵而诱发，畏风、常喜裹头，可加羌活、防风、藁本辛温散寒；痛剧则加制川乌、细辛温经通络以增强祛风止痛之效。

方解： 方中重用甘温补气兼有升提之功的黄芪，辅以党参、白术、炙甘草健脾益气，以收补中益气之效；升麻鼓动中焦阳气升发；川芎、白芷、刺蒺藜止头痛效果明显；熟地、白芍滋阴养血，阿胶、当归补血生血，避免温燥伤阴；半夏降气和胃，又防升散太过。诸药合用，共奏益气养血、升清降浊、祛风止痛之功效。

（二）专方治疗

1. 枕清眠安汤

方药： 生龙骨、生牡蛎各 30g，珍珠母 30g，炒酸枣仁 30g，沙参 20g，白芍药 25g，远志 15g，当归 15g，白术 15g，栀子 10g，菖蒲 10g，五味子 10g，柴胡 10g，细辛 5g，川芎 15g，牛膝 25g。

主治： 肝郁气滞血瘀头痛。

2. 芎参五白汤

方药： 川芎 20g，丹参 20g，白芍 15g，白芷 5g，白僵蚕 10g，白菊花 10g，白芥子 6g。

主治： 偏头痛，证属痰瘀阻络、上扰清窍。

3. 头痛自拟方

方药： 川芎 15g，柴胡 6g，细辛 3g，白芷 6g，僵蚕 9g，甘草 6g，天麻 15g，蜈蚣 2 条，白芍 25g，当归 15g。

主治： 头痛，证属气虚血瘀、风邪侵袭。

4. 偏头痛自拟方

方药： 川芎 30g，柴胡、羌活、全蝎、当归各 10g，白芥子、白芷、白芍、藁本、黄芩、香附各 15g，蜈蚣 2 条，细辛、甘草各 3g。

主治： 偏头痛。

5. 芎葛汤

方药： 川芎 9g，葛根 15g，白芍 10g，当归 10g，柴胡 10g，郁金 10g，白芥子 10g，藁本 8g，川牛膝 10g，甘草 6g。

主治： 气滞血瘀头痛。

6. 芎桂二夏汤

方药： 川芎 15~50g，桂枝 10g，夏枯草 15~50g，半夏 10~15g，细辛（后下）6~15g，元胡 15g，牛蒡子 10g，薄荷 5g。

主治： 风热侵袭脑络头痛。

7. 芎菊汤

方药： 菊花 60g，川芎、葛根、川牛膝、合欢皮、夜交藤、炒枣仁各 30g，防风、白芷、白芥子各 15g，蝉蜕 10g，甘草 6g。

主治： 风邪侵袭脑络头痛。

8. 芎麻止痛汤

方药： 川芎 10g，当归 10g，天麻 6g，白芍 15g，生地黄 10g，柴胡 10g，木香 6g，陈皮 10g，

菊花 10g，丹参 10g，甘草 6g。

主治： 瘀血化热头痛。

9. 芎牛琥珀汤

方药： 川芎 20~30g，牛膝 30~45g，琥珀（冲服）5~10g，蔓荆子 10~15g，僵蚕 5~10g，生石决明（先煎）20~50g。

主治： 痰阻血瘀头痛。

10. 芎七芍芷汤

方药： 川芎 15g，白芷 12g，三七 6g，白芍 30g，菊花 10g，蔓荆子 10g，生地黄 20g，僵蚕 6g，地龙 10g，甘草 6g。

主治： 痰阻血瘀头痛。

（三）单方验方

（1）桑叶、菊花、川芎、白英各 12g，川椒 6g，生石膏 30g，细辛 3g。水煎服，日 1 剂。治偏头痛。

（2）石决明 30g，杭菊、白蒺藜、川芎各 9g，钩藤 15g。水煎服，日 1 剂，连服 3~5 剂。治偏头痛。

（3）生川乌 21g，南星 15g。共研末，每次 3g，白开水冲服，日 1 次。治偏头痛。

（4）夏枯草 90g，香附 60g，甘草 120g。共研末，每次 4.5g，日 2 次，白开水冲服。治前额及眉棱骨疼痛。

（5）菊花 6~10g，决明子 10g。开水冲泡，代茶饮。治肝阳上亢头痛。

（6）山羊角（研末）1 个，天麻 10g，川芎 9g。水煎服。治头痛。

（7）玫瑰花 4~5 朵，蚕豆花 9~12g。将上 2 味用开水同泡，代茶频饮。治疗肝风头痛。

（8）香附子 3g，川芎 3g，茶叶 3g。上药共为粗末，沸水冲泡，代茶频饮。治疗肝气郁滞所致的慢性头痛。

（四）中成药

（1）七叶神安片：每次 50~100mg，每日 3 次或睡前服 100mg。适用于抑郁虚烦，心神不宁之肝气郁结头痛。

（2）小柴胡冲剂：每次 1 包，每日 2 次。适用于经期发作的肝郁气结型头痛。

（3）太极通天液：每次 1 支，每日 3 次，15 天为 1 个疗程，可连服 3 个疗程。适用于气血亏虚、瘀滞脉络，或兼夹风寒之头痛。

（4）正天丸：每次 1 包，每日 3 次，15 天为 1 个疗程。适用于气血亏虚夹瘀之头痛。

（5）全天麻胶囊：每次 2~3 粒，每日 3 次，15 天为 1 个疗程。适用于肝阳上亢、肝肾亏虚型之头痛。

（6）六味地黄丸：每次 6~8g，每日 3 次。适用于肝肾阴虚型之头痛。

（7）杞菊地黄丸：每次 6~8g，每日 3 次。适用于肝肾阴虚型之头痛。

（8）金匮肾气丸：每次 6~8g，每日 3 次。适用于肾阳不足型之头痛。

（9）正脑灵：每次 5 片，每日 3 次，15 天为 1 个疗程。适用于瘀血阻络之头痛。

（10）当归素片：每次 100mg，每日 3 次，1 个月为 1 个疗程。适用于瘀血阻络之头痛。

（11）清开灵注射液：60ml 加入 5% 葡萄糖注射液 500ml 静滴，每日 1 次，10 天为 1 个疗程。适用于肝阳上亢、肝火上炎，或兼夹风热证之头痛。

（12）当归素粉针剂：100mg 溶于 5% 葡萄糖注射液 500ml 静滴，每日 1 次，10~15 天为 1 个疗程。适用于气血亏虚、瘀血阻络之头痛。

（13）盐酸川芎嗪注射液：120~160mg 加入 5% 葡萄糖注射液 500ml 静滴，每日 1 次，10 天为 1 个疗程。适用于瘀血阻络型之头痛。

（14）葛根素注射液：400mg 加入 5% 葡萄糖注射液 500ml 静滴，每日 1 次，10~15 天为 1 个疗程。适用于风火上犯、风痰上扰、瘀血阻络型之头痛。

（五）针灸治疗

1. 针灸疗法的选择

毫针疗法对多数头痛具有良好的疗效，但要提高疗效，缩短疗程，往往需要根据病情选用适宜的针灸方法。如感受风寒者，毫针配合温针或艾灸可加强疏风散寒的效果；气虚清阳不升者，可配合艾灸百会、足三里以升举阳气；头痛久治不愈，如无热象，也可配合艾灸或温针以温通经络，提高疗效。

2. 常用基本穴

太冲、合谷、风池、百会、太阳、印堂、头维、曲池。

百会在头部，前发际正中直上 5 寸，两耳尖连线的中点处，有息风醒脑、升阳固脱的作用，为治疗头痛的要穴。风池位于胸锁乳突肌与斜方肌之间，平风府穴处。有疏风通络、镇静止痛、安神催眠之功。太冲位于足背侧，第一、二跖骨结合部之前凹陷处，可平肝息风、健脾化湿，为镇静镇痛要穴。合谷位于手背第一、二掌骨之间约平第二掌骨中点处，与太冲穴合称四关穴，为镇静镇痛安神的要穴。太阳在眉梢与外眼角之间，向后约一横指的凹陷处，可清热祛风，止头痛除烦躁。曲池在肘横纹外侧端，当尺泽与肱骨外上髁连线中点处，可疏风清热，通络止痛，镇静安神。印堂位于两眉头中间，有镇静安神、活络疏风的作用。头维位于额角发际上 0.5 寸，有息风镇静、止痛明目的作用。

3. 辨证选穴

（1）外感头痛

①风寒头痛：加风门、昆仑、外关；或加用灸法。

方义：风门、昆仑疏调太阳经气，散风寒，解表郁，外关疏经通络，诸穴共奏疏风散寒止痛之效。

②风热头痛：加列缺、后溪、大椎。

方义：列缺通肺气；后溪、大椎泄热解表。

③风湿头痛：加中脘、足三里、阴陵泉、丰隆、三阴交。

方义：中脘为胃经之募穴，又为腑会；丰隆为胃经之络穴，足三里为胃经合穴，与三阴交相配可健中焦以运化水湿，助阴陵泉祛风胜湿，使上扰清空之浊邪下行，则头痛自愈。

（2）内伤头痛

①肝郁头痛：加行间、膻中、肝俞。

方义：行间为肝经荥穴，肝俞为肝经俞穴，二者配合，疏肝解郁；膻中为气会，可调节一身气机。

②肝火上炎：加大椎、肩井、行间。

方义：大椎、肩井祛风清热，配合肝经荥穴行间，共奏清泻肝火之功。

③肝阳上亢：加中封、阳辅、三阴交、太溪、阳陵泉。

方义：中封、阳辅分别为肝、胆经之经穴，又为清利肝胆之对穴，配足少阴肾的太溪与足少阳胆经之阳陵泉，是治疗肝阳上亢头痛的特效穴。

④痰浊上泛：加阴陵泉、中脘、丰隆、上星。

方义：丰隆为胃之络穴，阴陵泉为脾经之合穴，中脘为胃经之募穴，三穴有健中州、化痰浊之功，上星透百会可醒神清脑，善治偏正头痛及昏蒙。

⑤瘀血头痛：加血海、地机、三阴交。

方义：血海、三阴交相配行气活血，佐地机通调经络止痛。

⑥气血两虚：加气海、关元、脾俞、三阴交、足三里。

方义：气海、关元皆为补气要穴，脾俞、足三里健脾益气，三阴交益气补血。

⑦肝肾阴虚：加肾俞、命门、关元、太溪、完骨、天柱。

方义：完骨、天柱益髓充脑，肾俞、命门、太溪补肾填精，关元为补气要穴，共疗肾阴亏虚之头痛。

（六）推拿治疗

1. 操作手法

按摩对头痛有较好的疗效，不仅对于慢性头痛，对外感头痛、血管神经性头痛、神经官能症性头痛亦常有迅速止痛的效果。治疗本病的手法分16步进行：

（1）揉太阳：以中指或食指揉太阳穴100次。太阳穴在眉梢与外眼角之间，向后约一横指的凹陷处，揉此穴可清热祛风，止头痛除烦躁。

（2）揉攒竹：以中指或食指揉攒竹穴100次。攒竹穴在眉头凹陷中，眶上切迹处，揉此穴可清热明目，活络散风。

（3）推坎宫：以两拇指自眉头向眉梢做分推36次。可醒脑明目，散风止痛。

（4）揉印堂：以中指或食指揉印堂（印堂位于两眉头中间）100次。有镇静安神，活络疏风的作用。

（5）开天门：两拇指罗纹面自眉心起，交替向上推至上星（位于头部前发际正中直上1寸）36次。可醒脑明目，宁心安神。

（6）提通天：两手掌按揉太阳穴数次，然后迅速提向通天（在头部，当前发际正中直上4寸，旁开1.5寸）3次。可活络通窍，清热散风。

（7）揉头维：以中指或食指揉头维（头维位于额角发际上0.5寸）100次。有息风镇静、止痛明目的作用。

（8）五指分梳：两手五指分开，从前发际梳向后发际66次。可行气活血，疏通经络，祛风定痛，安神养脑。

（9）点击头部：两手五指微曲成梅花形，以两手指端上下交替轻击头部100次。有安神养脑，疏通气血的作用。

（10）叩头部：两手相合，五指微曲，用小指侧叩击头部100次。有消除疲劳，疏通经络的作用。

（11）搓胆经：两手除拇指外的其余四指分别揉搓两耳上部胆经循行部位（即耳以上的侧头部）100次。可疏通经络，行气活血。

（12）揉风池：以指揉风池100次。风池位于颈后发际凹陷中（胸锁乳突肌与斜方肌上端之间的凹陷处），可明目开窍，镇静安神。

（13）拿颈项：沿膀胱经颈部循行部位，从上向下，拿揉6次。可镇静止痛，开窍提神。

（14）拿肩井：拿肩井3次。肩井位于肩部，大椎（第7颈椎棘突下）与肩峰端连线的中点上。可通调周身气血，振奋阳气。

（15）擦颈项：以小鱼际横擦颈项部，以透热为度。

（16）叩肩背：以虚掌叩击肩背部。

2. 辨证加减

侧头部痛者加揉率谷（耳尖直上入发际1.5寸）；前额部痛者加上星（头部前发际正中直上1寸）、阳白（瞳孔直上，眉上1寸）各揉100次。头痛重者，可屈指点按风池10次，常有立竿见影之效。胁痛口苦者加揉阴陵泉；睡眠不宁者加揉内关；腰酸，肾精亏损加揉太溪；腰痛疲软者加揉腰眼（在腰部，当第4腰椎棘突下，旁开约3.5寸凹陷中）；遗精带下者加揉关元；心悸怔忡者加揉神门、大陵；食欲不振者加揉中脘；胸闷者加揉膻中；恶心欲吐者加揉内关。

3. 自我推拿

（1）外感头痛：揉太阳100次，揉曲池（左右）各100次，揉合谷（左右）各100次，拿天柱（哑门穴旁开1.3寸）、风池50次，拿肩井（左右）各10次。

（2）肝阳头痛：揉百会、太阳各100次，分抹胆经，按揉肩髃、曲池、太冲各100次，擦涌泉，以透热为度。

4. 推拿禁忌证

头痛伴有喷射样呕吐者；头痛伴有颈项僵直者；头痛伴有高血压危象者；头痛伴有出血体质者；

头痛伴有昏蒙者。

（七）其他

1. 耳针法

选枕、额、脑、神门。可选用王不留行籽压丸或耳穴埋针法。顽固性头痛可在耳背静脉点刺放血治疗。

2. 刺络拔罐法

选大椎及背腧穴刺络放血加拔罐。用于治疗外感头痛．

3. 穴位注射法

用 1% 盐酸普鲁卡因或维生素 B_{12} 注射液，注射风池，每侧 0.5~1.0ml，每日或隔日 1 次。适用于顽固性头痛。

五、名医专家经验方

（一）天麻钩藤饮加减治疗伤神头痛与肝郁头痛（董国立）

1. 治疗肝郁头痛

组成：选用天麻、钩藤、生石决明、夜交藤四味，加全蝎、蜈蚣、僵蚕、蔓荆子、白芷、菊花、柴胡、川芎、半夏、防风、细辛、甘草等。

功效：肝郁头痛，症见头痛而眩，心烦易怒，睡眠不宁，恶心欲吐，口苦舌红，脉弦有力，血压偏高等。水煎服。

方解：天麻平肝息风，治头痛头眩；钩藤清热平肝息风，治血压偏高；生石决明平肝潜阳，治疗头痛；夜交藤养心安神，祛风活络以治神经衰弱失眠。这四味药均能归肝经，首先选用，但恐其药力仍不能上达于颠顶病位，故加全蝎、蜈蚣、僵蚕之均能归肝经者以息风止痉、散结通络止痛，菊花清上治头风，蔓荆子入肝清利头目，白芷散瘀止痛，柴胡疏肝解郁，细辛通窍止痛，川芎散瘀活血行气，使气通则不痛、气行则不瘀，颠顶之脉络流通，瘀阻消散，不仅头痛可以治愈，偏高血压亦徐徐而降。用上方曾治疗"肝郁头痛"数十例，均获得满意疗效。本方亦可加藁本祛风治偏正头痛；加白附子、南星、半夏等祛风散结化痰，止痉止痛；加防风、荆芥、羌活等祛风散瘀。总之不离开能上达颠顶辛开之药，临证选用不受限制。

2. 治疗伤神头痛

组成：在前方基础上减钩藤、生石决明、白附子、防风、荆芥、羌活等药，加何首乌、枣仁、远志。

功效： 伤神头痛，症见头痛头晕，遇劳更甚，恶心食欲不振，神疲乏力，精神不集中，记忆减退，失眠多梦，脉细弱等。水煎服。

方解： 何首乌平补肝肾，以治神衰，枣仁养心安神以治多梦，远志宁心安神祛痰开窍。用补益，而不以补益为主；用安神，而不以安神为重，而是以开郁通窍为急务，灵窍得通，机关得利，失眠健忘，头痛头眩症状可除。

（二）芎归散（李寿山）

适应证： 头痛。

组成： 全当归 10~30g，川芎 15~50g，细辛 3~9g，蜈蚣 1~3 条（研末冲服更佳）。

用法： 水煎服，痛甚者日服 3 次。

功效： 本方用于临床颇有效验。有注射盐酸哌替啶头痛不解者，服本方豁然而愈。此方收效之因有二：一则药少而精，针对性强。方中主药川芎，辛温味薄而气雄，功擅疏通，上行头目，下行血海，气行血活，故瘀血之垒可被攻破；当归养血活血，通经止痛，辅川芎增强止痛之效，并抑川芎辛窜太过之弊。细辛、蜈蚣虽为佐使之药，但方中不可无，乃本方行军破敌之先行，止痛收效之上品。二则量大而专，有的放矢。世人以为川芎辛温香窜不可过用，其实不然，顽证痼疾，犹如敌营堡垒，不用足量炸药，乃隔靴搔痒。李氏用川芎最小量起于 15g，以后递增，对头痛剧烈者，经常用至 50g 以上，实践中并无伤阴香窜之弊。当然与当归性柔而润，防止副作用有关。此君臣佐使配伍之妙也。另外"细辛不过钱"之说，亦不足信。李氏用细辛止痛，最少起于 3g，递增至 9g，并无不良反应。蜈蚣有毒，人皆畏之，但治瘀血头痛，确有祛风镇痉，搜风通窍，逐瘀止痛之效。每剂药用 3 条，并无毒性反应，故大胆用之，效如桴鼓。

（三）化裁六味辛芷良方（郑荪谋）

适应证： 肝阳上亢内伤偏头痛。

组成： 北细辛 2.5g，香白芷 3g，熟地黄 18g，粉丹皮 6g，山药 15g，茯苓 9g，山茱萸 9g，泽泻 9g，怀牛膝 9g，珍珠母（先煎）24g 或磁石（先煎）18g。

用法： 先煎珍珠母或磁石 15 分钟，再掷入诸药同煎，取水 750ml，煎至 500ml，分 2 次服，日服 1 剂。久痛者加川芎 3g；头晕者加向日葵 1 朵；经期便秘者加紫草。

功效： 适用于肝肾阴虚、肝阳上亢之头痛。阳虚及外感头痛者忌服。

方解： 本方源自古方。昔明代周慎斋曾用六味地黄汤加白芷、细辛治一女"噎鲠"。乃病在于上，取之于下意也，深受启迪。自思本证之头痛，系下虚上实之证，肝肾阴虚，精华之血不能朝会于高巅；阴虚生热，浮火上炎，扰乱清空，诸痛乃生。仿周慎斋治"噎鲠"方意，取六味地黄汤下滋肝肾之阴以图本，又因高巅之上，惟风药可达，故入细辛、白芷，取其味轻而升，祛痛力雄。引诸药上行于高巅之上。复加珍珠母重镇，配以怀牛膝下行，使肝肾之气归元，其奏滋水涵火之功。真阴充沛，髓海盈实，阴平阳秘，头痛自除。

（四）钩蝎散治疗偏头痛（朱良春）

组成： 全蝎、天麻、紫河车、地龙、川芎等份组成，共研极细末，胶囊装盛，利于服用。

用法： 每服 4g，发作时每日服 2~3 次，不发时每间日服 1 次，连服 2 周，可以得到巩固。阴虚明显而见口干、舌红、脉弦数者，另用川石斛、麦冬各 6g 泡茶送服药粉，可以养阴生津。

功效： 全蝎善于息风定痛，并有开瘀通络之效；天麻不仅息风定惊，尤善治头风、头痛，故张元素谓其"治风虚眩晕头痛"，兼有"通血脉"之功；地龙清热平肝、活血通络，《本草纲目》用其治头风；川芎活血止痛，王好古盛赞其能"搜肝气、补肝血、润肝燥，补风虚"；"久痛多虚"，故又佐以补气血、益肝肾之紫河车。如此融为一炉，相辅相成，其收效颇佳。

六、名医专家典型医案

（一）施今墨医案——血虚头痛

傅某 女，22 岁。

初诊： 病已年余，始于用脑过度，头痛而胀，尤以枕部为甚，气短，急躁易怒，大便数日一解，全身乏力，月经不调，量少色淡，面色白，舌苔薄白，脉象沉软。

辨证： 月经不调，量少色淡，是属血亏，真血虚耗，心失主辅，故有心跳气短，血不养肝，则急躁易怒，头痛而胀，大便数日一解，非属热结，乃属肠枯不润，气虚不达之象。

治法： 养血助心，疏肝活络。

处方： 紫贝齿（先煎）10g，紫石英（先煎）10g，醋柴胡 5g，火麻仁 15g，黄菊花 10g，柏子仁 10g，酒川芎 5g，生熟地各 6g，砂仁 5g，北细辛 1.5g，醋柴胡 5g，杭白芍 10g，蔓荆子 5g，鹿角胶（兑服）6g，炙黄芪 10g，油当归 10g，白蒺藜 15g，何首乌 10g，炒远志 10g，炙甘草 3g。

二诊： 服药 3 剂，头胀痛减轻，精神稍好，用脑多时即烦急易怒，心跳气短，大便已解但不畅，前方去黄芪，加白薇 6g。

三诊： 去年连诊 2 次，服药有效，但因出差，年余始返北京。现仍头痛发胀，性情急，厌烦嚣，喜独处，恶音声，大便不畅，食欲不振。

处方： 紫贝齿（先煎）10g，紫石英（先煎）10g，朱茯神 10g，朱寸冬 6g，火麻仁 10g，生龙骨 10g（先煎），生牡蛎（先煎）10g，厚朴花 5g，玫瑰花 5g，炙甘草 3g，旋覆花 5g，赭石 10g，月季花（后下）5g，代代花（后下）5g。

四诊： 前方服 5 剂，除食欲增加之外，效不甚显，余症如旧，又增睡眠不佳，每夜只能睡 4~5 小时。

处方： 磁珠丸 6g，秫米 12g，醋柴胡 5g，杭白芍 10g，油当归 10g，酒川芎 5g，生龙骨（先煎）10g，生牡蛎（先煎）10g，砂仁 5g，生熟地各 6g，北细辛 1.5g，旋覆花 6g，赭石 10g，全瓜蒌 18g，薤白头 10g，炙甘草 3g，青皮炭 5g，陈皮炭 5g，火麻仁 12g。

五诊：服药 6 剂，睡眠好转，心神安宁，不甚烦急，大便通畅，食欲增加，惟头痛未减。

处方：陈橘红、陈橘络各 5g，白蒺藜 12g，酒川芎 5g，黄菊花 10g，冬桑叶 6g，云茯苓、云茯神各 10g，香白芷 3g，炒远志 6g，生龙骨（先煎）10g，生牡蛎（先煎）10g。

六诊：前方服药 8 剂，头痛见好，又因出差 1 个多月，未能继续治疗，头痛又复如前，大便也不通畅，四肢酸麻。

处方：紫贝齿、紫石英各 10g，生龙骨（先煎）12g，生牡蛎（先煎）12g，冬桑叶 6g，炒远志 3g，酒军炭 6g，酒川芎 5g，朱茯神、寸冬各 10g，油当归 10g，桑寄生 18g，火麻仁 15g，沙蒺藜、白蒺藜各 10g。

七诊：连服 10 剂，症状都已减轻，除过劳时头痛心跳之外，一切接近正常。

处方：六诊处方之剂量加 2 倍，冉加柏子仁、酸枣仁各 30g，共为细末，炼蜜为丸，每丸重 10g。早、晚各服 1 丸，白开水送服。

按语：本案属血虚头痛，恙由用脑过度，暗耗阴血，血不上荣，脑失所养而致，遂有头痛、健忘。累及心肝，故有心跳、烦躁之表现。养血助心，疏肝活络，理应效果显著。就诊 2 次服药不满 10 剂，即停药出差 1 年之久，由于治疗不能持续，又复旅途劳累，病势只有加重，岂有自愈之理？回京就诊，又服 19 剂再度出差，如此波折仍能取得良好效果，皆因辨证明确，守方有法。贫血而大便干燥者，多属肠失滋润蠕动无力，并非热象实证，血充气达，便即润畅，无须通泻之剂。

（二）张琪医案——瘀血头痛

李某 男，43 岁。

初诊：1998 年 11 月 1 日。患者头痛病史 10 年，多家医院治疗效果不显，诊断为血管神经性头痛，近 1 年加剧，偏于右侧，睡眠不实，形体肥胖，多梦纷扰，耳鸣健忘，心烦，舌紫暗，苔腻，脉沉。

辨证：证属久病入络，脉络瘀阻，血瘀气滞痰凝。

治法：活血化瘀，行气涤痰。

处方：血府逐瘀汤合散偏汤化裁。

当归 20g，赤芍 20g，生地黄 20g，桃仁 20g，川芎 25g，夏枯草 25g，红花 15g，柴胡 15g，枳壳 15g，白芥子 15g，香附 15g，白芷 15g。

二诊：1998 年 11 月 15 日。服上方 7 剂，头痛明显减轻，仅觉头微痛不适，效不更方。

三诊：1998 年 11 月 22 日。服上方 6 剂，症再减，但不断有交叉痛出现，舌紫，脉沉，仍睡眠不佳，心烦，前方加祛风安神养心之品。

处方：生地黄 30g，当归 20g，桃仁 20g，赤芍 20g，柴胡 20g，川芎 20g，菊花 20g，酸枣仁 20g，红花 15g，白芥子 15g，远志 15g，夏枯草 25g，郁李仁 15g。

四诊：1998 年 12 月 16 日。服上方 16 剂，头痛未作，睡眠好，现有轻度腹泻，上方去郁李仁，加白术 15g，服 7 剂。1 年后随访未复发。

按语：本例属瘀血头痛。头痛日久，舌紫暗或有瘀斑，脉沉或沉涩多属血瘀，患者体胖苔腻，故证属血瘀夹痰湿，以血府逐瘀汤与散偏汤化裁取效。方中川芎上行头目，功擅辛散通络，为头痛要药；白芥子燥湿化痰，为治痰之要药，散偏汤中二药相伍为痰瘀合治之剂。散偏汤出自《辨证录》

卷二方，方书云："偏头痛一证，多因肝风上攻，病久邪入于脑络，经络瘀阻，则不免气滞痰凝，偶因寒暑，郁怒所触，则举发正常。"此方妙在重用川芎、佐白芷使其辛窜走头，香附行气，白芥子涤痰，柴胡入少阳之经，使其直达病所，发挥其疏导经络作用。夏枯草清肝散络，痰瘀化热者用之可平肝清热；菊花清利头目，与活血化瘀药合用相得益彰，故收效甚捷。现代药理研究证实，川芎内含生物碱、川芎嗪，具有明显的扩张脑血管、缓解脑血管痉挛、增加脑血流量作用，从而使脑内血液循环正常。

（三）陆小左医案——肝阳上亢

陈某 女，51岁，银行职员。

初诊：2011年3月31日。头痛头晕1年，加重半年。患者述一年前因工作问题生气劳累，开始出现血压升高，头胀痛，头晕，时血压为155/85mmHg，之前无高血压病史，平素血压为110/70mmHg左右。后经西医治疗服降压药后缓解。半年前因情绪不畅，又见血压升高，收缩压达155mmHg，头胀痛，头晕，右侧头痛明显，面红目赤，颜面发热，服中西药均未见缓解，西医诊断脑缺血，纳可，寐可，便秘20余年，小便可，无口渴喜饮。腿部胀痛不适，脚底疼痛。舌红尖有点刺，苔薄黄，脉沉弦。

辨证：肝郁化热，肝阳上亢，肝风上扰清窍。

治法：补气养血，疏肝平肝，息风止痛，行气通便。

处方

（1）内服药：白芍25g，天冬20g，玄参15g，龟甲（先煎）15g，代赭石30g，生龙骨30g，生牡蛎30g，生麦芽20g，牛膝30g，生甘草10g，柴胡10g，白芷10g，天麻15g，钩藤30g，大黄10g，丹参15g，砂仁10g，黄芪30g。7剂，水煎服，每日1剂，分早晚2次使用。

（2）平肝安神外用方2剂泡脚，以平肝潜阳息风。

（3）针灸1个疗程，扶正安神通任。

（4）耳针调平，调和营卫，通络安神止痛。

二诊：2011年4月7日。头胀痛、头晕明显减轻，大便可，纳可，偶见食后腹胀，近日失眠，多梦，睡眠清浅，日间嗜睡乏力，舌红苔薄黄，脉沉弦。

处方：初诊内服方加白术15g，磁石30g，首乌藤30g，健脾和中，镇静安神。7剂，水煎服，每日1剂，分早晚2次使用。针灸1个疗程。其余维持原诊疗方案。

三诊：2011年4月14日。头痛明显改善，现偶有右侧头部胀痛，头晕，甚或低头时加重，伴恶心呕吐，气短乏力，双腿沉重乏力，左脚底仍疼痛，食后见胁肋胃脘胀痛，纳可，二便可，仍睡眠不佳，多梦，舌红苔薄黄，尖有点刺，脉沉弦。血压100/70mmHg。

处方：二诊方去大黄、檀香，加葛根20g，增黄芪至60g，补气扶正，除烦安神。7剂，水煎服，每日1剂，分早晚2次使用。其余维持原诊疗方案。

四诊：2011年4月21日。诸症改善良好，偶有气短，喜静，仍多梦，纳可，胁肋胀痛，嗳气，脚底疼痛稍有缓解，大便燥结，小便黄，舌暗红尖红甚，苔薄黄，血压100/80mmHg。

处方：三诊方加大黄10g，檀香10g，元胡15g，郁金15g，香附15g，疏肝行气通便。7剂，水煎服，每日 1 剂，分早晚 2 次使用。其余维持原诊疗方案。

五诊：2011 年 4 月 28 日。感觉良好，头痛头晕未再发作，气机顺畅，情绪佳。为巩固疗效，针灸治疗 1 个疗程，以观其变，嘱多食新鲜水果蔬菜，禁油腻辛辣之品，情绪不可过激。

两月后随访，患者已愈。

按语：患者忧郁恼怒，情志不遂，肝失条达，气郁阳亢，阳亢风动，脑窍受扰，此为经络不畅，不通致痛，年龄较大，气血不足，脑窍失于濡养，此为不荣。故发头痛、头晕，血压升高，面红目赤，颜面发热。气机郁滞，不能宣达，通降失常，传导失职，糟粕内停，大便秘结，气滞血脉，气血不得濡养下肢，故见腿部胀痛，脚底疼痛，内服中药治疗使用柴胡、白芍调畅肝经，龟甲、生龙牡、代赭石、天麻、钩藤平肝潜阳，镇静安神，天冬、黄芪、牛膝补养肝肾，大黄、砂仁行气泻腹通便。平肝安神外用方水煎外洗平肝潜阳，结合针刺、耳针治疗，扶助正气，调畅经络，改善症状，多向调节，增强疗效。

七、预防与调护

（1）注意气候的影响，在天气变化的时候注意避风寒、保暖，不要暴晒淋雨，防止诱发致病。

（2）注意睡眠规律，劳逸结合，注意眼睛的调节，保持安静的环境。

（3）积极戒烟，注意室内通风，避免接触过敏原等。

（4）避免服用一些可诱发头痛的药物如避孕药、硝酸甘油、组织胺、利血平、肼苯达嗪、雌激素等。

（5）外感头痛应膳食清淡、慎用补虚之品。宜食有助于疏风散邪的食物，如葱、姜、豆豉、藿香、芹菜、菊花等。风热头痛者宜多食绿豆、白菜、萝卜、芹菜、藕、百合、生梨等具有清热作用的食物。内伤头痛虚证者以补虚为主，宜食大枣黑豆、荔枝、龙眼肉、鸡肉、牛肉、龟肉、鳖肉等滋补肝肾，补益气血的食物。内伤头痛的实证，治以攻邪，属痰湿、瘀血者，宜食有健脾除湿或活血化瘀作用的食物，如山药、薏苡仁、橘子、山楂、红糖等。

（6）头痛的患者，应禁食火腿、干奶酪等保存过久的食物，少吃牛奶、巧克力、乳酪、酒类、咖啡、茶叶等食物。

（陆小左）

参考文献

［1］史宇广，单书健．当代名医临证精华：头痛眩晕专辑［M］．北京：中医古籍出版社，1992．

［2］单书健，陈子华．古今名医临证金鉴：头痛眩晕卷［M］．北京：中国中医药出版社，1999．

［3］宋祖黉．当代名医证治汇粹［M］．石家庄：河北科学技术出版社，1990．

［4］吕景山．施今墨医案解读［M］．北京：人民军医出版社，2009．

［5］张佩青．国医大师临床经验实录：国医大师张琪［M］．北京：中国医药科技出版社，2011．

［6］胡广芹，刘洪宇．形神兼治针药并施：陆小左学术经验集萃［M］．北京：中国中医药出版社，2012．

［7］吴复苍，阚湘苓．常见病遣方用药规律［M］．北京：人民军医出版社，2015．

［8］方药中，邓铁涛，李克光，等．实用中医内科学［M］．上海：上海科技出版社，1985．

类风湿关节炎

Rheumatoid
Arthritis

一、概述

　　类风湿关节炎简称"类风湿病"，是一种以关节滑膜炎症病变为主的慢性全身性自身免疫性疾病。关节病变呈对称性、多发性，易反复发作，好发于手足小关节。在早期或急性活动期发病关节多呈红肿热痛和活动障碍，晚期则出现关节虫蚀样破坏、强直或畸形，可简单概括为"一疼、二肿、三虫、四直"，并有骨与骨骼肌萎缩。在整个病程中，可伴有发热、贫血、体重减轻、血管炎和皮下结节等病变，同时亦可累及心、肺、肾、神经及眼等脏器。本病为常见病、多发病，我国 RA 发病率为 0.32%~0.36%，目前临床尚无特效的治疗方法。本病好发年龄在 25~55 岁，其中女性发病率比男性高 3~5 倍。类风湿病最佳治疗时间是在患病后 3~6 个月内，关节不可逆损伤一般都会发生在患病后 2 年内。大多数情况下，本病不致影响人的生命，但少数患者，可造成严重残疾，使患者的劳动能力部分或完全丧失。有学者研究指出，本病能使患者寿命缩短 5~10 年。

类风湿关节炎归属中医"痹证"范畴，临床上一般按"骨痹""顽痹"进行辨证论治。中医学对"痹证"的治疗积累了丰富的经验，早在《内经》就对痹证的病因病机、证候分类和转归预后作了系统的论述，明确指出"风、寒、湿三气杂至，合而为痹也。"汉代张仲景《金匮要略·中风历节病脉证并治》首载"历节病"之名，其病以"历节痛，不可曲伸""其痛如掣""诸肢节疼痛，身体魁羸，脚肿如脱"为主要临床特征，与晚期类风湿关节炎症状极为相似，所记载的乌头汤、桂枝芍药知母汤等，至今仍为临床常用的有效方剂。《金匮要略》中记载"病者一身尽痛，日晡所剧者，名风湿"，第一次提出了"风湿"病名。此后历代医家见仁见智，对痹证的成因有了进一步的认识，如清代李用粹《证治汇补》论痹之成因："由元精内虚而三气所袭，不能随时祛散，流注经络，久而成痹"；并进一步指出"湿热痰火郁气死血流经络四肢，悉能为麻为痹"。同时代的汪文绮的《杂症会心录》在探讨痹证的病因病机时也云："肝肾为病，筋失于荣养，虚火乘于经络"，"医家概以外邪为治，病势渐增，阴液暗耗，虚虚之祸，有不可胜言矣。"均对后世研究痹证开拓了思路。近几十年，类风湿病的防治引起了医学界的广泛关注。在我国，中西医结合防治本病无论在辨证论治、专病专方方面，还是在单味药的研究和应用上，都取得了显著的成绩。

二、病因病机

（一）中医（见图1）

1.病因

类风湿关节炎在临床表现、治疗难度以及预后上均不同于一般痹证，故中医临床上称其为"顽痹"或"骨痹"。在病因病机上，感受外邪侵袭同时，多强调与机体正气不足有关。正气不足是指卫气不固、荣血不足、气血虚弱、肝肾亏损等，外邪侵袭为风寒湿热之邪气。在病变发展过程中可以出现停痰留瘀，痰瘀可以互结，也可与外邪相合，阻闭经络，深入骨骺，而致痼疾。

2.病机

基本病机是体虚感邪，客于经络，痹阻气血，痰瘀胶结，盘踞骨骺等。

本病多有先天禀赋不足而致营卫、气血不足，脏腑经络组织功能低下。或因劳倦过度，伤及营卫气血，导致阳气不足，腠理空虚，卫外不固，邪毒留注经络、关节、肌肉；或因房事过度、耗伤肾气，而致肝肾虚损，筋骨脆弱，复受风寒湿热之邪侵袭，与气血相搏痹阻关节，气血津液运行不畅，可导致停痰留瘀、痰瘀胶结，如油裹面，留注关节发为顽痹。

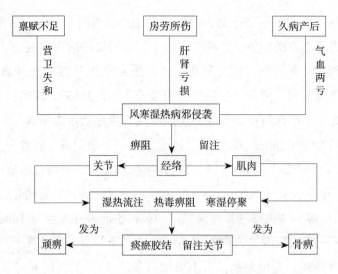

图1 类风湿关节炎发病中医病机

（二）西医

1. 病因

本病的病因尚未明确，但近年来的研究表明其发生与自身免疫、遗传、感染、内分泌紊乱等因素有关。

（1）免疫因素：许多研究均支持免疫发病，如骨骼组织中有大量淋巴细胞和浆细胞浸润，滑液中有变性的 IgG 和类风湿因子组成的免疫复合物等。类风湿关节炎患者血清 RF 呈阳性率越高，则病情相对更加严重。

（2）遗传因素：家谱调查结果表明，本病直系亲属有较高的易感性。已知人类白细胞抗原（HLA）是一个重要的遗传基因系统，患者中 HLA-DW4 近 70% 阳性。

（3）感染因素：认为链球菌、类白喉杆菌、支原体、EB 病毒等，为类风湿病原体。有学者曾在动物身上用感染的方法制造出类风湿关节炎模型，但在临床上尚未得到证实。

（4）内分泌失调：多见于女性，口服避孕药的女性中发病率较低，妊娠期病情常缓解，肥胖症患者类风湿关节炎发病率较高，更年期出现发病高峰，均提示该病与内分泌因素有关。

（5）其他因素：寒冷、潮湿、疲劳、营养不良、创伤、精神因素等常为本病发病的诱因。

2. 病变机制

类风湿关节炎的病理改变首先发生在关节滑膜，然后累及软骨和关节周围组织等，多数患者有血管炎的病变，并可累及全身结缔组织。病变初期表现为急性或亚急性关节滑膜炎症，日久不愈可出现滑膜增生肥厚，肉芽组织形成，继续发展形成为血管翳。由于血管翳含水解酶，可促使关节软骨破坏，软骨下骨韧带肌腱中的胶原基质受侵蚀，造成关节软骨、骨和关节囊的破坏，关节面互相融合，形成纤维性或骨性关节。关节附近的肌肉和皮肤逐渐萎缩，骨骼有脱钙和骨质疏松等表现。

三、诊断要点与鉴别诊断

（一）诊断依据

1. 临床表现

类风湿病的发病形式大致可见到三种，即隐渐发病、急性发病以及介于两者之间的中间型发病，以隐渐发病为多，可占60%~70%。临床表现大体分为全身症状、关节症状以及关节外表现。

（1）全身症状：患者常表现为疲乏无力，食欲不振，体重减轻，肌肉萎缩，四肢麻木，手指发凉，贫血等，部分患者可出现发热等症状。

（2）关节症状：以多关节对称性肿痛，伴有晨间关节僵硬为特征，局部表现为肿胀、疼痛、活动受限等。

①晨僵：关节晨僵是指患者在清晨睡醒后出现关节僵硬、活动不灵活的现象，严重时可有全身僵硬感，起床后经活动或温暖后可减轻或消失。这是本病的特征性症状，是重要诊断依据之一。晨僵持续时间和程度可作为评价病情活动和观察病情变化的重要指标。

②疼痛：是本病最突出症状，也是所有患者活动期所必有的临床表现。疼痛的程度与个体耐受性有关，并受情绪、气候、环境等因素的影响。其特点是活动时加重，活动后减轻。临床上的疼痛可分为触痛、活动痛（受累关节活动时才觉得痛）、自发痛（关节处于安静状态下也有疼痛，甚至从睡眠中痛醒）。明显的触痛与自发痛，提示该患者处在急性炎症期，或病变发展较快且较严重。

③肿胀：作为炎症指标之一，也是本病比较突出的症状。关节肿胀多为关节周围均匀肿胀，多呈对称性，局部一般不红，呈常色。炎症活动时也可见局部出现发红或触之有发热感，皮肤呈微紫色。

④活动障碍：是常见的体征之一。在早期，由于炎症疼痛和组织肿胀可引起活动障碍，若肿痛缓解，关节可以恢复正常。病变到了晚期，由于肌肉萎缩、粘连，骨关节内纤维组织增生，出现骨性融合或畸形，则关节功能不能复常。

⑤关节畸形或强直：是疾病晚期关节改变最坏的结果。由于关节的稳固性及关节周围的肌肉萎缩，韧带及关节被破坏，使关节出现某种特有的畸形，如有特征性的鹅颈畸形、扣眼畸形等。

（3）关节外表现：由于本病属全身性疾病，故其病变不仅局限于关节，病程中还可累及其他组织与器官。常见的并发症有：类风湿结节、类风湿性血管炎、心脏损坏、肺损坏、眼损害等。

①类风湿结节：大约20%~25%的患者在关节隆突部及常易受压磨损部位出现皮下结节。结节小如绿豆，大如蚕豆，数目1至数个不等。结节的出现，提示病变呈持续活动。

②类风湿性血管炎：由于免疫复合物在血管壁沉积，引起血管的炎症和沉积，临床上称之为类风湿性血管炎，也称恶性类风湿关节炎。临床分为两型：一是周围血管炎，表现为指（趾）的坏死、甲床瘀斑；二是累及内脏多器官的全身性血管炎，表现为发热、白细胞增多、肢体坏死、各种内脏损坏等，预后多不良。

③心脏损坏：心脏损坏可发生于心包膜、心肌以及瓣膜，引起心包炎、心肌炎或瓣膜闭锁不全。但多数患者的心脏损坏较轻，临床上一般无症状，尸检及超声波检查阳性率较高，明显的症状主要见于类风湿关节炎高度活动时。

④肺损坏：肺损坏的表现为慢性间质性肺炎、类风湿性胸膜炎。主要原因为长期不明原因的发热、咳嗽、咳痰、呼吸困难、胸痛、肺部啰音等，抗生素治疗无效而使用激素疗效显著。

⑤眼损害：表现为巩膜外层炎、巩膜炎、虹膜炎、虹膜睫状体炎、结膜炎和色素层炎等。一般疗法与抗生素无效，肾上腺皮质激素治疗效果显著而迅速。

2. 诊断标准

日前类风湿关节炎仍采用的是 1987 年修订的美国风湿病协会（ARA）类风湿关节炎的诊断标准，具备以下 7 条中 4 条或 4 条以上可诊断为类风湿关节炎：① 晨僵至少 1 小时（≥6 周）；② 3 个以上关节肿胀（≥6 周）；③ 手关节或掌指关节近端指间关节肿胀（≥6 周）；④ 对称性关节肿胀；⑤ 手指关节 X 线改变；⑥ 皮下类风湿结节；⑦ 类风湿因子阳性。2009 年美国风湿病学会（ACR）和欧洲抗风湿病联盟（EULAR）制定了新的类风湿关节炎分类标准，更加注重类风湿关节炎的早期诊断，但总体来说临床较少使用。该标准对关节受累情况、血清抗体检查结果、滑膜炎持续时间和急性时相反应物 4 个部分进行评分，总得分 6 分以上即可诊断类风湿关节炎。废除了原标准中晨僵、皮下结节、对称性关节炎及 X 线平片等项。

附：2009 年美国风湿病学会 / 欧洲抗风湿病联盟类风湿关节炎分类标准

A：受累关节

1 个大关节（0 分）；2~10 个大关节（1 分）；1~3 个小关节（有或没有大关节）（2 分）；4~10 个小关节（有或没有大关节）（3 分）；超过 10 个关节（至少 1 个小关节）（5 分）。

B：血清学（至少需要 1 项结果）

类风湿因子和抗瓜氨酸化蛋白抗体阴性（0 分）；类风湿因子和抗瓜氨酸化蛋白抗体，至少有一项低滴度阳性（2 分）；类风湿因子和抗瓜氨酸化蛋白抗体，至少有一项高滴度阳性（3 分）。

C：急性期反应物（至少需要 1 项结果）

C 反应蛋白和红细胞沉降率均正常（0 分）；C 反应蛋白或红细胞沉降率异常（1 分）。

D：症状持续时间

＜6 周（0 分）；≥6 周（1 分）。

评分在 6 分或以上者可以诊断为类风湿关节炎。

（二）鉴别诊断

类风湿关节炎表现形式多样，尤其是病变早期缺乏特异症状和体征，与许多其他风湿性疾病相类似。因此，早期诊断比较困难，需要与多种关节疾病相鉴别，如风湿性关节炎、痛风等。具体鉴别见表 1。

表1　类风湿关节炎鉴别表

疾病名称	鉴别诊断	
	鉴别依据	临床表现及实验室检查
类风湿关节炎	（1）隐匿性或急性发病 （2）四肢关节或脊柱关节出现肿胀疼痛 （3）不同程度的关节活动障碍	（1）发病以青年女性为主 （2）对称性的小关节肿胀疼痛 （3）类风湿因子检查阳性 （4）X线典型的类风湿改变
强直性脊柱炎		（1）男性青年好发 （2）主要侵犯骶髂关节和脊柱 （3）HLA-B27阳性 （4）脊柱可呈竹节样改变
增生性关节炎		（1）好发于40岁以上患者 （2）以负重关节受累为主 （3）发病关节常不对称 （4）X线可见关节边缘有唇样增生
痛风		（1）好发于40岁以上 （2）95%以上为男性患者 （3）第一跖趾关节红肿热痛为主 （4）高尿酸血症
风湿热		（1）好发于青少年 （2）常急性发病 （3）四肢大关节肿痛为主 （4）血清抗链球菌溶血素"O"阳性 （5）X线检查无阳性改变

四、中医治疗

类风湿关节炎的治疗至今尚无特效疗法，但若采用中西医结合的综合治疗，多数患者能够取得一定效果。治疗目的在于尽快控制关节及其他组织炎症、减轻疼痛、缓解症状，同时尽可能维持关节功能和预防关节畸形。

（一）治疗原则

1. 祛邪活络，缓急止痛

痹之为病或轻，或重，甚有恶候，因此，治疗上应善抓主症，分清层次。以祛邪活络、缓急止痛为其大法。对于风胜者以散风为主，当中病即止，不可多用，以防风燥之剂伤阴、燥血、耗气；寒胜者在散寒的同时，须结合助阳之品，使其阳气充足，鼓舞正气，则血活寒散，滞通痹畅而病愈；

湿胜者，在渗湿化浊的同时，需佐以健脾益气之品，使其脾旺能胜湿，气足无顽麻；热胜者，以清泄郁热为主，佐以活血通络，但须防苦寒伤阳、滞湿之过；病久入络者，倡用活血化瘀及虫类药物，搜剔宣通络脉，但防耗伤正气，须配以扶正药物。

2. 培补肝肾，化痰祛瘀

痹证日久不愈，易致气血耗伤，胶着经络，伤及脏腑，故在祛邪通络的同时，常需配合益气活血、滋补肝肾、扶正祛邪之品，方可取得较好的疗效。痹久"湿凝为痰、血停为瘀"，痰瘀胶结。痹阻经络，故祛瘀消痰之法应予以充分重视，并适当采用虫类药，痰瘀深入骨骱，非虫类之品搜风通络不能除也。

（二）辨证分型

1. 寒湿痹阻

主症：肢体关节疼痛，以小关节为主，晨僵，关节屈伸不利，昼轻夜重，遇寒则剧，得热痛减，伴畏寒肢冷，面白唇淡，舌质淡苔白腻，或边有齿痕，脉沉细或濡缓。

治法：温经散寒，祛湿通络。

方药：乌头汤加减。乌头、制附子、肉桂、细辛、芍药、木瓜、黄芪、五加皮、路路通、生甘草。

方解：麻黄发汗宣痹，乌头祛寒止痛；芍药、甘草缓急舒筋；黄芪益气固卫，助麻黄、乌头温经止痛，又可防麻黄过于发散；白蜜甘缓，解乌头之毒。诸药配伍，能使寒湿之邪微汗而解，则病邪去疼痛止。

加减：肿胀者加生薏苡仁 15~30g、云苓 10~15g；肌肉萎缩者加熟地 10~15g、党参 10~15g。

2. 湿热痹阻

主症：关节或肌肉局部红肿、疼痛、有沉重感，触之灼热或有灼热感，口渴不欲饮，伴有胸脘痞闷，面色萎黄，大便不畅，小便黄少，舌红苔白腻或黄腻、脉濡数或滑数。

治法：清热除湿，宣痹通络。

方药：二妙散合防己黄芪汤加味。黄芪、黄柏、苍术、白术、威灵仙、川萆薢、生薏苡仁、茯苓、桑枝、地龙、秦艽、防己。

方解：黄芪补气祛湿利水，散邪固表，为君药。臣以苍术苦温燥湿健脾，防己、萆薢苦泄辛散，祛风除湿，利水消肿。白术、茯苓补脾燥湿，既助黄芪补气固表，又助防己祛湿利水，为佐药。地龙、威灵仙祛风除湿，通络除痹止痛；桑枝通利关节。

加减：热重于湿者加虎杖 30g、土茯苓 30g；兼有胸脘胀闷、恶心呕吐加藿香梗 15g、半夏 15g、黄芩 10g。

3. 热毒痹阻

主症：关节肌肉疼痛较剧，手不可近，关节局部发红，活动受限，或兼有发热，口渴心烦，口苦咽干，大便干燥，小便赤黄，舌质红或绛，苔黄少津，脉洪大或滑数。

治法：清热解毒，活血化瘀。

方药：犀角地黄汤加减。犀角（或水牛角）、生地、赤芍、白芍、丹皮、土茯苓、地龙、银花、银藤、白花蛇舌草、生甘草、大黄。

方解：犀角清热凉血为君药，生地以助犀角清热凉血为臣药；赤白芍与辛苦微寒之丹皮共为佐药，清热凉血，活血散瘀；配伍特点是养血活血与凉血并用，使热清血宁而无耗血动血之虑，凉血止血又无冰伏留瘀之弊。

加减：肺胃热盛而毒血症状不明显者，可减犀角，加生石膏 30g、栀子 15g；口渴咽干较甚者加玉竹 15g、沙参 15g；便结不下、津枯液亏者加全瓜蒌 15g、柏子仁 15g。

4. 痰瘀痹阻

主症：关节肌肉疼痛呈不对称性，疼痛多呈刺痛，甚至关节变形，屈伸受限，肿胀关节呈棱形，按之稍硬，局部皮肤呈紫暗色，舌质紫暗或瘀斑，舌苔白腻，脉象沉涩。

治法：活血化瘀，化痰通络。

方药：阳和汤合桃仁四物汤加减。熟地、鹿角片、炮姜、肉桂、麻黄、白芥子、桃仁、红花、当归、赤芍、白芍、生甘草、独活。

方解：方中重用熟地大补营血为君药；鹿角片生精补髓，养血温阳为臣药；炮姜破阴和阳，肉桂温经通脉，白芥子消痰散结，麻黄调血脉，通腠理，桃仁、红花、赤芍、白芍、当归养血活血，均以为佐药；生甘草清热解毒调和诸药为使药。诸药合用，血瘀得行，痰湿得化，脉络得通。

加减：肿胀较剧者加皂刺 15g、䗪虫 10g；上肢痛甚者加片姜黄 15g、桂枝 10g；下肢痛甚者加牛膝 15g、宣木瓜 15g。

5. 气血不足

主症：关节疼痛日久不愈，疼痛呈酸痛，时轻时重，关节拘挛不利，或肌肉时有痉挛，兼有面黄少华，短气乏力，自汗心悸，肌肉萎缩，食少便溏，舌质淡，脉象濡弱或细微。

治法：益气养血，通络止痛。

方药：防己黄芪汤合四物汤加减。生黄芪、熟地、炒白术、防己、当归、鸡血藤、川芎、赤芍、白芍、威灵仙、豨莶草、细辛、生甘草。

方解：黄芪补气祛湿利水，散邪固表，熟地大补营血，二者共为君药。白术助黄芪健脾益气之功，当归、鸡血藤、赤芍、白芍养血活血，助熟地之效，均为臣药。佐以防己、威灵仙祛风除湿通络；豨莶草助防己祛湿之力，通利关节；甘草为使药，调和诸药。

加减：便溏者加肉豆蔻 10g、生薏苡仁 30g；气虚明显者加党参 15g。

6. 肝肾两虚

主症：关节肿胀，疼痛，昼轻夜重，病变关节僵硬，活动受限，腰膝酸软无力，足跟疼痛，兼见有面色㿠白，头昏耳鸣，畏寒肢冷，自汗，小便清长，夜尿多，脉沉细弱，舌质淡、苔薄白。

治法：滋补肝肾，祛寒除湿。

123

方药：独活寄生汤加减。人参、茯苓、独活、秦艽、防己、防风、细辛、当归、熟地、白芍、桑寄生、牛膝、杜仲、枸杞、黄芪、炒白术、甘草。

方解：牛膝、杜仲、熟地黄补益肝肾、强壮筋骨，独活、桑寄生祛风除湿，养血和营，活络通痹共为君药；当归、芍药养血活血，人参、茯苓、甘草益气扶脾，使气血旺盛，助于祛风湿，均为臣药；佐以细辛以搜风散寒止痛，以秦艽、防风祛周身风寒湿邪。诸药合用，标本兼顾，扶正祛邪。

加减：寒象甚者，加干姜 10g、鹿角片 15g；脾虚湿胜者，加生薏苡仁 30g、木瓜 15g。

（二）专方治疗

1. 化瘀通痹汤（《痹症治验》）

方药：当归 18g，丹参 30g，鸡血藤 21g，制乳香、没药各 9g，元胡 12g，香附 12g，透骨草 30g。水煎服。偏寒者，加桂枝、川乌、制草乌、细辛；偏热者，加败酱草、丹皮；气虚者加黄芪；久痹，骨节肿大变形者，加穿山甲、乌梢蛇、地龙、蜈蚣、全蝎、制马钱子。

主治：治瘀血型痹证，局部有外伤史，疼痛如针刺、刀割感，固定不移，压痛明显，局部皮色紫暗，或顽痹不愈，或关节肿大变形，肌肤甲错，或舌质紫暗，有瘀斑，脉弦涩。

2. 宣痹汤（《温病条辨》）

方药：防己 15g，杏仁 15g，滑石 15g，连翘 9g，山栀 9g，薏苡仁 15g，半夏（醋炒）9g，晚蚕沙 9g。水 8 杯，煮取 3 杯，分温 3 服，痛甚加片姜黄 6g、海桐皮 9g。

主治：温热痹，寒战热炽，骨节烦疼，面目萎黄，舌色灰滞。

3. 除湿益痹汤（《类证治裁》）

方药：苍术、白术、茯苓、羌活、泽泻、陈皮各 3g，甘草 1.5g，姜汁、竹沥各 3 匙。水煎服。

主治：湿痹身重酸痛，疼有定处，天阴即发。

（三）单方验方

（1）清风藤 15g、汉防己 10g，水煎服。

（2）五加皮 10g、银花藤 30g，水煎服。日两服，用治热痹疼痛。

（3）徐长卿 24~30g、猪瘦肉 200g、老酒二两，水煎服，日服二次。

（4）生地 120g，水煎服，每日水煎代茶频服。

（5）湿痹方：带节麻黄 1g、西芪皮 5g、丝瓜络 10g、伸筋草 10g、附子 2g、白芍 5g、炙甘草 5g、白术 5g、千年健 5g，水煎服。主治湿痹足疼，步履维艰。

（6）松节 30g、乳香 30g，上药慢火炒令焦，研细，服 3~6g，热木瓜酒调下。用治脚转筋挛急疼痛者。

（7）全蝎研粉，每日晨服 4 分。用治痹痛，对于肢体麻木亦可见效。

（四）中成药

（1）雷公藤多苷片：每次 2 片，每日 2~3 次，饭后服。

（2）昆明山海棠片：每次 2 片，每日 3 次，饭后服。

（3）正清风痛宁片：片剂：每次 50~100 mg，每日 2~3 次口服；针剂：每次 50~100mg，每日 1~2 次肌内注射，疗程 3~12 月。

（4）顽痹冲剂：每次 2 袋，每日 3 次。具有补肝肾，强筋骨，祛风散寒，除湿通络的作用。

（五）针灸治疗

针灸辅助治疗，调节滑膜细胞，可抑制滑膜分泌炎症相关免疫因子的作用。

常用选穴：颈部关节取大椎、风池、风府、天柱；肩关节取肩髃、肩髎；肘关节取曲池、曲泽、足三里；腕关节取阳池、外关、阳溪、腕骨；指关节取八风、八邪、合谷；脊柱关节取大椎、身柱、腰阳关、腰俞；髋关节取环跳、秩边；膝关节取膝眼、阳陵泉、膝阳关、梁丘、犊鼻；踝关节取昆仑、丘墟、照海、解溪。配以阿是穴联合治疗。

实证以泻法为主，寒邪偏胜者可用艾灸或深刺留针，疼痛剧烈者可用隔姜灸；湿邪偏胜者可针灸并用，或兼用温针、麦粒灸和拔罐法。虚证以补法为主，虚寒型者可加用艾灸或温针灸。每日或隔日 1 次，15~20 次为 1 个疗程。可有效改善患者临床症状，缓解疼痛，提高生活质量。

（六）推拿治疗

推拿通过不同形式的操作方法可刺激人体经络穴位或特定部位，具有调节阴阳、通经络、畅气血、滑利关节、强筋健骨的作用，起到消瘀、行滞、散肿、止痛的功效，并能增进局部营养，改善血液循环，防止肌肉萎缩或废用，改善关节活动功能，对本病有一定疗效，临床上可根据病情酌情选用。

常用穴位：大肠俞、环跳、承扶、委中、足三里等。

手法共百余种，如按法、压法、点法、摩法、推法、拿法、擦法、搓法、掐法、揉法、振法、抹法、抖法、摇法、拍击法、捏法等。依据具体情况，可选一种或几种综合应用。疗程：每天 1~2 次，每次 15~20 分钟，直至病情缓解。

（七）其他

1. 外治法

（1）药棒法：在特制的木棒上蘸上配好的药液，在人体适当的穴位上进行叩击，使拘挛之筋脉舒缓，闭阻之经脉通畅，达到气血流通，通则不痛。

药液配制：由川乌、草乌、三七、细辛、乳香、没药等药物组成，用市售白酒浸泡，7 天后，取滤液使用。

扣击方法： 选7寸至1尺5寸长的木棒一根，根据使用部位要求不同，其外型、长短不同。以右手拇指和食指第二关节及中指第三关节横纹处握棒为宜。右手劳宫穴紧贴棒尾，以腕力使棒对准穴位进行扣击，操作宜稳。

扣击选穴： 根据患者受累的关节不同而选穴。选穴原则以痛为俞，由点及面，局部取穴和循经取穴相结合，或经筋结聚处取穴。常用穴位有肩髃、肩髎、巨骨、秉风、臑臑、肩贞；肘部取曲池、肘髎、天井、手三里、少海、支正；腕部取腕骨、阳溪、阳池、神门、养老、太渊、外关；髋部取环跳、居髎、承扶；手指取各指关节处，称为指边穴；膝部取犊鼻、阳陵泉、膝眼、鹤顶、照海、阴谷、委阳、宾中、膑缘；踝部取丘墟、解溪、昆仑、跟平。痛者加肾俞、足三里；发热加丰隆、大椎；痛甚加曲池、肾俞、阿是穴等。

扣击手法： 实证应予重扣、快扣，频率为每分钟200次左右；虚证应予轻扣、慢扣，频率为每分钟90次左右。

（2）熏洗法：利用药物煎汤，趁热在皮肤或患处进行熏蒸、淋洗的治疗方法。它是借中药渗透力和热力，通过皮肤作用于肌体，促使腠理疏松，经络调和，气血通畅，从而达到治疗目的。

①手熏洗法：先选定药物纱布包裹，准备好脸盆、毛巾、布单。将煎好的药汤乘热倾入脸盆，患者先把手臂搁于盆口上，上覆布单不使热气外泄。待药液不烫手时，把患手浸于药液中洗浴。熏洗完毕后用干毛巾轻轻擦干，避风。

②足熏洗法：先选定药物纱布包裹，准备好木桶（以高、细的木桶为宜）、小木凳、布单、毛巾。将煎好的药汤乘热倾入木桶，桶内置一只小木凳，略高出药液面。患者坐在椅子上，将患足搁在桶内小木凳上，用布单将桶口及腿盖严，进行熏疗。待药液不烫足时，取出小木凳，把患足浸在药液中泡洗。根据病情需要，药液可浸至踝关节或膝关节部位。熏洗完毕，用毛巾擦干皮肤，注意避风。

处方： 透骨草15~30g，红花10~15g，五加皮10~20g，白芷10~15g，川芎10~20g，海桐皮10~20g，鸡血藤10~20g，赤芍10~20g，伸筋草10~15g，桑枝10~15g，白花蛇舌草15~30g。

上方加水共煎30分钟，按上法熏洗患部，每日1~2次，每次20~30分钟。

（3）外敷法：将药物敷在体表的特定部位来治疗疾病的一种方法。如果所用药物属于干品，不含汁液，就将药物研为细末，然后加入适量的调和剂（醋、酒等），调成干湿适度的糊状敷用；如果所用药物本身含有汁液，就将药物捣成糊状使用即可。

处方一： 川乌、草乌、生南星、附子各30g，炮姜、赤芍各90g，肉桂、白芷各15g，细辛12g。把上药共研为细末，装瓶中备用。用时根据患部面积取适量药物，用热白酒调成糊状，敷在患处，厚约0.5厘米。再覆盖上油纸，用纱布包扎固定。每天换1次药，重者换2次。本方对风寒湿痹急性发作者适宜，热痹者禁用。

处方二： 生半夏30g，生栀子仁60g，生大黄15g，桃仁15g，红花10g。上药同研为细末，用醋调成糊状，敷于患处。本方适用于关节红肿热痛之热痹。

处方三： 复方雷公藤散剂：雷公藤45g，赤芍15g，丹参15g，透骨草15g，伸筋草15g，老鹳草20g，黄芥子15g，防己20g。将适量药粉用酒和醋各一半调湿成药泥状，摊在塑料布上厚约0.2厘米，外敷于肘、膝关节周围，再用绷带包扎上下端，要扎紧，以防药液外溢，每次敷 24 小时，隔日 1 次。散剂外敷对于关节炎活动期红肿热痛有显著疗效。

2. 穴位注射

用复方当归注射液或骨宁注射液进行穴位注射。可选阿是穴或根据病变部位选穴。一般主穴酌选肩髃、曲池、臂中、合谷、环跳、足三里等。配穴一般遵循以下规律：指关节取八邪，腕关节取阳溪，肘关节取曲泽，肩关节取肩髃，髋关节取风市，膝关节取膝眼，踝关节取昆仑，趾关节取八风，脊椎取华佗夹脊。每次注射 2~6 个穴位，每穴 2ml，隔日 1 次。

3. 康复疗法

积极合理地进行康复医疗，有利于保持或恢复肢体关节功能，达到缓解疼痛，消除肿胀，改善功能障碍，预防及纠正关节畸形的目的。可以根据患者的不同病期，采用不同方法，具体有理疗、体疗、按摩、日常生活活动作训练、康复器械的应用等。

五、名医专家经验方

（一）通痹汤（娄多峰）

适应证： 痹证之邪实寒证。

组成： 当归 18g，丹参 18g，鸡血藤 21g，海风藤 18g，透骨草 21g，独活 18g，香附 21g，地风皮 18g。

用法： 水煎服，日 1 剂，早晚分服。

功效： 祛风散寒除湿，活血养血通络。

（二）除蒸理顽汤（李志铭）

适应证： 阴虚有热之痹证关节肿胀疼痛。

组成： 青蒿 30g，地骨皮 20g，生黄芪 15g，防己 15g，防风 12g，羌活、独活各 12g，乌梢蛇 15g，白术 12g，钩藤 15g，桑寄生 30g，地风皮 15g，地龙 12g，当归 12g，红花 8g，元参 15g，雷公藤 10~15g。

用法： 水煎服，日 1 剂，早晚分服。

功效： 滋阴清热，祛风通络止痛。

（三）补肾祛寒治顽汤（焦树德）

适应证： 肾虚热痹。

组成： 川断、熟地各 12~15g，补骨脂、淫羊藿、桂枝、赤芍、白芍各 9~12g，制附片 6~12g，骨碎补 10g，独活、牛膝、知母各 9g，苍术 6g，威灵仙 12g，防风、炙山甲各 6~9g，伸筋草 20~30g，麻黄 3g，松节 10~15g。

用法： 水煎服，日 1 剂，早晚分服。

功效： 补肾清热、疏风化湿、活化散瘀、强筋壮骨。

六、名医专家典型医案

（一）娄多峰医案——寒湿痹

张某 女，56 岁，家庭妇女。全身关节肿痛 36 年，手畸残 6 年。

1956 年 6 月产后数日拉风箱，旬日手指关节剧烈肿痛，满月时已波及全身多个关节。当地县医院诊为"产后身痛"，给激素可暂缓症状，10 年后双手指梭形改变，20 年后双手典型鹅颈样类风湿手。现全身多关节肿痛、酸困、僵硬，四肢及下颌关节为甚，张口困难，生活失理。肢体畏寒怕冷，倦乏无力。情绪悲观。舌淡暗。苔薄白，脉弦细涩。

辨证： 血瘀邪凝。

治法： 养血活血，益痹通络。

方药： 当归 30g，丹参 30g，鸡血藤 30g，炒山甲 12g，桂枝 12g，独活 20g，千年健 30g，木瓜 18g，香附 30g，川牛膝 30g，陈皮 15g，甘草 9g。

按语： 笔者认为瘀血顽痰凝结，以虫类药搜风剔络，破瘀涤痰，与此同时，病久正气虚弱，应适当扶正固本。以当归、丹参、鸡血藤活血养血为主，辅以炒山甲行血止痛；独活、千年健、木瓜、桂枝、川牛膝为祛风除湿散寒之平剂，祛邪而不伤正；陈皮、甘草共为佐使。该方养血活血、益痹通络，缓缓调之。

（二）路志正医案——湿热痹

马某 女，27 岁，1982 年 10 月 8 日因全身关节疼痛麻木 4 年，加重 2 个月来诊。

病患于 4 年之前小产后，诸关节疼痛，久治不效。来诊前化验血沉 46 毫米 / 小时，类风湿因子阳性，拟诊类风湿关节炎。现症：全身关节麻木疼痛，颈腰僵硬，两踝剧疼，步履艰难，需人搀扶，勉能稍行，形瘦体弱，气微声嘶，手握无力，不能持物，咽干口苦，纳呆，眠差梦多，大便稀，日二三行，小便黄赤短涩，唇如涂丹，舌尖红赤，有瘀点，苔黄厚而干，脉沉弦小数。

病机： 素禀不足，加之小产失血，百脉空虚，风寒湿邪侵袭，郁久化热，灼津耗液，胶结不解，以致身体日衰，病势日增。

治法： 宣泄湿热。

方药： 拟宣痹汤。连翘 9g，赤小豆 15g，晚蚕沙（布包）15g，防风、防己各 9g，炒桑枝 15g，赤芍、白芍各 9g，海桐皮 9g，生地 12g，草薢 9g，独活 6g，茵陈 12g，麻黄 3g，苍术 10g。5 剂。

按语： 本例患者素体虚弱复感外邪，路氏以防己为主药，清利湿热，宣通经络；草薢、茵陈助防己利湿清热之功；赤小豆、晚蚕沙、海桐皮祛湿化浊；桑枝、独活、防风疏风通络；加赤白芍、生地养阴血，连翘清郁热。

七、预防和调护

（一）预防

1. 防范风寒与潮湿环境的因素

感受风寒、潮湿是诱发本病的重要因素。要根据体质避免汗出当风，接触凉水，坐卧湿地，做到"虚邪贼风、避之有时"。

2. 防治感染

有些患者是在扁桃体炎、咽喉炎、鼻窦炎等感染性疾病发生后发病，因此感染也可能与发病有关，所以应预防和控制感染病灶。

3. 早期诊断与早期治疗

对怀疑有关节疼痛症状的患者，应及时到医院诊治，以获得早期诊断与治疗，控制病情发展，降低致残率和避免劳动能力的丧失。

（二）调护

1. 精神调护

临床上发现有些患者在发病前有明显的精神刺激，如心情压抑、过度悲伤等，发病后的不良情绪波动又往往加重病情的发展。因此医者必须引导患者对本病有正确的认识，减轻精神负担，面对疾病积极配合治疗。

2. 生活护理

由于疾病的原因，会给患者生活带来诸多的不便，不论是医护人员或是家属都要给予热情的帮助和指导。对肢体功能丧失卧床不起者，要防止褥疮的发生。对关节功能障碍、行动不便的患者，要注意防止跌仆。饮食要有节制，要注意营养。

3. 功能锻炼

坚持功能锻炼，有针对性地进行关节功能恢复训练。可以通过保健体操、慢跑、脚踏自行车等进行功能恢复训练，除此之外中国传统养生功，如太极拳、五禽戏等，通过导引、行气、吐纳舒筋活血，长期传统锻炼可以起到保护关节、有效改善关节活动，预防和减缓关节畸形的作用。锻炼强度应以活动后关节无新增明显不适感为宜。这样可以尽可能地避免出现僵直，防止肌肉萎缩，促进机体血液循环，改善局部营养状态，振奋精神，保持良好的体质。

（应森林）

参考文献

[1] 唐建武. 病理学[M].2版.北京：科学出版社，2012：227.

[2] 孙韬，熊峰，王春霞. 抗瓜氨酸蛋白抗体诊断类风湿关节炎的研究进展[J]. 风湿病与关节炎，2014，5（3）：5-7.

[3] Alsalahy MM, Nasser HS, Hashem MM, et al. Effect of tobacco smoking on tissue protein citrullination and disease progression in patients with rheumatoid arthritis[J]. Saudi Pharmaceutical Journal, 2010, 18（2）：75-80.

[4] Vossenaar ER, Van Venrooij WJ. Citrullinated proteins: sparks that may ignite the fire in rheumatoid arthritis[J]. Arthritis research and therapy, 2004, 6（3）：107-111.

[5] Farid SS, Azizi G, Mirshafiey A. Anti-citrullinated protein antibodies and their clinical utility in rheumatoid arthritis[J]. International journal of rheumatic diseases, 2013, 16（4）：379-386.

[6] 王国华. 类风湿关节炎免疫发病机制研究进展[J]. 中国组织化学与细胞化学杂志，2010，19（3）：19-22.

[7] 黄嘉，黄慈波. 类风湿关节炎的诊断治疗进展[J]. 临床药物治疗杂志，2010，8（1）：1-5.

[8] 中华医学会风湿病学分会. 类风湿关节炎诊断和治疗指南[J]. 中华风湿病学杂志，2010，14（4）：265-269.

[9] 娄高峰，娄玉钤. 娄多峰论治风湿病[M]. 北京：人民卫生出版社，2007.

[10] 路志正. 路志正医林集腋[M]//李俊德. 国医大师医论医案集. 北京：人民卫生出版社，2009.

崩漏

Metrorrhagia
and
Metrostaxis

一、概述

（一）定义

崩漏是指经血非时暴下不止或淋漓不尽，前者谓之"崩中"，后者谓之"漏下"。

崩与漏出血情况虽不同，然二者常交替出现，且其病因病机基本一致，故概称崩漏。

崩漏是因肾—天癸—冲任—胞宫生殖轴的严重紊乱，引起月经周期紊乱，"非时而下"，经量紊乱，或多，或少，或淋漓不断。

（二）特征

本病属妇科常见病，也是疑难急重病证。"疑"指崩漏虽属月经病，却不在行经期出血，《景岳全书》称其为"经乱之甚也"；"难"指难于获得疗效，发病机制复杂，因果相干，气血同病，多脏受累；"重"指崩漏耗伤大量气血，甚至可导致失血性休克。

（三）崩与漏的关系

（1）共同点：均不在行经期间出血，即"非时而下"。

（2）不同点："崩"来势急，出血量多，病情较重；"漏"来势缓，出血量少，病情较轻，单位时间出血少。

（3）相互转化："崩为漏之甚，漏为崩之渐"。久漏不止，病势日进而成崩；血崩日久，气血大衰而成漏。

（四）与西医关系

崩漏作为一个症状，可出现在以下各类疾病中。

（1）内分泌疾病：如功能失调性子宫出血，多见于青春期、更年期。①无排卵型：周期紊乱，出血时多时少，甚至长短不一，或短时停经，大量出血。②有排卵型：因黄体发育不全致月经先期；因黄体萎缩不全致经期延长。

（2）与妊娠有关的疾病：如先兆流产、不全流产、药物流产。

（3）与炎症有关的疾病：如阴道炎、宫颈炎、宫体炎、内膜炎、盆腔炎。

（4）肿瘤：如子宫肌瘤、卵巢肿物、宫颈癌。

（5）与创伤有关：外伤。

（6）全身性疾病：如血小板减少症、肝硬化。

二、病因病机

（一）中医

1.脾虚

素体脾虚，或劳倦思虑、饮食不节损伤脾气；或脾虚血失统摄，甚则虚而下陷，冲任不固不能制约经血发为崩漏。如《妇科玉尺》云："思虑伤脾，不能摄血，致令妄行。"

2.肾虚

（1）肾气虚：先天肾气不足；少女肾气未盛、天癸未充；房劳、多产损伤肾气；久病、大病穷必及肾；七七之年肾气渐衰，天癸渐竭，肾气虚则封藏失司，冲任不固，不能制约经血，子宫藏泻失常发为崩漏。

（2）肾阳虚：素体阳虚，命门火衰，或久崩久漏，阴损及阳，阳不摄阴，封藏失职，冲任不固，不能制约经血而成崩漏。

（3）肾阴虚：素体肾阴亏虚，或多产、房劳耗伤真阴，阴虚失守，虚火动血，子宫藏泻无度，遂致崩漏。

3. 血热

素体阳盛血热或阴虚内热；七情内伤，肝郁化热；内蕴湿热之邪，热伤冲任，迫血妄行，发为崩漏。

4. 血瘀

七情内伤，气滞血瘀；或热灼、寒凝、虚滞致瘀；或经期、产后余血未净而合阴阳，内生瘀血；或崩漏日久，离经之血为瘀。瘀阻冲任、子宫，血不归经妄行，遂成崩漏。

崩漏为病，可概括为虚、热、瘀的机制，但由于脏腑相生相克，脏腑、气血、经络密切相关，又病程日久，崩漏的发生和发展常气血同病、多脏受累、因果相干，错综复杂。

无论病起何脏，"四脏相移，必归脾肾"，"五脏之伤，穷必及肾"，以致肾脏受病。肾有肾气、肾阴、肾阳之分。阴虚阳搏成崩，病本在肾水阴虚，由此不能济心涵木，而成为心、肝、肾同病之崩漏。崩漏日久，失血耗气伤阴，离经之血为瘀，均不同程度地存在气阴虚夹瘀的病机。

崩漏病本在肾，病位在冲任，变化在气血，表现为子宫藏泻无度。

（二）西医

1. 无排卵型功能失调性子宫出血

无排卵型功血是由于单一雌激素刺激而无孕激素拮抗，子宫内膜不受限制地增生而引起的雌激素撤退性出血或突破性出血。来自机体的内外因素，精神过度紧张、恐惧、忧伤、环境与气候骤然变化，全身性疾病、营养不良、贫血及代谢紊乱均可通过大脑皮层和中枢神经系统影响下丘脑－垂体－卵巢轴的相互调节功能，最终发生功能失调性子宫出血。

无排卵型功能失调性子宫出血多发生于青春期和围绝经期妇女，但二者发病机制不完全相同。

青春期： 下丘脑和垂体的调节功能未臻成熟，它们和卵巢间尚未建立稳定的周期性调节。此时虽有一批卵泡生长，但发育到一定程度即发生退行性变而无排卵，形成闭锁卵泡。

围绝经期： 由于卵巢功能衰退，卵泡几乎已耗尽，剩余卵泡对垂体促性腺激素的反应性低下，雌激素分泌量锐减，对垂体的负反馈变弱，促性腺激素水平升高，发生无排卵功血。

2. 雌激素撤退性出血

在单一雌激素的持久刺激下，子宫内膜发生诸如单纯型增生、复杂型增生等，若有一批卵泡闭锁，雌激素水平可突然下降，内膜失去支持而剥脱出血。

雌激素突破性出血有两种类型：低水平雌激素维持在阈值水平，可发生间断少量出血，内膜修复慢使出血时间延长；高水平雌激素维持在有效浓度，则引起长时间闭经，因无孕激素参与，内膜增厚而不牢固，而发生自发急性突破出血，血量汹涌。由于内膜血管缺乏螺旋化，不发生节段性收缩和松弛，子宫内膜不能同步脱落，使一处修复，另一处又脱落出血，造成出血量多，时间长不能自止。由于多次组织的破损活化了血内纤维蛋白溶酶，引起更多的纤维蛋白溶解加重了出血。

三、诊断要点与鉴别诊断

（一）诊断要点

1. 病史

（1）年龄：与崩漏发病密切相关。

（2）月经史：指以往月经的周期、经期、经量有无异常；有无崩漏史。

（3）避孕史：指有无口服避孕药或其他激素；有无宫内节育器及输卵管结扎术史等。

（4）有无内科出血病史。

2. 临床表现

月经周期紊乱；行经时间超过半月以上，甚或数月断续不休；亦有停闭数月又突然暴下不止或淋漓不尽；常有不同程度的贫血。

3. 检查

根据病情需要选做 B 超、MRI、宫腔镜检查，或诊断性刮宫、基础体温测定等。

（1）妇科检查：应无明显的器质性病变；但如发现子宫颈息肉、子宫肌瘤应按该病论治。

（2）辅助检查：排除生殖器肿瘤（子宫肌瘤、子宫内膜癌、卵巢肿瘤）、炎症（子宫内膜炎、子宫肌炎、宫颈息肉、宫内膜息肉、盆腔炎）、全身性疾病（再生障碍性贫血、血小板减少）引起的阴道出血。

（二）鉴别诊断

1. 月经失调

	周期	经期	经量
月经先期	有，缩短	正常	正常，或多或少
月经过多	正常	正常	过多如崩
经期延长	正常	延长似漏	或多或少
月经先后无定期	或先或后	正常	正常
崩漏	同时严重失调		

2. 经间期出血

崩漏与经间期出血都是非时而下，但经间期出血发生在两次月经中间，颇有规律，且出血时间仅 2~3 天，不超过 7 天自然停止。而崩漏是周期、经期、经量的严重失调，出血不能自止。

3. 赤带

赤带与漏下的鉴别要询问病史和进行检查，赤带以带中有血丝为特点，月经正常。

4. 胎产出血

与妊娠早期的出血性疾病胎漏、胎动不安、异位妊娠相鉴别，询问病史，做妊娠试验和 B 超检查可以明确诊断。与产后病出血恶露不绝相鉴别，可询问病史，从发病时间恶露不绝发生在产后可作鉴别。

5. 生殖器肿瘤出血

临床可表现如崩似漏的阴道出血，通过妇科检查或结合 B 超、MRI 检查或诊断性刮宫可以明确诊断以鉴别。

6. 生殖系炎症

如宫颈息肉、宫内膜息肉、子宫内膜炎、盆腔炎等，其临床常表现漏下不止，通过妇科检查或诊断性刮宫或宫腔镜检查以助鉴别。

7. 外阴外伤出血

如跌仆损伤、暴力性交等，询问病史和妇科检查可鉴别。

8. 内科血液病

如再生障碍性贫血、血小板减少，在阴道出血期可由原发内科血液病导致血量过多，甚则暴下如注，或淋漓不尽。通过血液分析、凝血因子的检查或骨髓细胞的分析不难鉴别。

四、中医治疗

（一）辨治原则

1. 辨证

（1）辨虚实：虚者：脾虚、肾虚；实者：血热、血瘀。

（2）辨出血期还是止血后：出血期：多见标证或虚实夹杂证；血止后：本证或虚证。

出血期，初辨其证之寒、热、虚、实：热证见经血非时暴下，量多势急，继而淋漓不止，色鲜红或深红，质稠者；虚证见经血非时暴下或淋漓难尽，色淡质稀；血瘀见经血非时而至，时崩时闭，时出时止，时多时少，色紫暗有块或伴腹痛者；寒证见经血暴崩不止，或久崩久漏，血色淡暗，质稀。

2. 治疗

崩漏的治疗，本着"急则治其标，缓则治其本"的原则，灵活掌握和运用塞流、澄源、复旧的"治崩三法"。

（1）塞流：即止血，用于暴崩之际，急当塞流止血防脱。

（2）澄源：即正本清源，亦是求因治本，是治疗崩漏的重要阶段。一般用于出血减缓后的辨证论治。切忌不问缘由，概投寒凉或温补之剂，或专事炭涩，致犯虚虚实实之戒。

（3）复旧：即固本善后，是巩固崩漏治疗的重要阶段。用于止血后恢复健康，根据不同年龄阶段选择不同的治法，调整月经周期，或促排卵。治法补肾、扶脾、疏肝，三经同调，各有偏重。

治崩三法，各不相同，但又不可截然分开，临证中必须灵活运用。塞流须澄源，澄源当固本，复旧要求因。三法互为前提，相互为用，各有侧重，但均贯穿辨证求因精神。

（二）辨证治疗

1.出血期辨证论治

（1）脾虚

主症：经血非时暴下不止，或淋漓日久不尽，血色淡，质清稀，面色㿠白，神疲气短，小腹空坠，四肢不温，面浮肢肿，纳呆便溏，舌质淡胖，边有齿印，苔白，脉沉弱。

治法：补气摄血，固冲止崩。

方药：固本止崩汤或固冲汤。

固本止崩汤（《傅青主女科》）。人参、黄芪、白术、熟地黄、当归、黑姜。

方解：方中人参、黄芪大补元气，升阳固本；白术健脾资血之源又统血归经；熟地滋阴养血，"于补阴之中行止崩之法"。黑姜引血归经，更有补火温阳收敛之妙；黄芪配当归含有"当归补血汤"之意，熟地配当归一阴一阳补血和血。全方气血两补，使气壮固本以摄血，血生配气能涵阳。气充而血沛，阳生而阴长，冲脉得固，血崩自止。

《傅青主女科》云："方妙在全不去止血，而惟补血，又不止补血，而更补气，非惟补气，而更补火。盖血崩而至于黑暗昏晕，则血已尽去，仅存一线之气，以为护持，若不急补其气以生血，而先补其血而遗气，则有形之血，恐不能遽生，而无形之气，必且至尽散，此所以不先补血而先补气也。然单补气，则血又不易生；单补血而不补火，则血又必凝滞，而不能随气而速生。况黑姜引血归经，是补中又有收敛之妙，所以同补气补血之药并用之耳"。

加减：气虚运血无力，易于停留成瘀，常加三七、益母草或失笑散化瘀止血。

固冲汤（《医学衷中参西录》）。白术、黄芪、煅龙骨、煅牡蛎、山茱萸、白芍、海螵蛸、茜草根、棕榈炭、五倍子。

方解：方中黄芪、白术健脾益气以摄血；煅龙骨、煅牡蛎、海螵蛸固摄冲任；山茱萸、白芍益肾养血，酸收止血；棕榈炭、五倍子涩血止血；茜草根化瘀止血，血止而不留瘀。全方健脾益气，固冲止血。

若暴崩如注，肢冷汗出、昏厥不省人事、脉微欲绝者，为气随血脱之危急证候，按急证方法补气回阳固脱。必要时输液、输血迅速补充血容量以抗休克。

（2）肾虚证

①肾气虚

主症：青春期少女或经断前后妇女经乱无期，出血量多，或淋漓不净，或由崩而漏，由漏而崩，色淡红或淡暗，质清稀，面色晦暗，眼眶暗，小腹空坠，腰脊酸软，舌淡暗，苔白润，脉沉弱。

治法：补肾益气，固冲止血。

方药：加减苁蓉菟丝子丸（《中医妇科治疗学》）。党参、黄芪、阿胶、熟地、肉苁蓉、覆盆子、当归、枸杞子、桑寄生、菟丝子、艾叶。

方解：方中肉苁蓉、覆盆子温补肾气；菟丝子补阳益阴，阴阳双补；熟地滋肾益阴，使肾气充盛，封藏密固以止崩；黄芪、党参补气摄血；阿胶、艾叶补血、固冲、摄血；枸杞子、桑寄生补肝肾；当归补血活血，引血归经；全方共奏补肾益气，固冲止血之功。若嫌当归辛温助动，走而不守，亦可去之。

②肾阳虚

主症：经乱无期，出血量多或淋漓不尽，或停经数月后又暴下不止，血色淡红或淡暗质稀，面色晦暗，肢冷畏寒，腰膝酸软，小便清长，夜尿多，眼眶暗，舌淡暗，苔白润，脉沉细无力。

治法：温肾益气，固冲止血。

方药：右归丸（《景岳全书》）。党参、黄芪、三七、制附子、肉桂、熟地、山药、山萸肉、枸杞、菟丝子、鹿角胶、当归、杜仲。

方解：方中熟地滋肾养血、填精益髓，配山萸肉、山药，取六味地黄丸中"三补"以生水；附子、肉桂温肾壮阳，补益命门，温阳止崩，又使水火互济；鹿角胶为血肉有情之品，补命火，温督脉，固冲任；菟丝子、杜仲温补肝肾；当归、枸杞子养血柔肝益冲任；加党参、黄芪补气摄血；寒凝则血瘀，加三七以化瘀止血。全方温肾益气，固冲止血。

③肾阴虚

主症：经乱无期，出血量少，淋漓累月不止，或停闭数月后又突然暴崩下血经色鲜红，质稍稠，头晕耳鸣，腰膝酸软，五心烦热，夜寐不宁，舌红，少苔或有裂纹，脉细数。

治法：滋肾益阴，固冲止血。

方药：左归丸合二至丸或滋阴固气汤。

左归丸（《景岳全书》）合二至丸（《医方集解》）。熟地、山药、枸杞、山萸肉、菟丝子、鹿角胶、龟甲胶、川牛膝、女贞子、旱莲草。

方解：方中熟地、山萸肉、山药滋补肝肾，为六味地黄丸中"三补"；龟甲胶补任脉之虚；鹿角胶补督脉之弱；枸杞子、菟丝子、二至丸补肝肾，益冲任；川牛膝补肝肾，又能活血。全方为壮水填精、补益冲任之剂，使肾阴足，奇经固，经血自止。

加减：肾阴虚不能上济心火，或阴虚火旺，烦躁失眠，心悸怔忡，可加生脉散以益气养阴，宁心止血。

滋阴固气汤（《罗元恺论医集》）。菟丝子、山茱萸、党参、黄芪、白术、炙甘草、阿胶、鹿角霜、何首乌、白芍、续断。

方解：方中山茱萸补肾益精；何首乌、白芍补血养血；阿胶滋阴补血、止血；菟丝子补阳益阴；鹿角霜温肾助阳，又收敛止血；续断补益肝肾；党参、黄芪、白术、炙甘草补气摄血。

（3）血热

①虚热

主症：经来无期量少淋漓不尽或量多势急，血色鲜红、面颊潮红，烦热少寐，咽干口燥，大便秘结，舌红，少苔，脉细数。

治法：养阴清热，固冲止血。

方药：上下相资汤（《石室秘录·燥证门》）。人参、沙参、玄参、麦冬、玉竹、五味子、熟地、山萸肉、车前子、牛膝。

方解：方中地黄、山萸肉滋肾养阴为君；人参、沙参益气润肺为臣；玄参、麦冬、玉竹增液滋水降火；车前子养肺强阴益精；牛膝补肝肾；方内含增液汤滋水，更有生脉散益气养阴止血，清心除烦安神。全方滋肾为主，而佐以润肺之药，上润肺阴，下滋肾水，子母相资，上下兼润，庶使精生液长，血生津还，共奏养阴清热、固冲止血之功。

②实热

主症：经来无期，经血突然暴崩如注，或淋漓日久难止，血色深红，质稠，口渴烦热，便秘溺黄，舌红，苔黄，脉滑数。

治法：清热凉血，固冲止血。

方药：清热固经汤（《简明中医妇科学》）。黄芩、焦栀子、生地黄、地骨皮、地榆、生藕节、阿胶、陈棕炭、龟甲、牡蛎、生甘草。

方解：方中黄芩、山栀清热泻火；生地、地榆、藕节清热凉血，固冲止血；地骨皮、龟甲、牡蛎育阴潜阳；龟甲又能补任脉之虚，化瘀生新；阿胶补血止血；陈棕炭收涩止血；生甘草调和诸药。诸药各司其职，集清热、泻火、凉血、育阴、祛瘀、胶固、炭涩、镇潜、补任、固冲多种止血法于一方之中，能收清热凉血、固冲止血之功。

加减：兼见心烦易怒，胸胁胀痛，口干苦，脉弦数，为肝郁化热或肝经火炽之证，治宜清肝泻热止血。上方加柴胡疏肝；夏枯草、龙胆草清泻肝热。兼见少腹或小腹疼痛，或灼热不适，苔黄腻者，为湿热阻滞冲任，上方加黄柏、银花藤、连翘、茵陈清热利湿，去阿胶之滋腻。

（4）血瘀

主症：经血非时而下或淋漓不断，量时多时少，时出时止或停闭数月又突然崩中，继之漏下，经色暗有血块，小腹疼痛或胀，舌质紫暗或尖边有瘀点，脉弦细或涩。

治法：活血化瘀，固冲止血。

方药：逐瘀止血汤或将军斩关汤

逐瘀止血汤（《傅青主女科》）。生地黄、大黄、赤芍、丹皮、当归尾、枳壳、龟甲、桃仁。

方解：从桃仁四物汤合桃仁承气汤加减化裁而成。生地重用，清热凉血，酒炒寓止于行；当归尾、桃仁、赤芍祛瘀止痛；丹皮行血泻火；大黄凉血逐瘀下滞，配枳壳下气，加强荡涤瘀滞之功；妙用龟甲养阴化瘀。

将军斩关汤（《中华名中医治病囊秘·朱南孙卷》）。蒲黄炭、炒五灵脂、熟军炭、炮姜炭、茜草、益母草、仙鹤草、桑螵蛸、海螵蛸、三七粉、萆薢、薏苡仁、黄柏、赤茯苓、丹皮、泽泻、通草、滑石。

方解：方中蒲黄炭、炒五灵脂祛瘀止血定痛；熟军炭清热祛瘀，一热一寒，一攻一守，炮姜炭通涩并举；益母草通涩之剂；仙鹤草、茜草活血化瘀而止血；桑螵蛸益肾摄冲；海螵蛸、三七粉化瘀止血之圣药。全方通涩并用，以通为主，寓攻于补，相得益彰。用于崩漏虚中夹实者，屡屡奏效。

2. 止血后治疗

（1）个体化治疗

崩漏止血后治疗是治愈崩漏的关键。临证中要求个体化治疗。①青春期患者，有两种治疗目标：一是调整月经周期，并建立排卵功能以防复发；二是调整月经周期，不强调有排卵。因青春期非生殖最佳年龄，可让机体在自然状态下逐渐健全排卵功能。②生育期患者：多因崩漏而导致不孕，治疗解决调经种子的问题。③更年期患者：解决因崩漏导致的体虚贫血；防止复发；预防恶性病变。

（2）辨证论治：寒热虚实均可导致崩漏，针对病因病机进行辨证论治以复旧；可参照出血期各证型辨证论治，但应去除各方中的止血药。

（3）中药人工周期疗法：由于"经本于肾"，"经水出诸肾"，月经病的治疗原则重在治本以调经。青春期、生育期患者的复旧目标，主要是调整肾—天癸—冲任—胞宫生殖轴，以达到调整月经周期或同时建立排卵功能。采用中药人工周期疗法：分别按卵泡期、排卵期、黄体期、行经期，设计以补肾为主的促卵泡汤、促排卵汤、促黄体汤、调经活血汤进行序贯治疗，一般连用 3 个月经周期以上，可望恢复或建立正常的月经周期。

（4）先补后攻法：根据月经产生的机制，以补肾为主，从止血后开始以滋肾填精，养血调经为主，常选左归丸、归肾丸、定经汤等先补 3 周左右，第 4 周在子宫蓄经渐盈的基础上改用攻法，即活血化瘀通经，多选桃红四物汤加香附、枳壳、益母草、川牛膝。可达到调整月经周期或促进排卵的治疗目的。

（5）健脾补血法：运用于更年期崩漏患者，尽快消除因崩漏造成的贫血和虚弱症状，可选大补元煎或人参养荣汤。

（6）手术治疗：适应于生育期和更年期久治不愈的顽固性崩漏，或已经诊刮子宫内膜送病理检查，提示有恶变倾向者。

（三）专方治疗

加减固冲汤：生黄芪 15g，党参 15g，炒白术 30g，熟地 15g，菟丝子 15g，蒲黄炭 10g，花蕊石 10g，白芍 10g，阿胶 10g，五倍子 10g，棕榈炭 10g，煅龙骨 15g，煅牡蛎 15g，三七粉 3g，血余炭 10g。主治崩漏因气虚血瘀导致出血量多，有血块，伴周身无力、气短懒言、舌质暗淡有齿痕、瘀斑，苔白，脉细无力。

（四）单方验方

（1）独参汤：高丽参 10g。水煎服。

（2）参附汤：高丽参 10g、熟附子 10g。急煎服。

（3）六味回阳汤：人参、制附子、炮姜、炙甘草、熟地、当归。

（4）田七末 3~6g。温开水冲服。

（5）云南白药 1 支。温开水冲服。

（五）中成药

宫血宁胶囊：每次 2 粒，日 3 次，温开水送服。

（六）针灸治疗（止血）

艾灸百会穴、大敦穴（双）、隐白穴（双）。

五、名医专家经验方

（一）育阴止崩汤（韩百灵）

适应证： 由于肝肾阴虚而致的月经先期、月经过多、崩漏、经间期出血等病。素体阴虚或早婚多产、房事不节而耗伤精血，阴虚内热，热扰冲任，迫血妄行而致月经先期、月经过多、崩漏、经间期出血等病。症见腰酸腰痛，腿软乏力，足跟痛，头晕耳鸣，健忘，潮热盗汗，手足心热，面红颧赤等证；舌红无苔或少苔，脉象弦细数。

方药组成： 熟地黄 10~15g，山茱萸 15~20g，山药 15~20g，川断续 15~20g，桑寄生 15~20g，海螵蛸 15~20g，牡蛎 20~30g，白芍 15~20g，阿胶（烊化）10~15g，龟甲 10~20g，炒地榆 20~50g，甘草 5~10g。

方药释义： 方中熟地黄、山茱萸、白芍、阿胶共为君药，其中熟地黄滋阴补肾，为补血之要药，《珍珠囊》记载：熟地黄 "大补血气不足，通血脉，益气力"，《本草纲目》曰：熟地黄 "填骨髓，长肌肉，生精血。补五脏内伤不足，通血脉，利耳目，黑须发，男子五劳七伤，女子伤中胞漏，经候不调，胎产百病。" 山茱萸入下焦，补肝肾、固冲任以止血，可治疗妇女肝肾亏损，冲任不固引起的崩漏及月经过多，《本草新编》谓：山茱萸 "补阴之药未有不偏者，胜者也未有山茱萸大补肝肾而不杂，既无寒热之偏，又无阴阳之背，实为诸补阴之冠。" 称其为补阴圣药；白芍收敛肝阴，养血柔肝，可治疗由肝失疏泄之月经不调崩中带下。阿胶有补血、滋阴之功效，为血肉有情之品，可治疗多种出血证，对出血而兼见阴虚、血虚证者尤为适宜，《神农本草经》云：阿胶 "主心腹内崩……女子下血，安胎。" 臣以山药，《本草纲目》云："益肾气，健脾肾。" 能补后天以助养先天；续断，《名医别录》："妇人崩中漏血，金疮血内漏……" 桑寄生滋补肝肾，养血而固冲任，牡蛎血肉有情之品，既能滋补肝肾，又能固精止血，《本草通玄》谓：龟甲 "大有补水制火之功，故能强筋骨，益心智……祛瘀血，止新血。"《药性论》云："君主之剂，治女子崩中。" 炒地榆入血分，因其性苦寒下降，可治疗多种血热出血证，尤善于治下焦之血，《本草正》言：地榆 "微苦微涩，性寒而降，既消且涩……治女人崩漏下血，月经不止。" 海螵蛸性咸涩微温，有收敛止血、固精止带、制酸止痛等功效，可治疗多种内外出血，治疗外伤出血时，可单用研末外敷，《神农本草经》："主女子赤白漏下经汁。"《本草品汇精要》："止精滑，去目翳。" 二者共为佐药，用以塞流，助君臣之药止血之力；甘草调和诸药，为使药。

功效： 滋阴补肾，固冲止血。

加减： 如出血量多者重用炒地榆，加棕榈炭以增大止血之力；有血条、血块者加炒蒲黄、三七以活血止血。

（二）清热固经丸（顾小痴）

适应证： 阴虚血热所致的月经过多、经期延长、崩漏、经间期出血。

方药组成： 炙龟甲 1.2kg，生地 6kg，丹皮 3.6kg，黄芩 3.6kg，黄柏 3.6kg，阿胶珠 4.8kg，地榆炭 6kg，生牡蛎 6kg，椿白皮 6kg，旱莲草 6kg，上药共为细末，炼蜜为丸，每丸重 9g，每日 2 次，每次 1 丸。

方药释义： 方中炙龟甲、生地、阿胶珠共为君药，益肾滋阴，且龟甲、阿胶为血肉有情之品，可填补真阴，壮水之主；地榆炭、生牡蛎收涩止血为臣药；丹皮、黄芩、黄柏、椿白皮清热凉血止血为佐；旱莲草入肾，滋阴止血为使。

功效： 滋阴清热，固经止血。

（三）滋阴固气汤（罗元恺）

适应证： 崩漏。可用于功能性子宫出血。

方药组成： 党参 12g，黄芪 15g，白术 9g，阿胶（烊化）6g，续断 9g，菟丝子 15g，首乌 12g，山萸肉 15g，鹿角霜 15g，白芍 9g，炙甘草 6g。水煎服，每日 1 剂，日服 2 次。

方药释义： 方中以党参、黄芪峻补气血；白术健脾益气；首乌、菟丝子、山萸肉补益肝肾；阿胶养血止血；白芍敛阴和营；续断通调血脉；甘草调和诸药。全方以补气为主，气足可以摄血；以滋阴养血为辅，血充则肝能藏血，血归正经，何崩之有。

功效： 滋阴，补气，摄血。

加减： 出血多者，加棕炭、赤石脂、益母草，重用参、芪，并艾灸隐白、大敦、三阴交，共收止血之效；血止后，加入枸杞、补骨脂、巴戟天、淫羊藿、杜仲等品，以增强补肾之功。

六、名医专家典型医案

（一）刘奉五医案

史某某 女，41 岁。

初诊： 1975 年 6 月 6 日。月经先后不定期，行经日久约 1 年余。

现病史： 以往月经正常，近 1 年来月经增多，色紫有血块，去年 8 月大出血 10 余天，以后月经频至，甚至一月二至，量多行经日久（10 余天）。今年 1 月因阴道大出血而行刮宫术，病理诊断为"子宫内膜增殖症"。以后月经闭止二月后，阴道出血淋漓不止约10余天。曾用黄体酮治疗，月经来潮时则淋漓不止，色黑紫，量偏多，有小血块。近两年来性情烦急易怒，伴有胸肋胀满，纳差，腹胀，腰酸痛，大便干，2至3日1次。末次月经为4月22日，至今又闭经54天。舌质淡红，脉弦滑。

西医诊断：功能性子宫出血。

中医辨证：脾肾不足，血热肝旺。

治法：健脾补肾，凉血疏肝。

方药：山药5钱，石莲3钱，菟丝子3钱，川断3钱，生熟地各3钱，白芍4钱，炒荆芥穗1.5钱，柴胡1.5钱，黄芩3钱，丹皮3钱，益母草2钱。

二诊：1975年6月26日。上方服3剂后月经来潮，行经4天，色红，血中等。因胸肋胀疼明显，前方加川楝子3钱，继服7剂。

三诊：1975年8月1日。药后按月行经两次，每次6天。继服前方5剂。

四诊：1975年9月27日。自6月19日至8月1日共服中药23剂，诸症消失，按时行经，血量减少，行经3~5天，正常行经已3次。停药观察，月经又按规律来潮2次，周期稍有提前（23~25天）。末次月经为9月24日。

（二）宋光济医案

陈某某 女，16岁，学生。

初诊：1979年8月30日。肾气不足，冲任亦亏，月经提前，一月数行，量多如冲，色暗红，或淋漓不尽，面色不华，腰酸肢寒，睡眠不佳，脉细沉，苔薄白。治拟温肾益气，养血固冲：熟地炭、炒怀山药、炙黄芪、夜交藤、炒赤石脂、陈棕炭各12g，杞子、菟丝子、炒阿胶、茯神各9g，陈萸肉6g，艾叶炭3g。5剂。

二诊：1979年9月6日。前方服后出血已止，睡眠转安，近来带多、苔薄白。治拟健脾化湿止带：西党参、炒白术、炙黄芪、金樱子、芡实、车前草各9g，白莲须、煅牡蛎各12g、炒陈皮、炙甘草各3g。5剂。

三诊：1979年9月30日。周期已准，带下量多，色微黄，大便干，脉细缓，苔薄腻。再拟健脾化湿，清热止带：西党参、车前草、白莲须、女贞子、鸡冠花、焦谷芽各9g，炒怀山药、煅牡蛎各12g，柴胡、川柏、炒陈皮各3g。5剂。

按：本例天癸虽至，肾气不充，闭藏失职，月经量多，腰酸肢寒，脉来沉细，故拟温肾益气。方用调冲汤加减，以熟地炭、杞子、菟丝子、陈萸肉峻补肝肾，黄芪、阿胶补气养血，茯神、夜交藤养血安神，陈棕炭、赤石脂、艾叶炭温肾止血，怀山药健脾益肾，共奉补肾调冲之功。

（三）韩百灵医案

吕某 女，21岁。

初诊：2011年9月28日。近3年经水淋漓不净，常常持续月余。患者于8月25日阴道下血月余不止，量不多，色淡红，伴腰部酸痛，倦怠无力，少气懒言，少食，头晕，记忆力差，面色无华，体型偏瘦，体毛及阴毛多；舌淡，苔薄白，脉沉细。17岁月经初潮，稀发，量少，曾服西药炔雌醇环丙孕酮（达英-35）治疗2年余，用药阶段月经正常，停药后月经仍不行。

辅助检查：血清性激素六项：FSH：4.22mU/ml，LH：18.35mU/ml，PRL：11.96ng/ml，E_2：70.16pg/ml，P：0.51ng/ml，T：85.37ng/dl。糖耐量及胰岛素，甲状腺功能均正常。超声示：子宫稍小；卵巢多囊样改变，左侧卵巢大小35mm×22mm，可见2~4mm大小卵泡13个，右侧卵巢大小37mm×24mm，2~5mm大小卵泡16个。

诊断：崩漏（多囊卵巢综合征）。

辨证：脾肾两虚，冲任亏虚所至。

治法：益肾健脾，固冲止血。

方药：熟地黄20g，山茱萸15g，煅杜仲15g，续断20g，桑寄生20g，黄芪20g，党参20g，山药15g，茯苓15g，白芍15g，阿胶10g，煅牡蛎15g，地榆炭50g，甘草5g。7剂，水煎服，每日1剂，早晚分服。

二诊：2012年10月13日。服药后3天血止，于10月9日受外界惊吓，复见阴道下血，现带血5天，量较多4天，手足不温，背部发凉；舌淡红，苔薄白，脉沉缓。

煅杜仲15g，续断20g，桑寄生20g，黄芪20g，党参20g，山药15g，茯苓15g，白芍15g，阿胶10g，煅牡蛎15g，地榆炭50g，巴戟天15g，艾叶炭15g，花椒10g，甘草5g。10剂，水煎服，每日1剂，早晚分服。

三诊：2012年12月12日。现手足不温明显好转，背部发凉消失。末次月经2012年11月18日，带血6天。考虑经期将近，予以补肾调经之药。

熟地黄20g，菟丝子15g，巴戟天15g，赤芍15g，益母草15g，香附10g，当归15g，党参15g，山药20g，炙甘草10g。10剂，煎服法同前。

结合月经周期规律性，运用以上二方加减化裁，患者坚持治疗半年，近3个月月经25~37天一潮，经期带血5~7天。体重增加3kg，面色近于常人，诸症消失。血FSH：3.71mU/ml，LH：8.92mU/ml，T：53.31ng/dl。停汤剂，改服育阴丸和归脾丸巩固1~2个月。避免惊吓、过劳，注意饮食调摄。3个月后再次随访，患者月经尚正常，体质得到明显改善。

按：多囊卵巢综合征是一种复杂的内分泌紊乱性疾病，临床表现多样化。本案患者体型偏瘦，月经初潮较晚并见腰部酸痛，怠倦无力，头晕，记忆力差，均为肾虚所致。"经水出诸肾"，肾主生殖，藏真阴而寓元阳，"五脏之阴气非此而不能滋，五脏之阳气非此而不能发"，无论是肾阴不足，还是肾阳虚损都致血走而崩也。《医学纲目》曰："调经之法，必先补肾。"临证中韩氏依据"肝肾学说"为理论依据，治疗月经失调从肾入手，运用百灵育阴止崩汤和归脾汤，并补先后二天，以后天养先天之法。补肾为先，补肾同时不忘健脾养血以保证气血生化有源。调补脾肾，调和阴阳，阴阳平和，月经复常。若单纯塞流，不予以澄源、复旧，恐难解燃眉之急。在止血过程中必须考虑到正本清源，标本兼顾的治疗原则。

七、预防与调护

（1）崩漏是可以预防的。重视经期卫生，尽量避免或减少宫腔手术；及早治疗月经过多、经期延长、月经先期等出血倾向的月经病，以防发展成为崩漏。

（2）崩漏一旦发生，必须遵照塞流、澄源、复旧的治崩三法及早治疗，建立正常的月经周期，以防复发。

（3）崩漏调护，首重个人卫生防止感染；调饮食，增营养，纠正因出血导致的贫血；适度劳逸，舒畅情怀。

（罗美玉）

参考文献

［1］张玉珍.普通高等教育"十一五"国家级规划教材：中医妇科学［M］.2版.北京：中国中医药出版社，2007.

［2］韩延华.韩氏女科［M］.北京：人民军医出版社，2015.

［3］北京中医医院，北京市中医学校.刘奉五妇科经验［M］.北京：人民卫生出版社，1977.

［4］浙江省中医药管理局.浙江省名中医临床经验选辑［M］.杭州：浙江科学技术出版社，1990.

［5］陈泽霖.名医特色经验精华［M］.上海：上海中医学院出版社，1987.

不孕症

Infertility

一、概述

夫妇同居，性生活正常，男方生殖功能正常，未避孕1年而未受孕者为不孕症，从未怀孕者为原发性不孕症，中医称之为"全不产"；曾有妊娠史者为继发性不孕症，中医称之为"断绪"（1991年，中国中西医结合学会妇产科专业委员会在第三届学术会议上修订不孕标准）。早在2000多年前，中医对本病已有了较为系统的认识。在中医古籍中，不孕症的病名除"全不产""断绪"之外还有"不孕""无子""绝产"等称谓。不孕症与夫妇双方都有关，其病变部位既可在生殖器官也可在脏腑经络。近年来不孕症患者呈逐年增长趋势，已成为影响人类发展与健康的一个全球性医学和社会学问题。因此，世界卫生组织宣布将不孕症与心血管病、肿瘤病列为当今影响人类生活和健康的三大主要疾病。

二、病因病机

（一）病因

不孕症的病因较为复杂，致病因素可单一出现亦或是复合出现，其病因可归为以下两大类。

1. 先天性缺陷

古代医家很早就认识到不孕症与夫妇双方都有关，提出了一部分患者的发病部位是夫妇一方或双方存在先天性或后天性生殖器缺陷。金元时期朱震亨曾在《格致余论·受胎论》中指出有真两性阴阳人和假两性阴阳人的存在："男不可为父，女不可为母，与男女之兼行者……其类不一。以女涵男有二，一则遇男为妻，遇女为夫；一则可妻而不可夫，其有女具男之全者。"而此种人因其生殖器的异常是不能正常怀孕的。又如明代万全在《广嗣纪要·择配篇》中提出"五不女"："一曰螺，阴户外纹如螺蛳样，旋入内；二曰纹，阴户小如筋头大，只可通溺，难交合，名曰石女；三曰鼓，花头绷急似无孔；四曰角，花头尖削似角；五曰脉，或经脉未及十四而先来，或十五六而始至，或不调，或无。此五种无花之器，不能配合太阳，焉能结仙胎也哉。"清代卢若腾的《岛居随笔》中提到"五不男"："人有五不男：天、犍、漏、怯、变也。天者，阳痿不用，古云天阉是也；犍者，阳势割去，寺人是也；漏者，精寒不固，常自遗泄也；怯者，举而不强，见敌不兴也；变者，体兼男女，俗名二形。""五不女"和"五不男"分别指男女双方先天性生理缺陷、生殖器官发育畸形或其他病变而无生育能力的五种病证。

2. 后天病理变化

（1）外感因素：六淫邪气中风、寒、湿之邪直中胞宫，致使胞宫功能失调，寒邪凝滞，血阻成瘀，湿邪阻滞气机，从而出现月经量少，经来不畅甚或闭经，及崩漏、带下等疾病，从而导致不孕。明代薛己在《薛氏医案》中提出"妇女之不孕，亦有因六淫七情之邪，有伤冲任"的观点。

（2）内伤情志因素：情志因素是内因，七情皆可影响受孕。七情之中，暴怒和忧思影响最大。暴怒伤肝，情志不舒，则肝失于疏泄，气机郁结，致气血不调，冲任不能相资，故难有子。而忧思伤脾，脾失健运，痰湿内生，气机不畅，胞脉受阻，则难以摄精成孕。

（3）体质因素：由于先天禀赋和后天差异形成不同的体质。不同的体质对不同疾病的敏感度不同，其中不孕与某些体质因素密切相关。如《丹溪治法心要·卷七》云："肥者不孕，因躯脂闭塞子宫，而至经事不行……瘦者不孕，因子宫无血，精气不聚故也。"肥胖之人多为痰湿型体质，痰湿内盛，痰湿闭塞胞宫，故不能成孕；瘦者体质多偏于阴虚体质，其阴虚内热，火热灼阴，血枯经少，阴精难聚，亦可致不孕；而素体阳虚之人，阳气虚弱，不能温煦胞宫，易致宫寒不孕等。

（4）其他因素：女子因房劳不节，孕产过多过频，可致肾气亏虚，耗伤气血，损伤冲任，导致不孕。或因暴饮暴食，肆食生冷，导致脾胃受损，运化无权，不能充养冲任，或导致内生痰湿，阻滞胞脉而致不孕。

（二）病机

不孕症发病是一个慢性过程，其病机有虚实之分。历代医家对不孕症的病机均有论述，其主要病机为冲任、胞宫、肾、肝的功能失调。

1. 脏腑功能虚损

（1）肾虚：肾为先天之本，藏精气而主生殖。①肾气不足：肾藏精，精化气，肾中精气主宰着人体的生长、发育与生殖。肾气虚，则冲任虚衰不能摄精成孕。②肾阳虚衰：肾阳虚衰，命门火衰，不能温煦胞宫，摄精成孕。③肾阴虚衰：肾阴不足，则生内热，内热生则扰冲任血海，难以受孕。故肾气不足、肾阳虚衰、肾精亏虚，均可导致不孕。

（2）肝郁：妇人平素情志不畅，精神抑郁，或性情急躁，暴怒伤肝，致肝的疏泄功能失常，以致肝郁气滞，气血失调，冲任不能相资，不能成孕。

2. 经络致病

《素问》云："督脉生病，女子不孕。"提出不孕与经络的联系。《格致余论》主"血海太热。"《女科经纶》引朱丹溪言"妇人久无子者，冲任脉中伏热也……内热则荣血枯。"经络之中，尤以冲任二脉最为重要。"冲为血海""冲为十二经脉之海"，能调节十二经的气血；"任主胞胎"，冲任损伤必然导致妇科诸疾。

3. 气血代谢异常

（1）血瘀：晋代医家皇甫谧《针灸甲乙经·妇人杂病》云："女子绝子，血在内不下，关元主之。"这是有关血瘀不孕的最早记载。血瘀气滞，经水失调，积于胞中；或令胞脉阻滞，则精难纳入，故难以受孕。

（2）痰湿：多见于肥胖之人，由于形体肥胖；或肆食膏粱厚味，损伤脾胃，失其健运之功，致使痰湿内生，气机不畅，胞脉受阻，不能成孕。

其中肾虚固然是导致不孕的根本原因，然而五脏相通，肝郁、痰湿、血瘀等因素均能影响肾脏功能，几种病机间亦可相互转化，或多种病因伴随出现，终而导致月经失调，胞络受阻以致不孕。

三、诊断要点与鉴别诊断

（一）诊断要点

从疾病定义上讲，对于不孕年限的界定是该病诊断的前提，未避孕未孕1年方可称之为不孕症。从疾病诊查上讲，通过男女双方全面检查找出不孕原因，是不孕症的诊断关键。女方检查步骤主要包括结婚年龄、性生活情况、月经史、既往史（如有无阑尾炎手术、妇科手术、甲状腺病、糖尿病等）、家族史、既往生育史以及男方健康状况。对继发不孕者尤其须要问清有无流产史、异位妊娠史、感染史等。此外，在体格检查中要注意第二性征的发育、内外生殖器的发育情况，有无畸形、包块、炎症、乳房溢乳等。

（二）鉴别要点

1.明确不孕与不育

不孕与不育不同，不孕是不能怀孕；不育是指能怀孕而不生育，即虽曾妊娠，但发生堕胎、滑胎、小产而告结局。不育的另一含义指男性不能生育。

2.鉴别原发与继发不孕

不孕有原发、继发之分，原发不孕是指婚后夫妇有效性生活12个月经周期以上不受孕者。继发不孕是指曾有过妊娠，而又有效性生活12个月经周期以上不能再次受孕者。

3.不孕症与暗产鉴别

暗产指早早孕期，胚胎初结而自然流产者。《叶氏女科证治·暗产须知》曰："惟一月堕胎，人皆不知有胎，但谓不孕，不知其已受孕而堕也"。相当于西医学的生化妊娠，此时孕妇尚未有明显的妊娠反应，或仅月经周期后错，一般不易觉察而导致之后就诊时误认为原发不孕，在早早孕期可以通过基础体温、早早孕试纸、血人绒毛膜促性腺素辅助检查明确诊断。

四、中医治疗

（一）辨证治疗

不孕症的辨证治疗要点在于辨明脏腑、经络气血、冲任、胞宫的状况。治疗重点是调理冲任、温肾暖宫、疏肝解郁、补益气血、燥湿化痰以及活血化瘀。

1.肾阳虚衰

主症： 婚久不孕，月经迟发，性欲冷淡，小腹冷痛，头晕耳鸣，腰膝酸软，夜尿频数，舌淡苔白，脉沉细弱。

治法： 温肾暖宫。

对此类肾阳虚衰、宫寒不孕的患者，治宜温肾暖宫，可佐以补心火之品。正如《傅青主女科·种子》所言："补心而即补肾，温肾而即温心，心肾之气旺，则心肾之火自生，心肾之火生，则胞胎之寒自散。而今胞胎既热，尚有施而不受者乎？"

方药： 温胞饮或右归丸。

温胞饮。人参、白术、巴戟天、补骨脂、杜仲、菟丝子、芡实、山药、肉桂、附子。

右归丸。熟地黄、制附子、肉桂、山药、山茱萸、菟丝子、鹿角胶、枸杞子、当归、杜仲。

2. 肝郁气滞

主症： 婚久不孕，月经或先或后，或经前腹痛，经前乳房胀痛，烦躁易怒，精神抑郁，舌暗红或有瘀斑，脉弦细。

治法： 疏肝解郁。

解肝气之郁，宣脾气之困，而心肾之气亦因之俱舒，所以腰脐利而任带通达，不必启胞脉之门，而胞脉自启，立"开郁种玉汤"治疗嫉妒不孕。

方药： 开郁种玉汤。白芍、香附、当归、白术、丹皮、茯苓、花粉。

3. 瘀阻胞宫

主症： 婚久不孕，月经多推后，经来腹痛，经色暗，有血块，舌质暗，苔薄白，脉弦细或细涩。

治法： 活血化瘀。

王清任善用活血化瘀之法治疗诸多疾病，其论治不孕亦获奇效。

方药： 少腹逐瘀汤。小茴香、干姜、延胡索、没药、当归、川芎、官桂、赤芍、蒲黄、五灵脂。

4. 痰湿瘀阻

主症： 婚久不孕，形体肥胖，月经经常推后，毛发稀疏，甚闭经不行，带下量多，头晕心悸，舌淡胖，苔白腻。

治法： 燥湿化痰。

朱丹溪首倡"躯脂满溢，闭塞子宫，宜行湿燥痰。"《傅青主女科》云："治法必须以泄水化痰为主。然徒泄水化痰，而不急补脾胃之气，则阳气不旺，湿痰不去，人先病矣"，提出补脾化痰治不孕之法。

方药： 苍附导痰汤。苍术、香附、陈皮、南星、枳壳、半夏、川芎、滑石、茯苓、神曲。

（二）专方治疗

1. 暖宫孕子丸

组成： 当归、白芍、川芎、熟地、阿胶、黄芪、续断、杜仲、香附、艾叶。

用法： 每服 8g，日服 2~3 次，温开水送服。

主治： 婚后久不受孕，经期后错，量少色淡，面色晦暗，腰酸腿软，性欲淡漠，小便清长，大便不实，舌质淡，苔薄白，脉沉细或沉迟。

2. 定坤丸

组成： 西洋参、白术、茯苓、熟地、当归、白芍、川芎、黄芪、阿胶、五味子、鹿茸、肉桂、艾叶、杜仲、续断、佛手、陈皮、厚朴、柴胡、香附、延胡索、丹皮、琥珀、龟甲、地黄、麦冬、黄芩

用法： 每服 1 丸，日服 2 次，温开水送服。

主治：婚后久不受孕，经期后错，量少色淡，面色晦暗，腰酸腿软，性欲淡漠，小便清长，大便不实，舌质淡，苔薄白，脉沉细或沉迟。

3. 妇科得生丸

组成：益母草、白芍、当归、羌活、柴胡、木香。

用法：每服1丸，日服2次，温开水送服。

主治：婚后久不受孕，经期先后不定，经期腹痛，量少色暗，夹有血块，经前乳房胀痛，精神抑郁，烦躁易怒，舌质正常或暗红，舌苔薄白，脉弦。

4. 十二温经丸

组成：吴茱萸、肉桂、当归、川芎、阿胶珠、白芍、麦冬、党参、生姜、半夏、牡丹皮、炙甘草。

用法：每服1丸，日服2次，温黄酒送服。

主治：婚后久不受孕，常有明显受寒史，经期后错，量少色暗，小腹常有冷感，喜温拒按，舌苔薄白，脉沉紧。

5. 二陈丸合越鞠丸

组成：陈皮、半夏、茯苓、甘草、生姜、香附、川芎、六神曲、栀子、枳壳、槟榔。

用法：每次服12g，日服2次，温开水或姜枣水送服。

主治：婚后久不受孕，形体肥胖，经期后错，甚或闭经，带下量多，质地黏稠，面色白，头晕心悸，胸闷恶心，舌苔白腻，脉滑。

（三）针灸治疗

针灸作为临床常用的治疗方法之一，在治疗妇科疾病中较常见。针灸既可以调经又可诱发排卵。对于肾虚、肝郁、血瘀等病机，可选用冲、任、督脉有关腧穴，肾、肝、脾经的腧穴共同治疗。常用穴位有三阴交、气海、太冲、关元、血海、归来、中极、大赫、脾俞、肾俞、命门、太溪、足三里等，其中以三阴交最常用，其次为气海、关元、子宫、血海、足三里、肾俞。

（四）其他

1. 中药敷贴

穴位敷贴法既具有穴位刺激作用，又能通过特定部位的吸收而发挥作用，从而达到治疗的目的。药物敷贴疗法，具有温煦气血、透达经络的直接作用，又能改善局部血液循环，还有利于炎症病灶的吸收，从而起到松解粘连、消散包块、活血祛瘀的作用。临床中采用生附子、透骨草、芒硝、桂枝各60g，丹参120g，吴茱萸、小茴香各5g，艾叶30g，路路通20g共为末，用白酒浸透、拌匀、装袋、蒸热置于关元穴上，保温热敷15~20分钟，从经来第一天开始，每晚1次，连续2周，配合中药内服，治疗输卵管阻塞性不孕症疗效较佳。

2. 灌肠法

将肛管或导尿管放置肛门内，将药物灌入直肠内，灌后保留 30~60 分钟，每天 1 次，10 天 1 个疗程，经期停用。用透骨草、皂角刺、土茯苓各 15g，威灵仙 12g，制乳香、没药、三棱、苦参各 9g，煎取 100ml 保留灌肠，配合中药辨证治疗输卵管病变所致不孕症效果尤佳。

五、名医专家经验方

（一）古代名医

1. 温经汤（张仲景）

东汉时期张仲景名方之一"金匮温经汤"又名"大温经汤"，在古今中医妇科广泛被应用，为一张多功能的方子。

组成：吴茱萸三两、当归二两、川芎二两、芍药二两、人参二两、桂枝二两、阿胶二两、生姜二两、牡丹皮二两、甘草二两、半夏半升、麦冬一升。上十二味，以水一斗，煮取三升，分温三服。

功效：主妇人少腹寒，久不受胎；兼治崩中去血，或月水来过多，及至期不来。

2. 补宫丸（《扁鹊心书》）

组成：当归二两、熟地二两、肉苁蓉二两、菟丝子二两、牛膝二两、肉桂一两、沉香一两、荜茇一两、吴茱萸一两、肉果一两、真血竭五钱、艾叶五钱。上为末，醋糊为丸，如梧桐子大，每服50 丸，酒或白汤送服。

功效：女人子宫久冷不孕，经事不调，致小腹连腰痛，面黄肌瘦，四肢无力，减食发热，夜多盗汗，赤白带下。

3. 乌鸡丸（张景岳）

组成：人参三两、怀生地三两、怀熟地三两、青蒿子三两、香附三两、鳖甲三两、白术二两、枣仁肉二两、枸杞二两、麦冬二两、云苓二两、地骨皮二两、丹皮二两、白芍二两、当归身二两半、川芎一两、甘草一两。

用法：先将上诸药备完听用；乃取丝毛乌骨白公鸡 1 只（约重 1 斤许者）扑倒，去毛、秽、头、足、肠杂不用，将鸡切作 4 块；先以鳖甲铺铜锅底，次入杂药，以免焦腐，渐加童便约斗许，煮至极烂，捞起晒干，为末，将鳖甲去裙，并鸡骨俱以原汁蘸炙至干，为末，同前药炼蜜为丸，如梧桐子大。

功效：妇人羸弱，血虚有热，经水不调，崩漏带下，骨蒸不能成胎者。

4. 养精种玉汤（傅山）

组成：大熟地 30g，当归 15g，白芍 15g，山萸肉 15g。

功效：肾亏血虚，身体瘦弱，久不受孕。

5. 开郁种玉汤（傅山）

组成：白芍 30g，香附 9g，当归 15g，白术 15g，丹皮 9g，茯苓 9g，天花粉 6g。

功效：妇人肝气郁结所致的不孕症。

6. 苍附导痰丸（万全）

组成：苍术、香附各 60g，陈皮、茯苓各 45g，枳壳、半夏、南星、炙甘草各 30g。

功效：开痰散结，祛湿解郁，行气活血。

7. 少腹逐瘀汤（王清任）

组成：小茴香 7 粒，干姜 6g，延胡索 3g，没药 6g，当归 9g，川芎 6g，官桂 3g，赤芍 6g，蒲黄 9g，五灵脂 6g。

功效：逐瘀荡胞，调经助孕。

（二）现代医家

1. 名老中医——韩冰

全国中医妇科名专家韩冰教授认为月经不调是引起不孕症最重要的因素之一，经本于肾，种子以补肾调经为要。月经的正常与否与肝肾功能失常及冲任功能失调密切相关。韩老旨遵前贤，十分重视肝肾功能在不孕症中的作用，以补肾调冲为治疗大法，在多年的临床实践中形成了配伍相对，形式独特的药对，药力专一，取效迅捷，随症加减，灵活运用，效果颇著。现就韩老治疗不孕症常用药对举隅简述如下：

（1）菟丝子＋覆盆子：二药相须，阴阳并补，肝肾同治，冲任得养，治疗肝肾不足、精血亏虚之不孕疗效显著。

（2）女贞子＋墨旱莲：古名二至丸，补肾养肝，凉血止血，凡妇科之肝肾阴虚的经期延长、经间期出血等所致的不孕之症皆可用之。

（3）续断＋桑寄生：两药合用，共奏补肝肾、调冲任之功，临床上对于因冲任不固、肝肾亏损引起的不孕症，功效奇捷，值得借鉴。

（4）沉香＋肉桂：两药配伍理气通络，温肾散寒，常用治寒凝痛经、宫寒不孕，亦用于输卵管阻塞不通之不孕。

（5）黄精＋制首乌：二者共奏补肾阴益精血之功，肾精充足，血海充盈，方能促进卵子生长以助孕。

（6）丹参＋鸡血藤："一味丹参，功同四物"，丹参活血调经而不伤血，与鸡血藤合用既能活血，又能补血，对血瘀、血虚之证均宜，用于治血虚夹瘀，血海不能按时满溢之月经量少，月经后期而致之不孕。

（7）鹿角霜＋紫石英：鹿角霜温通督脉，紫石英引气血下行，温肾养肝暖宫，二药合用，补肾壮阳，固摄冲任，又温肾养肝，调经暖宫，用于女子虚寒经闭，宫冷不孕。

此外，韩冰教授根据肾气不足，瘀血内停，湿浊继生及癥瘕形成的不孕症拟成妇痛宁，其药物组成为三棱、莪术、血竭、丹参、穿山甲、皂角刺、海藻、鳖甲、薏苡仁等。三棱、莪术、血竭、丹参、穿山甲、皂角刺等活血化瘀，海藻、鳖甲等软坚散结，薏苡仁渗湿，全方组成结构严谨，随症加减，疗效显著。韩冰教授结合自己多年的临床经验，灵活加减。兼肾虚者，予肉苁蓉、巴戟天、鹿角霜等补肾化瘀；偏肝郁气滞者，酌加柴胡、乌药、香附、橘核等理气化瘀；寒凝血瘀者加用桂枝、细辛等温经通络、化瘀止痛；兼挟痰湿者常以川贝、皂刺、山慈菇等化痰湿、散瘀结。

2. 天津哈氏——哈孝贤

哈氏医学第四代传人哈孝贤在不孕症治疗中顺应周期，以承阴阳，将月经周期分为四期调理。

（1）经后期：用滋肾柔肝、养阴补血之品，以充血海，益冲任，药用熟地黄、山萸肉、枸杞子、阿胶、菟丝子、白芍、麦冬、当归等。

（2）氤氲期：在滋阴补血的基础上，育肾通络，加仙茅、淫羊藿、紫石英等以助阳运气，加王不留行、路路通、鸡血藤、刘寄奴等以通络活血，为受孕创造先决条件。

（3）排卵后期：常用桑寄生、炒杜仲、菟丝子、续断等温肾益精之品，使阳气充盛，如若受孕，更可固肾安胎。

（4）经前及月经期：此期如未受孕，多用逍遥散加减，因势利导，使经行畅达；如已受孕，则继以寿胎丸方加减以固肾安胎。

3. 江湾蔡氏——蔡小荪

蔡氏妇科蔡小荪教授认为肾气不足、冲任亏损是不孕症的主要病机。临床上采用周期疗法，根据月经周期，设孕Ⅰ、孕Ⅱ为基本方。孕Ⅰ方：云苓12g，生、熟地各9g，怀牛膝9g，路路通9g，炙甲片9g，公丁香2.5g，淫羊藿12g，石楠叶9g，制黄精12g，桂枝3g，以育肾通络促排卵。孕Ⅱ方：云苓12g，生、熟地各9g，石楠叶9g，紫石英12g，女贞子9g，狗脊12g，淫羊藿12g，仙茅9g，胡芦巴9g，鹿角霜9g，肉苁蓉9g，以育肾培元健黄体。每于月经净后开始服孕Ⅰ方7剂；约至排卵期换服孕Ⅱ方8剂，经行时可随症调治。通过育肾周期疗法，促使月经规律，抓住时机以受孕。

4. 浦东王氏——王辉萍

王氏妇科的王辉萍教授认为不孕症肝肾不足为本，而气滞、血瘀、痰湿等为标，治疗以调补肝肾为主，用加减定经汤，疏肝肾之气，补肝肾之精。药用菟丝子20g，熟地12g，当归12g，白芍10g，柴胡12g，淫羊藿15g，巴戟天15g，山萸肉12g，丹皮12g，广木香10g为基本方。对于气血亏虚为主的患者，治疗以益气养血、活血通经，药用党参12g，黄芪15g，当归15g，白芍12g，川芎8g，丹参12g，桃仁12g，怀牛膝15g，广木香10g为基本方，使后天生化有源，冲任满盈，月事按时而下。

5. 海派名医——庞泮池

海派中医妇科名家庞泮池教授有治疗不孕症的三大法宝，即：通管、促卵、健黄体。

（1）通管：所谓"通管"即输卵管再通治疗，自拟通管汤：当归9g，熟地9g，赤芍9g，白芍9g，川芎9g，桃仁12g，红花9g，生茜草9g，海螵蛸12g，制香附12g，路路通9g，石菖蒲9g，生薏苡仁12g，皂刺9g，败酱草15g，红藤15g。活血化瘀通络，常服久服，缓图其功。

（2）促排卵：排卵功能障碍是不孕症常见病因，庞教授认为主要病机是肾虚，治疗当补肾调冲。方以四物汤养血和血，加黄精、菟丝子、杜仲、肉苁蓉、淫羊藿补肾促排卵；紫石英、石楠叶温阳暖宫；茺蔚子、泽兰叶、王不留行子、牛膝活血通经。

（3）健黄体：黄体功能不足不利于受精卵的着床与生长，易造成不孕或先兆流产。庞教授认为其病机是脾肾不足、精血亏少，排卵期阴阳转化不及，即能摄精也难成孕。方取以圣愈汤为基础，加菟丝子、肉苁蓉、黄精、泽兰叶、茺蔚子，酌用当归、川芎、香附等药活血而不伤胎。

六、名医专家典型医案

（一）韩冰教授验案——肝肾亏虚

徐某 女，29岁。

初诊：2012年2月6日。结婚3年，夫妻生活规律，未避孕未孕。平素月经规律6~7/28~30天，量少，色红，少许血块，痛经（-），孕产史G1P0（2009年人流1次）。LMP：2012.1.22。性激素六项（M3）：FSH 6.54 mIU/ml，LH 1.57 mIU/ml，E2 23.00 mIU/ml，PRL 11.43 mIU/ml，P 0.30 mIU/ml，T 0.57 mIU/ml。B超及妇科检查无异常，男方精液常规正常。刻下：腰酸，夜寐安，二便调，舌淡暗，苔薄白，脉弦细。

西医诊断：继发性不孕。

中医诊断：不孕，肝肾亏虚证。

治法：补肝肾，调冲任，益精血。

处方：菟丝子30g，覆盆子15g，补骨脂15g，巴戟天10g，石斛20g，黄精30g，何首乌30g，丹参30g，鸡血藤30g，月季花10g，橘叶10g，鹿角霜15g，紫石英30g。

二诊：2012年2月20日。患者前1日月经来潮，经量较前明显增多，色红，无血块，腰痛明显好转，舌红略暗，苔薄白，脉沉。考虑患者正值经期，平素肝肾亏虚，精血不足，治以四物汤加减。

处方：熟地20g，当归10g，川芎10g，丹参30g，赤芍20g，桂枝10g，干姜6g，鸡血藤30g，橘核20g，荔枝核20g，益母草30g，月季花10g，鹿角霜15g。

三诊：2012年2月27日。LMP：2012年2月19日，6日净，量可，色红，无血块，舌红，苔薄白，脉略沉。患者正值经后期，阴生阳长，治疗以平补肝肾阴阳为主。

处方：菟丝子30g，覆盆子15g，巴戟天10g，补骨脂15g，石斛20g，何首乌30g，黄精30g，丹参30g，鸡血藤30g，紫石英30g，紫河车10g。

随证加减治疗6个月，患者月经逾期未至，查血HCG 123 mIU/mL，停经50天查B超示：宫内早孕，可见胎心胎芽，电话随访至患者顺产一子，母子体健。

按：以上遣方用药是韩老治疗不孕症长期实践的经验总结和精华所在，尤其其中药对的应用，体现了中医药配伍的特色，具有丰富的内涵，为临床不孕症的治疗用药拓宽思路，值得我们借鉴学习。

（二）哈孝贤教授——肝郁肾虚

刘某 女，30岁。

初诊：2014年1月22日。夫妻生活规律，未避孕未孕1年余。13岁初潮，平素月经规律5~6/26~28天，量少色黑，少许血块，痛经不明显，孕产史G1P0（2012年人流1次）。LMP：2014年1月12日。患者诉排卵期前后数日常小腹疼痛难忍。外院输卵管造影示：左侧输卵管通并远端粘连，右侧输卵管排出通畅。刻下：腰酸，腹隐痛，口干，尿频，带下多，舌红、苔白腻，脉沉滑。

西医诊断：盆腔炎，左侧输卵管远端轻度粘连，不孕症。

中医诊断：不孕，肝郁肾虚证。

治法：益肾养阴，疏肝通络。

处方：桑寄生30g，杜仲15g，生、熟地各15g，桑螵蛸30g，刘寄奴15g，麦冬30g，石斛15g，北沙参30g，半夏15g，黄连片9g，竹茹9g，豆蔻9g，穿山甲9g，皂角刺15g，丝瓜络9g，路路通9g。

二诊：2014年2月2日。患者服上剂后，排卵期腹痛减轻，尿频除，带下减少，口干缓解，舌淡红、苔薄白，脉沉细滑。治拟疏肝调冲。

处方：丹参30g，怀牛膝20g，皂刺15g，刘寄奴15g，石斛20g，北沙参30g，柴胡9g，香附9g，青皮9g，路路通15g，鸡血藤15g，王不留行15g，穿山甲9g。

三诊：2014年2月13日。LMP：2014年2月9日。刻诊：经将截，腹痛不甚，少量赤带，舌淡红、苔薄白微腻，脉沉滑。拟滋阴调冲通络。

处方：女贞子15g，墨旱莲15g，熟地30g，麦冬30g，北沙参30g，石斛20g，白豆蔻9g，王不留行15g，鸡血藤15g，皂刺15g，黄连6g。

四诊：2014年2月21日。服药后无不适，腰酸，脉沉滑，舌淡红、苔薄。拟益肾通络。

处方：当归15g，川芎9g，柴胡9g，杜仲15g，寄生30g，续断15g，路路通15g，鸡血藤30g，王不留行15g，白芥子15g，穿山甲9g，皂刺15g。循此法，加减调理4月。

五诊：2014年7月6日。患者月经逾期未潮，查血HCG：191.64 mIU/ml，黄体酮22.29 ng/ml，诉腰酸，乳房轻胀，便溏，舌红、苔薄白，脉滑数。拟益肾健脾，清热安胎。

处方：菟丝子30g，炒白术15g，太子参15g，杜仲炭15g，寄生30g，续断15g，黄芩6g，黄连6g，藿香9g，砂仁6g，阿胶珠15g。

守方调治至孕12周，逐渐减药至停药。后电话随访顺产一男婴，母子体健。

按：经前与经期哈老师善用疏肝通络、滋阴调冲治法，因势利导，重在调理气血，使经血畅行；月经将尽，血海空虚，则重在滋养肝肾，佐以活血通络；排卵后期，阴极化阳，则治以益肾通络、顺应阴阳之变。受孕后血清HCG、黄体酮值稍低、腰酸，有流产之虞，以寿胎丸加减化裁、健脾益肾、清热安胎，后顺利分娩，结局良好。

七、预防调护

中华医学博大精深，尤其针对疑难杂症的治疗，经验丰富，治疗效果明显，而"求嗣"文化作为西医学中的疑难杂症，中医在治疗中有着很大的优势，且重视"未病先防"。

（一）预防

（1）遵循求嗣之道。在选择婚配、年龄、交合等方面应符合"求嗣"之道。

（2）治疗痼疾。在种子前期先调月经，以及治疗各种相关疾病，尤其是带下病。

（二）调护

1. 畅达情志

通常患者心理压力大，心理承受力差，患者和家属间经常出现矛盾，因此，需加强对病患的心理疏导工作，例如：向病患及家属做好解释工作，消除他们的顾虑，减轻病患的烦恼，使病患保持情绪舒畅，夫妻感情和顺。

2. 加强锻炼

应劝导病患加强体育锻炼，强化体质，以增强肌体抗病能力。以此达到促进病患身心健康的目的，以提高中医治疗的疗效。

3. 调控饮食

应叮嘱病患，注意加强营养。要求病患的饮食营养全面，不可偏食、挑食。同时，饮食需有规律并保持节制，不可暴饮暴食，不可吸烟、饮酒。对于体形肥胖的患者，应严格控制脂肪和糖含量较高的食物的摄入，还需配合运动采取相关的减肥措施，但不能服用减肥药物，以免引发内分泌失调。

4. 规范习惯

对病患的日常生活习惯加以规范，叮嘱病患注意以下几点：应注意经期卫生，保持外阴清洁，每日以温开水清洗外阴，不可随意用洗液冲洗阴道以免破坏阴道的自然防御功能；经期不可过于劳累，不可过于紧张，不可有性生活，注意保暖；夫妻生活有节，以免耗伤肾精；建议日常监测基础体温，掌握排卵日期，利于受孕。

（王　卫）

参考文献

［1］田代华. 校勘学［M］. 北京：中国医药科技出版社，1995.

［2］李经纬，余瀛鳌，蔡景峰，等. 中医大词典［M］.2 版. 北京：人民卫生出版社，2004.

［3］薛己. 薛氏医案［M］. 北京：中国中医药出版社，1997.

［4］傅青主. 傅青主女科［M］. 北京：人民卫生出版社，2006.

［5］寇金矛，寇峥. 针刺治疗无排卵性不孕症 50 例临床观察［J］. 中医学报，1997，12（4）：45-46.

［6］班旭，何川. 内外合治输卵管阻塞性不孕症 86 例［J］. 北京中医药，1996，15（1）：33-34.

［7］贝润浦. 治疗输卵管病变所致不孕 150 例报告［J］. 中医杂志，1992，33（5）：37-38.

［8］韩延华，白兰，姚天天. 傅青主从脏腑论治不孕症之探析［J］. 辽宁中医杂志，2011，38（2）：267.

［9］徐瑾，罗玲英，吴铁荣. 二至丸的临床应用与剂量关系研究［J］. 亚太传统医药，2011，7（1）：132.

［10］常暖，韩冰，李同玺，等. 妇痛宁治疗子宫内膜异位症临床和实验研究［J］. 中医杂志，1997，38（8）：488-490.

［11］马平仲，吴颖秀. 韩冰教授治疗子宫内膜异位症伴发不孕的临床经验［J］. 湖南中医药导报，1998，4（7）：13.

［12］王桂萍，玄明实. 哈孝贤治疗不孕症经验［J］. 中医杂志，2014，55（3）：195-196.

［13］张亚楠，黄素英，胡国华. 海派中医妇科流派调经助孕经验浅述［J］. 四川中医，2012，30（6）：33-34.

反复呼吸道感染

Recurrent
Respiratory
Tract
Infection

一、概述

反复呼吸道感染是小儿常见疾病之一，临床凡一年内发生上、下呼吸道感染的次数超出正常范围，称为反复呼吸道感染。上呼吸道感染包括鼻炎、咽炎、扁桃体炎；下呼吸道感染为支气管炎、毛细支气管炎及肺炎等疾病。本病一年四季均可患病，以冬春气温变化剧烈时尤易反复，夏天有自然缓解的趋势，一般到学龄期前后感染次数明显减少。发病年龄多见于6个月~6岁的小儿，其中1~3岁的幼儿更易患病。若反复呼吸道感染日久不愈，易发生慢性鼻炎、咳嗽及肾炎、风湿病等疾患，严重影响小儿生长发育与身心健康。相当于中医古代医籍中的"自汗易感"，近年来常称为"易感儿"或"反复呼吸道感染"（简称"复感儿"）。

中医药防治本病，强调辨证施治，内治外治结合，重点在"防"，在改善小儿体质、增强抗病能力方面具有一定优势，并越来越受到人们重视。

二、病因病机

（一）中医

小儿反复呼吸道感染多因禀赋不足、喂养不当、用药不当、调护失宜、素禀体热等。本病病机责之于虚实两端：虚为正气不足，卫外不固；实为邪热内伏，遇感乃发。

1. 禀赋不足，体质虚弱

先天禀赋不足，如父母体弱多病或妊娠时患病，或早产、多胎、胎气孱弱，生后腠理疏松，肌肤娇嫩，不耐邪气侵袭，一感即病。

2. 喂养不当，脾胃受损

人工喂养、母乳不足，过早断奶或换乳不慎、辅食添加不当或偏食、厌食，营养不良，饮食精微摄取不足，脾胃虚弱，生化无力，肺脾气虚，外邪易趁机侵袭；或恣食生冷寒凉、肥甘厚腻之品，伤其脾胃，损伤正气，易感外邪而发病。

3. 调护失宜，不耐寒热

患儿缺少户外活动，日照不足，肌肤柔弱，卫外不固，对气候突变适应能力弱，感冒随即发生。或家长未能根据天气变化或季节交替，及时为患儿添减衣被，调护失宜，故易发病，或他人感染，一染即病。

4. 用药不当，损伤正气

外感之后过服解表之剂，损伤阳气，卫阳受损，表卫气虚，营卫不和，营阴不守而汗多，卫阳不固而易感，故易反复感邪。

5. 素禀体热，遇感乃发

平素嗜食肥甘厚腻、辛辣炙煿之品致肺胃蕴热或胃肠积热，或热病之后，余邪未清，或久居湿地，湿热内蕴，或素体热盛，邪热留伏，一旦外邪侵袭，新感易受，留邪内发，则生本病。

总之，本病的发病有虚实之分：小儿脏腑娇嫩，肌肤薄弱，易感外邪，虚者主要责之于肺、脾、肾之气阴亏损，正气不足，卫外不固，加之喂养不当、调护失宜，一遇外邪侵袭即可发病。实者主要责之于肺胃，患儿嗜食辛辣肥甘厚腻或热病余邪未清，邪热留伏于肺胃，或积于胃肠，如感外邪，则易见外寒内热之证。若反复呼吸道感染久病不愈，正气受损日益严重，患儿抵抗力不断下降，则易变生他病。

（二）西医

反复呼吸道感染的形成与小儿本身的呼吸系统解剖生理特点及免疫功能尚未成熟密切相关。其中，反复上呼吸道感染的常见病因还包括：微量元素、维生素缺乏，环境污染，被动吸烟，慢性上呼吸道病灶，如鼻炎、鼻窦炎、扁桃体、腺样体肥大等。反复下呼吸道感染特别是反复肺炎的患儿多数存在基础疾病，包括先天性或获得性呼吸系统解剖异常、吸入、先天性心脏病、免疫缺陷病和原发性纤毛运动障碍等。

三、诊断要点与鉴别诊断

（一）诊断要点

根据年龄、潜在的原因及部位不同，将反复呼吸道感染分为反复上呼吸道感染和反复下呼吸道感染，后者又可分为反复气管支气管炎和反复肺炎（表1）。

表1　反复呼吸道感染判断条件

年龄（岁）	反复上呼吸道感染（次/年）	反复下呼吸道感染（次/年）	
		反复气管支气管炎	反复肺炎
0~2	7	3	2
2^+~5	6	2	2
5^+~14	5	2	2

注：①两次感染间隔时间至少7天以上。②若上呼吸道感染次数不够，可以将上、下呼吸道感染次数相加，反之则不能。但若反复感染是以下呼吸道为主，则应定义为反复下呼吸道感染。③确定次数需连续观察1年。④反复肺炎是指1年内反复患肺炎2次，肺炎需由肺部体征和影像学证实，2次肺炎诊断期间肺炎体征和影像学改变应完全消失。

临床诊断该病，应注意寻找发病原因，如护理不当，缺乏锻炼，迁移住处，入托幼机构起始阶段，环境污染，微量元素缺乏或其他营养成分搭配不合理等。对于反复肺炎患儿，除考虑致病微生物外，需认真寻找反复肺炎的基础病变，如原发性免疫缺陷病（原发性抗体缺陷病、细胞免疫缺陷病、联合免疫缺陷病、补体缺陷病、吞噬功能缺陷病以及其他原发性免疫缺陷病等）、先天性肺实质异常、肺血管发育异常、先天性气道发育异常、先天性心脏畸形、原发性纤毛运动障碍，囊性纤维性变、气道内阻塞或管外压迫、支气管扩张、反复吸入。临床宜详细询问病史，注意患儿体质辨识，根据病情需要进行免疫学、胸部X线、微量元素检测及耳鼻喉科检查，必要时选择肺功能、支气管镜，肺部CT和气道、血管重建显影等检查。

（二）鉴别诊断

与鼻鼽鉴别。"鼻鼽"为中医病名，西医称"变应性鼻炎"或"过敏性鼻炎"，临床以突然和反复发作的鼻痒、鼻塞、流清涕、喷嚏频频为主要特征，可伴眼痒等眼部过敏症状。其发病常与接触蒿草、花粉等异物有关，多具过敏体质及变应性鼻炎家族史。

四、中医治疗

（一）辨证治疗

1. 辨证要点

本病主要以八纲辨证及脏腑辨证为主，临证首辨虚实，继辨脏腑。

（1）辨虚实：若患儿形体瘦弱或虚胖，常见多汗气短、倦怠乏力、纳差便溏、面色少华，或生长发育迟缓等症者，多属虚证；若素体热盛，平素嗜食肥甘厚味，常见口臭或口舌易生疮、手足心热、大便干结者，多属实证。

（2）辨脏腑：正虚者，以肺、脾、肾之气阴虚损为主。若见自汗、气短懒言、声音变低者，多为肺虚；面黄少华、倦怠乏力、食欲不振、腹胀便溏者，多属脾虚；生长发育迟缓、骨骼不坚甚则畸形者，常为肾虚。偏气虚者，面黄少华，气短乏力，语声低微，舌淡嫩，边有齿痕，脉细无力；偏阴虚者，低热盗汗，手足心热，口干咽燥，舌红少津，脉细数。

邪实者，以肺胃积热证居多，常见咽微红，口臭或口舌易生疮，手足心热，腹胀，便干，苔厚或黄，脉滑数。

2. 治疗原则

本病以虚证为主，治疗以补虚为要，临床强调把握用药时机，或健脾补肺，或益气养阴，或温补脾肾；若属实证者，多以清泻肺胃为主。该治疗原则用于反复呼吸道感染患儿没有出现急性呼吸道感染症状期间，治疗期间如果出现呼吸道感染，应根据不同的疾病，结合患儿体质特点，给予相应治疗。

3. 证治分类

（1）肺脾气虚

主症： 反复外感，气短，多汗，唇口色淡，面黄少华，纳呆食少，大便不调，舌质淡红，脉细无力或指纹淡。

辨证： 本证多见于后天失调，喂养不当，乏乳早断之小儿，或者久病耗气者，临床以反复外感，气短多汗，面黄少华，纳差，大便不调为特征。

治法： 健脾益气，补肺固表。

方药： 玉屏风散加味。黄芪、防风、白术、党参、山药、牡蛎、陈皮、甘草。

方解： 黄芪甘温，内补脾肺之气，外可固表止汗；白术、党参、山药健脾益气，助黄芪以加强益气固表之功；防风走表而散风邪，合黄芪、白术以益气祛邪；牡蛎敛表止汗；陈皮健脾化痰；甘草调和诸药；全方含补中寓疏、散中寓补之意。

加减： 汗多者加五味子；纳少厌食者，加鸡内金、焦三仙；便溏者，加炒薏苡仁、茯苓；便秘者，加生大黄、枳壳。

（2）营卫失调

主症：屡受外邪，反复感冒，恶风畏寒，平素汗多，汗出不温，肌肉松弛，面色少华，四肢欠温，舌质淡红，苔薄白，脉无力或指纹淡紫。

辨证：本证多见于素体肺气虚、卫阳不足的小儿，或感邪后治疗不当，过服解表发汗药，汗出过多而伤阳，以致卫阳不固，营阴外泄，外邪易侵。临床以喂养不当，乏乳早断之小儿，或者久病耗气者，临床以恶风畏寒，平素汗多，汗出不温为特征。

治法：扶正固表，调护营卫。

方药：黄芪桂枝五物汤加味。黄芪、芍药、桂枝、生姜、大枣、生龙骨、生牡蛎。

方解：黄芪甘温补气，补在表之卫气；桂枝散风寒而温经通痹；芍药养血和营而通血痹；生姜辛温，疏散风邪；大枣甘温、养血益气；生龙骨、生牡蛎固表止汗。

加减：兼有咳嗽者加百部、杏仁、款冬花；身热未清者加青蒿、连翘。

（3）气阴两虚

主症：反复外感，面色潮红，手足心热，或低热，盗汗或自汗，口干，神疲乏力，纳呆食少，大便偏干，舌质红，苔少或花剥，脉细数，或指纹淡红。

辨证：本证多见于素体阴虚，或屡感热病、嗜食辛热燥性食品伤阴者。临床以面色潮红，口干，大便偏干为特征。

治法：养阴润肺，益气健脾。

方药：生脉散加味。人参、麦门冬、五味子、白术、北沙参、生牡蛎。

方解：人参甘温，益元气，补肺气，生津液；麦门冬甘寒养阴清热，润肺生津；人参、麦冬合用益气养阴；五味子酸温，敛肺止汗，生津止渴；白术健脾益气；北沙参养阴清肺，益胃生津；生牡蛎固表止汗。

加减：偏气虚者，加黄芪；纳差加砂仁、鸡内金；大便干结加瓜蒌仁、柏子仁；盗汗低热加地骨皮、牡丹皮。

（4）脾肾两虚

主症：反复感冒，甚则咳喘，面白无华，肌肉松弛，多汗易汗，睡眠欠安，食少纳呆，大便溏泄，立、行、齿、发、语迟，或鸡胸龟背，腰膝酸软，形寒肢冷，夜尿多，舌苔薄白，脉数无力。

辨证：本证多因先天禀赋不足，后天调养失调。临床以面白无华，肌肉松弛，生长发育迟缓，腰膝酸软，形寒肢冷为特征。

治法：温补肾阳，健脾益气。

方药：金匮肾气丸加味。地黄、茯苓、山药、山茱萸、牡丹皮、泽泻、桂枝、附子、人参、甘草、白术。

方解：地黄、山茱萸补益肾阴而摄精气；山药、茯苓健脾渗湿；泽泻泄肾中水邪；牡丹皮清肝胆相火；桂枝、附子温补命门真火；白术、人参健脾益气；甘草调和诸药。

加减：五迟者加鹿角霜、补骨脂、生牡蛎；汗多者加黄芪、煅龙骨；低热者加鳖甲、地骨皮；

阳虚者加鹿茸、紫河车、肉苁蓉。

（5）肺胃积热

主症： 反复外感，咽微红，口臭、口舌易生疮，汗多而黏，夜寐欠安，手足心热，大便干结，舌质红，苔厚或黄，脉滑数。

辨证： 本证多见于平素嗜食肥甘辛辣食品或素体内热者。临床以口臭、口舌易生疮，大便干结为特征。

治法： 清泻肺胃。

方药： 凉膈散加减。连翘、栀子、黄芩、淡豆豉、薄荷、桔梗、牛蒡子、芦根、大黄、朴硝、竹叶、生石膏、甘草。

方解： 黄芩、栀子苦寒泄降，清泻胸膈邪热；连翘、薄荷辛凉轻清，清散心胸邪热；淡豆豉解肌发表，宣郁除烦；桔梗宣肺气；牛蒡子疏散风热；芦根清热生津，除烦；大黄、芒硝、生石膏泻火通便，引邪热下行；竹叶清心利尿，导热外出；甘草清热润燥，调和诸药。

加减： 口舌生疮加栀子、通草；口臭者加黄连、山楂；脘腹胀者加枳壳、莱菔子。

（二）中成药

（1）玉屏风口服液：用于肺脾气虚证，1岁以下每次5ml，2~5岁5~10ml，5岁以上10ml，每日3次，口服。

（2）槐杞黄颗粒：用于气阴两虚证，1~3岁每次5g，3~12岁10g，每日2次，口服。

（3）童康片：用于肺脾两虚证偏脾气虚者，每次3~4片，每日4次，嚼碎后吞服。

（4）龙牡壮骨颗粒：用于脾肾两虚证，2岁以下每次5g，2~7岁每次7g，7岁以上每次10g，每日3次，冲服。

（5）清降片：用于肺胃积热证，1~3岁每次3片，每日2次；3~6岁每次4片，每日3次；6岁以上每次6片，每日3次，口服。

（三）针灸治疗

（1）耳压法：取穴肺、脾、大肠、肾、咽喉、气管、内分泌、皮质下、神门、脑干、耳尖（放血）。先将耳廓皮肤用75%酒精棉球消毒，取0.4cm×0.4cm方形胶布，中心贴1粒王不留行籽，对准耳穴贴压，用手轻按片刻，6日为1个疗程。

（2）穴位注射法：双侧足三里穴位注射黄芪注射液。常规注射消毒，得气后注射，每次每穴0.2~0.3ml。隔3~4天注射1次，1周2次，4周为1个疗程。

（四）推拿治疗

（1）捏脊疗法：操作时用双手的中指、无名指和小指握成半拳状，食指半屈，拇指伸直对准食指前半段，然后顶住患儿皮肤，拇、食指前移，提拿皮肉。自尾椎两旁双手交替向前，推动至大椎两旁，算作捏脊 1 遍。每次反复捏 6 遍。每天捏 1 次，每周治疗 5 天，4 周为 1 个疗程。

（2）四时捏脊疗法：在捏脊基础上，春季加揉按肝俞、肺俞；夏季加揉按心俞、小肠俞；秋季加揉按肺俞、大肠俞；冬季加揉按肾俞、膀胱俞。

（3）四时辨证捏脊疗法基本处方：四时捏脊、按揉风池、头面四大手法（开天门、推坎宫、运太阳、揉耳背高骨）。

①肺脾气虚证加补肺经、擦肺俞、运内八卦、补脾经、揉足三里。

②气阴两虚证加揉气海、补肺经、补脾经、揉二马、清天河水、推天柱骨。

③脾肾两虚证加补脾经、补肾经、揉三阴交、揉涌泉、推三关。

④营卫失调证加补肺经、补脾经、揉肾顶、揉外劳宫、推三关。

⑤肺胃积热证加清肺经、清胃经、退六腑、顺时针摩腹、揉膊阳池。

（五）中药外敷

应用白芥子 3 份，细辛 2 份，甘遂 1 份，皂荚 1 份，五倍子 3 份，冰片 0.052 份，共研细末。每次 1~2g，姜汁调成糊状，贴敷于穴位上，以双侧肺俞为主穴，配合大椎、膈俞等其他穴位，外用胶布固定，每年的初伏、中伏、末伏以及一九、二九、三九的前 3 天，各治疗 1 次，共 6 次。

五、名医专家经验方

（一）抗感至宝口服液（李少川）

适应证：小儿反复呼吸道感染肺脾气虚证。

组成：藿香、厚朴、陈皮、半夏、六曲、扁豆、柴胡、前胡、桔梗、枳壳、羌活、独活、川芎、赤芍、升麻、葛根。

用法：3 岁以下每次 6ml，3~6 岁每次 10ml，6 岁以上每次 20ml，每日 3 次，1 个月为 1 个疗程。

（二）防感合剂（江育仁）

适应证：小儿反复呼吸道感染营卫失调证。

组成：桂枝、黄芪、甘草、白芍、干姜、大枣等。

用法：3 岁以下每次 10ml，3~6 岁每次 15ml，6 岁以上每次 20ml，每日 2 次，2 个月为 1 个疗程。

（三）健益方（虞坚尔）

适应证：小儿反复呼吸道感染肺脾气虚证。

组成：生黄芪、炒白术、防风、法半夏、陈皮、茯苓、黄芩、甘草、地龙、车前子、辛夷。

用法：每日 1 剂，水煎取汁 100ml，早晚分服。

（四）壮尔颗粒（王雪峰）

适应证： 小儿反复呼吸道感染气阴两虚证。

组成： 生黄芪、生地黄、太子参、丹参、香菇、甘草。

用法： 6 岁以下者每次 4g，每日 2 次；6 岁以上者每次 8g，每日 2 次，连用 1 个月为 1 个疗程。

（五）参芪固本汤（韩新民）

适应证： 小儿反复呼吸道感染肺脾气虚证。

组成： 党参、炙黄芪、白术、防风、山药、百合、百部、陈皮、炙甘草。

用法： 每日口服 1 剂，3~4 岁每日服用煎剂 60~100ml，5~14 岁每日服用煎剂 100~150ml，服药时间为 1 个月。

（六）纳气敷脐散方（王力宁）

适应证： 反复呼吸道感染肺脾气虚证、气阴两虚证。

组成： 吴茱萸、胡椒、五倍子、丁香、苍术等。

用法： 贴敷于神阙穴。

（七）防感香囊（韩新民）

适应证： 小儿反复呼吸道感染肺脾气虚证。

组成： 苍术、白术、石菖蒲、白芷、细辛、冰片。

用法： 昼间置于胸前贴身口袋，夜间放置于枕边，每 10 日更换 1 次，连续使用 4 次。

六、名医专家典型医案

李少川医案——肺脾气虚

王某 男，3 岁 8 个月。

初诊： 2004 年 2 月 1 日。患儿平素面黄形瘦，纳差便干。一年内感冒 8 次，肺炎 2 次。患儿为早产儿，气候稍变则易感，诊时流涕咳嗽，晨起、夜间为重，时觉脐周腹痛，舌质淡红，舌苔薄黄，脉浮细弱。

诊断： 反复呼吸道感染，属肺脾气虚证。

辨证： 脾失健运，肺失宣肃，卫外不固。

治法： 疏解清化，调理脾胃。

处方：藿香 5g，羌活 3g，独活 3g，柴胡 5g，前胡 6g，枳壳 5g，桔梗 6g，半夏 5g，川芎 3g，陈皮 5g，云苓 5g，川朴 5g，赤芍 5g，升麻 5g，葛根 3g，六曲 5g，甘草 3g，7 剂。煎汤分次频服，2 日 1 剂。

二诊：2005 年 2 月 5 日。咳止纳增，腹痛消失，大便尚结，脉细无力。前方加熟军 3g，继以调理。

三诊：2005 年 3 月 6 日。患儿家属代诉，以上方调服 2 个月，胃纳大开，体质渐壮。共服药 40 余剂，近 1 年未患感冒。

按语：患儿肺脾气虚则体弱易感，肺脾气虚的关键是脾虚，脾气不足，母病及子，则肺脾两虚。在治疗上勿见脾虚补脾，肺虚补肺，而是要从整体出发，调整机体气机运化，既要顾及太阳之表、少阳之枢，又要注意到阳明肠胃之里。总而言之为脾虚宜健不宜补，肺虚宜疏不宜固。

本方系《幼科铁镜》天保采薇汤化裁而成，方中藿香、厚朴、陈皮、半夏、六曲芳香化浊，和胃健脾；柴胡、前胡、桔梗、枳壳疏解少阳，宣通肺气；羌活、独活，用其辛苦微温之气，以顾少阴肾经，解太阳之表；川芎、赤芍活血行气，适用于久病入血，气机不畅；葛根、升麻能升发脾胃清阳之气，可升清降浊，调和营卫。

七、预防与调护

（一）预防

（1）注意环境卫生，避免污染，室内空气要流通，适当户外活动，多晒太阳，按时预防接种。

（2）感冒流行期间不去公共场所。家中有人感冒时可用食醋熏蒸室内：每立方米空间用食醋 2~5ml，加水 1~2 倍，置容器内，加热至全部气化。每日 1 次，连续 3~5 日。

（3）避免接触过敏物质。

（二）调护

（1）饮食合理，富于营养，不偏嗜饮食。

（2）避风寒，勿吹冷风，汗出较多时，及时擦干，洗澡时尤应注意。

（李新民）

参考文献

［1］马融，韩新民．中医儿科学［M］．2版．北京：人民卫生出版社，2012．

［2］汪受传，俞景茂．全国高等中医药院校研究生规划教材：中医儿科临床研究［M］．北京：人民卫生出版社，2009．

［3］赵顺英，胡仪吉，陈慧中，等．反复呼吸道感染的临床概念和处理原则［J］．中华儿科杂志，2008，46（2）：108-110．

［4］马融．李少川．儿科经验集［M］．北京：人民卫生出版社，2013．

［5］马融，王萍芬，郑玉梅，等．防感合剂防治小儿反复呼吸道感染的临床研究［J］．中西医结合杂志，1991，11（10）：592-594．

［6］张志巧，虞坚尔．虞坚尔辨治小儿疾病验案举隅［J］．上海中医药杂志，2011，45（10）：16-17．

［7］宋铁玎，李红，王雪峰，等．壮尔颗粒治疗小儿反复呼吸道感染50例临床观察［J］．中医杂志，2006，47（12）：917-919．

［8］刘成全，韩新民．参芪固本汤加防感香囊治疗儿童反复呼吸道感染68例临床观察［J］．中国中医急症，2013，22（6）：900-901．

［9］陈炜，王力宁，杨岩．王力宁教授中医调理防治小儿反复呼吸道感染的经验［J］．中国中西医结合儿科学，2010，2（6）：491-493．

Chronic Obstructive Pulmonary Disease

慢性阻塞性肺疾病

I. Overview

Chronic Obstructive Pulmonary Disease (COPD) is a disease characterized by persistent airflow limitation, and it can be prevented and treated. The airflow limitation progressive development is related to the aggravation of chronic inflammatory reaction of the airway and lung tissue on harmful gases or harmful particles such as tobacco and smoke. Acute exacerbation and complications affect the severity of the disease and the prognosis of the individual. Chronic inflammatory reaction can lead to the destruction of the lung parenchyma which leads to pulmonary emphysema, and damage the normal repair and defense mechanisms which leads to small airway fibrosis. The clinical manifestations of COPD include: dyspnea, chronic cough, chronic expectoration, wheezing and chest tightness. The above symptoms may be aggravated suddenly. COPD belongs to "cough", "dyspnea", "lung distension", etc. in TCM in most cases.

II. Etiology and pathogenesis

i. Etiology

1. Chinese Medicine

(1) Invasion of exogenous pathogenic factors: The patient is infected with exogenous cold and invaded in lungs; skin and pore are blocked from exterior, and lungs are blocked from interior; failure of lung qi in dispersion and blocked qi movement will lead to cough and dyspnea. If the patient has lung heat exuberance, or exterior pathogen is not removed and heat is reserved in the body, the patient is external cold and interior heat; the heat can not be discharged, and the gasification of lungs is decreased, causing cough and dyspnea. When the wind and heat attack lung, lung Qi is blocked and qi movement is disordered, cough and dyspnea will occur. The pathogenic heat hurts body fluids, gathers to form phlegm, and blocks qi movement, so that dyspnea with cough arises.

(2) Improper diet: The uncooked and cold food is eaten immoderately, which stays in the body; fatty and salty food is eaten, so phlegm and heat are produced in the body; drinking excessive alcohol or eating meat or fish or stimulating food lead to dysfunction of spleen in transportation, and interior stay of phlegm-dampness. The phlegm-dampness invades lungs and blocks lung qi, so the airway is blocked, so that this disease attacks.

(3) Weakness due to chronic disease: Symptoms like long-term dyspnea, chronic cough, chronic expectoration, etc. can not be healed for a long time, thus causing the weakness. The lung deficiency leads to weakened defensive qi, so exterior pathogens can attack the body easily, as a result inducing the onset and aggravation of this disease. Lung and kidney promote each other. Long-term lung deficiency can not benefit the kidney, and kidney deficiency will also occur. The kidney does not receive qi and the breath is short and hard, as is said in *Jing-yue Complete Works*: "severe injury of five zang-fu organs will reach the kidney". The disorder of child-organ affecting the mother organ or spleen deficiency and dysfunction of spleen in transportation result in undissolved dampness turbidity. It gathers and forms phlegm. Next, the phlegm-dampness stays in lung, the dispersing and descending function of lung is decreased, causing this disease.

2. Western medicine

(1) Smoking: Smoking is an important pathogenic factor. The case rate of chronic bronchitis in smokers is 2-8 times higher than that of non-smokers. The longer the smoking year is, the greater the amount of smoking will be, then the higher the case rate of COPD will be. Chemical substances in tobacco, such as tar, nicotine and hydrocyanic acid, can damage the epithelial cells in airway and the ciliary movement, and then reduce the purification capacity of airway. Those substances can promote the proliferation of bronchial mucus glands and goblet cells, increase mucus secretion, and stimulate the parasympathetic nerve so that the bronchial smooth muscle contracts and the airway resistance increases. Besides, those substances can increase the oxygen free radicals, induce the neutrophile granulocyte to release protease, destroy the lung elastic fibers, and induce the formation of pulmonary emphysema.

(2) Occupational dusts and chemicals:As to exposure to occupational dusts and chemicals, such as smoke, allergen, industrial waste gas and indoor air pollution, too high density or too long exposure time is likely to produce COPD unrelated to smoking.

(3) Air pollution: The harmful gases in the air such as sulfur dioxide, nitrogen dioxide, chlorine can damage the airway mucous epithelium, decrease the clearance function of cilia, increase the mucus secretion, and add conditions of bacterial infection.

(4) Infection: Infection is one of the important factors in the occurrence and development of COPD. Viruses,

bacteria and mycoplasma are the important factors in the acute exacerbation of this disease. Thereinto, viruses are mainly influenza virus, rhinovirus, adenovirus and respiratory syncytial virus and so on. Bacterial infections are often secondary to viral infections. Common pathogens are usually streptococcus pneumoniae, hemophilus influenza, Moraxella catarrhalis and staphylococcus.

(5) Others: Organic factors, such as immune function disorder, airway hyperreactivity and increase of age, and environmental factors, such as climate, are related to the occurrence and development of this disease. For example, the hypoadrenocorticism, cellular immune function and lysozyme activity decreasing in old people can easily lead to the repeated infection of respiratory tract infection. Cold air can stimulate the gland to increase mucus secretion, then the ciliary motility weakens, the mucosal blood vessels contract, and local blood circulation is unsmooth, thus leading to secondary infection.

ii. Pathogenesis

1. Chinese Medicine

COPD is triggered by long-term lung disease, recurrent onsets, delayed healing, loss of treatment and improper treatment. The diseased region is mainly at the lung, then affecting spleen and kidney functions. Likewise, the spleen or kidney dysfunction can also cause the decreased dispersing and descending function of lung, leading to dyspnea with cough.

Lung is in charge of qi and breath, opening into the nose and being related to skin; their essence lies in hair; lung is directly connected with the celestial qi, so the exogenous pathogenic factors invade from mouth, nose, skin and hair, attacking lung firstly in most cases. Furthermore, lung is in high position which is the top of zang-fu organs, and link with all vessels, so lesions of other zang-fu organs are easy to influence the lungs. No matter exopathic disease or internal injuries or other visceral lesions are likely to attack or influence lungs, causing dysfunction of lung qi. The lung qi adverse rising leads to cough; abnormal ascending and descending leads to asthma; durable dysfunction of lung qi will cause lung deficiency; the function of governing qi becomes abnormal.

Kidney is the congenital origin, and governs water and the inspiration of qi. Therefore, although human's breath is governed by lung, its root is in the kidney, so there is a saying: "the lung is the governor of qi and the kidney is the root of qi". The relationship between lung and kidney is known as mutual promotion between mental and water. Both coordinate to adjust the respiratory movement. If the lung qi is deficient for a long time so as to hurt the kidney qi, the kidney fails to control respiring qi, or the essence of kidney is deficient, the kidney can not keep and control qi, so qi floats above. Both cases may cause cough and asthma, and the symptom becomes aggravated after physical activities.

The spleen is the root of acquired constitution, and the source of blood and qi formation. The supply and distribution of essential substances from water and cereals depends on the dispersing and descending of lung qi. The protracted disease leads to lung deficiency, namely an offspring steals its maternal principle, thus causing dysfunction of the spleen in transport, fatigued limbs and lack of strength, less diet and loose stools, emaciation, sallow complexion and other symptoms. In the case of dysfunction of the spleen in transport, dampness fails to transform and gathers to form phlegm. The phlegm blocks the qi movement, causing cough and dyspnea. Therefore, there is a saying: "the spleen is the source of phlegm and the lung is the reservoir of phlegm".

The pathological nature of COPD contains deficiency and excess. The excess lies in lung; the invasion of exogenous pathogenic factors or phlegm obstruction causes dysfunction of lung qi. The deficiency is due to lung, spleen and kidney, especially deficiency of qi. The dysfunction of the spleen in transport and failure of kidney in control and keep can arise impairment disoder of dispersing and descending function of the lung. The deficiency symptom is infected with exogenous pathogenic factors again, or chronic illness of the excess hurts the healthy qi, from lung to spleen and kidney. The disease condition shows mixture of deficiency and excess.

The main pathological products of COPD are phlegm and blood stasis. The production of phlegm at first is blame to the abnormal ascending and descending of lung qi, as well as the failure of qi movement. What's more, the lung is the upper source of fluids; the lung fails to regulate the water passage, so fluids stop and gather to form phlegm. The dysfunction of lung influences spleen, the child-organ consumes the mother-organ, and the spleen fails in transport, therefore the internal dampness generates and gathers to form phlegm. The patients with COPD suffer from chronic cough and deficiency of lung qi. The lung qi fails to link all vessels to the heart, so the blood flow is sluggish and blood stasis appears. The mixture of phlegm and blood stasis makes the disease more refractory.

COPD is a chronic, recurrent, unstable and lingering disease, which is especially seen in elderly and frail patients. Since their bodies lack healthy qi and their viscera functions decline gradually, this disease is hard to be cured. In clinical practice, if the deficiency leads to yin and yang dissociation, dissociated yang coming to the body surface, and qi ascending counterflow, or if the excess leads to pathogenic qi blocking lung, stifling oppression in the chest, respiratory distress, etc., they are all critical signs, and must be treated in no time.

2. Western medicine

(1) Inflammatory mechanisms: Chronic inflammation of airway, lung parenchyma and pulmonary vessels is the characteristic changes of COPD. Neutrophil granulocytes, macrophages, T lymphocytes and other inflammatory cells are involved in the development of COPD. The activation and aggregation of neutrophil granulocytes is an important link in the inflammatory process of COPD. The release of various bioactive substances such as neutrophil elastase results in chronic hypersecretion of mucus and destroys the lung parenchyma.

(2) Protease-antiprotease imbalance mechanism: Proteolytic enzymes have a damaging effect on tissues; the antiprotease may inhibit elastase and many other proteases, among which $\alpha 1$-antitrypsin ($\alpha 1$-AT) is the most active. The balance of protease and antiprotease is the main factor to prevent the normal structure of lung tissue from injury and damage. Too much protease or deficiency of antiprotease can lead to the damage of tissue structure and cause pulmonary emphysema.

(3) Oxidative stress mechanism: Many studies have shown the increased oxidative stress in patients with COPD. Oxides mainly include superoxide anion, hypochlorous acid and nitric oxide, etc. Oxides can influence and destroy many biochemical macromolecules such as proteins, lipids and nucleic acids, cause cell dysfunction or cell death, and do damage to the extracellular matrix. Oxides can also give rise to the imbalance of protease and protease, promote the inflammatory response, such as the activation of transcription factor NF-kB which can be involved in the transcription of multiple inflammatory mediators, for example, IL-8, TNF-α, inducible nitric oxide synthase (NOS) and epoxide hydrolase.

(4) Other mechanisms: For example, autonomic dysfunction, malnutrition, temperature change may be involved in the occurrence and development of COPD.

The above inflammatory mechanism, protease-antiprotease imbalance mechanism, oxidative stress mechanism and autonomic dysfunction take effect together, and lead to two major lesions: firstly, small airway diseases including small airway inflammation, small airway fibroplasia, small airway lumen mucus plug, etc., significantly increase the small airway resistance. Secondly, pulmonary emphysema reduces the normal traction force of the alveolus pulmonis to the small airway, and makes the small airway easy to collapse. Meanwhile, the pulmonary emphysema obviously decreases the alveolar elastic recoil. The combined action of small airway disease and pulmonary emphysema leads to the characteristic persistent airflow limitation of COPD.

III. Key points of diagnosis and differential diagnosis

i. Key points of diagnosis

(1) The patients have a history of many years of chronic lung disease. Their conditions are recurrent,

lingering, refractory and unstable.

(2) The main clinical manifestations are mainly dyspnea, cough and expectoration. Opening the mouth and lifting the shoulders; the nasal ala flapping, fullness in chest, pant that will be aggravated after physical activities, severe cough and so on can be seen.

(3) This disease is generally induced by exogenous pathogenic factors. Emotional stimulation or overstrain can also induce this disease.

(4) The continuing airflow limitation in the pulmonary function test is the essential condition to diagnose COPD. After the inhalation of bronchial dilation agent, $FEV_1/FVC<0.70$ is the limit to confirm the presence of persistent airflow limitation.

ii. Differential diagnosis

1. Identification of COPD and cough

The main manifestation of cough is only coughing, and is not accompanied by dyspnea. Coughing, phlegm and wheezing are often seen together in COPD; COPD is recurrent, unstable, and is often caused by recurrent attacks of chronic cough.

2. Identification of COPD and asthma

Asthma also shows dyspnea, coughing and expectoration. In most cases, it is caused by prolonged chronic cough developing to cough and asthma, with varying degrees. The difference between asthma and COPD is that asthma attacks intermittently and suddenly and can be relieved rapidly. There is wheezing sound in the throat with mild coughing or no coughing.

IV. TCM therapy

i. Syndrome differentiation and treatment

1. Wind attacking the lung

Main symptoms: coughing and wheezing, white and dilute phlegm, aversion to cold with fever, no sweat, nasal congestion, watery nasal discharge, soreness of body, thin and white tongue fur, floating and tight pulse.

Therapeutic method: to ventilate lung qi, dispell wind and relieve cough.

Prescription: Zhi Sou San. Platycodon Root, Fi neleaf Schizonepeta Herb, Tatarian Aster Root, Processed Stemona Root, Willowieaf Rhizome, Liquorice Root, Dried Tangerine Peel.

Prescription analysis: Platycodon Root can disperse lung qi, purge fire and dissipate cold; Fi neleaf Schizonepeta Herb can dispel wind-dampness, refresh oneself and relieve the sore throat; Tatarian Aster Root can tonify deficiency, harmonize the middle, eliminate phlegm and relieve cough; Stemona Root can moisten lung and relieve cough; Willowieaf Rhizome can clear phlegm and stop coughing; Dried Tangerine Peel can harmonize the middle, remove stagnation and eliminate phlegm; Prepared Liquorice Root can relieve the sore throat, relieve cough and coordinate the drug actions of a prescription.

Modification: dried flower spike of Fi neleaf Schizonepeta Herb, Divaricate Saposhnikovia Root, Fermented Soybean are added for patients with severe wind-cold; Honeysuckle Flower and Hogfennel Root are added for patients with wind-heat; Great Burdock Achene, Platycodon Root, unprepared Liquorice Root and Jindeng are added for patients with pharyngalgia; Biond Magnolia Flower, Siberian Cocklebur Fruit and Small Centipeda

Herb are added for patients with nasal obstruction; Periostracum Cicada and Belvedere Fruit are added for patients with pharyngeal itching and allergy; Mulberry Leaf and Loquat Leaf are added for patients with dry pharynx; Skullcap Decoction, Coptis and Raw Gypsum are added for patients with internal heat; Heartleaf Houttuynia Herb and Dandelion are added for patients with much yellow phlegm.

2. External cold and internal heat

Main symptoms: dyspnea with cough, short of breath in case of more severe condition. Flaring of the nares, viscous phlegm, disturbance of coughing and expectorating, irritancy, sweating or no sweat, persistent feverish body, thirst, thin and yellow tong fur, slippery and rapid pulse.

Therapeutic method: to ventilate lung by pungent-cool medicines, clear heat and relieve dyspnea.

Prescription: Ma Huang Xing Ren Gan Cao Shi Gao Tang. Bitter Apricot Seed, Gypsum and Licorice Decoction. Ephedra, Bitter Apricot Seed, Prepared Liquorice Root and Gypsum.

Prescription analysis: Ephedra can ventilate lung and relieve dyspnea; Gypsum is sweet-cold and can clear lung heat and promote fluid production; Bitter Apricot Seed is bitter and can descend the lung qi and relieve cough and dyspnea; Prepared Liquorice Root can protect stomach qi and coordinate the drug actions of a prescription.

Modification: Fi neleaf Schizonepeta Herb and Perilla Leaf are added for patients with severe pathogenic factors from the exterior, aversion to cold without sweating; for patients with heavy lung heat, the dosage of Gypsum should be increased, or White Mulberry Root-Bark, Baical Skullcap Root, Common Anemarrhena Rhizome, Heartleaf Houttuynia Herb and Dandelion should be added; for patients with much phlegm and rapid breathing, Pepperweed Seed and Loquat Leaf are added; for patients with thick and yellow sputum and chest tightness, Snakegourd Fruit, Fritillary Bulb, Baical Skullcap Root and Platycodon Root are added.

3. External cold and internal fluid retention

Main symptoms: ecphysesis, shortness of breath, qi counterflow, fullness and oppression in the chest and diaphragm, cough, less phlegm and difficulty in expectorating, white and spumous phlegm. No thirsty or liking hot drinks in the case of thirsty, cold body with the fear of cold that occurs easily when it is cold or a cold is caught. Dark complexion, white and slippery tongue fur, tight stringy pulse or floating pulse.

Therapeutic method: to ventilate lung and dispel cold, resolve phlegm and relieve dyspnea.

Prescription: She Gan Ma Huang Tang or Xiao Qing Long Tang. Blackberrylily Rhizome, Ephedra, Fresh Ginger, Manchurian Wildginger, Tatarian Aster Root, Common Coltsfoot Flower, Chinese Date, Pinellia Tuber, Chinese Magnoliavine Fruit, Ephedra, Peony, Manchurian Wildginger, Dried Ginger, Prepared Liquorice Root, Cassia Twig, Chinese Magnoliavine Fruit, Pinellia Tuber.

Prescription analysis: Ephedra and Blackberrylily Rhizome can ventilate lung, relieve dyspnea, resolve phlegm and relieve sore throat; Dried Ginger, Manchurian Wildginger and Pinellia Tuber can warm lung, resolve fluid retention and descend adverse qi; Tatarian Aster Root and Common Coltsfoot Flower can resolve phlegm and relieve cough; Chinese Magnoliavine Fruit can convergence lung qi; Chinese Date and Liquorice Root can regulate stomach.

Modification: Biond Magnolia Flower and Siberian Cocklebur Fruit are added for patients with nasal obstruction and watery nasal discharge. Raw Gypsum and Baical Skullcap Root are added for patients with heat manifestations and dysphoria. Apricot Seed, Blackberrylily Rhizome and Common Coltsfoot Flower are added for patients with wheezing due to retention of phlegm in throat. Indian Bread and Chuling are added for patients with edema.

4. Phlegm-heat obstructing lung

Main symptoms: coughing and rapid breathing, dyspnea with rapid respiration, red face, chest pain and chest tightness, yellowish green phlegm with fishy smell, dry mouth and throat, red tongue, greasy and yellow tongue fur, slippery and rapid pulse.

Therapeutic method: to clear lung, resolve phlegm, remove blood stasis and discharge pus.

Prescription: Wei Jing Tang. Phragmites Stem, Coix Seed, Snakegourd Fruit Seed, Peach Seed.

Prescription analysis: Phragmites Stem is sweet-cold and floating, and it can clear lungs and purge heat; Snakegourd Fruit Seed can resolve phlegm and discharge pus; Peach Seed can activate blood circulation and dispel stasis; Coix Seed can clear lungs and eliminate toxicant swelling.

Modification: Honeysuckle Flower, Baical Skullcap Root, Golden Thread, Raw Gypsum and Heartleaf Houttuynia Herb are added for patients with exuberant pathogenic heat; Pericarpium Trichosanthis and Turmeric Root Tuber are added for patients with chest tightness; Pinellia Tuber, Apricot Seed, Thunberg Fritillary Bulb, Tabasheer, Bile Arisaema and Platycodon Root are added for patients with much phlegm; Immature Orange Fruit, Officinal Magnolia Bark and Radish Seed are added for patients with abdominal distension; Chinese Angelica, Sichuan Lovage Rhizome, Frankincense and Myrrh are added for patients with chest pain; Perilla Fruit, Pepperweed Seed and Apricot Seed are added for patients who can not lie flat.

5. Deficiency of lung qi

Main symptoms: cough and asthma, weakness, shortness of breath that will be aggravated after physical activities, thin phlegm, low timid voice, mental and physical fatigue, pale complexion, anemophobia and spontaneous perspiration, pale tongue with white tongue fur, and feeble pulse.

Therapeutic method: to tonify lung qi, consolidate exterior and stop coughing.

Prescription: Yu Ping Feng San. Divaricate Saposhnikovia Root, Milkvetch Root and White Atractylodes Rhizome.

Prescription analysis: Milkvetch Root can tonify spleen qi and lung qi, consolidate exterior and stop sweating. White Atractylodes Rhizome can invigorate spleen, tonify qi and consolidate exterior. Divaricate Saposhnikovia Root can release exterior and disperse wind, tonify qi and eliminate pathogens.

Modification: Aster, Hogfennel Root and Willowieaf Rhizome are added for patients with heavy cough; Fructus Tritici Levis, Concha Ostrear Preparata and Ephedra Root are added for patients with heavy spontaneous perspiration; Perilla Leaf is added for patients who are weak and easy to get cold; Mulberry Leaf and Loquat Leaf are added for patients with dry throat; Baical Skullcap Root, Golden Thread and Raw Gypsum are added for patients with internal heat.

6. Deficiency of spleen qi

Main symptoms: coughing and wheezing, shortness of breath, fatigued limbs and lack of strength, less diet and loose stools, emaciation, sallow complexion, enlarged tongue body with teeth prints, deep and weak pulse.

Therapeutic method: to invigorate spleen and tonify qi, resolve phlegm, relieve cough and dyspnea.

Prescription: Shen Ling Bai Zhu San. Pulp of Lotus Seed, Coix Seed, Villons Amomum Fruit, Platycodon Root, Hyacinth Bean, Indian Bread, Ginseng, Prepared Liquorice Root, White Atractylodes Rhizome and Common Yam Rhizome.

Prescription analysis: White Atractylodes Rhizome, Ginseng and Indian Bread can invigorate spleen, tonify qi and eliminate dampness. Common Yam Rhizome and Pulp of Lotus Seed can invigorate spleen, tonify qi and relieve diarrhea. Hyacinth Bean and Coix Seed can invigorate spleen and eliminate dampness. Villons Amomum Fruit can wake up spleen and harmonize stomach, move qi and resolve food stagnation. Platycodon Root can ventilate lung and promote qi, dredge and regulate water passage, and load drugs upwards. Prepared Liquorice Root can invigorate spleen, harmonize stomach, and coordinate the drug actions of a prescription

Modification: Pinellia Tuber and Apricot Seed are added for patients with much phlegm; Immature Orange Fruit, Officinal Magnolia Bark and Radish Seed are added for patients with abdominal distension; Dried Ginger and Cassia Bark are added for patients with interior cold and abdominal pain.

7. Deficiency of kidney qi

Main symptoms: coughing and wheezing, more exhalation than inhalation, shortness of breath, heavier wheezing after physical activities, soreness of the waist and the knees, tinnitus, frequent urination at night, cough with enuresis, pale white complexion, fatigued spirit and lack of strength, pale tongue, and weak, deep and slow pulse.

Therapeutic method: to tonify kidney, improve qi reception and relieve dyspnea.

Prescription: Qi Wei Du Qi Wan. Chinese Magnoliavine Fruit (prepared), Asiatic Cornelian Cherry Fruit (prepared), Indian Bread, Tree Peony Root Bark, Prepared Rehmannia Root, Common Yam Rhizome, Oriental Waterplantain Rhizome.

Prescription analysis: Prepared Rehmannia Root can nourish kidney yin; Asiatic Cornelian Cherry Fruit and Common Yam Rhizome can tonify liver, replenish spleen, and produce essence and blood; Oriental Waterplantain Rhizome and Indian Bread can promote diuresis and eliminate dampness, and prevent Rehmannia Root from being too greasy; Tree Peony Root Bark can clear liver and discharge heat; Chinese Magnoliavine Fruit can tonify kidney, arrest seminal emission with astringents and prevent enuresis.

Modification: Dried Tangerine Peel, Pinellia Tuber, Perilla Fruit and Willowieaf Rhizome are added for patients with much phlegm; Heterophylly Falsestarwort Root shall be added for patients who cough and wheeze and are going to collapse with beads of sweat; Tokay Gecko and Chinese Caterpillar Fungus are added for patients with soreness in waist and heavier short breath; Perilla Fruit, Pepperweed Seed and Apricot Seed are added for patients who can not lie flat.

ii. Single ingredient prescriptions and proved prescription

(1) Smash the Stemona Root and take its natural juice, which is boiled into paste with the same amount of white honey. Twice per day; one spoon each time. It applies to chronic cough.

(2) 60 g of pearl power and a little Natural Indigo are mixed with Sesame Oil. Take 8 times, twice per day. It is used for acute cough.

(3) Baical Skullcap Root, Snakegourd Peel and Heartleaf Houttuynia Herb are decocted in water. 3 times per day. It applies to heat-phlegm cough.

(4) Tendrilleaf Fritillary Bulb, pear juice and crystal sugar are decocted in water. It applies to cough due to yin-deficiency.

(5) 25g of Branches of Stem and Leaf of Japanese Ardisia; 15g of Gypsum; 12g of Platycodon Root; 9g of Dried Earthworm; 30g of honey; 5g of one pig gall; Liquorice Root. Decoct them in water. It is used for dyspnea due to excess or heat.

(6) 3g of Red Ginseng and 20 grains of Chinese Magnoliavine Fruit (pro dosi) are grinded to powder. Twice per day. It is used for dyspnea due to deficiency.

(7) 6g of Ginseng, 2 pieces of Walnut Fruits (removing shell but not peel), 5 pieces of Fresh Ginger and 2 Chinese Dates are decocted in water. It is used for dyspnea due to deficiency.

(8) 15g of Ginseng, one pair of Tokay Gecko (stir-fried), 30g of Apricot Seeds, 30g of Tendrilleaf Fritillary Bulb, 30g of Human Placenta are grinded to fine powder. Take 3g each time and twice or 3 times each day. It is used for dyspnea due to deficiency.

iii. Chinese patent medicine

1. Dissipating cold, relieving cough and dyspnea

(1) Tong Xuan Li Fei Pill: take orally. Big Honey Pill, 2 pills at a time, twice or 3 times per day. It can resolve superficies and dispel cold, ventilate lung and relieve cough. It is used for treating cough and expectoration caused by wind-cold attacking lung.

(2) Zhi Sou Qing Guo Pill: for oral using. 2 pills at a time, twice per day. It can ventilate lung, resolve phlegm, and relieve cough and dyspnea. It is used for cough with profuse sputum, fullness and oppression in the chest and diaphragm, shortness of breath, dyspnea, dry mouth and throat and other symptoms caused by wind-cold affecting lung.

(3) Dong Wan Zhi Ke Granules: taken after being mixed with warm water. One bag at a time and 3 times per day. It can dispel wind and cold, ventilate lung and relieve cough. It is used for syndrome of wind-cold attacking lung, whose symptoms are cough, thin and white phlegm, pharyngeal itching, aversion to cold, fever, etc. It also applies to the symptoms above caused by acute bronchitis.

(4) Xiao Qing Long Mixture:for oral using. 10-20 ml at a time; 3 times per day. Shake it well before using. It can resolve superficies, resolve fluid retention, and relieve cough and dyspnea. It is used for treating wind-cold and retained fluid, aversion to cold with fever, no sweating, dyspnea with cough and thin phlegm.

2. Heat-clearing, relieving cough and dyspnea

(1) Qing Fei Xiao Yan Pill: for oral using. 60 grains at a time; 3 times per day. 40 grains at a time for children at 6-12 years old; 30 grains at a time for children at 3-6 years old; 20 grains at a time for children at 1-3 years old; 10 grains at a time for infants within 1 year old. It can clear lung, resolve phlegm and relieve cough and dyspnea. It is used for heat phlegm obstructing lung, whose symptoms include cough and asthma, distending pain in the chest and hypochondrium, yellow and thick phlegm. It is also used for treating upper respiratory tract infection, acute bronchitis, chronic bronchitis and pulmonary infection.

(2) Zhi Sou Ding Chuan Pill: for oral using. 10 grains at a time; twice or 3 times per day. It can clear lung heat and relieve dyspnea with cough. It is used for treating fever, thirst, cough with yellow phlegm, short breath and chest tightness.

(3) Ke Xin Kang Pian: for oral using. 3-4 tablets at a time; 3 times per day. It can descend qi, relieve dyspnea, clear lung and resolve phlegm. It is used for treating cough due to lung heat and cough caused by tracheitis.

(4) Xiao Chuan Ning Granules: taken after being mixed with boiled water. Take 5g at a time for children under 5 years old, 10g for children at 5-10 years old, 20g for children at 10-14 years old. Adults can increase dosage as appropriate or follow doctor's advice, and take twice per day. It can ventilate lung and relieve cough, clear heat and relieve dyspnea. It is used for treating cough due to lung heat.

(5) Ji Zhi Syrup: for oral using. 20-30 ml at a time; 3 or 4 times per day. 5 ml at a time for children within 1 year old; 7 ml each time for children at 1-3 years old; 10 ml each time for children at 3-7 years old; 15 ml each time for children above 7 years old; 3-4 times per day. It can clear heat, resolve phlegm, ventilate lung and relieve cough. It is used for treating cough due to the infection with exogenous wind-heat. The symptoms are fever, aversion to cold, fullness and oppression in the chest and diaphragm, cough and sore throat. It also applies to symptoms above caused by acute bronchitis and chronic bronchitis.

(6) Ling Yang Qing Fei Pill: taken after being mixed with boiled water. One pill each time; 3 times per day. It can clear lung, relieve sore throat, clear pestilence and relieve cough. It is used for treating exuberant lung-stomach heat and the infection with seasonal pathogen. The symptoms are fever and dizziness, sore limbs, cough with profuse sputum, swelling and pain in throat, epistaxis and hemoptysis, dry mouth and tongue.

(7) Qing Jin Zhi Sou Hua Tan Pill: for oral using. Take 6g each time and 23 times per day. It can clear lung, resolve phlegm and relieve cough. It is used for treating cough with yellow phlegm, disorder of chest and diaphragm, sore throat, hoarseness and dry stools caused by exuberant phlegm due to lung-heat.

3. Resolving phlegm and relieving dyspnea

(1) An Sou Hua Tan Pill: for oral using. One pill each time; twice per day. It can clear lung, resolve phlegm, moisten lung and relieve cough. It is used for treating cough with exuberant phlegm, shortness of breath, thirst and dry throat, chronic cough due to overexertion, bloody phlegm, which are caused by lung heat due to yin deficiency.

(2) Bai Ke Jing Syrup: for oral using. 5 ml each time for children at 1-2 years old; 10 ml each time for children at 3-5 years old; 20-25 ml each time for adults; 3 times per day. It can clear heat, resolve phlegm and relieve cough and dyspnea. It is used for cough and expectoration caused by affection of exogenous wind-heat. It also applies to the symptoms above caused by common cold, acute or chronic bronchitis, and pertussis..

(3) Chuan Bei Zhi Ke Syrup: for oral using. Take 15 ml at a time and 3 times per day. It can relieve cough and expel phlegm. It is used for treating cough due to lung heat, and abundant phlegm with yellow color.

(4) Chu Tan Zhi Sou Pill: for oral using. 2 pills each time; twice per day. It can clear lung, reduce fire, remove phlegm and relieve cough. It is used for treating cough and reserved flow of qi yellow and sticky phlegm, sore throat and dry stools caused by lung heat due to exuberant phlegm.

(5) Fei Li Ke Capsule: for oral using. Take 3-4 grains each time and 3 times per day. Or take it according to doctor's advice. It can relieve cough and dyspnea, clear heat and and remove toxin, normalize qi and expel phlegm. It is used for treating cough and phlegm, disturbance in respiration, acute and chronic bronchitis. It also applies to the above symptoms caused by pulmonary emphysema.

(6) Xie Bai Syrup: for oral using. Take 10 ml at a time for children above 1 year old, 5 ml for children within 1 year old, and take twice per day. It can ventilate lung and clear heat, resolve phlegm and relieve cough. It is used for treating common cold with cough, abundant phlegm and full chest, thirst and dry tongue, stuffy nose.

(7) Xiao Chuan Pill: for oral using. Take 10g at a time and twice per day. It can relieve cough and dyspnea. It is used for chronic cough and chronic asthma due to excessive phlegm.

(8) Ju Hong Tan Ke Liquid: for oral using. 10-20 ml at a time and 3 times per day. It can regulate qi, resolve phlegm, moisten lung and relieve cough. It is used for cough, asthma and phlegm caused by turbid phlegm obstructing lung; It also applies to above symptoms caused by common cold, bronchitis, pharyngolaryngitis, etc.

4. Tonifying lung and relieving dyspnea:

(1) Bu Fei Pill: for oral using. One pill each time; twice per day. It can tonify lung and tonify qi, and relieve cough and dyspnea. It is used for deficiency of lung qi, short breath, dyspnea with cough, low coughing sound, dry cough with sticky phlegm, etc.

(2) Shen Bei Ke Chuan Pill: for oral using. 40 pills each time; 3 times per day. It can invigorate spleen and resolve phlegm, tonify lung and replenish kidney, relieve cough and dyspnea. It is used for treating patients with chronic bronchitis which has the symptoms of cough and asthma due to deficient cold.

(3) Ren Shen Bao Fei Pill: for oral using. 2 pills at a time; 2-3 times per day. It can tonify qi, replenish lung, relieve cough and dyspnea. It is used for treating consumptive disease, chronic cough, shortness of breath and other symptoms caused by deficiency of lung qi and body fluid depletion.

(4) Yu Ping Feng Capsule: for oral using. 2 pills at a time; 3 times per day. It can tonify qi, consolidate superficial resistance and stop sweating. It is used for treating patients with unconsolidation due to superficies deficiency, spontaneous sweating, aversion to wind, white complexion or patients who are easy to be infected with wind pathogen due to weak health.

5. Improving qi reception and relieving dyspnea

(1) Chuan Tai Granules: taken orally after being mixed with warm water. 4 times per day and 3g each time. It can ventilate lung, relieve dyspnea, replenish lung and expel phlegm. It is used for syndrome of superficies cold and interior heat during an acute attack of bronchial asthma. The symptoms are ecphysesis, throat wheezing, fullness in chest and hypochondrium, cough and sticky phlegm sometimes with cold body, general fever, vexation, bodily pain, thirst, etc.

(2) Xie Fei Ding Chuan Tablets: take 5 tablets each time orally and twice per day. It can purge lung and improve qi reception, and relieve cough and dyspnea. It is used for dyspnea with cough caused by obstruction of lung qi and failure of kidney to receive qi.

(3) Gu Shen Ding Chuan Pill: for oral using. 1.5-2.0g each time; 2-3 times per day. It can warm kidney, improve qi reception, invigorate spleen and promote diuresis. It can be taken before omens of disease, and can prevent recurrence of chronic asthma. One course of treatment for 15 days. It applies to chronic bronchitis, pulmonary emphysema, bronchial asthma, deficiency-type dyspnea in the elderly due to deficiency of spleen and kidney and deficiency of lung qi and kidney qi.

(4) Jin Shui Bao Capsule: take 3 grains each time orally and 3 times per day. It is used for patients with chronic renal insufficiency. For them it shall be taken 6 grains each time and 3 times per day, to tonify lung and kidney, replenish essence and qi. It treats deficiency of lung and kidney, deficiency of essential qi, chronic cough

and deficiency-type dyspnea, fatigued spirit and lack of strength, insomnia and forgetfulness, soreness in the waist and the knees, irregular menses, impotence and premature ejaculation. It applies to patients with chronic bronchitis, chronic renal insufficiency, hyperlipidemia and liver cirrhosis who show the above symptoms.

(5) Bai Ling Capsule: taken orally. Specifications: ① 5-15 gains at a time; ② 2-6 grains at a time; 3 times per day. Chronic renal insufficiency: 10 grains each time and 3 times per day, One course of treatment for 8 weeks. The capsule can tonify lung and kidney, and replenish essential qi. It is used for treating cough, asthma, hemoptysis and back pain caused by deficiency of lung and kidney; as well as the adjuvant treatment of chronic bronchitis, etc.

6. Invigorating spleen and resolving phlegm

(1) Shen Ling Bai Zhu San: take 6g each time orally and 3 times per day. It can invigorate spleen and tonify qi. It is used for weariness, lack of strength, less diet and and loose stools.

(2) Chen Xia Liu Jun Pill: for oral using. Take 6g of Water-honey pill, 9g of small honey pill, one pill of big honey Pill at a time, for twice or 3 times a day. It can tonify spleen and invigorate stomach, regulate qi and resolve phlegm. It is used for weak spleen and stomach, less diet and indigestion, abdominal distension and chest distress, qi deficiency and abundant phlegm.

iv. Acupuncture and moxibustion therapy

1. Acupuncture

Main points are BL 13 (double), GV 14, BL 12 (double) and EX-B1. LU 5 and LU 9 are coordinated for patients with heavier cough; LI 4 and ST 36 are coordinated for patients who are weak and easy to catch a cold; ST 36, CV 12, ST40 and BL 20 are coordinated for patients with abundant phlegm; CV 22 and CV 17 are coordinated for patients with qi counterflow due to accumulation of phlegm; BL 23, CV 4 and KI 3 are coordinated for patients with failure of kidney in controlling and receiving; TF (4), PC 6 and BL 15 are coordinated for patients with palpitation. The lifting and thrusting method and the twirling method are adopted when needling GV 14, CV 12, LU 5, CV 4, BL 13, BL 12, BL 15 and BL 23. The lifting and thrusting method is secondary to the twirling method when needling LI 4, LU 9, PC 6, LU 10 and KI 3. Slight lifting, thrusting and twirling method is adopted to needle CV 22; the needle is not retained after the arrival of qi. The lifting and thrusting method and the twirling method are adopted when needling ST 36. During the acute exacerbation, the needling manipulation is performed once a day. In stable period, the needling manipulation is performed once a day or every other day; the needles are retained for 30 min every time and are manipulated every 10 min. Reinforcing method for deficiency and reducing method for excess are taken according to specific disease conditions. Namely, weakened body resistance appears in stable period mostly, so the reinforcement method should be adopted in the needling manipulation; during the acute exacerbation, excessiveness of pathogen or deficiency-excess in complexity usually appears, therefore the reduction method or neutral reinforcement and reduction should be adopted in the needling manipulation. 10 times of needling manipulation is a course of treatment. The patients shall rest for 3-5 days between 2 needling manipulations, and then receive another one or two courses of treatment.

2. Moxibustion

Main points: CV 22, BL 13, LU 7 and CV 4. EX-B1, LU 5 and ST 40 are added for patients with excess syndrome and phlegm-heat syndrome; BL 13, BL 23, CV 22, BL 43 and ST 36 are added for patients with deficiency syndrome and cold syndrome. The patients with qi deficiency and yang-deficiency shall have moxibustion or acupuncture and moxibustion simultaneously, and the selection of points is as above. The mild-warm moxibustion with moxa stick is taken as the principal therapeutic method, and conducted during the needle-retaining period or after the needles have been drawn out. Each point takes 5-10 min, until local flush appears. Moxibustion is performed once every day; 10 times are a course of treatment.

3. Fire cupping

BL 13, GV 12, BL 12 and TE 5 are selected when the patients are infected with wind-cold pathogen; GV 14, BL 12, BL 13 and LI 11 are selected when the patients are infected with wind-heat pathogen. Larger cupping jars or wide mouth glass bottles are used on the points. If the patients are thin, small cupping jars can be used. The cupping jars are retained about 10 min.

4. Manipulation of dermal needle

Selection of points: governor vessel on neck and back, bladder meridian, both sides of the throat. Method: use 75% alcohol to sterilize local parts, then use dermal needles to tap and insert the selected points slightly or moderately; once a day, 10 times for a course of treatment.

v. Others

1. Auricular plaster therapy

Selection of points: CO (14), CO (16), TG (2p) and CO (7). Antiasthmatic point is added for patients with heavier asthma; the spleen point is added for patients with abundant phlegm. Method: firstly use 75% alcohol to sterilize one ear, then put a vaccaria seed on the corresponding point and stick it well with a tape of 0.4×0.4 (cm); press it slightly until the patients feel burning and painful in auricular. The patients are advised to press the points slightly 3-5 times every day. Two ears are applied alternately. Paste it once every 4 or 5 days and 5 times for a course of treatment.

2. Point application

The main points are BL 13, BL 23, GV 14, BL 43 and EX-B1, etc. Drug composition: Ephedra, White Mustard Seed and Yanhusuo (20g for each); Gansui Root and Manchurian Wildginger (10g for each). The above drugs are grinded to fine powder, and added with 0.6g of Musk, finally stirred evenly with fresh ginger juice. Operational method: the patients should have routine sterilization at the selected acupoints first by taking sitting pose, and make the drug into round cakes with a diameter of around 1.5cm and a thickness of around 0.5cm. Stick the round cakes on the above points and fix it with a tap of 4×4 (cm). The application time is 4-6 h for adults, and 2-3 h for children in dog days or in coldest days of winter. The drug is applied every 10 days, and Chinese medicine is often taken simultaneously.

V. Empirical prescription of famous physicians and experts

(1) Fei Shen Ke Chuan Fang (Meng Shujiang)

Indication: cough with dyspnea and asthma, deficiency of lung and kidney, chronic bronchitis with deficiency-excess in complexity, and pulmonary emphysema.

Prescription: 4g of Ephedra, 9g of Apricot Seed, 3g of Liquorice Root, 9g of Rhizoma Pinellinae Praeparata, 6g of Dried Tangerine Peel, 10g of Indian Bread, 9g of Chinese Angelica, 12g of Prepared Rehmannia Root.

Usage: decocted with water.

Function: to ventilate lung and resolve phlegm, relieve cough and dyspnea, tonify and replenish lung and kidney.

Note: Chronic bronchitis and pulmonary emphysema belong to the scope of TCM cough and dyspnea. This syndrome is caused by deficiency of lung and kidney which results in phlegm-dampness and interior excess, and induced by new pathogenic Qi. Therefore, it shows dual exterior and interior disease and deficiency-excess in complexity. There is an old saying that kidney is treated in normal condition, and lung is treated in occurrence. If this syndrome is treated with general formulas of relieving cough, resolving phlegm and relieving asthma, although momentary effect can be obtained, it is always difficult to get the satisfactory effect. This prescription is modified from Six Gentlemen Metal and Water Decoction of Zhang Jingyue. In the prescription, Ephedra and Bitter Apricot Seed can ventilate lung and resolve phlegm, and Ephedra also has the effect of opening lung, relieving exterior and relieving dyspnea. Pinellia Tuber and Dried Tangerine Peel can regulate Qi and resolve phlegm to normalize Qi and descend phlegm. Indian Bread can invigorate spleen and resolve dampness. Phlegm is generated from spleen deficiency and transformed from dampness, it is not only used to invigorate spleen to avoid the source of phlegm, but also remove dampness to resolve phlegm. Indian Bread is compatible with Pinellia Tuber and Dried Tangerine Peel, called Decoction of Two Old Ingredients. It is compatible with Chinese Angelica to harmonize blood, or compatible with Prepared Rehmannia Root to tonify kidney and receive Qi, so as to treat the root cause. This prescription can be used to treated chronic cough and dyspnea that cannot be cured after many times of treatment, and always has a better therapeutic effect. Especially, insist on taking this medicine at the beginning of winter and before the occurrence of this disease, the conditions can be greatly relieved.

(2) Fei Re Ke Chuan Fang (Ma Ruiting)

Indication: cough and asthma due to lung heat caused by the following reasons. For example, exterior pathogen involves in interior to damage lung, so that the lung fails in purification and descending astringing. As well, the lung metal is tormented by the up-flaming ministerial fire, insulting in Qi counterflowing due to lung heat.

Composition: 12g of unprepared Coix Seed, 6g of unprepared Liquorice Root, 12g of Debark Peony Root, 9g of Tree Peony Root Bark, 12g of Unprocessed Rehmannia Root, 9g of Guangzhou Orange Red, 9g of Bitter Apricot Seed Brain, 9g of Rhizoma Pinellinae Praeparata, 9g of Thunberg Fritillary Bulb, 9g of Chinese Arborvitae Kernel, 25g of Fresh Reed Rhizome, 12g of Coastal Glehnia Root.

Usage: decocted with water.

Function: to calm gallbladder and smooth liver, clear and descend lung and stomach, resolve phlegm and relieve cough.

Note: Cough and asthma due to lung heat include acute or chronic pneumonia and other cough and asthma syndromes caused by pulmonary dryness-heat dyspnea. Pneumonia belongs to the scope of cough and asthma due to lung heat or seasonal febrile disease according to in TCM. This disease is acute. As to it, both interior and exterior can be infected with pathogens so heat exists in dual exterior and interior. In addition, Qi and fire rush upward, stagnation and exuberance of lung heat appears, thus immediately causing fever, cough and asthma as well as chest distress and pain once the disease onset. For some patients, this disease is acute and rapidly changes. When the state of the disease is serious, some symptoms will appear, including delirious speech and delirium, stupor and groping of the air, finding clothes and touching the bed, dysphoria. Specific to above conditions, it should be treated cooperating with western medicine. If the patient has cough and asthma gurgling with phlegm, droops head and closes eyes, and sounds as swallow saw, it prove that he is in a serious state and the point of death. At this time, the western medicine should be used to hope save the patients' life from death. The lung is the house of heart which is the residence of the spirit, if the house is burnt, the spirit is out of hiding, necessarily resulting in swinging soul and spiritual dispersing. The heart governs blood vessel, sovereign and ministerial fire is burning hot, the heat damages nutrient-blood, which will essentially endanger heart. Therefore, patients with serious condition show unconsciousness, delirious speech and other heart meridian syndromes. This is inward invasion of pericardium by heat. Ye Tianshi called it "the upper attack of warm pathogen starting from lung, reversed transmission to pericardium". Hence, Chinese Arborvitae Kernel is used in this prescription to nourish heart, strength heart to prevent collapse or Chinese Magnoliavine Fruit and Asparagus Cochinchinensis are added to clear and astringe lung Qi and also prevent collapse.

VI. Typical medical records from famous experts

i. Medical records of Ding Ganren

Zhu Zuo record: new cold results in phlegm-fluid retention macerated in the lung, additionally occurrence of cough and dyspnea, feeling cold and fear of cold, thin and greasy tongue fur, and thread and slippery pulse. It is similar to phlegm-fluid retention in Golden Chamber and should be harmonized with warm medicine.

Cinnamomum Wilsonii (eight fen), Indian Bread (three qian), Rhizoma Atractylodis Macrocephalae (five qian), Prepared Liquorice Root (five fen), Rhizoma Pinelliae (two qian), Orange Red (one qian), Sweet Apricot Seed (three qian), Processed Radix Polygalae (one qian), Processed Fructus Perillae (five qian), Inula Japonica (bag, five qian), Radish Seed (stir-fried, milled, two qian), Balanophyllia sp (one qian). (one qian = 3.72 g, one fen = 0.372 g)

Exterior is invaded by sudden cold, and then phlegm-fluid retention is gathered inside to make bronchus blocked in the lung, so that the purification and descent are out of control. As a result, serious asthma and cough occur. Hence patients cannot lie down day and night, showing physical cold and fear of cold, eating less and nausea, with white and greasy tongue fur and stringy and slippery floating pulse. Modification of Minor Green-Blue Dragon Decoction is proposed to sooth and release exogenous pathogenic factors and warm and resolve phlegm and fluid retention.

Stir-frying with honey Ephedra (four fen), Cinnamomum Wilsonii (eight fen), Indian Bread (three qian), Rhizoma Pinelliae (two qian), Chinese Magnoliavine Fruit (four fen), Light Dried Ginger (four fen), processed Perilla Fruit (two qian), Sweet Apricot Seed (three qian), Prepared Common Monkshood Daughter Root (one qian), Balanophyllia sp (one qian), Xiaohou Zijin Pill (additional swallowing, taking two days continuously, two pills.) (one qian = 3.72 g, one fen = 0.372 g)

The second diagnosis: Taking two doses of Minor Green-Blue Dragon Decoction, asthma and cough are relieved greatly on the day, but worsen at night, showing less eating and nausea, thin and greasy tongue fur and thready and slippery pulse. Yin exuberance is at night and fluid retention pathogen seizes yang position and blocks Qi movement. Descending of lung and stomach impairs control and then warm and resolvefluid retention pathogen to purify and descend lung Qi.

Cinnamomum Wilsonii (eight fen), Indian Bread (three qian), Rhizoma Pinelliae (two qian), Orange Red (one qian), Chinese Magnoliavine Fruit (four fen), Light Dried Ginger (four fen), Processed with water Radix Polygalae (five fen), Sweet Apricot Seed (three qian), Processed Perilla Fruit (five qian), Inula Japonica (bag, five qian), Prepared Common Monkshood Daughter Root (one qian), Balanophyllia sp (one qian). (one qian = 3.72 g, one fen = 0.372 g)

The third diagnosis: asthma and cough are relieved at night, nausea is also stopped. Only the root of phlegm and fluid retention has been a long time, and it is difficult to be resolved immediately. Spleen is the source of phlegm and lung is the container of phlegm. Prescription of regulating spleen and purifying lung and warming and resolving phlegm and fluid retention is proposed.

In original prescription, Inula Japonica and Milkwort Root are removed, but Rhizoma Atractylodis Macrocephalae (five qian) and stir-fried Malaytea Scurfpea Fruit (five qian) are added. (one qian = 3.72g)

ii. Medical records of Wu Peiheng

Zheng ××, female, 25 years old, who was from Yunnan province, has got married. She had chronic asthma for more than fourteen years and she was pregnant for over four months at that time. She lived in Kunming military region××hospital and invited me for diagnosis on October 9, 1959. With regard to her history of disease, she was easy to get disease once being infected with wind-cold due to the weakness at the young age. Besides, her improper adjustment of medicine and food makes the wind-cold hide in interior, and inversely ascend to lung with dampness-phlegm. Therefore, she often had cough and asthma, which are more serious in cold weather. The disease has been for many years and turned into chronic asthma finally. The syndromes are cough, shortness of breath and dyspnea, much white phlegm, discomfort in throat, and sometimes occurrence of wheezing, pale complexion with less polishing, green black ocular orbit and lips. Eating less without drinking, short and unclear urine, especially serious asthmatic cough at night, difficulty to lie down and sleep. White slippery thick greasy tongue fur, cyan tongue body, tstringy and slippery pulse, which is weak and powerless when being pressed heavily. This is because wind-cold is in lung and stomach, and long-term cough results in lung and kidney Qi deficiency, as a result yang cannot operate due to its insufficiency, and cold-dampness as well as phlegm and fluid is blocked. Xiaoqinglong Decoction and Prepared Common Monkshood Daughter Root should be used to lift lung-cold, tonify kidney to improve Qi reception and warm and resolve phlegm-dampness .

100g of Prepared Common Monkshood Daughter Root, 10g of Debark Peony Root, 10g of Ephedra, 6g of Herba Asari, 30g of Dried Ginger, 20g of Cassia Twig, 5g of Chinese Magnoliavine Fruit, 10g of Pinellia Tuber, 10g of Liquorice Root.

After taking two doses of decoction in above prescription, large amount of clear white phlegm are expectorated. Chest distress, shortness of breath and asthma cough all have been relieved. Patients can sleep for four or five hours, eating more, whose lip and tongue are turned into red with slight cyan, and half of thick greasy white fur has been removed. Although the above prescription is effective, yang Qi is not sufficient. Cold-dampness and phlegm and fluid retention have not been purified, and it should continue to be treated with formula of warming, resolving, opening and lifting. In this prescription, Ephedra, Pungent Formula and Cassia Twig should be added in combination of Sini Decoction and Decoction of Two Old Ingredients.

200g of Prepared Common Monkshood Daughter Root, 40g of Dried Ginger, 30g of Indian Bread, 15g of Rhizoma Pinellinae Praeparata, 10g of Guangdong Dried Tangerine Peel, 8g of Herba Asari, 10g of herba ephedrae (stir-frying with honey), 10g of superior Cinnamon Bark (milled, and soaked in water), 10g of Liquorice Root.

After taking the above prescription, asthma and cough are both relieved. Keep using the prescription for treatment, modifying the herbs and their dosages according to the syndrome. After taking over twenty doses, asthma and cough are gradually relieved. After taking another more than ten doses, the disease is cured while the pregnancy goes on well. She gave birth to a child until full term. Both mother and child are healthy after delivery.

Note: It was said that if women were pregnant, Gall of Garter Snake, Prepared Common Monkshood Daughter Root and Pinellia Tuber are forbidden, which is not true. Although unprepared Gall of Garter Snake, Prepared Common Monkshood Daughter Root and Pinellia Tuber are toxic and cannot be taken, the toxicity can be eliminated if they are prepared properly by the way of processing of materia medica and decocting method, and then they are applied in accordance with disease, it is no harmful even to pregnant women. If women are pregnant and suffer from the disease, fetal Qi will be easily damaged and insecure. The prescription is prescribed in the light of the syndrome to make sure that pathogen is eliminated and fetus is safe. This is the essential of calming and securing fetus. As said in *Internal Classic*: "Treating the pregnant women with toxics……if there is a disease cause, then the toxics will not do harms to the mother, nor the fetus." It means medicines should be used according to the disease. When there is a medicine, the medicines work on the disease, therefore, the pregnant woman will not get hurt, nor the fetus. I had several decades of clinical practice and benefited a lot based on the thinking for root causes and much verification in practice. (*Medical Records of Wu Peiheng*).

iii. Medical Records of Zhao Shaoqin

Mr. Qi, male, is 47 years old. Preliminary diagnosis: he had asthma and cough for more than 10 years, which would occur when meeting cold. He had much clear phlegm, even couldn't lie down in serious condition. Recently due to catching a cold, asthma and cough occurs again and is serious at night. Tongue is white and fur is greasy and neat, pulse is deep and stringy, and tight and rapid when being pressed. In the case of mutual contention of cold and fluid retention and reversed flow of qi, asthma and cough attacks. Cold-fluid retention should be warmed and resolved to relieve dyspnea. He receives Minor Green-Blue Dragon Decoction method.

6g of Ephedra, 6g of Cinnamon Twig, 10g of Pinellia Tuber, 3g of Manchurian Wildginger, 10g of Debark Peony Root, 6g of Dried Ginger, 6g of Prepared Liquorice Root; seven fu in total.

The second diagnosis: after medication, dyspnea with cough is relieved and the amount of phlegm is reduced. The pulse is still deep and stringy, while tongue is white and moistening. The previous method is used to advance and retreat.

3g of Ephedra, 6g of Cinnamon Twig, 10g of Pinellia Tuber, 3g of Manchurian Wildginger, 6g of Dried Ginger, 10g of Debark Peony Root, 6g of Prepared Liquorice Root, 10g of Bitter Apricot Seed, 10g of inula japonica; seven fu in total.

The third diagnosis: After taking Minor Green-Blue Dragon Decoction twice, he ate less with much phlegm, white tongue and moistening fur, whose asthma and cough are gradually calmed and pulse is not so deep. The method of ventilating lung and resolving phlegm is still used.

10g of Perilla Leaf, 10g of Bitter Apricot Seed, 10g of Thunberg Fritillary Bulb, 10g of Radish Seed, 6g of White Mustard Seed, 6g of Stir-fried Orange Fruit, 10g of Platycodon Root, 10g of Charred Triplet, 10g of Pinellia Tuber, 10g of Dried Tangerine Peel. After taking seven doses. For the decoction, the patient stops coughing and wheezing and eats more. Cold and cool diet is forbidden. Sports exercise is done to strength constitution, in order to prevent from the cold and the disease recurrence.

Note: Main manifestation of chronic asthmatic bronchitis is recurrent asthmatic cough and profuse phlegm. This disease often reappears or aggravates due to catching a cold or wind-cold. The pathogenesis is internal fluid retention and external cold, which is said in *Internal Classic*: "physique cold and drinking or eating cool food can harm the lung. Two cold interacts, and the middle and exterior are both harmed, hence, Qi flow is reversed and rises". Since the pathogenesis is external cold and internal fluid retention, Minor Green-Blue Dragon Decoction of Zhongjing should be used to disperse external cold and resolve cold and fluid retention. It will be effective after patients who have this disease take this decoction. Cold-natured medicines cannot be taken due to inflammation. Cold and cool diet is forbidden, such as cold drink or raw or cold food as well as melon and fruit. After recovery, recurrence shall be prevented. It is most important to prevent from the cold and eating cold and cool food for prevention method. Patients themselves shall do more exercises strengthen constitution and improve ability of disease resistance. Medicines of invigorating spleen-stomach and assisting digestion are given in priority. If spleen-stomach is invigorated, phlegm-dampness will not be generated. If Original Qi is secure, exogenous pathogenic factors will be difficult to invade, which is the fundamental method. (*Zhao Shaoqin's Clinical Recipe Cases Selection*)

VII. Prevention and aftercare

1. Pay attention to season and climate to prevent common cold.

In cold season or days with the changing weather, the winter protection and keeping warm, actively prevent the attack of the cold, chronic bronchitis, bronchial asthma and other pulmonary diseases shall be paid attention to. It shall be avoided being affected by exogenous pathogenic factors, to prevent inducing or aggravating emphysema. Cold-resistance exercise should be insisted, which can improve the ability of patients against wind-cold.

2. Spicy or irritant food, raw or cold food and greasy food shall be avoided.

Diet shall be light. Digestible food with high protein, high calorie, high vitamin, low salt shall be appropriate. Food of tonifying and replenishing lung yin and invigorating spleen shall be added. Patients with turbid phlegm obstructing lung shall avoid having raw or cold food, greasy and thick flavor food and sweetmeat; patients with lung Qi deficiency shall avoid having cold and cool food, but can eat food of warming and tonifying lung Qi, such as mutton and pig lung. Patient with lung heat and yellow phlegm shall not eat spicy, greasy food and other food assisting fire and producing phlegm.

3. Smoking and drinking alcohol are forbidden. Irritant gas, dust, pollen and animal shall be avoided.

Give up smoking to avoid smoke dust. Irritation of harmful gas and bad factors on respiratory tract shall be prevented. Allergic patients shall keep away from allergen, for example, irritant gas, dust, pollen and animal and other sensitizing agents.

4. Overwork, hunger and emotion irritation shall be avoided.

Pay attention to combination of exertion and rest and have a regular living. Don't be too tired. Patients shall be encouraged to be positive in prevention and treatment, coordinate with the doctor, establish confidence in conquering the disease, keep relaxed mood and avoid rage.

5. Medicine nursing

The medicines are used correctly following the doctor's advice, in order to avoid arbitrarily taking medicines that cause cough and dyspnea as side effects. Traditional Chinese medicines of tonifying lung and replenishing kidney shall be taken when they are warm in the morning or at night with an empty stomach. They should be taken for many times with less volume when the patient coughs and wheezes. When insomnia or dysphoria appears, the medicines cannot be used arbitrarily without the approval of the doctor.

(XING Shuli)

References

[1] Global strategy for the diagnosis, management and prevention of chronic obstructive pulmonary disease(updated2015)[EB/OL].[2015-01].http://www.goldcopd.org/guidelines-global-strategy-for-diagnosis-management.html.

[2] Li JS, Li SY, Yu XQ. Guideline about diagnosis and treatment of TCM on chronic obstructive pulmonary disease (2011 edition) [J]. Journal of traditional Chinese medicine 2012, 53(1):80-84.

[3] Sun LP, Xu S, Zhang NZ. TCM research progress on chronic obstructive pulmonary disease [J]. Clinical Journal of Traditional Chinese Medicine, 2012, 24(4):368-370.

[4] Liu SZ, Zhang YZ, Xing SL. Clinical observation of "COPD" treated with Ear Points application method [J]. Journal of Emergency in Traditional Chinese Medicine, 1992, 1(1):40-41.

[5] Yang J. Meng Shujiang—— Book series of hundreds of TCM clinicians of Chinese hundreds of years [M]. Beijing: China Press of Traditional Chinese Medicine, 2001.

[6] Sun QX. Therapeutic experience collection of Ma Ruiting [M]. Beijing: China Press of Traditional Chinese

Medicine, 2011.

[7] Ding GR. Medical records of Ding Ganren [M]. Shanghai: Shanghai Science and Technology Press, 1960.

[8] Wu SY. Medical records of Wu peiheng [M]. Kunming: Yunnan People's Publishing House, 1979.

[9] Peng JZ, Yang LZ. Selected clinical cases of Zhao Shaoqin [M]. Beijing: Academy Press, 1996.

Chronic Heart Failure

慢性心力衰竭

I. Overview

Chronic heart failure is a kind of complex clinical syndrome that results from ventricular filling or impaired ejection which are caused by any abnormal situations of the structure or function of the heart. The main clinical manifestations of the chronic heart failure are dyspnea, malaise (limited activity tolerance) and fluid retention (pulmonary congestion and peripheral edema). And these manifestations are described with the terms of the "palpitations", "fearful throbbing", "dyspnea", "edema", "phlegm-fluid retention", "chest impediment", "abdominal mass" and so on in Traditional Chinese Medicine.

Heart failure is the severe or final stage of various heart diseases, with the features of high incidence and death rate. The survival rate of 5 years of heart failure is similar to that of malignant tumor, and the death rate of the patients in severe cases is 50% within 1 year. According to the epidemiological investigation in China, in the past 40 years, resulting from the increase of astogeny and risk factors of cardiovascular diseases, the death rate of heart failure in China has increased by 6 times and the morbidity has reached around 0.9%. According to retrospective investigations towards 10,714 cases of heart failure hospitalizations at 42 hospitals in some parts of China, it is found that coronary heart disease ranked the first of the disease cause of heart failure, followed by hypertension, and the morbidity of rheumatic valvular heart disease was reduced; The death rate of heart failure of each age group was higher than that of other angiocardiopathies occurring in the same period. The main causes of death were left heart failure (59%), arrhythmia (13%) and sudden death (13%) in turn. According to the statistical report released by American Heart Association (AHA) in 2005, there were 5 million heart failure patients and the annual growth of the disease was 550 thousand. European Society of Cardiology (ESC) conducted a survey in 51 countries and found that among ordinary people, the total incidence of the heart failure was 2%-3%, but the number was 10%-20% among aged people of 70-80 years old. The incidence of heart failure continues to increase in recent years and is becoming the most common cardiovascular disease in the 21th century.

II. Etiology and pathogenesis

i. Chinese Medicine

The etiology and pathogenesis of the heart failure are related to viscera loss, yin-yang disharmony and disorder of Qi and body fluid metabolism. The external causes are mainly pathogenic wind, cold, damp and heat, and the internal causes mainly are improper diet, internal injury due to seven emotional disorder, congenital deficiencies, senile decay and aeipathia. The clinical practice and research towards the disease cause and pathogenesis based on the disease at present have been through a long exploring time. According to document analysis, expert inquiry and relevant epidemiological investigation, it was found that the etiology of chronic heart failure is mainly about deficiency in origin and excess in superficiality. The deficiency in origin includes Qi deficiency, yin deficiency and yang deficiency, and excess in superficiality includes blood stasis, dampness and retention of phlegm and fluid. The disease location is in heart, involving lung, spleen, kidneys, liver and organs of Sanjiao.

1. Qi deficiency, yin deficiency, yang deficiency as basement

Inner Canon of Huangdi: records that "If the qi of the Hand Shaoyin disappeared, the channel will be blocked. If the channel blocked, the blood flow will stoped." "The heart qi deficiency will lead to continuous dyspnea." These descriptions are all related to the symptoms of chronic heart failure. The main pathogenesis is the deficiency of heart Qi. The heart governs blood and vessels, so if with deficiency of heart Qi, weak heart beat, slow blood flow or blood stasis happen, the heart failure will be caused. The heart Qi will be stimulated relying on the warmth of the heart yang. If the heart yang deficiency occurs, it cannot help lung metal in the upper jiao, and warm the spleen earth in the middle jiao and the kidney water in the lower jiao then the symptoms of oppression in chest, asthma, abdominal distension and edema will happen; only when the heart yang is vigorous, will the heart Qi be abundant, and then the blood transporting will be in normal state. Because of the mutual rooting between yin-yang, yin injury in yang because of prolonged illness. or the impairment of yin during the process of diureses in the treatment and insufficient dietary sources in the case of yin deficiency in protopathy happening before the illness, the patients will also suffer from the lack of Qi and yin and the losses of yin and yang.

2. Blood stasis, water-dampness and phlegm-turbidity as signs

Vomiting Blood of *Theory of blood* records: "Qi is the commander of blood, and the blood runs with it", so the Qi deficiency will cause the weakness in blood transportation and finally lead to blood stasis. If the Qi deficiency lasts for a long time, yang qi will be damaged, and the warming and propelling function of yang qi will be weakened. Hence, there will come pathological states that Qi fails to help and promote water movement and transformation and finally the water will be accumulated and form the humidity or phlegm even edema, showing the symptoms such as cough, expectoration or edema. If the phlegm is detained in vessels, the blood flow will be inhibited, which will cause blood stasis. In *Water qi Disease* of *Jin Synopsis of the Golden Chamber*, Zhang Zhongjing has put forward "Blood stasis will cause edema", if the water cannot be expelled and accumulated, the meridian Qi and blood running will be interfered. In addition, the blood stasis and water-dampness affect each other. Blood stasis, water-dampness and phlegm-turbidity intertwine cach other, which can become the new pathology for further stage of the illness. The chronic heart failure is caused by deficiency and then develops to excess, and the two are mingled to each other, which becomes a vicious circle.

3. The disease location is at heart, involving lungs, spleen, kidneys, liver and organs of sanjiao

The disease location is at the heart, but is not limited to it. The five zang viscera are organically integrated, which not only do their own work but also cooperate with each other physically in order to accomplish the physiological function. They affect each other in pathology and the illness happening in one organ will lead to the outset of the illness in another organ. On the one hand, because of "the heart is the great governor of the zang-fu viscera", if the heart yang is in deficiency, the heart blood does not flow and the blood vessels are inhibited, then the channels in five zang-organs will lose nourishments, and after a long term, the four zang-organs of lung, spleen, kidney and liver will all be damaged. On the other hand, the imbalance of lung, spleen, kidney, liver and Sanjiao will be harmful to the heart. Lungs are in charge of Qi, breath, vessels, down and waterway, and if the lung Qi is in deficiency or the lung Qi fails in purification, the heart vessel will be inhibited and the symptoms like chest distress will happen; the spleen is the source of Qi and blood, the hub for transporting the fluid, so the deficiency of spleen will lead to the origin lack of Qi and blood, the fluid transport stopping and becoming water-dampness, which will foster the heart water, and then the symptoms of abdominal distension, anorexia and vomiting will happen; kidneys are the congenital foundation, containing the Yuan-yin and Yuan-yang inside. The heart takes kidney as fundamental, and the heart Qi and heart yang are produced from the kidneys, the kidney Qi and kidney yang can warm the heart. The heart governs the internal heat, and the kidney governs the internal water, so the two will cooperate with each other, with mutual rooting of yin and yang as well as coordination between water and fire. If the kidney yang is in deficiency, the disturbance of Qi transformation happens, causing the edema, even or rapid respiration and palpitation due to pathogen attacking heart and lung. The liver governs storage of blood, and free flow of Qi. If liver dysfunction and the disturbance of Qi movements happen, it will lead to Qi-stagnation and blood stasis, with hepatomegaly, modern depression and other symptoms. "Sanjiao are the channels that primordial Qi runs in and out, up and down, which govern three Qi to run through the viscera. ", "Sanjiao are the channels of water liquid running, and the beginning and ending of the Qi". If Sanjiao Qi is blocked, the water cannot be expelled without flowing, so the abdominal distension will occur and Qi will be full, and it is difficult to urinate, and finally the water distention will happen.

ii. Western Medicine

1. Etiology

(1) Myocardial dysfunction: the myocardial damages that are caused by myocardial infarction, myocarditis, cardiomyopathy, myocardial toxicity or myocardial fibrosis; myocardial metabolic abnormalities that are caused by vitamin B1 deficiency, ischemia or oxygen deficit.

(2) Cardiac overload: the volume overload that is caused by valvular insufficiency, arteriovenous fistula, ventricular septal defect, severe anemia and hyperthyreosis; pressure overload that is caused by hypertension, coarctation of the aorta, aortic stenosis, pulmonary hypertension and pulmonary stenosis.

2. Precipitating factors

According to epidemiological analysis, about 60% - 90% of heart failure cases have precipitating factors, and the common precipitating factors include infection, arrhythmia, over-exertion, pregnancy and childbirth, pulmonary embolism, disturbances of water and electrolyte balance, acid-base imbalance and malpractice.

III. Key points of diagnosis and differential diagnosis

i. Key points of diagnosis

Referred to *Chinese Heart Failure Diagnosis and Treatment Guidelines 2014*, the diagnosis of chronic heart failure (CHF) should take medical history, symptoms, signs and auxiliary examination into consideration. Based on left ventricular ejection fraction (LVEF), CHF can be divided into heart failure of reduced ejection fraction (HF-REF) and heart failure of preserved ejection fraction (HF-PEF). Generally speaking, HF-REF refers to the traditional systolic heart failure, and HF-PEF refers to the diastolic heart failure. Some heart failure patients have both of symptoms. LVEF is one of the important indexes of classification and prognosis in CHF patients.

1. The clinical assessment of CHF patients

(1) Medical history, symptoms and signs: The detailed history-taking and physical examination can provide references. The heart failure patients go to hospital for one of the following three reasons: decreased exercise tolerance, fluid retention and other cardiogenic or non-cardiogenic diseases which all show corresponding symptoms and signs. During the clinical reception, doctors shall evaluate volume status and vital signs, monitor the weight change of the patients, estimate the jugular venous pressure, and check whether there are edemas, paroxysmal nocturnal dyspnea or orthopnea.

(2) The routine examination of heart failure: Two-dimensional echocardiography and doppler ultrasonography; electrocardiogram; laboratory examination; biomarkers: If it is determined that plasma natriuretic peptides [B natriuretic peptide (BNP)]<35ng/L and N-terminal pro-B type natriuretic peptide (NT-proBNP) <125ng/L, it will not support the diagnosis of CHF. Other biomarkers include myocardial damage (cTn), fibrosis (Soluble ST2; Galectin-3), the sign of inflammation, oxidative stress, neural hormone disorder and myocardial and matrix remodeling; chest x-ray.

2. The diagnosis criteria of chronic HF-PEF

(1) The following two aspects shall be taken into full consideration when diagnosing.

① The main clinical manifestations: the patients have typical symptoms and signs of heart failure; the patients show normal or slightly decreased LVEF number (≥ 45%), and the left ventricle is normal; patients have related structural heart diseases (such as left ventricular hypertrophy and left atrial enlargement) and (or) diastolic dysfunction; patients don't have valvular disease after being examined by echocardiography, and pericardial disease, hypertrophic cardiomyopathy and limit (invasive) cardiomyopathy can be excluded. The LVEF standards of the disease have not been yet unified. The number of LVEF between 41%-49% can be called criticality HF-PEF, and the population characteristics, treatments and prognosis are all similar to HF-REF, which indicates that it will be better to take LVEF>50% as clinical diagnosis standard. Besides, the number of LVEF of some patients has been decreased to ≤ 40%, and its clinical prognosis will be differ from patients who has LVEF persistent reservation.

② Other factors to be considered: the factors shall accord with epidemiologic features of the disease; the major patients are aged people and women, heart failure patients whose disease causes are hypertension or previous history of high blood pressure for a long time. And some patients will also have diabetes, obesity or atrial fibrillation; BNP and (or) NT-proBNP determinations have reference value but are in dispute. If the determination result shows slight or medium increase, or at least is in the "grey number district", the result will can be referred to during diagnosis.

(2) Auxiliary examination: Because echocardiographic parameters used for diagnosing left ventricular

diastolic dysfunction are not inaccurate, with poor repeatability, cardiac structure and function shall be comprehensively evaluated in conjunction with all of two-dimensional ultrasound and doppler parameters. Early diastolic myocardial velocity of mitral annulus (e ') can be used to assess myocardial relaxation, and E/e ' value is associated with left ventricular filling pressure. Echocardiography evidences of left ventricular diastolic dysfunction may include e ' reduction (e' average <9cm/s), E/e ' value increase (>15), E/A disorders (>2 or < 1), or a combination of these parameters. At least 2 anomalies and (or) atrial fibrillation increase the likelihood of diagnosis of left ventricular diastolic dysfunction.

ii. Differential diagnosis

(1) Bronchial asthma should be distinguished from left-sided cardiac failure. The paroxysmal nocturnal dyspnea caused by left-sided cardiac failure can be called "cardiac asthma", which shall be distinguished from bronchial asthma. The former disease is common among aged people who have the medical history of hypertension or chronic valvulopathy, and the latter one is more common among adolescents with allergic history; the patients who have the former disease shall sit up when the disease happens, and for patients of severe cases, there will be dry wet rale in their lungs and some will even cough. When the latter disease happens, typical wheezing sounds can be heard in both of two lungs of the patients, and after coughing the white phlegm, the symptom of dyspnea can be often relieved. Determining the plasma BNP levels will be helpful to make differential diagnosis of cardiac asthma and bronchial asthma.

(2) When diseases of hydropericardium and constrictive pericarditis happen, symptoms of distention of jugular vein, hepatomegaly and edema of lower extremity caused by blocked vena cava will occur. Doctors shall make differential diagnosis based on medical history and cardiac and peripheral vascular signs of patients and then the disease can be affirmed by adopting echocardiography.

(3) Cirrhotic ascites accompanied by lower limb edema shall be distinguished from chronic right-sided heart failure. Except that basic signs of heart disease are helpful in distinguishing, distention of jugular vein or other body signs of blocked superior vena cava will not happen during the treatment of non-cardiogenic hepatic cirrhosis.

(4) Symptoms of edema and ascites that are caused by right-sided heart failure shall be distinguished from those caused by renal edema, pericardial asthma and cirrhosis. Renal edema appears more at eyelid or loose parts of facial tissue and the symptoms will become more severe after the patients get up in the mornings. Therefore it is different from the edema due to gravity. Ascites of pericardial diseases and cirrhosis are often more obvious than peripheral edema.

IV. TCM therapy

i. Syndrome differentiation and treatment

Because CHF is a kind of chronic progressive disease, once the disease happens, even though there is no new cardiac damage, and the patients are still in the clinical stabilization stage, the disease itself can develop continuously too. Therefore the CHF is a kind of disease with features of slow development and acute exacerbation, during the development of the disease, naturally showing the alternation of aggravating and mitigating of the disease. Once the symptoms inducing the exacerbation of the CHF exist, such as infection, arrhythmia, high blood pressure, electrolyte disturbance, too much and too fast infusion and emotional excitement, the patients will enter exacerbation period. And the clinical manifestations will include chest breath, rapid respiration, reduced exercise tolerance, difficulty in lying down, breath with difficulty, cough, edema of lower limbs, or even dropsy of chest and ascites, which will lead to the decrease of the life qualities of patients. From the perspective of traditional Chinese medicine, the clinical manifestations of the CHF in exacerbation period are mainly the manifestation excess syndrome pathogenesis characteristics such as blood stasis, water-dampness and phlegm turbidity. Among them, the major symptom is edema, and the root deficiency symptoms of Qi deficiency, yang deficiency and yin deficiency will be accompanied at the same time. However, in catabasis period, manifestation excess syndrome such as blood stasis, water-dampness and turbid phlegm will be relieved apparently, and the main pathogenesis characteristics include Qi deficiency, yang deficiency and yin deficiency. Because of the features of low development and acute exacerbation, the patients with severe conditions have to be treated in the hospital. Because the clinicians "concern more about hospitalization while pay less attention to extramural hospital treatment"at present, in addition, the patients and their families often "concern more about the treatments in the exacerbation period and pay less attention to the treatment in catabasis period", patients always go to the hospitals only when the disease becomes severe and leave the hospital when the symptoms are relieved. What's more, there is a lack of reasonable treatment after leaving the hospital, thus causing the situation of repeated attack and repeated hospitalization. Hence, it is actually in accordance with the major feature "deficiency in root and excess in manifestation" of CHF acknowledged by traditional Chinese medicine to divide the CHF into the exacerbation period and catabasis period, showing the principle of "symptomatic treatment in acute condition while radical treatment in chronic case" in traditional Chinese medicine in treating diseases

1. The exacerbation period of the CHF

The classification of exacerbation period of CHF is based on excess in manifestation, and separated treatment of cold and heat is conducted according to the eight-principle syndrome differentiation and classification is made combining with Qi-blood-liquid-fluid pattern identification. Based on the different natures of bodies of patients, the exacerbation period of CHF can be divided into cold stasis and water condensation type and heat stasis and water condensation type. In the exacerbation period, because the symptom of water stasis cannot be avoided, blood stasis, water-dampness and phlegm turbidity will become the main disease pathogenesis characteristics. However, due to the different natures of cold and heat, the TCM therapies will be different. The clinical diseases are nothing more than cold and heat, so doing the classification according to the cold and heat shows the treating principle of "heat the cold and freeze the heat". The goals of treatment in exacerbation period: rapidly relieve the symptoms of heart failure and control the outset of the CHF. The principles of treatment: the keys are on edema alleviating and inducing dieresis, lung draining and relieving asthma, clearing heat and dispelling phlegm and activating blood and removing blood stasis, which can show the principle of treatment of "Relieving the manifestation in an urgent case", and at the same time, the significant Chinese medicine therapy of "symptomatic treatment in acute condition while radical treatment in chronic case" shall be obeyed and the root deficiency symptom of the patient shall be given the same consideration, treated with replenishing Qi, warming yang, tonifying yin and generating liquid. It can reflect the principle of "eliminate pathogen and reinforce healthy Qi" and achieve "eliminate pathogen with no harm to healthy Qi".

(1) Cold stasis and water condensation

Main symptoms: wheezing cough and propped breathing, impossible of lying on the back, coughing foamy phlegm; edema of lower limbs or whole body, and the edema will be sunken when pressed, patients with severe conditions will have swelling of vulva; difficulty of urination, palpitations and hard breath, and the symptom will become severe if the patients do activities; the light and fat tongue texture, white and smooth tongue fur, weak or slow sunken and thin pulse.

Therapeutic method: warm yang and excrete water, excrete sediments and activate blood.

Prescription: Zhen Wu Tang and Ling Gui Zhu Gan Tang. Milkvetch Root, Tangshen, Prepared Common Monkshood Daughter Root, Cassia Twig, Cortex Acanthopanacis, Rhizoma Alismatics, Indian Bread, White Atractylodes Rhizomeme, Semen Lepidii, Cortex Mori, Plantain Seed, Chinese Lobelia Herb, Hirsute Shiny Bugleweed Herb, Liquorice Root.

Prescription analysis: the property of Prepared Common Monkshood Daughter Root is of heat, for tonifying fire and assisting yang; Cassia Twig can warm meridian and invigorate pulse, reinforce yang and transform Qi; Milkvetch Root and Tangshen can tonify middle and replenish Qi. And if four medicines are combined, they can activate yang Qi, warm and resolve water-dampness. Semen Lepidii and Cortex Mori can purge lung and relieve dyspnea, induce dieresis, dispel water-dampness in upper jiao; Indian Bread can invigorate spleen and induce diuresis with bland drugs. White Atractylodes Rhizomeme can invigorate spleen, dry dampness, make the middle jiao transport fluently and let the water dampness be dispelled automatically; Cortex Acanthopanacis can warm kidney and dispel dampness. Rhizoma Alismatics, Plantain Seed and Chinese Lobelia Herb can drain damp and relieve stranguria. Hirsute Shiny Bugleweed Herb can induce diuresis and activate blood to make the water way in lower jiao more fluent. Prepared Liquorice Root can invigorate spleen, invigorate the middle-warmer, harmonize the drugs in order to warm yang and promote dieresis, and excrete feculence and activate blood.

Modification: patients who often cough and have much phlegm can adopt Arisaema with Bile and Caulis Bambusae to dry dampness and resolve phlegm; patients who suffer from cough breathing and cannot lie down can adopt Radix Peucedani and rhizome Cynanchi, Semon Ginkgo and Platycodon Root to ventilate lung and regulate Qi; the patients who suffer from nausea and vomit can adopt Ginger, Evodia Rutaecarpa and Pinellia Ternata to lower the adverse flow of Qi, warm the stomach and resolve vomit. Or they can adopt Fructus Amomi, Dried Tangerine or Orange Peel and Eupatorium to remove dampness to restore normal functioning of the stomach; patients who have the symptom of having water sound in epigastric oppression or stomach can adopt Fructus Aurantii Immaturus and Ginger to dispel phlegm and water stasis; patients who have Qi stagnation and abdominal distension can use areca and areca peel; people who have hepatosplenomegaly can remove blood stasis and eliminate stagnated food by using turtle shell, Rhizoma Sparganii and Curcuma Zedoary; people who have uropenia or anuresis symptoms can use Polyporus and Fourstamen Stephania Root.

(2) Heat stasis and water condensation

Main symptoms: cough and propped breathing, difficulty in lying down, cough phlegm while coughing and the thick phlegm or both yellow and thick phlegm; edema in lower limbs or whole body, and the edema that will be sunken when being pressed, swelling of vulva that will appear in the patient with severe condition; palpitations and breathe hard that will become severe if the patients do activities, chest tightness and short of breath; abdominal distension and anorexia, dry mouth and thirsty, difficulty of urination; pale red or pale purple tongue, thick or yellow tongue fur, as well as slippery and rapid pulse.

Therapeutic method: clear heat and activate blood, purge the lung and induce dieresis.

Prescription: modified Ji Jiao Li Huang Tang. Stephania tetrandra, Si Chuan Pepper Accounts, Pepperweed Seed, Rhubarb, White Mulberry Root-bark, Citron Fruit, Hedyotis, Chinese Lobelia Herb, Shiny Bugleweed Herb, Rhizoma Alismatics, Plantain Seed, Indian Bread, White Atractylodes Rhizomeme, Liquorice Root.

Prescription analysis: Stephania Tetrandra can clear heat, induce diuresis, and dispel the damp-heat of bladder in lower jiao. Si Chuan Pepper Accounts, Hedyotis Diffusa and Chinese Lobelia Herb can clear the heat, remove the dampness and eliminate the steam in stomach; Shiny Bugleweed Herb, Rhizoma Alismatics and Plantain Seed can help activate blood, dispel heat and osmotic diuresis; Semen Lepidii and White Mulberry Root-bark can purge the lung, relieve asthma and induce diuresis; Indian Bread and White Atractylodes Rhizomeme can tonify spleen and separate the wetness. Rhebarb can clear the heat and relax the menstruation. Citron Fruit can relieve inflation. Liquorice Root can harmonize all the drugs. The whole prescription can clear the heat and activate the blood, and purge the lung and induce diuresis.

Modification: patients who have lung heat and acute asthma can adopt Mufangji and Gypsum to clear heat and remove dampness; patients who have much phlegm can use Tendrilleaf Fritillary Bulb, Bile Arisaema, Tabasheer and Heartleaf Houttuynia Herb to ventilate the lung and resolve phlegm; hemoptysis patients can adopt Japanese Thistle Root, Field Thistle Root and Chinese Arborvitae Twig and Leaf; patients who often vomit can use Bamboo Shavings and Fresh Ginger to relieve phlegm and vomiting; patients with severe abdominal distension can adopt Magnolia Obavata, Radish Seed, Areca and Semen Pharbitidis; patients who suffer from hard and dry stool can use Rheum Officinale, areca and oriental arborvitae to loosen the bowels to relieve constipation; patients who have uropenia or anuresis problems can use Talc, Chuling, Chinese Waxgourd Peel and waxgourd seed to free urine and clear lower heat.

2. The catabasis period of the CHF

In the catabasis period of CHF, the symptoms of excess in manifestation are controlled or relieved and then the symptoms of deficiency in root become the main clinical manifestation. The division method of the catabasis period of CHF is based on the symptoms of deficiency inroot, and the main pathogenesis characteristics are Qi deficiency, yin deficiency and yang deficiency. During this period, the doctors can adopt separation treatment of yin and yang based on eight-principle syndrome differentiation and combine with Qi-blood fluids syndrome differentiation. According to the different features of deficiency of yin and yang of the body, the catabasis period of the CHF can be divided into the type of deficiency of both Qi and yin, internal blockage of the blood stasis and the type of the deficiency of both Qi and yang, internal blockage of the blood stasis. The blood stasis in the catabasis period of the CHF is the pathogenesis characteristic that will occur throughout the whole period, so there will only be the differences of degree compared with exacerbation period. However, resulted from the difference of yin deficiency and yang deficiency, the clinical disease is nothing more than yin and yang. And the classification of yin and yang fully shows the treatment principle of "Nourish yin when yin deficiency happens and tonify yang when yang deficiency happens". The treatment of the catabasis period of the CHF shall be concentrated on the balance of the Qi and blood of yin and yang and regulating visceral functions. And based on Qi and blood, yin and yang syndrome differentiation, the treating process shall be conducted on syndrome differentiation of Sanjiao such as heart, lung, spleen, kidney and liver. And the treating purposes are to strengthen the disease - resistant ability of patients, promote the repair of tissues, improve the life ability and reduce the possibility of relapse. Once the state of disease aggravates, the patient will enter the exacerbation period. The treatment principle shall be concentrated on replenishing Qi and warming yang, nourishing yin and generating fluid and balancing the Qi and blood of yin and yang and regulating visceral functions, which shows the principle of "prime treatment in chronic case". And meanwhile, the doctors shall treat the disease according to the treatment method of Chinese medicine as "symptomatic treatment in acute condition while radical treatment in chronic case", and also pay attention to the patients' symptoms of blood stasis, water-dampness and phlegm-turbidity and adopt the treatment methods of activating blood and resolving stasis, purging lung and relieving dyspnea, inducing diuresis and alleviating edema, which shows the principle of "strengthening healthy qi to eliminate pathogens" to achieve strengthening the body resistance while eliminating pathogenic factors. In the catabasis period, the Chinese Medicine prevention and treatment characters of "preventing disease from exacerbating" as "treatment based on syndrome differentiation, holistic medicine, complex interventions, dynamic adjustment " to achieve the overall effect level of preventing the patients entering the exacerbation period, regaining the Qi transformation funcation of viscera and improving the CHF.

(1) Deficiency of both Qi and yin, the internal blockage of blood stasis

Main symptoms: rapid respiration and breathlessness and the symptom will become severe if the patients do activities; palpitations and flusteredness-fluster, tired and unwilling to move, sweating in the case of movement; insomnia and dreamfulness, shortness of breath and fatigue, spontaneous sweating or night sweat; dysphoria in chestpalms-soles, dry mouth and thirsty, dark red of faces, red tongue body and lack of tongue fur, weak fine rapid pulse or knotted and intermittent pulse.

Therapeutic method: tonify Qi and activate blood, nourish yin and receive Qi.

Prescription: modified Sheng Mai San. Tangshen, Dwarf Lilyturf Tuber, Chinese Magnoliavine, Unprocessed Rehmannia Root, Milkvetch Root, Red Peony Root, Chinese Angelica, Asiatic Cornelian Cherry Fruit, Fragrant Solomonseal Rhizome, Pepperweed Seed, Indian Bread, Plantian Seed.

Prescription analysis: Ttangshen is sweet in taste, and neutral in nature, which can tonify middle and replenish Qi, quench thirst, invigorate spleen and nourish lungs, nourish blood and promote fluid; Ophiopogon tastes sweet and is of cold drug property, which can nourish yin and clear heat, moisten lung and promote fluid; Tangshen and Dwarf Lilyturf Tuber together can achieve the function of tonifying Qi and nourishing yin better; Chinese Magnoliavine tastes sour and is warm in drug property, and it can help astringe lung and achieve hidroschesis, promote fluid and quench thirst. If all these three drugs are taken together that one for repairing, one for moistening, and one for astringing, they can tonify Qi and nourish yin, promote fluid and quench thirst, and can recover Qi and promote fluid, stop sweating and preserve yin, fulfill Qi and complete pulse; Unprocessed Rehmannia Root, Red Peony Root, Chinese Angelica and Fragrant Solomonseal Rhizome can promote fluid and nourish yin, tonify blood, activate blood; Milkvetch Root can help strengthen tonifying Qi; Asiatic Cornelian Cherry Fruit tastes sour and can astringe and promote fluid; Pepperweed Seed can drain lung and resolve asthma, achieve diuresis; Indian Bread can invigorate spleen and excrete dampness and drain dampness; Plantian Seed can enter kidneys and bladder meridian to achieve excreting dampness and diuresis. The whole prescription can tonify Qi and activate blood, nourish yin and improve Qi.

Modification: in terms of patients who have obvious asthma in the case of movement, the dosages of Tangshen and Milkvetch Root are increased; in the case that palpitations and insomnia are serious, Mother-of-pearl, raw Dragon's Teeth and Spine Date Seed are added to soothe the nerve and calm palpitations; for the patients with steaming skin, especially in the late afternoon, as well as yin deficiency and tidal fever, Starwort Root and Chinese Wolfberry Root-bark and Turtle Shell are added to nourish yin and bring fever down; in the case of patients with heat damage to yin fluid and vexation and thirst, Pollen and Reed Rhizome are added to clear heat and generate fluid; with regard to patients with obvious sweating, Light Wheat is added to constrain sweat; if stomach reception is not good enough, Villous Amomum Fruit, Common Yam Rhizome, Jiao San Xian and fried Chicken's Gizzard-Skin can be added; as to patients with diarrhea, Gordon Euryale Seed, fried Common Yam Rhizome and Lotus Seed can be added; in the case of patients with severe blood stasis, Chinese Angelica, Salvia Root and Cortex Moutan are added; in the case that patients have the symptom of hemoptysis, Ophicalcite and Panax Notoginseng Powder are added;

(2) Deficiency of both Qi and yang, internal blockage of static blood

Main symptoms: rapid respiration and breathlessness that aggravates in the case of movement, thin phlegm; palpitations and fluster, fatigue and laziness to move, sweating and aggregated respiration in the case of movement; insomnia and dreamfulness, shortness of breath and fatigue, spontaneous sweating or night sweat; mental fatigue and anorexia, abdomen fullness and distention; grey and white face, mouth and lip cyanosis, cold limbs, clear urine, pale and enlarged tongue body, white and greasy or water slippery tongue fur, thread and sunken or knotted and intermittent pulse.

Therapeutic method: reinforce healthy Qi and activate blood and warm yang and remove blood stasis.

Prescription: modified Bao Yuan Tang. There are Tangshen, Milkvetch Root, Morinda Root, Cassia Bark, Indian Bread, Plantain Seed, Peperweed Seed, Salvia Root, Epimedium Herb, Dodder Seed and Radix Acanthopanacis.

Prescription analysis: Tangshen and Milkvetch Root tonify middle and replenish Qi, Morinda Root, Epimedium Herb and Cassia Cinnamon Bark warm and tonify kidney yang. Dodder Seed is sweet and warm, which can mildly reinforce liver and kidneys. Indian Bread invigorates spleen and eliminates dampness, Peperweed Seed promotes urination and diuresis, Salvia Root activates blood and removes blood stasis, and Radix Acanthopanacis is used to tonify Qi and coordinate each medicine. The whole prescription replenishes Qi and activates blood, warms yang and removes blood stasis.

Modification: in terms of patients with kidney deficiency and serious respiration, Human Placenta and Gekko can be added; in the case of patients with much phlegm and gasp, Rhizoma Pinelliae and Perilla-seed are added; for the patients with yang deficiency, fear of cold and obvious cold limbs, Prepared Common Monkshood Daughter Root, Dodder Seed, Common Curculigo Rhhizome and Fructus Psoraleae and the like are added to warmly reinforce kidney yang; in the case of patients with yang collapse, Prepared Common Monkshood Daughter Root and Dried Ginger are added to restore yang and rescue from collapse; for the patients with palpitations and fluster, Spine Date Seed and stir-baked Milkwort Root are added; in the case that patients suffer from obvious blood stasis, Sichuan Lovage Rhizome, Peach Seed and Safflower are added; for the patients with constipation, Desertliving Cistanche is added; if knotted and intermittent pulse occurs, Prepared Liquorice Root, raw Bone Fossil of Big Mammals and raw Oyster Shell can be added;

ii. Specific prescription treatment

Common basic prescription used by Professor Shi Dazhuo from China Academy of Chinese Medical Sciences for treating CHF is: 10g of Ginseng, 30g of raw Milkvetch Root, 15g of Cassia Twig, 30g of Salvia Root, 30g of Hirsute Shiny Bugleweed Herb, 30g of Motherwort Herb, 30g of Plantain Seed and 30g of Rice Bean. The whole prescription replenishes Qi and warms yang, activates blood and promotes urination. It usually has a good efficacy on treating CHF.

iii. Single ingredient prescription and proved prescription

Peperweed Seed between 6 g and 10g is decocted, and patients take one dose a day; patients take Peperweed Seed powder 1-2g once after mixing with water, 3 times a day. It can be used to treat heart failure.

iv. Chinese patent medicine

(1) Qi Li Qiang Xin Capsule: 4 capsules for one time, and 3 times a day. It can replenish Qi and warm yang, activate blood and dredge collaterals, and induce diuresis and reduce swelling, and be used for the patients with the syndrome of yang qi deficiency as well as collaterals stasis and water retention who suffer from mild and moderate CHF syndrome due to coronary heart disease and hypertension.

(2) Bu Yi Qiang Xin Pian: 4 tablets for one time, and 3 times a day. It can replenish Qi and nourish yin, activate blood and induce diuresis, and be used for CHF of deficiency of both Qi and yin and blood stasis and water retention type with fluster, short breath, lack of strength, oppression in chest, chest pain, pale complexion, sweating, dry mouth, swelling, mouth and lip cyanosis and the like due to coronary heart disease and hypertension (heart function grades Ⅱ ~ Ⅲ).

(3) Shen Fu Qiang Xin Pian: 2 tablets for one time, and 2-3 times a day. It can replenish Qi and support yang, tonify heart and induce diuresis, and be used for the heart-kidney yang deficiency patients with some symptoms for CHF like palpitations, short breath, oppression in chest and rapid respiration and swelling in face and limbs.

(4) Qi Shen Yi Qi Di Pill: 1 dose for one time, and 3 times a day. It can replenish Qi, dredge collaterals, activate blood and relieve pain, and be used for chest impediment of Qi deficiency and blood stasis. Symptoms include oppression in chest, chest pain, short breath and lack of strength, palpitations, spontaneous sweating, lusterless complexion, enlarged tongue with teeth mark, dim or dark purple tongue texture or the tongue texture with stasis maculae, sunken or deep wiry pulse. In modern times, it is commonly used for treatment of asymptomatic heart failure or heart failure after infarction in recovery period clinically.

v. Acupuncture and moxibustion therapy

1. Body needle

Main points: PC 6, PC 5, HT5, HT 8, BL 15, TF (4) and ST 36. In the case of patients with edema, CV 9, ST 28, GB 34 and GV7 and CV 2, or SP 6, KI 5, BL 58, KI 7 and BL 23 are added; two groups of points can be alternatively used. For the patents who cough with much phlegm, LU 5 and ST 40 are added; in the case of patients with belching and abdominal distension, CV 2 is added; for the patients with palpitations and egersis, LI 11 is added; with regard to the patients who breathe heavily and couldn't lie down, BL 13, LI 4, CV 17 and CV 22 are added.

2. Moxibustion method

BL 15, Gv 20, CV 8, CV 4, Philtrum, PC 6 and ST 36 are selected. In terms of asthma and suffocation, BL 13 and Bl 23 are added; in the case that the patients suffer from edema, ST 28, BL 22 and SP 9 are added. 3~5 points are selected each time, and each point is cauterized with moxa stick for 15~20 min, until flush skin presents. Moxibustion is conducted once a day.

vi. Massage treatment

Soft massage towards centrality has certain efficacy on the patients with mild heart failure in early period.

vii. Others

1. Ear acupuncture

Points of heart, lung, kidney, HT7, AH (6a), EX-B1 and CO (18) are taken, and 3~4 points are selected each time. Needles are imbedded, or points are pressed with CowHerb Seed.

2. Point injection

It is reported that application of Milkvetch Root Injection in ST 36 and Shenfu Injection in PC 6 has obvious efficacy on treating CHF, and they can significantly improve heart functions.

3. Others

Some points like BL 15, CV 17 and PC 6 are taken to paste, and lines are embedded; Chinese material medicine in CV 8 with ultrasonic induction therapy; Chinese Medicine foot massage, and so on.

V. Empirical prescription of famous experts

i. Tiao Xin Yin Zi (Zhang Qi)

Indication: heart failure due to heart yang exhaustion and stagnation and obstruction of blood collaterals.

Components: 15g of Ginseng, 25g of Milkvetch Root, 20g of Liquorice Root, 50g of Wheat, 5 Red Dates, 15 g of Prepared Common Monkshood Daughter Root (fired early), 15 g of Cassia Twig, 15 g of Dwarf Lily-turf Tuber, 15 g of Chinese Magnoliavine Fruit, 15 g of Safflower, 20 g of Salvia Root, 30g of Suberect Spatholobus Stem and 15g of Red Peony Root of 15 g.

Application: water decoction, 1 dose a day.

Efficacy: to replenish Qi and warm yang, and activate blood and dredge collaterals.

ii. Wen Yang Yi Xin Yin (Zhang Qi)

Indication: heart failure due to yang deficiency of heart and kidney, water pathogen attacking heart and stagnation and obstruction of blood collaterals.

Components: 15 g of Ginseng and 15 g of Prepared Common Monkshood Daughter Root, 20g of Indian Bread, 15g of White Atractylodes Rhizomeme, 20g of White Peony Root, 15 g of Cassia Twig and 15 g of Fresh Ginger, 20 g of Oriental Waterplantain Rhizome and 20 g of Salvia Root, 15g of Safflower, 20g of Peperweed

Seed and 15g of Red Tangerine Peel.

Application: water decoction, 1 dose a day.

Efficacy: to replenish Qi, warm yang, and induce diuresis

iii. Wen Yun Yang Qi Fang (Yan Dexin)

Indication: heart failure whose main kind is yang deficiency of heart Qi.

Components: 15g of Prepared Common Monkshood Daughter Root, 9g of stir-baked Ephedra Herb, 4.5 g of Manchurian Wildginger, 9 g of Pollen Typhae (wrap-boiling), 15g of Salvia Root and 15g of Kudzuvine Root.

Application: water decoction, 1 dose a day.

Efficacy: to warm yang Qi.

iv. Xin Qi Huo Xue Fang (Yan Dexin)

Indication: heart failure whose main kind is stagnation and obstruction of heart blood.

Components: 9g of Peach Seed, 9g of Safflower, 9g of Red Peony Root, 9g of Chinese Angelica, 9g of Sichuan Lovage Rhizome, 12g of Unprocessed Rehmannia Root, 4.5g of Chinese Thorowax Root, 6g of Orange Fruit, 9g of Radix Achyranthis Bidentatae, 6g of Platycodon Root, 2.4g of Rosewood and 15g of Milkvetch Root.

Application: water decoction, 1 dose a day.

Efficacy: to move Qi and activate blood.

VI. Typical medical records from famous experts

i. Medical record of Du Wuxun——— heat stasis and water coagulation

Hao ×, female, 78 years old, the body shape of hers is above the average. She accepted preliminary diagnosis on October 24th, 2011. She had a disease history of chronic cough for 8 years. Her symptoms happened when the season was changing and she would suffer from asthma, suffocated, tired and became severe when she prostrated. The symptoms include asthma, heavy sweat, being disable to prostrate at nights, xerostomia or bitter taste in mouth, the sticky coughed phlegm, wheezing due to retention of phlegm in throat, abdominal distension, anorexia and dry stool as once in every 3-4 days, difficulty in sleeping at nights, cyanosis finger nail, blue jaundice of lips, swelling of both upper and lower limbs (++), dark red tongue, yellow and thick tongue fur, rolling and rapid pulse. Physical examination: gloomy complexion, jugular vein distention, the heart rate was 106 times/min, with regular heartbeat, rales heard at the bottoms of both lungs, liver touched 2cm under the rib, and blood pressure: 130/100mmHg.

Diagnosis in Western Medicine: CHF; pulmonary heart disease.

Diagnosis of TCM: dyspnea, with the syndrome of the heat stasis and water coagulation

Therapeutic method: clear heat and activate blood, purge lung and induce diuresis

Prescription: modified Ji Jiao Li Huang Wan. 15g of Hanfangji, 9g of Si Chuan Pepper Accounts, 30g of Pepperweed Seed, 12g of Rhubarb, 12g of Baical Skullcap Root, 30g of Heart-leaf Houttuynia Herb, 30g of Indian Bread, 15g of Largehead Atractylodes Rhizome, 30g of White Mulberry Root-bark, 30g of Plaintain Seed, 15g of Oriental Water-plantian Rhizome, 30g of Hedyotis, 15g of Chinese Lobelia Herb. 1 dose per day. It was decocted with water for two times and reserve the juice for 300mL, and taken eparately in the morning and evening, and 7 doses were taken totally.

Secondary diagnosis was on November 1, 2011. The symptoms of asthma and suffocation were relieved, sometimes with cough, the little amount of urine, with dry stool. Patient still had yellow and thick tongue fur, swelling of both upper and lower limbs (+). Blood pressure: 120/80mmHg. The prescription made in the preliminary diagnosis was changed as the amount of Rhubarb and Baical Skullcap Root increased to 15g. Other 7 doses of medicine shall be taken.

Third diagnosis was on November 8, 2011. Patient did not have apparent symptoms of asthma and suffocation in resting state, sometimes had hardness of breath or lacking in strength, cyanosis of lips and fingernails and the apparent reliving of swelling of both upper and lower limbs. Ordinary stool and urine, with dark red tongue, yellow thin tongue fur. The prescription made in the secondary diagnosis was changed as adding 30g of Danshen Root, 30g of Milkvetch Root and the patient took other 6 doses. Then, the patient continued to take more than 10 doses to achieve consolidation therapy.

Note: The symptoms of CHF commonly include cough, asthma, phlegm, stasis, edema and palpitate. And the clinical manifestations are the symptoms of deficiency-excess in complexity, vigorous pathogenic factors and health Qi deficiency, heat and cold mingled. Therefore it is a kind of emergency and severe case that can not be treated easily. The common syndrome of the disease is the intertie of phlegm, heat, water and stasis. Doctor Du obeyed the treatment principle based on syndrome differentiation and chose the modified Ji Jiao Li Huang Wan for treatment by clearing heat and resolving phlegm, inducing diuresis and relieving stasis. Resulting from that the patient's body shape was above the average all along, with phlegm-dampness accumulation, her spleen lacked the health transporting, with gastrointestinal stasis, Qi movement repression, impede circulation of Qi and blood, internal stop of blood stasis and heat was produced after the stasis for long time, the disease happened. The disease belongs to heat stasis and water coagulation in the acute stage of CHF and the treatment shall be concentrated on the modified Jijiaoli Yellow Pill. In the prescription, the Pepperweed Seed tastes bitter and has the drug property of cold, and it can dispel phlegm and relieve asthma, purge lung and induce diuresis; the Hanfangji tastes bitter and has the drug property of cold, and it is good at going downwards, inducing diuresis and relieving edema; Si Chuan Pepper Accounts tastes bitter and has the drug property of cold, and it can relieve Qi and induce diuresis and lead other drugs to go downwards to reach the lesion; Rhubarbcan induce diuresis and relieve turbid, activate blood and invigorate pulse. White Mulberry Root-bark is added to purge lung and relieve asthma, Indian Bread Largehead Atractylodes Rhizome Oriental Water-plantian Rhizome Plaintain Seed and Chinese Lobelia Herb to induce diuresis and relieve edema, Hedyotis, Baical Skullcap and Root Heart-leaf Houttuynia Herb to clear heat and remove toxin. The whole prescription can help to activate blood and induce diuresis, clear heat and remove toxin, purge lung and relieve asthma. When the patient accepted the secondary diagnosis, she had the symptoms of un-relieved yellow thick tongue fur, dry stool and un-relieved fever, so the amount of Rhubarb and Baical Skullcap Root were added to strengthen the treatment of clearing heat and relieving internal fire. On the third diagnosis, the patient sometimes had the symptoms of hard breath, lack of strength, still cyanosis of lips and fingers, so Danshen Root and Milkvetch Root were added to activate blood and resolve stasis, tonify Qi and consolidate the origin. The prescription is concentrated on the mechanism of disease of the mixture of phlegm heat and water stasis of CHF, so all the drugs were modified in order to strengthen the functions of resolving phlegm and relieving asthma, tonifying Qi and activating blood, inducing diuresis and relieving edema. By combining all the drugs, it can achieve ventilating the upper jiao, mediating middle jiao and draining the lower jiao, perfusion of viscera, taking both symptom and root into consideration, eliminating pathogen and reinforcing healthy Qi and eliminating pathogen with no harm to healthy Qi. By harmonizing yin and yang, adjusting circumfluence, the viscera can recover healthy state and finally the disease can be cured.

ii. Medical record of Sun Guangrong —— edema due to yang deficiency and qi deficiency and blood stasis

Mr. Hou, male, 81 years old, preliminary diagnosis was on March 7, 2014. The patient showed wheezing & oppression in chest, which would be more serious in movement for more than 2 months; the exacerbation of state of an illness lasted for one week. The patient was pushed into the ward by people with wheelchair. He had a cold in January, 2014, after that he began to cough and show short breath, wheezing & oppression in chest, swelling of lower limbs and often palpitations. The exacerbation of symptom began a week ago. He showed palpitations in movement, with fullness in chest and hypochondrium as well as the bottom of the heart. He coughed and had foam-like thin sputum. It was difficult for him to lie on the back sometimes with dripping cold sweat. His both lower limbs showed pitting edema. He showed poor appetite and oliguria, pale and enlarged tongue, water slippery tongue fur and sunken pulse without force. Physical examination: orthopnoea; pale complexion; lips of mild cyanosis; distention of jugular vein; heart rate of 100 times/min; regular heart rhythm; Fine Crackles heard in each direction of two lungs. X-ray DR slice showed: pleural effusion of two chests (about 800 ml). Tuberculous pleuritis was excluded after the check of The Institute of Tubercosis Prevention and Control. He has suffered from diabetes for many years, coronary heart disease and hypertension.

Diagnosis in Western Medicine: heart failure grade II ; cardiac pleural effusion. Diagnosis of TCM: gasp syndrome according to tongue vein syndrome. Syndrome differentiation: edema due to yang insufficiency; Qi deficiency and blood stasis.

Therapeutic method: tonify Qi and activate blood; warm yang and promote diuresis.

Prescription: Zhen Wu Tang combined with Tiao Qi Huo Xue Yi Xie Tang (self-prepared, consisting of: Milkvetch Root, Ginseng, Salvia Root) modification: 20 g of Radix Aconiti Lateralis Preparata (decocted earlier), 20g of Fresh Ginger, 20g of White Peony Root, 15g of White Atractylodes Rhizome, 30g of Poria, 30g of Oriental Waterplantain Rhizome, 20g of Ginseng, 60g of Milkvetch Root, 30g of Salvia Root, 30g of Pepperweed Seed, 10g of Chinese Date, 15g of Raw Pinellia, 20g of Fructus Trichosanthis, 10g of Dried Ginger, 10g of Chinese Magnoliavine Fruit, 10g of Manchurian Wildginger, 10g of Liquorice Root. 3 doses, decocted with water of 500 ml, taken in warm state in three times of early, middle and late; 1 dose taken every day.

Urine volume of the patient increased significantly, which reached 1,500ml every day after he took 3 doses of prescription above. Wheezing & oppression in chest of the patient were improved and he was able to lie on the back. The food intake was improved; the patient showed no palpitations and sweating; swelling of lower limbs was improved. The pulse became a bit strong. The patient continued to take 3 doses according to original prescription with same decocting and dosing methods. The swelling would disappear after the sixth dose was taken. X-ray DR slice showed: pleural effusion of two chests was about 400 ml. It was considered that there were oppression in chest, expectoration, short breath and other symptoms, 6g of Officinal Magnolia Bark and 6g of Pericarpium Citri Reticulatae were added to the prescription above to relieve chest stuffiness, regulate vital energy, eliminate dampness and resolve phlegm, while 9g of Perillaseed was added to descend Qi and relieve a cough. Cough stopped after five doses again; the patient showed oppression in chest and asthma after high activity level; however, the other symptoms were all improved. Pale tongue and tongue fur were both improved; X-ray DR slice showed: pleural effusion of two chests was absorbed completely. The prescription was changed to 10g of tag (decocted earlier), 10g of fresh ginger, 20g of White Peony Root, 15g of White Atractylodes Rhizome, 15g of Poria, 15g of Oriental Waterplantain Rhizome, 20g of Ginseng, 60g of Milkvetch Root, 30g of Salvia Root, 10g of Dwarf Lilyturf Tuber, 10g of Chinese Magnoliavine Fruit, 10g of Dodder Seed, 10g of Common Curculigo Rhizome and 10g of Malaytea Scurfpea Fruit. The patient took medicine for one week, after that all symptoms were resolved, the heart rate was 85 times/min and the food intake was normal with urine and stool self regulating.

Note: The patient showed oppression in chest and asthma; it was difficult for him to lie on the back; the disease would be more serious in movement; sweating, edema of lower limbs, pale complexion, cyanosis of mouth and lip, pale, enlarged and gloomy tongue, water slippery tongue fur as well as sunken and weak pulse occurred; therefore, the disease can be diagnosed as eduma with syndrome of due to yang deficiency and syndrome of Qi deficiency and blood stasis. Heart governs sovereign fire while kidney governs life fire; sovereign fire and life fire are interdependent and mutually promoted. Ultimate source of heart failure is yang Qi insufficiency and sovereign life fire decline; swelling will occur if there is yin constipation; blood stasis will occur if there is not blood circulation depending on Qi flow. Heart failure cannot drive the movement of blood, so blood stasis happens and water stops. When water pathogen attacking heart and lung, oppression in chest, asthma and palpitations will occur. Sweating occurs due to Qi deficiency astringent therapy weakness; therefore, treatment method of heart failure is to warm yang, promote urination-induce diuresis and move Qi to disperse stagnation; Ginseng, Milkvetch Root and Salvia Root can replenish Qi and activate blood, move Qi, resolve stasis and promote blood circulation; Pepperweed Seed and Chinese Date are able to excrete water, purge lung and strengthen heart; The whole prescription is able to warm yang, promote diuresis and strengthen heart, replenish Qi and activate blood, resolve stasis and dispel phlegm, which completely conforms to the pathogenesis, therefore it has good effects.

VII. Prevention and aftercare

As the trend of population aging in China was increasingly obvious in recent years, the incidence of CHF has increased day by day. Therefore, strengthening the daily aftercare for patients, delaying disease progression and preventing acute exacerbation are of great advantage for prolonging survival time and improving the quality of life of patients.

i. Control of risk factors

(1) Hypertension. According to Framingham Heart Study, hypertension leads 39% of men with hypertension and 59% of women with hypertension to heart failure; however, control of hypertension can make new morbidity of heart failure reduce by about 50%. Patients with hypertension shall control hypertension actively to make the blood pressure value reach the standard in the long time.

(2) Diabetes. Clinical observation showed that the morbidity and mortality of diabetes combined with heart failure are 4 to 8 times more than those of non-diabetic patients. In addition to macroangiopathy and microangiopathy, diabetes also can cause the changes of myocardial structure and function. Insulin resistance and hyperinsulinemia can make the heart wall and blood vessel wall thicken, thus accelerating progress of heart failure and especially resulting in decline of simple diastolic function. Therefore, diabetes patients shall actively treat the primary disease and complication to prevent the occurrence of heart failure.

(3) Change of life style. Cultivation of healthy living habits, regular daily life, moderate diet, regular life, proper exercise, smoking cessation and abstinence, prevention of obesity and hyperlipidemia and the like can effectively reduce the occurrence of heart failure. When the body is in activity, heart rate will quicken and oxygen consumption will increase. Therefore, rest and activity shall be properly arranged. The activity is limited to not feeling fatigue and not aggravating symptoms; participation in heavy physical labor as well as working and learning for long time shall be avoided by all means; active rest and ample sleep shall be ensured. The principle of "dynamic" shall be followed and appropriate activity shall be conducted to prevent phlebothrombosis or pulmonary embolism in catabasis.

(4) Avoidance of the use of cardiotoxicity drugs. The risk of cardiotoxicity and organ function of patients shall be fully assessed before deciding to use such drugs and after drug use; special attention shall be paid to accumulated dose of drugs, variety and dosage form and method of administration; heart function detection shall be enhanced to prevent the occurrence of cardiotoxicity and heart failure as soon as possible.

ii. Prevention of CHF exacerbation

(1) Prevention of fluid retention. Excessive sodium salt and water intake can not only cause water retention in the body but also enhance neuromuscular excitability, thus aggravating heart load. Therefore, moderate salt and water intake shall be proper; heart failure patients are informed that they shall measure weight every day regularly.

(2) Various infections (especially the upper respiratory tract and pulmonary infection), pulmonary infarction, arrhythmia [especially atrial fibrillation (AF) with the rapid ventricular rate], electrolyte imbalance and acid-base imbalance, anemia, renal function damage, excessive salt intake, excessive intravenous fluids supplement, application of drugs damaging myocardium or heart function and the like all can cause deterioration of heart failure, which shall be dealt with or corrected timely.

Toxicity or bacterial infections can directly or indirectly damage myocardial contractility and reduce the cardiac function; among them, the upper respiratory infection is most common; rheumatism activity is the main inducement of rheumatic heart disease and heart failure, which is often associated with respiratory tract infection. For serious arrhythmia, especially frequent arrhythmia, heart failure, cardiac shock and even death may occur due to excessively fast heart rate, increased cardiac workload, short ventricular end diastole, stroke volume reduction, lower blood pressure, myocardial ischemia and the like.

(3) Regular drug taking. Insufficient drugs or premature discontinuation and the like all can cause or aggravate heart failure.

iii. Psychological stimulation

Emotional excitement may cause vegetative nerve functional disturbance and sympathetic nervous excitement. Increased catecholamine secretion may cause accelerated heart rate and elevation of blood pressure, thus increasing myocardial oxygen consumption and aggravating heart load. Therefore, well psychological adjustment must be conducted for all sorts of heart disease patients; their fear and nervous psychology and pessimism shall be eliminated; anti-anxiety or antidepressant medicines can be used appropriately when necessary.

(DU Wuxun)

References

[1] Chinese Society of Cardiology, Editorial Board of Chinese Journal of Cardiology. Chinese Heart Failure Diagnosis and Treatment Guidelines 2014[J]. Chinese Journal of Cardiology, 2014, 42 (2) : 98-122.

[2] Chinese Society of Cardiology. Retrospective Investigation for CHF Hospitalization Cases of Parts of China in 1980, 1990 and 2000 [J]. Chinese Journal of Cardiology, 2002 (30): 450-454.

[3] Lu ZY, Zhong NS. Internal Medicine. 7th ed. Beijing: People's Medical Publishing House, 2008:170.

[4] Dickstein K, Cohen-Solar A, Filippatos G,et al.ESC Guidelines for the diagnosis and treatment of acute and CHF 2008 The Task Force for the Diagnosis and Treatment of Acute and CHF 2008 of the European Society of Cardiology.Developed in collaboration with the Heart Failure Association of the ESC (HFA) and endorsed by the European Society of Intensive Care Medicine (ESICM) [J].Eur J Heart Fail, 2008, 10 (10): 933-989.

[5] Cui XL, Mao JY, Wang XL, et al. Heart failure TCM Syndrome Epidemiological Survey Design [J]. Beijing Journal of Traditional Chinese Medicine, 2009, 28 (3): 179-181.

[6] Cai H, Mao JY, Wang Q, et al. Literature Analysis for TCM Syndrome Differentiation of CHF [J]. Sichuan Journal of Traditional Chinese Medicine, 2011, 29 (7): 22-25.

[7] Cai XL, Mao JY, Wang XL, et al. Expert Investigation Analysis for TCM Syndrome of Heart Failure [J]. Acta Universitatis Traditionis Medicalis Sinensis Pharmacologiaeque Shanghai, 2009, 23 (2): 31-33.

[8] Cai XL, Mao JY, Wang XL, et al. Expert Investigation Analysis for TCM Treatment Medication of Heart Failure [J]. Chinese Patent Medicine, 2009, 31 (9): 1431-1433.

[9] Jessup M, Abraham WT, Casey DE, et al. 2009 focused Update: ACCF/AHA guidelines for the diagnosis and management of heart failure in adults: a report of the American College of Cardiology Foundation/American Hearl Association Task Force on Practice Guidelines: developed in collaboration with the International Society for Heart and Lung Transplantation [J]. Circulation, 2009, 119: 1977-2016.

[10] Arnold JM, Liu P, Demers C. et al. Canadian Cardiovascular Society consensus conference recommendations on heart failure 2006: diagnosis and management[J]. Can J cardiol, 2006, 22: 23-45.

[11] Paulus WJ, Tschope C, Sanderson JE, et al. How to diagnose diastolic heart failure: a consensus statement on the diagnosis of heart failure with normal left ventricular ejection fraction by the Heart Failure and Echocardiography Associations of the European Society of Cardiology[J].Eur Heart J,2007,28:2539-2550.

[12] Zhang KQ, Sun Q. Experience summary of Shi Dazhuo on chronic cardiac insufficiency treatment [J]. Chinese Archives of Traditional Chinese Medicine, 2003, 21(1):29.

[13] China Association of Chinese Medicine. Diagnosis and treatment guidelines for common diseases of Chinese medicine internal medicine (Western medicine disease part) Heart Failure [J]. Chinese Medicine Modern Distance Education of China, 2011,9(18):147.

[14] Xie YP, Chen FP, Huang GM, et al.clinical observation of treatment of CHF with Milkvetch Root injection and ST 36 acupoint injection [J]. Practical Clinical Journal of Integrated Traditional Chinese, 2014, 14(4):5-6.

[15] Fang JZ, Xia YF, Huang QC, et al. Observation of index (such as ICAM –1) effect of Traditional Chinese medicine acupoint injection on patients with CHF [J]. People's Military Surgeon, 2013, 56(10):1192-1193.

[16] Sun YY, Wu ST, Jiang DY, et al. Experience introduction of congestive heart failure treatment of Zhang Qi [J]. Liaoning Journal of Traditional Chinese Medicine, 2006, 33 (11): 1394-1395.

[17] Yan X, Zhou WB, Yang ZM, et al. Summary of heart failure treatment experience of Professor Yan Dexin [J]. Journal of Practical Traditional Chinese Internal Medicine, 2003, 17 (6): 447.

[18] Liu H. Some experiences about difficulty miscellaneous disease treatment by the regulating Qi, activating blood and suppressing pathogenic factor Decoction of master of Traditional Chinese Medicine, Sun Guangrong [J].Guangming Journal of Chinese Medicine 2015, 30 (4): 695-696.

中风　　Stroke

I. Overview

Stroke is a disease whose main clinical manifestations are brain ischemia and hemorrhagic damage. It is also called stroke or cerebrovascular accident, which can be divided into two kinds, namely hemorrhagic stroke (cerebral hemorrhage or subarachnoid hemorrhage) and ischemic stroke (formation of cerebral infarction, cerebral thrombosis). Clinically, cerebral infarction is most common. Stroke has high incidence and mortality, and sequelae of stroke always remains. Patients tend to be young. It is one of the most important fatal diseases in the world.

According to TCM, stroke is believed as a disease whose basic pathogenesis is that disorder of Qi and blood results from asthenia of healthy Qi, diet, emotion and over-strain internal injury and the like, so that wind, fire, phlegm and stasis are produced, finally brain vessel is blocked or blood spills outside of cerebral vein. The main clinical manifestations of stroke are sudden faint and unconsciousness with deflection of angle of mouth, sluggish speech or mutism and hemiplegia, or deflection of angle of mouth and hemiplegia only. As it is characterized by acute onset, quick changes and various symptoms, just like wind that is mobile and changeable, it is also named as stroke or apoplexy and divided into two kinds, one kind is stroke involving channel and collateral, the other kinds is stroke involving zang-fu viscera. The disease is mostly seen in middle aged and elderly people, and occurs in all seasons. However, it is most common in winter and spring. In terms of prevention, treatment and rehabilitation of the disease, traditional Chinese medicine owns obvious efficacy and advantages. For hemorrhagic and ischemic cerebrovascular diseases, syndrome differentiation and treatment in this section can be referred to.

II. Etiology and pathogenesis

Head is "confluence of all YANG channels". The essence and blood in five zang-organs and Qi in six-fu organs are injected upward to brain. For the occurrence of stroke, its locations are heart and brain, and it is relevant to liver and kidney. It is a severe syndrome with upper excess and lower deficiency as well as imbalance of yin and yang.

i. Etiology

There are many causes of stroke. Its occurrence is a complex pathological process by many factors, in which wind, fire, phlegm and stasis are the main causes. Patients usually suffer from Qi and blood deficiency and heart, liver and kidney dysfunction. Then, the disease is induced by accumulating damage of internal injury, dietary irregularities, damage by emotion, invasion of exogenous pathogenic factors and so on. The pathogenesis of stroke is complex, but can be summarized as deficiency (yin deficiency, blood deficiency), fire (liver fire, heart fire), wind (liver wind, external wind), phlegm (wind phlegm, damp phlegm), Qi (Qi counterflow, Qi stagnation) and blood (blood stasis). Basic pathogenesis is the imbalance of yin and yang and the counterflow of Qi and blood, and main pathological natures are deficiency in origin and excess in superficiality. Liver-kidney yin deficiency as well as Qi and blood deficiency are the pathopoiesia root causes, and wind, fire, phlegm, Qi and stasis are pathopoiesia incidents, and the two can be in a mutual cause-effect relation.

ii. Pathogenesis

Stroke is sorted into stroke involving channel and collateral and stroke involving zang-fu viscera. If there is phlegm in liver wind, the wind crosses leap into meridians, and Qi and blood can't nourish body because of blood vessel stagnation, then mild symptoms in stroke involving channel appeared, the manifestations are hemiplegia and deviation of eye and mouth without disturbance of consciousness; if phlegm-fire and wind cause mental confusion and disordered Qi and blood flow upward to brain, then the meridians are damaged, blood spills, and stasis blocks brain collaterals, then severe syndrome in zang-fu viscera are seen, the manifestations are sudden syncope and unconsciousness.

In early period of onset, pathogenic Qi rises suddenly, phlegm-fire and wind are exuberant, and Qi and blood flow upward, so the focus is on the excess in superficiality; if the condition suddenly deteriorates, healthy Qi is quickly defeated under vicious attack of pathogenic factors, so the main pathogenesis is healthy Qi deficiency, even healthy Qi collapse. In the later stage, healthy Qi is not recovered, and pathogenic Qi is left only, then sequelae can be left.

1. Fire transformation to wind in emotions of depression and anger

Extreme changes of five emotions and exuberant heart fire can trigger endogenous wind. If people usually are depressed or get angry, emotion is gloomy, then liver Qi is constrained and fire is transformed from depressed Qi; with violent rage, liver Yang has a sudden hyperactivity, so that heart fire is caused. Qi and fire both rise, and Qi and blood upwells to brain, and mind is blocked, then sudden fall and unconsciousness are led; or internal injury is excessive for a long time, Yin essence is secretly consumed, deficiency fire internally burns, and water fails to nourish wood, thus deficiency of liver-kidney yin is triggered. Again, emotions are injured, liver yang has a sudden hyperactivity, Qi and blood is reversed upward, and heart and spirit confuse, thus stroke is triggered. Young adults with exuberant yang Qi and excessive heart and liver fire can also suffer from the disease suddenly for transformation of yang hyperactivity into wind resulting from rage.

2. Phlegm turbidity caused by intemperate diet

When people overfeed greasy food and glycol wine, spicy and fried and scorch products, or eat too much or too less, or overdrink alcohol, spleen loses its transportation function, and dampness pathogen internally remains which accumulates to phlegm. Phlegm is pented in body, which blocks the meridians and causes seven orifices. Or, phlegm dampness produces heat, wind fire and phlegm-heat are excessive, thus liver wind intrudes into meridians, disturbs with phlegm and blocks mind, then people are suddenly dizzy and fall, and suffer from hemiplegia.

3. Overstrain and excessive desires as well as accumulation of internal injury

Exhaustion causes malnutrition in body and spirit, yin deficiency and blood deficiency, transformation to wind from deficient yang and wind-fire fusion. Or, if people indulge in desires, it will damage essence, trigger heart fire, and consume kidney water, then water can't control fire. Or, people are aged with weak physique, liver-kidney yin is deficient, and liver yang is hyperactive, that wind stir, so that Qi and blood inverse which causes mental confusion, then the disease suddenly happens.

4. External wind attacking to physique due to Qi and blood insufficiency

Old age with aeipathia can cause insufficient Qi and blood and empty channels. In abrupt change of climate, pathogenic factors of wind enter channel and collateral, therefore Qi and blood are blocked, and muscles lose nourishment; or, phlegm and dampness are usually excessive, physique is strong and Qi is weak, and external wind induces internal wind, phlegm and dampness block the meridians, so that deviation of eye and mouth occurs.

5. Blood stasis

Qi stagnation and obstructed circulation of blood or Qi deficiency and feeble blood circulation or blood accumulation in upper part for rage or contracting stagnation for cold or yin fluid injury for heat and the like can cause sluggish blood circulation, and blood stasis forms. In terms of pathogenesis of the disease, blood accumulation in upper part for rage or Qi deficiency and blood stasis is the most common.

III. Key points of diagnosis and differential diagnosis

i. Key points of diagnosis

1. Inducements

Onset is mostly relevant to inducements like emotional disorder, improper diet or tiredness.

2. Age

The disease mostly happens to the people aged more than 40

3. Pre-symptoms

Some symptoms such as dizziness, headache and numbness of one side of limbs.

4. Clinical manifestations

Mostly, onset of the disease is quite acute with clinical manifestations like sudden faint and fall, unconsciousness, hemiplegia, hemianesthesia, deviation of eye and mouth and inarticulateness. Dizziness, hemianesthesia, deviation of eye and mouth and hemiplegia are seen in mild symptoms.

5. Clinical examination

Stroke is similar to acute cerebrovascular diseases in western medicine. Clinically, examinations of cerebrospinal fluid and fundus, CT and MRI and the like can be conducted according to specific situation.

ii. Differential diagnosis

1. Facial paralysis

Facial paralysis can occur in different ages, often accompanied with postauricular pain. Clinically, there is no hemiplegia or disturbance of consciousness. Main manifestations are muscle paralysis on face in one side, deviation of eye and mouth and drool at the corner of mouth, or accompanying barylalia. The disease is mostly caused by blockage of Qi and blood in the meridians.

2. Dizziness

Fall caused by severe dizziness is similar to faint and fall in stroke, but there are no symptoms like hemiplegia, unconsciousness and deviation of tongue and mouth. However, it shall be noted that dizziness is differentiated with the manifestations of pre symptoms of stroke clinically.

3. Syncope

In syncope, unconsciousness time is short, and coldness of limb is often accompanied. Most patients are able to revive by selves without hemiplegia, deviation of tongue and mouth, inarticulateness, and so on.

4. Epileptic syndrome

Severe symptoms of epilepsy can also be sudden fall down and unconsciousness. After revival, patients have no symptoms like hemiplegia and deviation of eye and mouth.

5. Convulsion syndrome

Onset of convulsion syndrome can be accompanied by unconsciousness, and it often happens after a long-time tic. The main symptoms are tic of limbs, stiffness of nape and neck. Whereas, there are no manifestations of hemiplegia and deviation of eye and mouth and the like.

6. Flaccidity-syndrome

Onset of flaccidity-syndrome is mostly slow. It is characterized by paralysis of the lower limbs or quadriplegia. Or, muscular atrophy and muscular twitching and cramp are mostly seen without unconsciousness.

IV. TCM therapy

i. Syndrome differentiation and treatment

According to condition and disease locations, stroke is clinically divided into stroke involving channel and collateral and stroke involving zang-fu viscera. The treatment of stroke involving channel and collateral shall focus on pacifying liver and extinguishing wind and resolving phlegm, dispelling stasis and dredging collaterals. With regard to the treatment of stroke involving zang-fu viscera, extinguishing of wind, clearing of fire, elimination of phlegm, open of orifices, relaxation of bowels and discharge of heat shall be followed for blockage syndrome; rescue of yin, revival of yang and relief of prostration shall be conducted for collapse syndrome; for the syndrome of internal block and external collapse, the methods of enlivening spirit and opening orifices as well as reinforcing healthy Qi and relieving prostration shall be both used. In rehabilitative period and sequela period, most symptoms belong to the syndromes of deficiency-excess in complexity. Healthy Qi shall be reinforced, and pathogen should be eliminated, and superficial manifestations and root causes should be both treated. These shall be applied with the methods of pacifying liver and extinguishing wind, resolving phlegm, dispelling stasis, nourishing liver and kidney, replenishing Qi and nourishing blood.

1.Stroke involving channel and collateral

The main symptoms are hemiplegia, stiff tongue and sluggish speech and deviation of corner of mouth. Generally, there is no mind disorder. Clinically, there are five syndromes□ syndrome of liver Yang hyperactivity and wind-fire upward disturbance, syndrome of meridians and collateral block due to wind-phlegm and blood stasis, syndrome of wind-phlegm invading upward due to phlegm-heat and excess in fu organs, Qi deficiency and blood stasis syndrome and stirring wind due to yin deficiency syndrome.

(1) Liver Yang hyperactivity and wind-fire upward disturbance

Main symptoms: hemiplegia, deviation of tongue and mouth and stiff tongue and sluggish speech or mutism. There are flushed face and red eyes, vertigo and headache, hemianesthesia, dysphoria and irritability, bitter taste in mouth and dry pharynx, stool constipation, dark urine, red or deep-red tongue, yellow or dry tongue fur and wiry, slippery but strong pulse.

Therapeutic method: to settle liver, extinguish wind, nourish yin and restrain yang

Prescription: modified Zhen Gan Xi Feng Tang. Radix Achyranthis Bidentatae, Daizheshi, Bone Fossil of Big Mammals, Oyster Shell, White Peony Root, Radix Scrophulariae, Gui Ban, Cochinchinese Asparagus Root, Virgate Wormwood Herb, Szechwan Chinaberry Fruit, Raw Malt and Radix Acanthopanacis.

Modification: in case that patients suffer from serious ascendant hyperactivity of liver yang, Tall Gastrodia Tuber and Uncaria are added to reinforce the efficacy of pacifying liver and extinguishing wind; for the patients with serious vexing heat, Fructus Gardeniae and Radix Scutellariae are added to clear heat and eliminate vexing heat. In terms of the patients with severe headache, Antelope Horn, Abalone Shell and Common Selfheal Fruit-spike are added to extinguish wind and clear yang; in case of patients with severe phlegm-heat, Arisaema with Bile, Bamboo Vinegar and Tendrilleaf Fritillary Bulb are added to clear phlegm-heat; if Deficiency of liver-kidney yin, fine and string-like pulse and red tongue texture occur, herbs for nourishing liver and kidneys like Rehmanniae Radix, Fleeceflower Root, Glossy Privet Fruit, Barbary Wolfberry Fruit and Yerbadetajo Herb are added; if bitter taste in mouth and red face, constipation, brown urine, yellow tongue coating and wiry and rapid pulse are seen, Turmeric Root Tuber, Chinese Gentian Root and Common Selfheal Fruit-spike and the like can be added to clear liver fire.

(2) Meridians and collateral block due to wind-phlegm and blood stasis

Main symptoms: hemiplegia, deviation of tongue and mouth and stiff tongue and sluggish speech or mutism. There are numb limbs or spasm of hand and feet, dizziness, dim tongue texture, white or yellow greasy tongue coating and wiry and slippery pulse.

Therapeutic method: to expel wind, nourish blood, promote blood circulation, resolve phlegm and dredge collateral.

Prescription: modified Da Qin Jiao Tang. There are Largeleaf Gentian Root, Incised Notopterygium Rhizome and Root, Doubleteeth Pubescent Angelica Root, Divaricate Saposhnikovia Root, Chinese Angelica, Debark Peony Root, Prepared Rehmannia Root, Sichuan Lovage Rhizome, White Atractylodes Rhizomeme, Indian Bread, Baical Skullcap Root, Gypsum and Rehmanniae Radix.

Modification: in case of old patients with weak body, Milkvetch Root is added to replenish Qi and reinforce healthy Qi. In case that vomit and much phlegm and greasy tongue coating and slippery pulse are serious, Radix Rehmanniae is removed, and Rhizoma Pinelliae, Nan Xing, Rhizoma Typhonii and Scorpioon are added to expel wind-phlegm and dredge collateral. If patients don't suffer from internal heat, Gypsum and Baical Skullcap Root can be removed. If turbid phlegm accumulates for a long time and transforms into heat, Indian Bread can be removed, and Bamboo Shavings and Immature Orange Fruit and the like can be added to clear heat and drying dampness. For the patients with blood stasis symptom, herbs for activating blood and expelling stasis like Peach Seed, Safflower and Sichuan Lovage Rhizome can be added.

(3) Wind-phlegm invading upward due to phlegm-heat and excess in fu organs

Main symptoms: hemiplegia, deviation of tongue and mouth and stiff tongue and sluggish speech or mutism. There are dizziness, hemianesthesia, sticky mouth with excessive phlegm, abdominal distention, dry stool and constipation, dull-red or dim tongue texture, yellow greasy or gray black tongue coating and wiry, slippery and large pulse.

Therapeutic method: to clear heat, resolve phlegm, regulate Qi and dredge fu organs.

Prescription: Da Cheng Qi Tang(*ShangHanLun*). There are Rhubarb, Immature Orange Fruit, Officinal Magnolia Bark and Sodium Sulfate.

Modification: if stool is unobstructed after patient taking drugs, then fu-qi is smooth, and phlegm-heat decreases, then condition recovers to an extent. The dosage of using yellow saltpetre in the method depends on the patient's condition and constitution. Generally, it is controlled about in range of 10~15g, depending on the effects of unobstructed stool and elimination of accumulated phlegm-heat. Excessive dosage is not allowed to avoid damaging healthy Qi. After fu-qi is smooth, herbs for clearing phlegm-heat, activating blood and dredging collaterals medicines shall be given, such as Bile Arisaema, Snakegourd Fruit, Salvia Root, Red Peony Root and Suberect Spatholobus Stem. If dizziness is severe, Gambir Plant Nod, Chrysanthemum Flower and Mother-of-pearl can be added. If red tongue texture, dry mouth and throat occur, and the patients are restless and suffer from pernoctation, it belongs to accumulation of phlegm-heat and serious damage to liquid. The medicines for nourishing yin, generating liquid and stabilizing spirit such as Fresh Rehmanniae Radix, Radix Adenophorea, Dwarf Lily-turf Tuber, Figwort Root, Indian Bread and Tuber Fleeceflower Stem can be added but not too much, or elimination of phlegm-heat will be disturbed.

(4) Qi deficiency and blood stasis

Main symptoms: hemiplegia, deviation of tongue and mouth and stiff tongue and sluggish speech or mutism. There are weak limbs, hemianesthesia, hand and foot swelling, palpitations and spontaneous sweating, short breath and lack of strength, loose stool, pale white complexion, dim tongue texture, thin and white or white greasy tongue coating, sunken and thready or thready and moderate, thready and wiry and thready and sluggish pulse.

Therapeutic method: to reinforce healthy Qi and promote blood circulation.

Prescription: modified Bu Yang Huan Wu Tang. There are raw Radix Astragalis, Angelica Tail, Sichuan Lovage Rhizome, Red Peony Root, Peach Seed, Safflower and Earthworm.

Modification: if hemiplegia is severe, Mulberry Twig, Pangolin Scales and Leech and the like are added to strengthen the effect of activating blood circulation and dredging collaterals, dispelling stasis and promoting tissue regeneration; in case of weak limbs, Chinese Taxillus Herb and Radix Achyranthis Bidentatae and the like can be added to nourish liver and kidneys; for the patients with unsmooth speech, Acorus calamus and Milkwort Root are added to clear phlegm and open orifices; in case of patients with hand and foot swelling, Indian Bread, Oriental Waterplantain Rhizome, Chinese Barley and Fourstamen Stephania Root can be added for promoting diuresis with drugs of tasteless flavor; for the patients with serious loose stool, Peach Seed is removed, and fried White Atractylodes Rhizomeme and Common Yam Rhizome are added to invigorate spleen.

(5) Stirring wind due to yin deficiency

Main symptoms: hemiplegia, deviation of tongue and mouth and stiff tongue and sluggish speech or mutism. There are numb limbs, contracture or wriggle, vexing heat and insomnia, dizziness and tinnitus, feverish feeling in palms and soles, red tongue texture, and scanty tongue coating or absence of tongue fur, and thready wiry and thready rapid pulse.

Therapeutic method: to nourish yin and extinguish wind.

Prescription: modified Da Ding Feng Zhu. There are Egg Yolk, Ass Hide Glue, Radix Rehmanniae, Dwarf

Lily-turf Tuber, White Peony Root, Gui Ban, Turtle Shell, Chinese Magnoliavine Fruit and Prepared Liquorice Root.

Modification: in case of patients with severe hemiplegia, Radix Achyranthis Bidentatae, Common Floweringqince Fruit, Earthworm, Centipede and Mulberry Twig and the like can be added; in case of patients with vexing heat in heart, Fructus Gardeniae and Radix Scutellariae are added to clear heat and eliminate vexing heat; when blood stasis syndrome such as dull-red tongue texture and sluggish pulse occur, Salvia Root, Suberect Spatholobus Stem, Peach Seed and Eupolyphaga and the like are added to activate blood circulation and dispel stasis; for the patients with serious unsmooth speech, Acorus calamus, Turmeric Root Tuber and Milkwort Root are added to produce sound and relive orifices.

2. Disease involving zang-fu viscera

Main symptoms are delirium, vague mind, somnolence or lethargy, even coma and hemiplegia. It is sorted into two syndromes, namely block and collapse.

(1) Block syndrome

Main symptoms: unconsciousness and trance, somnolence or lethargy, even coma and hemiplegia. Lockjaw, tonic spasm of limbs, polypnea, wheezing due to retention of phlegm in throat, anuria and constipation, yellow and greasy tongue coating and large and rapid pulse.

1) Phlegm-fire and stasis blockage

Accompanying symptoms: red facial complexion and fever sensation of body, heavy breath and halitosis, disturbance and restless, yellow and greasy tongue coating.

Therapeutic method: to extinguish wind, clear fire, eliminate phlegm and open orifices.

Prescription: Ling Jiao Gou Teng Tang (*Tong Su Shang Han Lun*). There are Antelope Horn, Uncaria, Mulberry Leaf, Tendrilleaf Fritillary Bulb, fresh Bamboo Shavings, raw Radix Rehmanniae, Chrysanthemum Flower, White Peony Root, Pine among the Indian Bread and raw Radix Acanthopanacis.

Modification: if phlegm-heat is blocked in airway and wheezing occurs due to retention of phlegm in throat, bamboo juice can be taken to eliminate phlegm and relieve convulsion; in case of liver fire exuberance, flushed face and red eyes and wiry and strong pulse, herbs for clearing liver and reliving shall be properly added, for instance, Chinese Gentian Root, Capejasmine, Common Selfheal Fruit-spike, Daizheshi and Magnetitum; if the patients suffer from fu excess and heat accumulation, abdominal distension and constipation and yellow and thick tongue fur, it is suitable to add raw Rhubarb, Anhydrous Sodium Sulphate and Immature Orange Fruit; for the patients with damage to fluid caused by phlegm-heat, dry and red tongue texture and yellow and dry tongue coating, it is suitable to add Radix Adenophorea, Dwarf Lily-turf Tuber, Dendrobium and Rehmanniae Radix.

2) Blockage of phlegm-turbidity and static blood

Main symptoms: pale facial complexion and dark lips, repose without restless, cool limbs, abundant phlegm-saliva, white and greasy tongue coating, deep, slippery and moderate pulse.

Therapeutic method: to resolve phlegm, extinguish wind, remove stasis and open orifices.

Prescription: Di Tan Tang (*Ji Sheng Fang*). There are Indian Bread, Ginseng, Radix Acanthopanacis, Red Tangerine Peel, Arisaema with Bile, Rhizoma Pinelliae, Bamboo Shavings, Immature Orange Fruit and Acorus Calamus.

Modification: if patients also suffer from stirring wind, Tall Gastrodia Tuber and Uncaria are added to extinguish internal wind; in case of patients with the symptoms of phlegm-turbidity and static blood transforming to heat, Radix Scutellariae and Golden Thread are added; if floating yang syndrome in patients, which belongs to condition deterioration, it is suitable to quickly give Shenfu decoction Bai Tong and Zhudanzhi decoctions for treatment.

(2) Collapse syndrome

Main symptoms: delirium, vague mind, somnolence or lethargy, even coma and hemiplegia. There is faint breathing, short breath, pale complexion, mydriasis, closed eyes and open mouth, flaccid paralysis limbs, excessive sweating and cold limbs, incontinence, greasy tongue coating and scattered pulse or weak pulse.

Therapeutic method: to tonify Qi, restore yang, rescue yin and relieve prostration.

Prescription: Shenfu decoction (*Fu Ren Liang Fang*) and Sheng Mai San (*Bei Ji Qian Jin Yao Fang*). There are Ginseng, Prepared Common Monkshood Daughter Root, Natural Lindigo, Radix Adenophorea and Chinese Magnoliavine Fruit.

Modification: in case of patients whose yang floats superficial for yin failing to astringing yang,, and fluid can't be internally kept, and excessive sweating appears, Bone Fossil of Big Mammals and Oyster Shell can be added to astringing sweating and restore yang; for the patients with damaged Yin essence, dry tongue and faint pulse, Fragrant Solomonseal Rhizome and Crystalline Leans are added to rescue yin essence.

3. Sequelae

(1) Hemiplegia

1) Blockage of collaterals due to Qi deficiency and blood stasis

Main symptoms: besides hemiplegia and weak limbs without strength, patients also suffer from hand and foot swelling in affected side, sluggish speech, deviation of eye and mouth, sallow or dim facial complexion, thin and white tongue coating, pale and purple tongue or deviated tongue, thready, sluggish and weak pulse and the like.

Therapeutic method: to tonify Qi, promote blood circulation, dredge meridians and collaterals.

Main prescription: modified Bu Yang Huan Wu Tang

2) Blockage of collaterals due to ascendant hyperactivity of liver yang

Main symptoms: stiffness and spasm in affected side, and headache and dizziness, reddish facial complexion and tinnitus, crimson tongue, thin and yellow tongue coating and wiry, hard and strong pulse are also seen.

Treatment principle: to pacify liver, restrain yang, extinguish wind and dredge collaterals.

Main prescription: modified Zhen Gan Xi Feng Tang or Tian Ma Gou Teng Yin.

(2) Unsmooth speech

1) **Wind-phlegm collateral blockage:** as wind-phlegm blocks upward and the meridians loses balance, stiff tongue and sluggish speech, numb limbs and wiry and slippery pulse occur. In terms of treatment, it is suitable to dispel wind and eliminate phlegm, and ventilate orifices and dredge collaterals. Therefore, Jie Yu Dan is the prescription. Tall Gastrodia Tuber, Scorpion, Bile Arisaema and Rhizoma Typhonii and the like in the prescription are used to pacify liver, extinguish wind and dispel phlegm; Milkwort Root, Acorus calamus and Chinese Eaglewood Wood and the like are applied to ventilate orifices and dredge collaterals; Incised Notopterygium Rhizome and Root is used to expel wind.

2) **Kidney deficiency and essence deficiency:** as kidney is deficient, essence Qi can't nourish upward, which leads to dull voice and aphasia, palpitations, short breath and soreness and weakness of waist and knees. In terms of treatment, it is suitable to nourish yin, tonifiy kidney and disinhibit orifices. Dihuangyinzi is the prescription. Cassia Bark and Prepared Common Monkshood Daughter Root are removed, and Peach Seed, Balloonflower and Indian Trumpetflower Seed are added to produce sound and facilitate orifices.

3) **Ascendant hyperactivity of liver yang, orifices blockage of phlegm:** Tianma Goutent decoction or liver-settling wind-extinguishing decoction can be offered, and Grassleaf Sweetflag Rhizome, Milkwort Root, Bile Arisaema, Tabasheer and Scorpioon are added to pacify liver and subdue yang, dispel phlegm and open orifices.

(3) Deviation of eye and mouth: It is mostly caused by wind-phlegm blockage in collateral. In terms of treatment, it is suitable to expel wind, dispel phlegm and dredge collateral, and the prescription is Qian Zheng San.

ii. Acupuncture and moxibustion therapy

1. Basic treatment

(1) Stroke involving channel and collateral

Therapeutic method: to restore consciousness and open orifices, nourish liver and kidney, and dredge meridians. Acupoints in hand jue yin meridian, governor meridian and Foot-Taiyin meridian are the priorities.

Main points: Neiguan (PC 6), Shuigou (GV 26), Sanyinjiao (SP 6), Jiquan (HT 1), Chize (LU 5) and Weizhong (BL 40).

Combinated points: in case of constrained liver yang, Taichong (LR 3) and Taixi (KI 3) are added; in case of wind-phlegm collateral blockage, Fenglong (ST 40) and Hegu (LI 4) are added; in case of phlegm-heat and fu excess, Quchi (LI 11), Neiting (ST 44) and Fenglong (ST40) are added; in case of Qi deficiency and blood stasis, Zusanli (ST 36) and Qihai (CV 6) are added; in case of yin deficiency and stirring wind, Taixi (KI 3) and Fengchi (GB 20) are added; in case of deflection of angle of mouth, Jiache (ST 6) and Dicang (ST 4) are added; in case of upper limb paralysis, Jianyu (LI 15), Shousanli (LI 10) and Hegu (LI 4) are added; for Lower limb paralysis, Huantiao (GB 34), Yinlingquan (SP 9) and Yanglingquan (GB 31) are added; with regard to dizziness, Fengchi (GB 20), Wangu (GB 12) and Tianzhu (BL 10) are added; with regard to talipes varus, Qiuxu (GB 40) and Zhaohai (KI 6) are added; in case that constipation occurs, Shuidao (ST28), Guilai (ST 29), Fenglong (ST40) and Zhigou (TE 6) are added; in case of diplopia, Fengchi (GB 20), Tianzhu (BL 10), Jingming (BL 1) and Qiuhou (EX-HN7) are added; for urinary incontinence and urinary retention, Zhongji (CV 3), Qugu (CV 2) and Guanyuan (CV 4) are added.

Manipulation: reducing method is used for Neiguan (PC 6); sparrow-pecking method is for Shuigou (GV 26), and watery eyeball for patient is the best; when Sanyinjiao (SP 6) is punctured, keep an angle of 45 between the needle and the skin along medial border of tibia and use needle tip to puncture to Sanyinjiao (SP 6) with reinforcing method; in puncturing of Jiquan (HT 1), perpendicularly insert the needle at 2 cun below Jiquan (HT1) along heart channel and avoid armpit hair, using lifting-thrusting reducing method until the patient has the feeling of numbness, distension and twitching; perpendicularly puncture Chize (LU 5) and Weizhong (BL 40) to make limbs suffer from twitch feeling.

Prescription significance: heart governs blood vessels. Neiguan (PC 6) is pericardial meridian point, which can regulate heart Qi and dredge Qi and blood. Brain is the house of primordial spirit. Governor channel enters collaterals and brain, and Shuigou (GV 26) is an acupoint on governor channel, which can restore consciousness and open orifices, regulate spirit and induce Qi. Sanyinjiao (SP 6), the intersection point of three yin channels of the foot, is able to nourish liver and kidney. Jiquan (HT 1), Chize (LU 5) and Weizhong (BL 40) are capable of dredge the meridians of limbs.

(2) Stroke involving zang-fu viscera

Therapeutic method: to restore consciousness, open orifices, open the blockage and stop collapsing. Hand jue yin and governor channel are the priorities.

Main points: Neiguan (PC 6) and Shuigou (GV 26).

Combination points: in case of blockage syndrome, twelve Jing points, Taichong (LR 3) and Hegu (LI 4) are added; in case of collapse syndrome, Guanyuan (CV 4), Qihai (CV 6) and Shenque (CV 8) are added.

Manipulation: the manipulation on Neiguan (PC 6) and Shuigou (GV 26) are the same as above. Use three-edged needle to prick twelve Jing points for bleedletting; reducing method is used on Taichong (LR 3) and Hegu (LI 4) to achieve strong stimulation. Moxibustion method of large moxa cone is applied to Guangyuan (CV 4) and Qihai (CV 6), and salt moxibustion method is used on Shenque (CV 8), until limbs become warm.

Prescription significance: Neiguan (PC 6) regulates state of mind, and Shuigou (GV 26) restores consciousness and opens orifices. Pricking Jing points for bleedletting can connect Qi of regular twelve channels, and regulate yin and yang. Taichong (LR 3) and Hegu (LI 4) are also operated to pacify liver and extinguish wind. Guanyuan (CV 4) is the intersection point of conception channel and three yin channels of the foot, and moxibustion on the point can support kidney yang. Shenque (CV 8) is the root of life, and owned by genuine Qi. It can replenish Qi, consolidate base, rescue yang and stop collapse with the acupuncture in CV 6.

2. Other treatments

(1) Scalp acupuncture: select MS6, MS8 and MS9 or AT (2), or temporal three-needle to horizontally prickle

under scalp with filiform needle, quickly twirl for 2~3 min, and retain the needle for 30 min. twirl the needles for 2~3 times during the retention of needle. Later, patients are encouraged to move limbs. For the patients with sleeplessness or dysphoria, MS1 is selected.

(2) Eye acupuncture: double upper energizer area and double lower energizer area are the main points, and Needles should be retained for 5~15 min.

(3) Electropuncture: select two corresponding point as a combination in the limb of affected side for acupuncture. After the arrival of qi by acupuncture,, electropuncture instrument is connected to, until muscle in patient slightly tremble. Each energization lasts for 20 min.

(4) Dermal needle: select corresponding meridians in limb of affected side, mainly meridian of yangming, and tap with pyonex. Slight acupuncture technique is applied, and flush skin in stimulation site is a reference.

V. Typical medical records of famous experts

1. Medical record of Zhang Boyu—ascendant hyperactivity of liver yang

Ms Huang, female, 54.

Preliminary diagnosis: on October 14, 1976.

Patient has medical history of hypertension. Ten days before, she suddenly suffered from stroke. She improves by rescue with integration of Chinese and western medicine. At present, her mind is clear and confused now and then, and she has hemiplegia in her right body, sluggish speech, constipation, small and thready pulse, red tongue texture and shortage of fluid. Kidney yin is deficient, water fails to nourish wood, wind yang stirs with phlegm-heat blockage which confuses heart spirit. Di Huang Yin Zi is offered.

Prescription: Rehmanniae Radix 18g, Coastal Glehnia Root 18g, Dwarf Lily-turf Tuber 15g, Dendrobium 18g (decocted earlier), sweet CistanchedeseuticolaMa 12g, Zhuyuanzhi 6g, Salvia Root 12g, fried Sophora Flower 12g, Tabasheer 9g, Turmeric Root-tuber 9g and fine Grassleaf Sweetflag Rhizome 9g, and there were six bags of medicine.

Secondary diagnosis: on October 20, the patient was conscious, right body could lightly move, and had food. However, her speech still was sluggish with red tongue and thready pulse. Wind-yang gradually was balanced, damage in kidney yin was not recovered, and phlegm-heat still had the possibility of transformation, the treatment should follow the original principle but with some modifications. Turmeric Root-tuber and Tabasheer were removed from the previous prescription, and Dadilong of 6g was added, and there were twelve bags of medicine.

Third diagnosis: on November 6, the movement of right body improved day by day, The symptom of sluggish speech is gradually improved, stool and urine were normal, and tongue was red and moistened with thready pulse. Damage in kidney yin recovered gradually, and wind yang and phlegm-heat also were balanced, and the doctor continued offering the medicine for regulating and reinforcing heart and kidneys.

Prescription: large Rehmanniae Radix 12g, Coastal Glehnia Root 18g, Dwarf Lily-turf Tuber 15g, Dendrobium 18g (decocted earlier), sweet CistanchedeseuticolaMa 12g, Radix Polygoni Multiflori Preparata 15g, Indian Bread 9g, Zhuyuanzhi 6g, Salvia Root 12g, fried date seed 9g, wheat in Jianghuai 30g and Radix Achyranthis Bidentatae 9g. There are fourteen bags of medicine.

Fourth diagnosis: on November 27. The patient could speak clearly, her right limb could move. The patient was capable of walking with cane. Her tongue was red and moistened, and pulse was thread and small. Apoplectoid stroke was in recovery, and the patient was still conditioned according to the previous method to promote recovery. Seven bags of medicines were given according to original prescription.

2. Medical record of Wang Qicai— —stroke involving channel and collateral

Ms Zhao, female, 72.

Preliminary diagnosis: on October 2, 1990. The patient had medical history of hypertension for over 20 years. When she go to the bathroom, she felt heart pain and dizzy, numbness in left limb, soreness and lassitude. Then she immediately slumped in the bathroom. However, she had no dysfunction of consciousness, aphasia, nausea or vomiting. Then she was sent to hospital for emergent rescue. Examination: myodynamia of upper and lower limbs in left side was in range of levels II ~ III , with the symptom of deflection of corner of mouth. Cerebral CT showed there was a 1.31cm×1.31cm high density region in right thalamus. The patient was transferred to acupuncture and moxibustion ward for treatment after observed and treated in emergency room. First acupuncture and moxibustion was given in Hegu (LI 4) in both sides, Dicang (ST 4) and Jiache (ST 6) in left side, Quchi (LI 11), Zusanli (ST 36), Yanglingquan (GB 34), Fenglong (ST 40) and Taichong (LR 3) to offer moderate stimulation, and needle movement and retention time was 30 min with language hint. After the needle was withdrawn, the patient was able to walk tens of meters with the assistance of her family members. After 5 times of treatment, she could walk with cane independently. The myodynamia of upper and lower limbs in left side was at level IV , only numb left corner of mouth, finger and toe ends existed. She recovered and left the hospital after 3 weeks. (Wang Qicai, Zhenyi Xinwu. Publishing House of Ancient Chinese Medical Book. 2001)

3. Medical record of Shi Xuemin— —stroke involving channel and collateral

Mr. Zhang, male, 67, a retired worker.

Preliminary diagnosis: on September 23, 1980, with admission No. 9456.

Chief complaint: Hemiplegia in left body with unsmooth speech for 13 days.

Medical history: the patient caught a cold in the nighttime of September 11, and suffered from hemiplegia in left body in the morning of the next day. He was conscious, with numb limbs and sluggish speech, and he couldn't walk. Then, he was sent to observation room of one hospital for observation. Lumbar puncture report: cerebrospinal fluid was colorless and transparent, and semi-quantitative test for glucose showed (+), then the disease was diagnosed as "cerebrovascular accident". Blood circulation promotion and anti-infection treatment were offered. After 12 days, the condition was stable. He had clear mind and deviation of eye and mouth, and his affected limb had no voluntary movements. His speech was unsmooth, and there were no headache and dizziness. Stool and urine were controlled. He denied that he had a medical history of hypertension previously. He was hospitalized in our department for treatment on September 23. Physical examination: blood pressure of 240/120 mmHg, pulse rate of 60 times/min, with consciousness and lean body, central facial paralysis in left side, unsmooth speech and symmetric pulse in bilateral internal carotid artery; muffled heart sound, A2> P2, regular heart rhythm, harsh breathing sound in the left lung; soft abdomen, low bowel sound; flaccid paralysis in left upper and lower limbs, physiological reflex (+), reflection of right palm jaw (+), and Babinski symptom (+); red tongue texture, yellow and greasy tongue coating and wiry and thready pulse.

Impression:

Chinese medicine diagnosis: stroke (stroke involving channel and collateral)

Western medicine diagnosis: hypertension, arteriosclerosis and cerebral thrombosis.

Syndrome differentiation: the patient was over sixty-four, whose healthy Qi was deficient, liver and kidney had been deficient with hyperactive liver yang, at the same time, he suffered from external wind and cold. It made intern wind disturb orifices, and orifices were closed, and mind was concealed, so that hemiplegia and deflection of mouth was seen. Wind pathogen made phlegm-dampness flow through collateral, then stiff tongue and sluggish speech occurred.

Treatment principle: to restore consciousness and open orifices, nourish liver and kidneys and dredge collaterals.

Selected points: Neiguan (PC 6), (GV 26), Sanyinjiao (SP 6), Jiquan (HT 1), Chize (LU 5), Weizhong (BL 40), Fengchi (GB 20), Shangxing (GV 23) and Baihui (GV 20).

Manipulation: first acupuncture Neiguan (PC 6) in both sides, insert the needle to 1cun, and rotate the needle with twirling and lifting-thrusting reducing method for 1 min. Then, puncture Rengzhong (GV 26), inserting the needle for 5 min with Sparrow-pecking reducing method. until eyeball is moisted or tears shed. The needle shall present 45°angle with skin in acupuncture of Sanyinjiao (SP 6) along rear edge of tibia, and insert needle to 1-1.5 cun with lifting-thrusting reinforcing method, so as to make lower limbs twitch for 3 times; perpendicularly puncture Jiquan (HT 1) to 1-1.5 cun with lifting-thrusting reducing method, and make upper limbs twitch for 3 times; operation of Chize (LU 5) and requirements for measurement are the same as those of HT 1; for Weizhong (BL 40), the acupoint should be located when supine position is adopted and straight legs are lifted. Insert needle to 1 cun with lifting-thrusting reducing method, and make lower limbs twitch for 3 times; for Fengchi (GB 20), puncture to laryngeal prominence, and insert needle to 2~2.5 cun with twirling reinforcing method in small amplitude and high frequency for 1 min. With regard to Shangxing (GV 23) and Baihui (GV 20), perform penetration acupuncture towards Baihui (GV 20) along scalp with twirling reinforcing method to achieve local soreness and distention.

Treatment procedure: after one-week treatment, the patient was able to straightly lift left lower limb for 40°, and bend and lift elbow of left upper limb to chest. The speech was clear. After two weeks, the patient could walk with assistance, then walk independently. Left upper limb was lifted over head. Only the grip strength of left hand was weak. About in four weeks, the patients had normal functions of four limbs and clear voice. The patient recovered and left the hospital.

VI. Prevention and aftercare

i. Prevention

(1) Reduction of the risk factors that possibly trigger stroke: the diseases that possibly cause stroke involving arteriosclerosis, diabetes, coronary heart disease, hyperlipemia, hyperviscosity, adiposis, cervical spondylosis and the like shall be as soon as possible treated.

(2) Notice of signal symptoms of stroke: some patients often have Pre symptoms like elevation and fluctuation of blood pressure, dizziness, headache, lethargy, abnormal character and numb and weak hands and foot. Once these symptoms are found, patients shall take measures to control them as soon as possible.

(3) Effective control of transient ischemia attack: when patients have pre symptoms of transient ischemia attack, they shall rest quietly, and go to a hospital to receive diagnosis and treatment timely, so as to prevent the development to cerebral thrombosis.

(4) Notice of the effects of meteorological factors: seasonal and climate changes will make the patients with hypertension have unstable emotion and fluctuation of blood pressure, and trigger stroke. The occurrence of stroke shall be prevented on the occasion. Patients shall adapt to the environmental temperature gradually, and the difference between indoor and outdoor temperatures shall not be large (especially for the aged). In addition, patients shall be slow in getting up and bending head to lace shoes and the like in daily life; bath time shall not be too long, and so on.

ii. Aftercare

(1)TCM have better treatment effects on stroke. Early intervention of acupuncture therapy has a better effect,, especially on recovery of limb movement, language and swallowing, and so on.

(2) In acute stage of stroke, when high fever, unconsciousness, heart failure, increased intracranial pressure, upper gastrointestinal bleeding and the like occur, integrated treatment shall be adopted.

(3) The patients who lie in bed with stroke shall turn over regularly, keeping dry skin and good blood circulation to avoid bedsore. Meanwhile, it is noted that unblocked respiratory tract shall be kept.

(4) During treatment and recovery, function exercise is helpful for the recovery of the movement function of the hemiplegic limb.

(5) Patients shall have more bland diet, and avoid or eat less greasy and spicy food, which can prevent wind generation due to heat accumulation, phlegm generation due to dampness accumulation.

(6) Usually, patients should keep relaxed and happy, and avoid the effects of bad emotions such as exasperation, depression, too much worry and sorrow.

(7) Prevention for the disease shall be focused. For people over 40, dizziness, headache and numb limbs often occur. Paroxysmal unsmooth speech, flaccid and weak limbs and the like occasionally happen. Pre symptoms of stroke should be alerted, and the prevention and treatment shall be strengthened.

(XU　Li)

References

[1] Department of Acupuncture and Moxibustion in The First Affiliated Hospital of TIANJIN UNIVERSITY OF TCM. Applied Chinese Acupuncture for Clinical Practitioners of Shi Xuemin [M]. Tianjin: Tianjin Science & Technology Press, 1990.

[2] Wang QC. Zhenyi Xinwu [M]. Beijing: Publishing House of Ancient Chinese Medical Book, 2011.

[3] Yan SY, Zheng PD, He LR. Medical records of Zhang Boyu [M]. Shanghai: Shanghai Scientific & Technical Publishers, 2003.

[4] Zhou ZY. Internal Medicine of TCM [M]. Beijing: China Press of Traditional Chinese Medicine, 2003.

[5] Shi XM, Dai XM, Wang J. Internal Medicine of TCM [M]. Beijing: China Press of Traditional Chinese Medicine, 2009.

[6] Zhang BL. Internal Medicine of TCM [M]. Beijing: People's Medical Publishing House, 2012.

[7] Shi XM. Acupuncture and moxibustion (bilingual school textbook) [M]. Beijing: Higher Education Press, 2005.

[8] Gao SZ. Acupunture and moxibustion therapy [M]. Shanghai: Shanghai Scientific & Technical Publishers, 2009.

[9] Wang QC. Acupunture and moxibustion therapy [M]. Beijing: China Press of Traditional Chinese Medicine, 2004.

Insomnia 失眠

I. Overview

Insomnia is also called "sleeplessness" and "inability to sleep" in Traditional Chinese medicine; it refers to a disease characterized by frequent sleep disorders. In *Inner Canon of Huangdi,* it is also called "inability to sleep" and "eyes unable to be closed". The location of disease lies in heart, and kidney, liver, spleen, stomach and gallbladder are closely related. Having no peace of mind is the main reason of the disease. The clinical manifestations are deficiency in sleep time and sleep depth. The less serious cases have difficulty in falling asleep or sleeping soundly; sometimes being asleep sometimes being awake, or they aren't able to fall asleep again after waking up. The serious cases can not sleep throughout the night, which often influences their normal work, learning, living and health. In order to improve people's awareness of the importance of sleep, the International Society for Mental Health and Neuroscience Fund has launched a global sleep and health programMarch 21 every year has been identified as "World Sleep Day". Thus it can be seen that insomnia has gradually become a global health problem.

In western medicine, insomnia can be the main clinical manifestation of neurosis, menopausal syndrome, chronic indigestion, depression, anxiety disorder, atherosclerosis and so on. In this case, these diseases can adopt syndrome differentiation and treatment by referring to the content of insomnia.

II. Etiology and pathogenesis

i. Chinese medicine

The occurrence of insomnia is mainly related to unconstrained diet, emotional disorders, imbalance between work and rest, weakness after disease, weakness due to old age, etc. The normal sleep usually relies on sufficient Qi and Blood, viscera harmony, yin and yang in equilibrium, so as to ensure ataraxia and peace sleep. If patients worry too much, their hearts and spleens will be hurt, Qi and Blood will be deficient, so the hearts can not be nourished and they will feel ill at case. If patients are weak due to chronic disease, and have symptoms of yin-blood deficiency, hyperactive fire due to yin deficienc, disturbance of effulgent fire, they will be ill at case. If the patients are terrified suddenly, his Qi in heart and gallbladder will be deficient, he will lack preservation of spirit, and be absent-minded, thus feeling ill at case. If patients are upset emotionally, depression of Qi generates fire, so liver fire rises and their heart fire is intense, finally spirit is disturbed and they feel upset and can not fall asleep. If diet hurts the spleen, the retained food is stagnated, long stagnation leads to heat, and the stomach is disturbed, thus the patients can not sleep well.

1. Etiology

In *Inner Canon of Huangdi*, it is considered that insomnia is caused by pathogenic Qi residing in internal organs, thus defense Qi flows in yang, and is unable to flow into yin. *Ni Diao Lun* of *Suwen* records "the disorder of the stomach leading to insomnia with restlessness". *Treatise on Cold Damage Diseases* of Zhang Zhongjing in Han Dynasty divided the etiology of insomnia into two types— external factors and internal injuries— and also put forward the opinion of "consumptive disease and dysphoria leading to sleeplessness". Li Zhongzi put forward knowledgeable opinions on the cause of insomnia: "there are about five causes of insomnia: one is Qi deficiency; another is yin deficiency; the others are phlegm stagnation, water retention and stomach disharmony". Dai Yuanli in Ming Dynasty put forward the theory of "for the elder, yang declines and they can not sleep" in *Asthenic Disease* of *Key to Diagnosis and Treatment* The of *Feng Tips Volumn XII* of Qing Dynasty presents "young people's kidney yin is strong, so they sleep deeply for a long time; the elder's yin Qi is weak, so they sleep light and are easy to wake up". This shows the etiology of insomnia is also related to the deficiency of yin and yang in kidney.

(1) Unconstrained diet: The patients eat and drink too much, and the retained food stays in the body, leading to the spleen and stomach injury. Thus the phlegm-dampness is generated in body and blocks in the middle. After a long time, phlegm-heat is produced and harasses the upper body, and the stomach-qi is disharmonic. Therefore, the patients cannot sleep well. In *Incapability of Supination* of *Comprehensive Medicine According to Master Zhang*, the etiology of insomnia is explained as "for the patients with slippery, rapid and forceful pulse and inable to lie down, there is phlegm fire stagnated for a long time and this is known as disorder of the stomach leading to insomnia with restlessness".

(2) Emotional disorders: Extreme emotions may result in the disorder of viscera function, thus leading to insomnia. In ordinary days, if the patients are unhappy or upset, the depressed anger will damage the liver; the liver qi is stagnated and transformed into fire; the fire disturbs the spirit; the disturbed spirit will lead to insomnia. Otherwise, as five emotions overact, internal heart fire is intense, and the heart spirit is disturbed, leading to insomnia. Or excessive laughter disturbs spirit and restless mind result in insomnia. What's more, if patients are terrified suddenly, they feel timid in heart-gallbladder and restless in mind, so they can not sleep at night. As is recorded in *Insomnia* of *Shen's Zunshengshu*: "timidity in heart and gallbladder and being easily startled when anything comes up would result in many ominous dreams, dysphoria and insomnia"; or patients may feel uneasy

and hard to sleep at night because excessive anxiety hurts hearts and spleens, so the nutrient blood is insufficient and unable to nourish heart. *Insomnia* of *Treatment of Different Kinds of Diseases* records: "worry impairing spleen, and deficiency of spleen blood are the reasons for insomnia for years".

(3) Imbalance between work and rest: Too much work hurts spleen, so does too much rest and little movement. Weakness of spleen and Qi, failure of transportation and transformation, and deficiency of the source of qi and blood formation will lead to impaired nourishment of heart, causing insomnia. *Insomnia* of *Jing Yue Complete Works* records: "people who think or work too much will certainly suffer from blood loss and no master of spirit. Therefore, they can not fall asleep." Thus it can be seen that the dysfunction of spleen in transportation and no reborn Qi and Blood will cause blood deficiency; impaired nourishment of spirit will cause insomnia.

(4) Weakness after disease: Prolonged illness causing deficiency of yin blood, old age and weakness lead to deficiency of heart blood, lack of nourishment of heart, uneasiness and insomnia, just as recorded in *Insomnia* of *Jing-Yue Complete Works*: "people without pathogen but with insomnia must be deficient in nutrient Qi; the nutrition mainly comes from blood, so with blood deficiency heart cannot be nourished in the case of blood deficiency, and deficiency of heart will make people out of their mind". The disease may be caused by body deficiency due to old age as well as deficiency of yin and yang. In the case of yin deficiency and excess of sexual intercourse, the kidney yin is damaged; yin is deficient in lower body and can not nourish the heart; water and fire is imbalanced; heart fire is stronger; exuberant fire and failure of the heart and kidney integration lead to absence and restlessness in mind. As "deficiency of true yin, essence and blood; non-interaction between yin and yang; these result in uneasy spirit" recorded in *Insomnia* of *Jing-Yue Complete Works*.

2. Pathogenesis

There are many disease causes of insomnia; however its basic pathogenesis is restless heart spirit, which is attributed to exuberance of yang with decline of yin and non-interaction between yin and yang. That is to say, yin deficiency cannot receive yang, or exuberance of yang cannot enter yin. The location of disease lies in heart, and liver, spleen, stomach, kidney and gallbladder are closely related. The heart governs the mind; the peaceful mind brings about good sleep and restless mind results in insomnia. Since the source of yin and yang, Qi and Blood derives from the essence of water and grain. The heart spirit is nourished when it goes to the heart; liver is soft when it hides in the liver; the gallbladder qi is strong and the spirit qi is peaceful when it is raised in gallbladder; generation and transformation are endless when it is governed by spleen; when it is regulated aptly, it transforms into essence, and hides in the kidney; the kidney essence links to the heart, and the heart qi links to the kidney; thus the yin essence is controlled, and the mind is peaceful.

The pathological nature of insomnia contains deficiency and excess. If liver depression forms fire, the phlegm-heat may disturb internally, or the heart fire is exuberant, the patients with restless heart spirit are mainly excess syndrome. Deficiency of heart and spleen; deficiency of Qi and Blood; water-fire imbalance, lack of preservation of spirit and restless spirit due to deficiency of heart qi and gallbladder qi, or non-interaction between heart and kidney belong to deficiency syndrome generally. If the disease history is long, it can be shown as deficiency-excess in complexity, or it may be caused by static blood.

The prognosis of insomnia is usually good. In the case of improper treatment or lack of treatment, the pathogenesis may be transformed. If the condition of patients with transformation of fire from liver depression worsens due to improper treatment, fire-heat hurts yin and consumes qi, in which case excess transforms into deficiency. The patients with deficiency of both heart and spleen eat and drink irregularly, their spleen and stomach are hurt further; the food is stagnated internally, and deficiency and excess coexist. The prognosis varies due to different conditions. The patients with short course of disease and simple conditions can see the effects faster; the patients with long course of disease and complex conditions are hard to receive quick results. If the course of disease extends due to improper treatment or lack of treatment, it is easy to produce emotional disease, making state of illness more complicated, and increasing the difficulty in treatment.

ii. Western medicine

Insomnia can be divided into primary and secondary insomnia according to the disease causes.

1. Primary insomnia

It usually lacks clear disease cause, or insomnia symptoms still exist after the exclusion of possible disease causes. It mainly includes 3 types: psychological and physiological insomnia, idiopathic insomnia and subjective insomnia. The diagnosis of primary insomnia lacks specificity index, mainly an exclusionary diagnosis. After the possible disease causes are excluded or cured, insomnia symptoms still exist, then it can be considered as primary insomnia. The disease causes of psychological and physiological insomnia can all be traced to the effect of one or several long-term events on the functional stability of the limbic system. The imbalance of the functional stability of the limbic system eventually leads to disorder of brain's sleep function and insomnia.

2. Secondary insomnia

It is often caused by physical disease, mental disorders, drug abuse and so on. It is related to sleep apnea syndrome, sleep movement disorders and etc.

Insomnia and other diseases often occur at the same time; sometimes it is difficult to determine the causal relationship between these diseases and insomnia. Therefore, the concept of comorbidinsomnia was raised in recent years to describe insomnia accompanied by other diseases.

III. Key points of diagnosis and differential diagnosis

i. Key points of diagnosis

1. Traditional Chinese Medicine

(1) The mild insomniacs have difficulty in falling asleep. They are easy to wake up after falling asleep, or cannot fall asleep after waking up, or sometimes fall asleep and sometimes awake, or can ot sleep well. These symptoms last for more than 3 weeks. The serious insomniacs do not sleep throughout the night.

(2) The patients may also have dizziness, headache, palpitation, amnesia, lassitude, restless heart spirit and dreaminess, etc.

(3) They generally have such histories of unconstrained diet, emotional disorders, weariness and excessive thinking, weakness after disease and etc.

(4) No other organic lesions were found to interfere with sleep through various system examinations and laboratory examinations.

2. Western medicine

(1) With typical symptoms of insomnia: sleep disorder is almost the only symptom, and other symptoms are secondary to insomnia, including difficulty in falling asleep, unsound slumber, dreaminess, waking too early, inability to sleep again after being awake, discomfort or fatigue after waking up, or somnolence during the day.

(2) The above sleep disorders happen at least 3 times every week, and last for more than 1 month.

(3) Insomnia brings about obvious distress, or reduction of efficiency of mental activities, or interference of social functions..

(4) It is not a part of the symptoms of any physical disease or mental disorder.

ii. Differential diagnosis

Insomnia shall be distinguished from temporary sleeplessness, physiological less sleep and sleeplessness caused by pain of other diseases. Insomnia simply refers to the main symptom of sleeplessness, and is manifested as persistent and severe trouble in sleeping. The temporary sleeplessness caused by temporary emotional effects or changes in living environment does not belong to morbid state. As for the elderly, less sleep and being awake early also belong to physiological state in most cases. If the patients suffer from sleeplessness due to other diseases, they shall focus on treating related disease causes.

1. Insomnia caused by mental factors

Mental stress, anxiety, fear, excitement, etc. can cause transient insomnia. The clinical manifestations are mainly difficulty in falling sleep and unsound slumber. The insomnia is relieved after the elimination of mental factors.

2. Insomnia caused by physical factors

The pain, itching, nasal congestion, difficulty in breathing, asthma, coughing, frequent urination, nausea, vomiting, abdominal distension, diarrhea, palpitations and other reactions caused by various somatic diseases can lead to sleep difficulties or light sleep. The insomnia can be improved after the relief of somatic diseases.

3. Physiologic factors

Changes of living and working environment, new arrival at a new place, unfamiliar environment, drinking strong tea and coffee and so on can lead to insomnia. The insomnia can be relieved after being out of uncomfortable environment or short-term adaptation.

4. Diffuse brain lesion

Insomnia is often the early symptom of diffuse brain lesion caused by chronic poisoning, endocrine diseases, dystrophy and dystrophy, cerebral arteriosclerosis and other factors. The manifestations are reduced sleep time, discontinuous sleep and restless sleep, as well as disappearance of deep sleep stage. Insomnia can be relieved with the relief of the diseases; insomnia will worsen when the condition is aggravated; sleepiness or consciousness disorder may appear when the condition is too severe.

IV. TCM therapy

i. Syndrome differentiation and treatment

1. Liver fire disturbing heart

Main symptoms: difficulty in falling asleep, sleeplessness and dreaminess; even pernoctation, anxiety and irritability, accompanied by dizziness and headache, red eyes, tinnitus, dry mouth with bitter taste, poor appetite, constipation, bloody urine, red tongue and yellow tongue fur, stringy and rapid pulse.

Therapeutic method: to soothe liver, purge fire, set heart and tranquilize mind.

Prescription: modified Long Dan Xie Gan Tang. Chinese Gentian, Cape Jasmine Fruit, Chinese Thorowax Root, Baical Skullcap Root, Unprocessed Rehmannia Root, Oriental Waterplantain Rhizome, Chinese Angelica, Akebia Stem, Plantain Seed, Unprocessed Liquorice Root, Unprocessed Bone Fossil of Big Mammals, Unprocessed Oyster Shell, and Magnetite.

Prescription analysis: this prescription has the function of clearing and purging liver-gallbladder excessive fire. It mainly applies to insomnia, dreaminess, dizziness, headache, red eyes and tinnitus caused by liver depression transforming into fire and flaming upward. Chinese Gentian, Baical Skullcap Root and Cape Jasmine Fruit can clear the liver and drain fire; Oriental Waterplantain Rhizome and Plantain Seed can clear dampness-heat and release stagnant fire; Chinese Angelica and Unprocessed Rehmannia Root can nourish yin and blood to avoid hurting yin when purging fire. Chinese Thorowax Root sooths liver and and relieves depression; Liquorice Root harmonizes the middle; Unprocessed Bone Fossil of Big Mammals, Unprocessed Oyster Shell and Magnetite set the heart and calm the mind.

Modification: Nutgrass Galingale Rhizome, Turmeric Root Tuber and Finger Citron are added for the insomniacs accompanied with chest tightness, rib-side distention and susceptible sigh to enhance the function of soothing liver and and relieving depression. A lot of Golden Thread and Medicinal Evodia Fruit shall be added for the insomniacs accompanied with poor appetite and belching with fetid odour with regurgitation of stomach acid to enhance the function of clearing liver and purging fire, harmonizing stomach and descending adverse Qi. The insomniacs accompanied with pernoctation, dizziness, headache, irritability and constipation shall use Angelica, Dang Gui Long Hui Wan instead of this prescription.

2. Phlegm-heat disturbing heart

Main symptoms: vexation and insomnia, chest tightness, epigastric fullness, belching, with bitter taste and bad smell in the mouth, dizziness, blurred vision, red tongue, yellow and greasy tongue fur, slippery and rapid pulse.

Therapeutic method: to clear and resolve phlegm-heat, strengthen the middle energizer and tranquilize mind.

Prescription: modified Huang Lian Wen Dan Tang. Golden Thread, Bamboo Shavings, Immature Orange Fruit, Pinellia Tuber, Dried Tangerine Peel, Liquorice Root, Fresh Ginger, Indian Bread, Dragon Teeth, Nacre and Magnetite.

Prescription analysis: this prescription has the functions of clearing heart, reducing fire, resolving phlegm and calming the middle. It mainly applies to vexation and insomnia, dizziness and dreaminess caused by phlegm-heat disturbing heart spirit. Pinellia Tuber, Dried Tangerine Peel, Immature Orange Fruit and Indian Bread can invigorate spleen, resolve phlegm, regulate Qi and harmonize stomach. Golden Thread and Bamboo Shavings can clear heart, reduce fire and resolve phlegm. Dragon Teeth, Nacre and Magnetite can relieve convulsion and tranquilize mind.

Modification: Ban Xia Su Mi Tang shall be added to invigorate spleen, harmonize stomach and descend Qi for the insomniacs accompanied with chest tightness, belching, abdominal distention, dyschesia, greasy tongue fur and slippery pulse. Medicated Leaven, Parched Hawthorn Fruit and Radish Seed are added to help digestion and harmonize the middle for the insomniacs accompanied with food stagnation, stomach disharmony, belching with fetid odour with regurgitation of stomach acid and abdominal swelling and pain. Meng Shi Gun Tan Wan is added to purge fire and remove phlegm for the insomniacs accompanied with abundant phlegm-heat, phlegm-fire disturbing heart spirit, pernoctation and constipation.

3. Exuberance of heart fire

Main symptoms: vexation and insomnia, dysphoria, mouth parched and tongue scorched, scanty dark urine, aphthae boil of the tongue, red tip of tongue, thin and yellow tongue fur, strong pulse or thready rapid pulse.

Therapeutic method: to clear heart, purge fire, tranquilize mind and clam heart.

Prescription: modified Zhu Sha An Shen Wan. Cinnabar, Golden Thread, Chinese Angelica, Unprocessed Rehmannia Root, Liquorice Root, Baical Skullcap Root, Cape Jasmine Fruit and Lotus Plumule.

Prescription analysis: this prescription has the functions of clearing heat, purging fire, relieving restlessness and tranquilizing mind. It mainly applies to dysphoria and sleeplessness as well as dysphoria and unrest resulting from heart fire hyperactivity.Cinnabar is used for tranquilization with heavy material; Golden Thread is bitter cold and can clear heart, clear fire and relieve restlessness. The mixture of Cinnabar and Golden Thread can work together to clear heat, clear fire, relieve restlessness, and to tranquilize mind with heavy material. Chinese Angelica nourishes blood and unprocessed Rehmannia Root nourishes yin ,which complements yin blood consumed by exuberant fire. Liquorice Root coordinates the drug actions of a prescription. Baical Skullcap Root, Cape Jasmine Fruit and Lotus Plumule can be added to enhance the function of clearing heart and reducing fire.

Modification: Fermented Soybean and Bamboo Shavings are added to ventilate the stagnated fire in the chest for the insomniacs accompanied with irritancy in chest, chest tightness and nausea. Rhubarb, Lophatherum Herb and Amber are added to lead fire downward and release heart spirit for the insomniacs accompanied with constipation and reddish urine.

4. Failure of descending of the stomach-qi

Main symptoms: dysphoria and insomnia, abdominal fullness and distention, belching with fetid odor and acid regurgitation, nausea and vomiting, dyschesia, foul defecation, constipation and abdominal pain, red tongue, yellow and greasy or yellow rough fur, stringy and slippery or rapid pulse.

Therapeutic method: harmonize stomach and resolve food stagnation, calm heart and tranquilize mind.

Prescription: modified Bao He Wan. Hawthorn Fruit, Medicated Leaven, Radish Seed, Dried Tangerine Peel, Pinellia Tuber, Indian Bread, Weeping Forsythia Capsule, Milkwort Root, Chinese Arborvitae Kernel and Tuber Fleeceflower Stem.

Prescription analysis: this prescription has the efficacy of promoting digestion, removing food stagnation, harmonizing stomach and tranquilizing mind. It mainly applies to the symptoms of abdominal fullness and distention, sometimes pain in abdominal distension and dysphoria and insomnia caused by food accumulation, retention and stagnation and failure of descending of the stomach-qi. Hawthorn Fruit can resolve greasy meat stagnation; Medicated Leaven can resolve accumulation of stale wine and food; Radish Seed can disperse stagnation of phlegm turbidity caused by food made from wheat; Dried Tangerine Peel, Pinellia Tuber, Indian Bread can regulate Qi and harmonize stomach, dry dampness and resolve phlegm; Weeping Forsythia Capsule can dissipate mass and clear heat; all drugs have the effect of promoting digestion and harmonizing stomach; Milkwort Root, Chinese Arborvitae Kernel and Tuber Fleeceflower Stem can be added to calm heart and tranquilize mind.

Modification: for patients concurrently with chest tightness and belching, and abdominal fullness and distention, Immature Orange Fruit and Orange Fruit are added to move Qi and resolve accumulation; for patients concurrently with stomach disharmony, nausea and vomiting, White Atractylodes Rhizome, Officinal Magnolia Bark and Nutgrass Galingale Rhizome are added to invigorate spleen and drain dampness, smooth middle and arrest vomiting; for patients concurrently with Qi depression and Qi stagnation, epigastric upset of distention of the stomach, and distention and pain in the chest and abdomen, Depression Resolving Harmony-Preserving Pills can be used to sooth liver and resolve depression, stimulate appetite and promote digestion.

5. Blood vessel stasis and obstruction

Main symptoms: insomnia and dreaminess, dysphoria, amnesia, hypomnesia, dry and bitter mouth, dizziness and headache, fatigue and lack of strength, dry stool, dark urine, dark red tongue, ecchymosis in tongue, yellow greasy or thin yellow tongue fur and fine and stringy pulse.

Therapeutic method: to activate blood and resolve stasis, calm heart and tranquilize mind.

Prescription: modified Xue Fu Zhu Yu Tang and Suan Zao Ren Tang. Chinese Angelica, Sichuan Lovage Rhizome, Red Peony Root, Peach Seed, Safflower, Radix Achyranthis Bidentatae, Chinese Thorowax Root, Platycodon Root, Orange Fruit, Unprocessed Rehmannia Root, Chinese Angelica, Spina Date Seed, Common Anemarrhena Rhizome, Indian Bread, Liquorice Root.

Prescription analysis: this prescription has the efficacy of dispelling stasis and invigorating pulse, nourishing blood and tranquilizing mind. It mainly applies to palpitation, amnesia and insomnia caused by deficiency of both heart and spleen caused by stagnation of blood stasis and clear yang failing to ascend. Chinese Angelica, Sichuan Lovage Rhizome, Red Peony Root, Peach Seed, Safflower can promote blood circulation circulation and resolve stasis; Radix Achyranthis Bidentatae can dispel stasis and stagnation to dredge blood vessel and conduct blood stasis descending; Chinese Thorowax Root can sooth liver and relieve depression, ascend and clear yang; Platycodon Root can open and relieve lung-qi, and carry the medicines upwards, combined with Orange Fruit, ascending and descending, combined with Orange Fruit, ascending and descending, to open chest and promote qi circulation and therefore promote blood circulation;Unprocessed Rehmannia Root and Chinese Angelica can nourish yin and moisten dryness to dispel stasis without damage to yin blood; Spina Date Seed, Common Anemarrhena Rhizome, Indian Bread can nourish blood and tranquilize mind; Liquorice Root can coordinate the drug actions of the prescription. The combination of all herbs can stringy and dispel stasis and stagnation, and release Qi and dispel depression, activate blood circulation without blood loss, and remove blood stasis to produce new blood; therefore, blood stasis is removed to tranquilize mind.

Modification: for patients with sleep difficulties, Tuber Fleeceflower Stem, Silktree Albizia Bark and Chinese Arborvitae Kernel are added to nourish heart and tranquilize mind; for patients with serious insomnia and severe palpitation, unprocessed Bone Fossil of Big Mammals, raw oyster shell and Nacre are added to tranquilize mind.

6. Deficiency of both heart and spleen

Main symptoms: sleep difficulties, dreaminess and restless sleep, palpitation and amnesia, mental weariness and poor appetite, dizzy vision, fatigued limbs, abdominal distension and loose stools, lusterless complexion, light tongue and thin fur, thin and weak pulse.

Therapeutic method: to invigorate spleen, benefit heart, nourish blood and tranquilize mind.

Prescription: modified Gui Pi Tang. Ginseng, White Atractylodes Rhizome, Liquorice Root, Chinese Angelica, Milkvetch Root, Milkwort Root, Spina Date Seed, Indian bread with Pine, Longan Aril, Common Aucklandia Root.

Prescription analysis: this prescription has an efficacy of invigorating spleen and nourishing heart, replenishing Qi and tonifying blood. It mainly applies to insomnia and amnesia, severe palpitation, yellowish complexion and reduced appetite caused by deficiency of both heart and spleen. Ginseng, White Atractylodes Rhizome, Liquorice Root can invigorate spleen and replenish Qi; Chinese Angelica, Milkvetch Root can tonify Qi and generate blood; Milkwort Root, Spina Date Seed, Indian Bread with Pine, Longan Aril, can tonify heart and spleen and tranquilize mind; Common Aucklandia Root can promote Qi circulation and sooth spleen.

Modification: for patients concurrently with serious insufficiency of heart blood, palpitation and amnesia, Prepared Rehmannia Root, Peony and Ass Hide Glue are added to nourish heart and blood; for patients concurrently with sleep difficulties, Chinese Magnoliavine Fruit, tuber fleeceflower stem, Silktree Albizia Bark, Chinese Arborvitae Kernel are added to nourish heart and tranquilize mind; for patients with serious insomnia and severe palpitation, unprocessed Bone Fossil of Big Mammals, Raw Oyster Shell, Amber powder are added to calm and tranquilize mind; for patients concurrently with gastral cavity depression and anorexia, greasy tongue fur, much White Atractylodes Rhizome is used, together with. Atractylodes Rhizome, Pinellia Tuber, Dried Tangerine Peel, Indian Bread, Officinal Magnolia Bark, to invigorate spleen and dry dampness, regulate Qi and dispel phlegm. Provided that the old early wakes during night sleep without dysphoria, which is due to insufficiency of Qi and Blood, much Chinese Angelica and Milkvetch Root are used to tonify Qi and Blood.

7. Disharmony between heart and kidney

Main symptoms: dysphoria and sleeplessness, sleep difficulties, palpitation and dreaminess, accompanied with dizziness and tinnitus, soreness and weakness of waist and knees, tidal fever and night sweating, dry throat and less fluid, men seminal emission, menstrual irregularities of women, red tongue and less fur, thready rapid pulse.

Therapeutic method: nourish yin and reduce fire, restore coordination between heart and kidney.

Prescription: modified Liu Wei Di Huang Wan and Jiao Tai Wan. Prepared Rehmannia Root, Pulp of Dogwood Fruit, Common Yam Rhizome, Oriental Waterplantain Rhizome, Indian Bread, Tree Peony Root Bark,

223

Golden Thread, Cinnamon Bark.

Prescription analysis: main function of Six-Ingredient Rehmannia Pills is mainly for kidney yin, and it is mainly used for syndrome of insufficiency of kidney yin, such as dizziness and tinnitus, soreness and weakness of waist and knees, and tidal fever and night sweating. Jiaotai Pills can clear heart and reduce fire, return fire to its origin and is mainly used for dysphoria and sleeplessness, nocturnal emission and seminal emission and other symptoms due to hyperactivity of heart and fire. Prepared Rehmannia Root can nourish yin and tonify kidney, supplement essence and replenish marrow; Pulp of Dogwood Fruit can tonify liver and kidney and astringe essence; Common Yam Rhizome can tonify spleen yin and also consolidate kidney. The combination of the three herbs can achieve the effect of tonifying kidney, liver and spleen. Oriental Waterplantain Rhizome can excrete dampness and drain kidney turbidity to reduce nourishing greasy of Prepared Rehmannia Root; Indian Bread can eliminate spleen dampness with bland medicinal to assist transportation of Common Yam Rhizome; Tree Peony Root Bark can clear deficient heat to restrict warm astringency of Pulp of Dogwood Fruit. Golden Thread can clear heart and reduce fire; Cinnamon Bark can return fire to its origin.

Modification: for patients concurrently with insufficiency of heart yin, Tian Wang Bu Xin Dan is added to nourish yin and blood, invigorate heart and tranquilize mind; for patients concurrently with dysphoria and insomnia, pernoctation, Cinnabar, Magnetite, Bone Fossil of Big Mammals and dragon teeth are added to settle and tranquilize mind; for patients concurrently with yin-blood deficiency and heart fire hyperactivity, Zhu Sha An Shen Wan is added.

8. Deficiency of heart qi and gallbladder qi

Main symptoms: insomnia and dreaminess, restless sleep, timidity and palpitation, susceptibility to fright in contacting matters, anxiety all the day, accompanied with shortness of breath and laziness to talk, easily frightening and fearing, spontaneous sweating out, fatigue and lack of strength, light tongue and white fur, fine, wiry and weak pulse.

Therapeutic method: tonify Qi and relieve convulsion, tranquilize mind and stabilize mind

Prescription: modified An Shen Ding Zhi Wan and Suan Zao Ren Tang. Spina Date Seed, Ginseng, Indian Bread, Liquorice Root, Indian bread with Pine, Milkwort Root, dragon teeth, Grassleaf Sweetflag Rhizome, Sichuan Lovage Rhizome, Common Anemarrhena Rhizome.

Prescription analysis: main function of Spirit-Tranquilizing and Mind-Stabilizing Pills is to relieve convulsion and tranquilize mind, and it is mainly used for symptoms of vexation and sleeplessness, shortness of breath and spontaneous sweating, lassitude and lack of strength; Spina Date Seed Decoction is used to nourish blood, clear heat and relieve vexation and used for symptoms of dysphoria and insomnia, anxiety all the day, susceptibility to fright in contacting matters. Ginseng, Indian Bread and Liquorice Root can tonify heart and gallbladder qi; Indian bread with Pine, Milkwort Root, Dragon Teeth and Grassleaf Sweetflag Rhizome can resolve phlegm,calm heart, relieve convulsion and tranquilize mind; Sichuan Lovage Rhizome can regulate blood and nourish heart; Common Anemarrhena Rhizome can clear heart and relieve vexation.

Modification: for patients concurrently with palpitation and sweating out, the syndrome is heart-liver blood deficiency. Ginseng is used more, Debark Peony Root, Chinese Angelica and Milkvetch Root are added to nourish liver blood; for patients concurrently with the syndrome of over-restricting of liver-wood to spleen-earth, showing the symptoms of chest tightness, preference for sighing, anorexia and abdominal distension, Chinese Thorowax Root, Dried Tangerine Peel, Common Yam Rhizome, White Atractylodes Rhizome are added to soothe liver and invigorate spleen; for patients concurrently with palpitation, fright and unrestlessness, Bone Fossil of Big Mammals, Unprocessed Oyster Shell and Cinnabar are added to settle and tranquilize mind.

ii. Single ingredient prescription and proved prescription

(1) 10g of Tuber Fleeceflower Stem and Unprocessed Rehmannia Root respectively and 6g of Dwarf Lilyturf Tuber are decocted in water and taken 1 time before noon break and sleep at night respectively. This is used for

insomnia caused by yin deficiency with effulgent fire.

(2) 2g of Lotus Plumule and 3g of Raw Liquorice Root. They are brewed with boiled water, and taken as tea for several times every day. This is used for dysphoria and insomnia caused by internal blazing of heart fire.

iii. Chinese patent medicine

1. Liver fire harassing heart

Chinese patent medicine: Long Dan Xie Gan Pill. 3-5g is taken every time and 2-3 times a day.

Prescription analysis: in this prescription, Rough Gentian, Baical Skullcap Root and Cape Jasmine Fruit can clear liver and purge fire; Oriental Waterplantain Rhizome, Akebia Stem and Plantain Seed can promote urination and clear heat; Chinese Thorowax Root can soothe liver and relieve depression; Chinese Angelica and Unprocessed Rehmannia Root can nourish blood, tonify yin and emolliate liver; Liquorice Root can regulate stomach.

In the case of effulgent fire in liver and gallbladder, vexation and restlessness, dizziness, tinnitus and deafness and hypochondriac pain, Liver-Draining and Mind-Tranquilizing Pills can be added. In the case of splitting headache, mad insomnia, abdominal distension pain and constipation, Angelica, Gentian and Aloe Pill can be used to purge fire and remove stagnation. For patients with emotional stress, dysphoria and irritability, modified Xiaoyao Pills can be used to soothe liver and relieve depression and also can improve sleep.

2. Phlegm-heat disturbing heart

Chinese patent medicine: Meng Shi Gun Tan Wan. 6-12g is taken every time and 1 time a day.

Prescription analysis: in this prescription, Chlorite Schist can be used to treat excess heat and dense phlegm; Rhubarb steamed with wine can eliminate phlegm and remove stagnation; Baical Skullcap Root is used to clear heat; Chinese Eaglewood Wood can relieve stagnation. Combination of four herbs is used as effective prescription of treating heat-phlegm.

In the case of phlegm-heat above clouding heart spirit, fright and unrest, Heart-Clearing and Phlegm-Rolling Pills can be added to relieve convulsion and stabilize mind, dispel phlegm and tranquilize mind; in the case of food accumulation at night,belching with fetid odour and acid regurgitation, abdominal distension pain, Immature Orange Fruit Stagnation-Removing Pills can be added to digest and evacuate, regulate stomach and stabilize mind. In the case of phlegm-heat clouding seven orifices, dizziness and heavy head as well as pernoctation, Bovine Bezoar Heart-Clearing Pills can be used to purge fire and eliminate phlegm, open orifices and tranquilize mind.

3. Intense heart fire

Chinese patent medicine: Zhu Sha An Shen Wan. 6g is taken every time and twice a day.

Prescription analysis: in this prescription, Golden Thread is used to purge fire with bitter cold, clear heart and eliminates vexation; Cinnabar can settle and tranquilize mind, and compatibility of two herbs can play the role of clearing heart fire, and have the efficacy of settling and tranquilizing mind; Chinese Angelica and Unprocessed Rehmannia Root can nourish yin and blood; Liquorice Root can coordinate the drug actions of the prescription.

In the case of heart fire hyperactivity and dysphoria and unrest, Bovine Bezoar Upper-Body-Clearing Pills can be added to clear heat and relieve dysphoria, relieve convulsion and tranquilize mind; in the case of palpitation and fidget, Spirit-Tranquillizing Mind-Stabilizing Pill can be added to tranquilize heart and mind. If exuberance of heart fire consumes heart and blood, not only being insomnia, amnesia, palpitation, flusteredness, but hand, foot and heart heat, mouth parched and tongue scorched and mouth and tongue sore, Celestial Emperor Heart-Tonifying Pills can be used to clear heat, nourish yin, settle and tranquilize mind.

4. Failure of descending of the stomach-qi

Chinese patent medicine: Bao He Wan. 6g is taken every time and twice every day.

Prescription analysis: in this prescription, Hawthorn Fruit can disperse greasy and thick taste stagnation; Medicated Leaven can disperse accumulation of wine and food; Radish Seed can disperse stagnation of cooked wheaten food and phlegm-turbidity; Dried Tangerine Peel, Pinellia Tuber and Indian Bread can invigorate spleen and dry dampness, relieve the chest and regulate Qi, harmonize stomach and descend adverse Qi; Weeping Forsythia Capsule can clear heat and dissipate mass; all the herbs have the efficacy of promoting digestion, harmonizing stomach, regulating Qi and descending adverse Qi.

In the case of abdominal fullness and distention and loss of appetite, Tongren Liver-Soothing Stomach-Regulating Pill can be used be to soothe liver and relieve depression, harmonize stomach and relieve pain; in the case of Qi-depression stagnation, distention in both rib-sides,belching with fetid odour and acid regurgitation, hiccup and vomiting, epigastric pain and stool disharmony, Depression Resolving Harmony-Preserving Pills can be used to soothe liver and resolve depression, stimulate appetite and promote digestion.

5. Blood vessel stasis and obstruction

Chinese patent medicine: Xue Fu Zhu Yu Capsules. 2.4g is taken every time and twice a day.

Prescription analysis: in this prescription, Peach Seed and Safflower can activate blood and resolve stasis; Chinese Angelica, Sichuan Lovage Rhizome and Red Peony Root can enhance the efficacy of activating blood and dispelling stasis; Radix Achyranthis Bidentatae can dispel stasis blood and dredge blood vessel, leading stasis blood descending; Chinese Thorowax Root can soothe liver and relieve depression, ascend and clear yang; Platycodon Root and Orange Fruit, one ascending and one descending, can relieve stagnation in the chest to promote Qi circulation and therefore promote blood circulation; Unprocessed Rehmannia Root can cool blood and clear heat, combining with Chinese Angelica, which can nourish yin and moisten dryness to make stasis blood dispelled without damage to yin; Liquorice Root can detoxify and coordinate the drug actions of a prescription. Combination of all drugs not only can be used to move blood and dispel stasis and stagnation, but relieve Qi and disperse depression, activate blood without blood loss, dispel stasis and produce the new, therefore, blood stasis is removed to tranquilize heart spirit.

In the case of insomnia and dreaminess, dysphoria, amnesia and hypomnesia, Spirit-Tranquilizing and Mind-Stabilizing Pills is used to activate blood and disperse stasis, calm heart and tranquilize mind.

6. Deficiency of both heart and spleen

Chinese patent medicine: Ren Sheng Gui Pi Wan. 1 pill is taken every time and twice a day.

Prescription analysis: in this prescription, Ginseng can powerfully tonify primordial Qi, restore pulse and relieve Qi desertion, tonify spleen and replenish lungs, promote fluid and tranquilize mind; White Atractylodes Rhizome can tonify spleen, replenish stomach, dry dampness and harmonize the middle jiao; Indian Bread can drain damp and excrete water, invigorate spleen and harmonize stomach, calm heart and tranquilize mind; Radix Astragali Preparata can replenish Qi and tonify middle jiao; Chinese Angelica and Longan Aril can tonify heart spleen, nourish blood and tranquillize spirit; Spina Date Seed can nourish liver, calm heart and tranquillize spirit; Milkwort Root can tranquillize spirit and promote intelligence; Common Aucklandia Root can regulate Qi and harmonize the middle jiao; Radix Glycyrrhizae Preparata can tonify Qi and nourish yin, activate yang and restore the pulse.

In the case of severe palpitation, amnesia and insomnia, dreaminess and easily fright, Spirit-Tranquilizing and Mind-Stabilizing pills can be used to nourish heart and tonify yin, tranquilize spirit and stabilize mind; in the case of withered yellow facial complexion, reduced appetite and body fatigue, Blood-Nourishing and Mind-Tranquilizing Pills can be used.

7. Non-interaction between heart and kidney

Chinese patent medicine: Liu Wei Di Huang Wan and Jiao Tai Wan. 1 pill is taken respectively every time and twice a day.

Prescription analysis: in this prescription, Prepared Rehmannia Root, Pulp of Dogwood Fruit and

Common Yam Rhizome are used together to achieve the effect of nourishing kidneys, liver and spleen; Oriental Waterplantain Rhizome can excrete damp and descend the turbid to reduce nourishing greasy of Prepared Rehmannia Root; Indian Bread can eliminate dampness of spleen with bland medicine to assist transportation of Common Yam Rhizome; Tree Peony Root Bark can clear deficiency heat to restrict warm astringency of Pulp of Dogwood Fruit; Cinnamon Bark can return fire to its origin, commonly used with Golden Thread to restore coordination between heart and kidney, regulate between water and fire and tranquilize heart and mind.

In the case of dysphoria and palpitation, nocturnal emission and seminal emission, Mind-Tranquilizing and Heart- Tonifying Capsules can be added to nourish yin, tonify heart and tranquilize mind; for patients with insomnia, amnesia and dizziness, Spina Date Seed Mind-Tranquilizing Solution can be used to nourish heart, tranquillize mind and promote intelligence.

8. Deficiency of heart qi and gallbladder qi

Chinese patent medicine: An Shen Ding Zhi Wan. 1 pill is taken every time and twice a day.

Prescription analysis: in this prescription, Ginseng is used for tonifying and replenishing heart and gallbladder qi; Indian Bread, Indian bread with Pine and Milkwort Root can calm the heart and tranquilize mind; Dragon Teeth and Grassleaf Sweetflag Rhizome can relieve convulsion, open orifices and tranquilize mind.

In the case of insomnia and amnesia, easily surprising and fearing, Tongren Baizi Yangxin Pills is added to nourish heart and tonify Qi; in the case of weak body of the old, insomnia and dreaminess, palpitation and lacking in strength, dry mouth and less fluid, Spirit-Tranquillizing and Brain-Strengthening Liquid can tonify Qi and nourish spirit, tranquilize mind and generate fluid.

iv. Acupuncture and moxibustion therapy

1. Liver fire disturbing heart

Main points: Anmian, LR 2, G B 44, GB 20 and HT7.

Adjunct acupuncture points: If hypochondriac pain is severe, LR 14 shall be an additional acupuncture point.

Prescription analysis: Anmian is an experience point for treating insomnia and has good effects on all kinds of insomnias. LR 2, spring point of liver meridian, has function of calming liver to reduce pathogenic fire. GB 44, a well point of gallbladder meridian, has effect of reduction gallbladder fire to relieve restlessness. GB 20 can be used to soothe and regulate liver and gallbladder. HT7 can calm heart and tranquilize mind, and if the mind is tranquilized, patient can fall asleep. LR 14 is sanative to soothe liver, reduce pathogenic fire and tranquilize mind.

Acupuncture technique: filiform needling and application of reducing method.

2. Phlegm-heat disturbing heart

Main points: Anmian, ST40, ST44, SP 4 and HT7.

Adjunct acupuncture points: If patient feels more dizzy, GV 20 and EX-HN 3 shall be additional acupuncture points.

Prescription analysis: Anmian is an experience point for treating insomnia. ST40 has function of clearing and transporting turbid phlegm. If combined with ST44, they can purge heat in spleen and stomach. SP 4 is sanative to invigorate spleen to transmit dampness. HT7, source point of heart, has effect of calming heart and tranquilizing mind. GV 20 and EX-HN 3 can be used for clearing heat and opening orifices.

Acupuncture technique: filiform needling and application of reducing method.

3. Intense heart fire

Main points: Anmian, HT7, HT 8, and PC 8.

Adjunct acupuncture points: If the boil of lips and tongue is severe, HT9 and SI 1 shall be additional acupuncture points.

Prescription analysis: Anmian is an experience point for treating insomnia. HT7, source point of heart meridian, has effect of tranquilizing and allaying excitement. HT 8, and PC 8 have effects of clearing and purging heart fire through reducing method. Bloodletting of HT9, well point of heart meridian, and SI 1, well point of small intestine meridian can clear and purge heart fire to avoid up-flaming with swift pricking blood therapy.

Acupuncture technique: filiform needling, application of reducing method and swift pricking blood therapy in HT9 and SI 1.

4. Failure of descending of stomach-qi

Main points: Anmian, CV 12, ST 36 and HT7.

Adjunct acupuncture points: If rib-side distention and stomachache are severe, LR 3 shall be an additional acupuncture point. If patients' symptoms also include abdominal fullness and distention, belching with fetid odor and acid regurgitation, as well as nausea and vomiting, PC 6 and SP 4 shall be added. In the case of ungratifying defecation, ST 25 shall be added.

Prescription analysis: Anmian is an experience point for treating insomnia. CV 12 and ST 36 have effects of invigorating spleen and harmonizing stomach as well as descending Qi and regulating middle jiao. HT7, source point of heart, has effect of tranquilizing and allaying excitement. LR 3 can play a role in soothing liver and regulating Qi. PC 6 and SP 4 have effects of harmonizing stomach and descending adverse Qi. ST 25 can recuperate stomach and intestines and promote digestion to relieve constipation.

Acupuncture technique: filiform needle pricking and application of reducing method or both reinforcement and reduction.

5. Blood vessel stasis and obstruction

Main points: Anmian, BL 17, SP 10, GV 20, GV 24 and HT7.

Adjunct acupuncture points: If patients' symptoms include amnesia and hypomnesia, EX-HN 1 shall be an additional acupuncture point. If patients feel dizzy and have a headache, GV 23 shall be an additional acupuncture point.

Prescription analysis: Anmian is an experience point for treating insomnia. BL 17 and SP 10 have effects of blood-activating, dredging collaterals and stasis-dispelling. GV 20 has the effect of dredging brain collateral. GV 24 and HT7 are effective to tranquilize and allay excitement. EX-HN 1 is used for nourishing brain and improving intelligence. GV 23 can play a role in dredging collaterals and relieving pain.

Acupuncture technique: filiform needle pricking and application of reducing method or both reinforcement and reduction.

6. Deficiency of both heart and spleen

Main points: Anmian, BL 15, HT7, ST 36, SP 6 and BL 20.

Adjunct acupuncture points: If patients' symptoms include epigastric tightness and anorexia, CV 12 shall be an additional acupuncture point.

Prescription analysis: Anmian is an experience point for treating insomnia. BL 15 and HT7, point combination of back transport point and source point, have effects of tonifying and replenishing Qi and blood of heart as well as nourishing heart and tranquilizing mind. ST 36 and SP 6 are important acupuncture points for invigorating spleen, replenishing Qi and nourishing blood. If combined with BL 20, they can support the acquired foundation to furnish the origin of producing Qi and Blood. CV 12 has the effect of invigorating spleen and harmonizing stomach.

Acupuncture technique: filiform needle pricking and reducing method, sometimes adding moxibustion.

7. Non-interaction between heart and kidney

Main points: Anmian, KI 3, HT7, BL 15, PC7, KI 6 and BL 62.

Adjunct acupuncture points: If patients' symptoms include waist soreness and asthenia, BL 23 shall be an additional acupuncture point.

Prescription analysis: Anmian is an experience point for treating insomnia. KI 3, source point of kidney meridian, is good at nourishing kidney yin and in the case of excessive water, the heart fire is not intense. When HT7, source point of meridian PC7, source point of pericardium meridian, and BL 15, back-shu point of heart, are used jointly, they are effective to descend heart fire as well as calm heart and tranquilize mind. BL 23 has the effect of strengthening waist and pine. KI 6 and BL 62, confluence points of eight extraordinary meridians, connect to yin heel vessel and yang heel vessel separately and are mainly in charge of sleeping. If function of yang heel vessel is exuberant, insomnia will appear. Therefore yin heel vessel and yang heel vessel will function coordinately through tonifying yin and reducing yang, then insomnia will be self-cured.

Acupuncture technique: KI 3, BL 15, BL 23 and KI 6 adopt reinforcing method; BL 62 applies reducing method; other points apply even reinforcing-reducing method.

8. Deficiency of heart-qi and gallbladder-qi

Main points: Anmian, BL 15, HT7, PC7, BL 19, GB 40, KI 6 and BL 62.

Adjunct acupuncture points: If patients eat less food and are weak, ST 36 shall be an additional acupuncture point.

Prescription analysis: Anmian is an experience point for treating insomnia. BL 15, PC7 and HT7 can warm and nourish heart qi to avoid distraction and keep spirit in interior. L 19 and GB 40 have effect of tonifying and replenishing gallbladder qi to avoid deficiency of fu-viscera with clear juice, thus palpitation due to fright fails to grow. ST 36 is applicable to transportation of spleen and stomach to accumulate spleen and stomach being origin of producing Qi and Blood. KI 6 and BL 62, confluence points of eight extraordinary meridians, connect to yin heel vessel and yang heel vessel separately and are mainly in charge of sleeping. If function of yang heel vessel is exuberant, insomnia will appear. Therefore, yin heel vessel and yang heel vessel will function coordinately through tonifying yin and reducing yang and insomnia will be self-cured.

Acupuncture technique: filiform needle pricking; reducing method for BL 62 and reinforcing method for other points.

v. Massage therapy

1. Head massage

① The physician applies grasping manipulation with hands about 10 times on both sides of patient's head. ② Patient's EX-HN 3 is manipulated for 1 minute, pushed forward straightly from EX-HN 3 to GV 24 for 5~10 times with two thumbs alternately, and kneaded from point to point from GV 24 to GV 20 along center of the head (governor vessel); then GV 20 is vibrated with finger for 1 minute. ③ The physician pushes with his thumbs of both hands from forehead and geisoma to EX-HN 5 for 3~5 times and vibrates EX-HN 5 with finger for 1 minute. ④ The patient's head is hit laterally; the temples and top of head are vibrated with palms for about 2 minutes. The above operations shall be to the extent as patients have deep penetration feeling as well as relaxed and comfortable feelings. The patients shall be treated once a day, and 15 consecutive days is one course of treatment.

2. Abdominal massage

① Abdomen is massaged for about 6 minutes, and the operation is manipulated anticlockwise and moves clockwise. ② CV 12, CV 8, CV 6 and CV 4 are knead or imposed one-finger-pushing manipulation method separately for 1 minute, and then are vibrated by fingers. Manipulation shall be soft. ③ Both palms are joint from blow rib to pubis, and then push horizontally from middle to both sides for 3~5 times. ④ Abdomen is vibrated by palms for about 1 minute. The patients shall be treated once a day, and 15 consecutive days is one course of treatment.

3. Back massage

① Both GB 21 are lifted and grasped for about 1 minute. It is advisable to make patients feel relaxed and comfortable. ② Governor vessel of back and Taiyang meridian on both sides shall be pushed straightly for about 10 times; the manipulation shall be deep and power and the speed shall be even and gentle. ③ Taiyang meridian of back is manipulated, and BL 15, BL 20, BL 21 and BL 23 shall be manipulated as key points. The strength shall not be stronger than partially sore and heavy. ④ Taiyang meridian on both sides of back shall be tapped alternately with palms. The patients shall be treated once a day, and 15 consecutive days is one course of treatment.

vi. Others

1. Ear acupuncture

Selection of points: AT (4), AH (6a), HT7, CO (15), CO (12), CO (13), CO (10), LO (4) and P (1).

Methods: The patient shall be treated once a day and each time 3~4 acupuncture points are selected and acupunctured with filiform needling. The needles are retained for 30 minutes. Or thumb-tack needle for subcutaneous embedding for twice a week or stick and press Cowherb Seeds for 2~3 times a week.

2. Cutaneous acupuncture

Selection of points: GV from neck to waist and the first lateral line of Taiyang Bladder Meridian of Foot.

Method: The selected acupuncture points are acupunctured with cutaneous needle from top to bottom till derma flushes. Once a week.

3. Cupping method

Selection of points: GV from neck to waist, the first and second lateral lines of back of Taiyang Bladder Meridian of Foot.

Method: The selected acupuncture points shall be slid cupping 1~twice a week from the top to bottom along back till derma flushes or subcutaneous part turns bruising.

4. Electric needle

Selection of points: EX-HN 1 and EX-H N 5.

Method: The selected acupuncture points shall be stimulated in lower frequency and each simulation lasts 30 minutes.

V. Empirical prescriptions of famous physicians and experts

1. Empirical prescription (Li Peisheng)

Components: 50g Chinese Magnoliavine Fruit, 50g Indian bread with Pine, 15g Silktree Albizia Flower and 15g Rhizoma Pinelliae Preparatum.

Application: decocted in water for an oral dose, one dose a day.

Efficacy: to nourish yin and warm yang as well as invigorate spleen and tranquilize mind.

2. Qian Yang Ning Shen Tang (Zhang Qi)

Components: 30g Honeysuckle Stem, 20g Cooked Date Seed, 15g Milkwort Root, 20g Chinese Arborvitae Kernel, 15g Poria, 20g Unprocessed Rehmannia Root, 20g Figwort Root, 25g Raw Oyster Shell, 30g Raw Sienna (grinded), 10g Sichuan Coptis Root and 20g Raw Bone Fossil of Big Mammals.

Application: decocted in water for an oral dose, one dose a day.

Efficacy: to nourish yin and subdue yang, clear heat and calm mind, nourish brain and tranquilize mind.

3. Gou Qi Zao Ren Tang (Peng Jingshan)

Components: 30g Barbary Wolfberry, 40g Cooked Date Seed and 10g Chinese Magnoliavine Fruit.

Application: They shall be put in the teacup and immersed with boiling water, one dose a day. The decoction shall be drunk frequently as tea or drunk 3 times a day and 50 ml for each time.

Efficacy: to nourish liver and kidney as well as nourish blood and tranquilize mind.

VI. Typical cases of famous physicians and experts

i. Medical record of Li Guilan——liver depression transforming into fire and fire harassing heart spirit

Ms Li, female, 61 years old.

Preliminary diagnosis: on October 5, 2009. Two years ago, the patient could not sleep soundly at night due to hard work together with gloomy mood. Her symptoms were sleep difficulties, dreaminess and restless sleep, with palpitation and fatigue sometimes. One month ago, the patient felt her insomnia became severe, and she only slept for two or three hours a day and suffered from dysphoria, a lack of strength and poor appetite. For fear of side effects of western medicine, she came here and resorted to TCM Therapy. Present symptoms: the patient was in her right mind, but in poor mental health and vexation. Her left side of head swelled with bad feelings and right rib-side distends and constrains. She couldn't sleep soundly at night and suffered from poor appetite, nausea as well as normal urination and defecation.

Syndrome differentiation: liver depression transforming into fire and fire harassing heart spirit.

Therapeutic method: to soothe liver and relieve depression as well as regulate nerves and tranquilize mind.

Prescription: 12g Chinese Thorowax Root, 12g Pinellia Tuber, 15g Skullcap, 30g Common Selfheal Fruit-Spike, 30g Spina Date Seed, 15g Silktree Albizia Bark, 15g Nacre, 15g Honeysuckle Stem, 3 slices of Fresh Ginger, 5 Chinese Dates and 10g Licorice. The prescription shall be decocted in water for oral dose and one dose a day.

Prescription of acupuncture and moxibustion: the main points take GV 20, EX-HN 1, GV 24, HT7, GB 20, LR 3, SP 6 and Anmian. Adjunct acupuncture points are LR 2 and PC 6. Manipulation: even reinforcing-reducing method is adopted to manipulate on GV 20, EX-HN 1, GV 24 and PC 6. Twisting and reinforcing method is used to manipulate on SP 6 and Anmian. Twisting and reducing method is chosen to operate on GB 20, LR 3 and LR 2. For each manipulation, retaining needle shall last 30 min. This prescription shall be used every other day.

Second diagnosis: on November 13, 2009. All symptoms of the patient were improved after a month's treatment. the patient came to a subsequent visit. She was then in her right mind, didn't complain any vexation, head swelling and right rib-side distending and her appetite increased. She could fall asleep faster and her sleeping time was prolonged. Her urination and defecation became normal, tongue body was red, and tongue fur was thin and white; her pulse was stringy. In order to further consolidate curative effect she continued to be treated with acupuncture and moxibustion and Chinese medicine for a week. After a week, all of her symptoms disappeared and never recurred.

Note: the brain is the extraordinary fu-viscera, and governs thoughts, emotions and decisions. All activities of spirit, consciousness, thoughts, emotions, memory and the like are dominated by brain. As recorded in *Biond Magnolia Flower Bar* of *Compendium of Materia Medica* "Brain is fu-viscera of mental activity". As it was said in *Insomnia* of *Jing-yue Complete Works* "Sleep probably lies in yin at root, and spirit plays a major role. If spirit is tranquilized, patient can fall asleep. Otherwise, patient can't fall asleep". Therefore, brain dysfunction can cause insomnia.

Professor Li thinks that lack of nourishment in the brain, liver failing to act freely, Qi-depression transforming into fire can disturb the upward heart spirit and then result in insomnia. During treatment, methods of needling and medicine shall be combined and its basic principle of treatment shall be aligning nerves and tranquilizing mind and soothing liver and relieving depression. EX-HN 1, GV 20, GV 24, GB 20, LR 3, PC 6, SP 6 and Anmian are selected to be used in needle insertion treatment. The operation shall be manipulated strictly in accordance with the manipulation quantification standard to insert needle on each point. GV 20 and EX-HN 1 are selected partially on brain and mainly used to negotiate up and below so as to regulate blood in the whole body and comfort Qi movement of brain. PC 6, confluence point of eight extraordinary meridians, the collateral point of pericardium meridian, connects directly with yin link vessel, contact ssanjiao meridian and can calm heart and tranquilize spirit, help astringent of yang ascending and make heart focused. If GV 24, governor vessel point, is manipulated with needle, it can produce the effect of soothing brain and tranquilizing spirit. SP 6, confluence point of three meridians of liver, spleen and kidney, can nourish liver and kidney, tonify yin-blood, harmonize stomach and descend turbid matters, and return fire to its origin so as to promote balance of Qi and Blood as well as yin and yang. GB 20 is a gallbladder meridian point and also is the confluence point of yang meridian, yang link and yang heel vessel. Heart is connected with gallbladder divergent channel and each yang meridian is held together by yang link vessel. So they have the effect of calming heart and tranquilizing spirit. LR 3, source point of liver meridian, can purge liver fire, calm liver yang and soothe liver and resolve depression. Anmian, extra point, has efficacy of tranquilizing spirit; when it is manipulated with needle, intracranial and extracranial vessel and neural mechanisms can be regulated. Coordinated with Chinese medicine decoction, the therapy can stabilize mind and tranquillize spirit as well as clear heart and remove worries.

ii. Medical record of Li Guilan——liver-stomach disharmony

Mr. Yang, male, 46 years old.

Preliminary diagnosis: on February 28, 2010. Because of the long-time hardworking, the patient had difficulty in falling asleep and after sleep he woke up easily and could hardly fall asleep again; as a result he only slept three or four hours a day. One month ago, due to high pressure from work and strain in brain, his insomnia recurred and he started to take sleeping pills which were effective at first but became less effective later. He dreamed a lot, felt vexation and slept for only 2~3 h a day. Moreover, his stomach and intestines became uncomfortable. For fear of drug fastness and side effects of western medicine, he came here and resorted to TCM Therapy. Present symptoms: the patient was in his right mind, but in poor mental health. He slept restlessly at night, had difficulty in falling asleep, and felt dizzy, moody and uneasy in chest; moreover, he also suffered from belching and acid regurgitation, dry throat and dry mouth, poor appetite as well as normal urination and defecation.

Syndrome differentiation: liver qi depression, upward adverse flow of stomach-qi and failure of descending of the stomach-qi.

Therapeutic method: to tranquilize spirit and resolve depression as well as invigorate spleen and harmonize stomach.

Prescription: 15g of Chinese Thorowax Root, 20g of Debark Peony Root, 20g of Chinese Angelica, 20g of Indian Bread, 20g of Raw Cape Jasmine Fruit, 15g of Turmeric Root Tuber, 20g of Szechwan Chinaberry Fruit, 30g of Salvia Root, 15g of Sichuan Lovage Rhizome, 40g of Spina Date Seed, 20g of Silktree Albizia flower, 20g of Grassleaf Sweetflag Rhizome, 20g of Tuber Fleeceflower Stem, 20g of White Atractylodes Rhizome, 12g of Villons Amomum Fruit, 20g of Coastal Glehnia Root, 15g of Radish Seed, 30g of Medicated Leaven, 15g of Chinese Magnoliavine Fruit and 10g of Liquorice Root. The prescription shall be decocted in water for oral dose and one dose a day.

Prescription of acupuncture and moxibustion: the main points take GV 20, EX-HN 1, GV 24, HT7, GB 20, LR 3, SP 6 and Anmian. Adjunct acupuncture points are LR 2, PC 6, ST 36 and CV 12. Manipulation: even reinforcing-reducing is applied on GV 20, EX-HN 1, GV 24, HT7 and PC 6. Twisting and reinforcing method is used to manipulate on SP 6, ST 36, CV 12 and Anmian. Twisting and reducing method is chosen to act on GB 20, LR 3 and LR 2. For each manipulation, retaining needle shall last 30 min. The prescription shall be used every other day.

Second diagnosis: on March 6, 2010. The patient said his sleeping situation was improved, but he still had difficulty in falling asleep and felt vexation sometimes. He still suffered from poor appetite, acid regurgitation but without nausea and mouth dry and his urination and defecation was normal, tongue body is red, tongue fur is thin and yellow, and pulse is small and wiry. The prescription of acupuncture and moxibustion is the one mentioned above during treatment, while the prescription of Chinese medicine shall add 15g of Milkwort Root on the basis of the above prescription.

Third Diagnosis: on April 2, 2010. When the patient came to visit again, his sleep had returned to normal, without uncomfortable symptoms. He had reached the criterion of cure.

Note: *Volume I* of *Experiential Prescriptions for Universal Relief* says "For healthy people, the spleen is pathogen resistant, so when they sleep, soul is in liver. If spirit is calm, one can fall asleep. Now pathogens attack liver, soul has no place to go, so during sleeping, soul floats as it isolates from its abode". Professor Li thinks that the liver governs free flow of Qi and can comfort Qi movement of brain, and lead normal catharsis. So ascending, descending, exiting and entering of Qi are in order; blood circulation becomes normal, and Qi and blood are harmonized, making people energetic, peaceful in mind and spirit. If brain and spirit are lack of nourishment and cannot govern liver, the liver will fail to act freely, liver Qi will be in long stagnation and easily transform into fire, just as Zhu Danxi said "excessive Qi can cause fire". Temper disturbs the heart, so the patients are absent-minded, leading to insomnia. At the same time, excessive working and thinking can damage spleen and stomach. If spleen is damaged, people eat less and have poor appetite. Moreover, earth loss and wood sparse, Qi stasis, failure of descending of the stomach-qi and liver-stomach disharmony can cause belching, acid regurgitation and poor appetite. *Inner Canon of Huangdi* says "If the stomach is disharmonious, one fails to sleep soundly", so it also can lead to insomnia. Appearances of depression of liver transforming into fire and consumption of yin are shown as red tongue body, dry throat and dry mouth, thin and yellow tongue fur as well as small and wiry pulse. During treatment, methods of needling and medicine shall be combined and the basic treatment principles are aligning nerves and tranquilizing mind, soothing liver and relieving depression, invigorating spleen and harmonizing stomach.

VII. Prevention and aftercare

(1) Pay attention to mental adjustment, and avoid adverse mental stimulation. *Inner Canon of Huangdi* records: "if one person can keep calm and serene, and he is indifferent to fame or gain, then genuine Qi in body will be engouh all the time, how will he be sick?". Therefore, one shall adjust psychology and emotions actively, have moderate joy and anger and keep a cheerful mind.

(2) The daily life shall be regular; avoid being too easy or too tired; develop good sleep habits.

(3) Create a good sleep environment. The bed should be comfortable; the light in the bedroom should be soft. What's more, try to reduce noise and remove all kinds of external factors that may affect sleep.

(4) Do not be too hungry or too full at dinner. Light and digestive food is suggested.

(5) Avoid drinking tea, Coca-Cola, coffee and other excessive exciting and stimulating drinks before sleep.

(6) In order to improve the sleep quality, it is advisable to take foot bath for 20 min in warm water, or to drink a cup of hot milk before sleep.

(7) For the patients whose insomnia is caused by other diseases, their primary affections shall be treated at the same time.

(8) The acupuncture and moxibustion therapy can yield better results in the afternoon or evening.

(9) Avoid long-term use of sedative hypnotic drugs which have side effects like dependency and addiction.

(10) Engage in appropriate physical activity or exercise. Strike a proper balance between work and rest. Strengthen the physique gradually.

(LI Guilan)

References

[1] Shi XM. "The 11th five-year plan" national planning textbook of Acupuncture and Moxibustion [M]. Beijing: China Press of Traditional Chinese Medicine, 2010.

[2] Wang H. "12th five-year" national planning textbook on acupuncture and moxibustion [M]. Beijing: Higher Education Press, 2013.

[3] Gao SZ. "12th five-year" national planning textbook on acupuncture and moxibustion therapy [M]. Beijing: China Press of Traditional Chinese Medicine, 2014.

[4] Wu MH. "12th five-year" national planning textbook on internal medicine of TCM [M]. Beijing: China Press of Traditional Chinese Medicine, 2014.

[5] Wang NN. Two cases of Professor Li Guilan treating insomnia syndrome with acupuncture and medicines for invigorating brain and regulating liver [J]. Modern Chinese Medicine, 2012, 32 (4): 1-2.

慢性萎缩性胃炎 Chronic
Atrophic
Gastritis

I. Overview

Chronic atrophic gastritis (CAG) is a common disease of the digestive system with pathologic features such as atrophy of the gastric mucosa and its glands, mucosal thinning, or intestinal dysplasia and metaplasia. CAG is common, frequently-occurring disease and difficult to treat. In 1978, CAG was classified by the World Health Organization as a precancerous condition for gastric cancer. With the development of understanding of the disease, we have realized the relationship between the disease and gastric cancer. The typical pattern of evolution of the disease is as follows: chronic gastritis → chronic atrophic gastritis → intestinal metaplasia → atypical hyperplasia → gastric cancer. Hence, treating and reversing CAG ranks a very significant place in preventing gastrointestinal cancer. At present, there is a lack of effective methods in treating CAG in Western medicine, where treatment according to mere symptoms and periodic check-ups has become the main method for treating the disease. Several clinical reports show that traditional Chinese medicine can be very helpful in relieving symptoms, promoting repsir of the gastric mucosa and preventing intestinal metaplasia. Based on clinical symptoms, the name of CAG in traditional Chinese medicine can be classified into "stomach mass", "stuffiness and fullness" and "stuffiness syndrome of deficiency type".

II. Etiology and pathogenesis

i. Chinese Medicine

Traditional Chinese medicine (TCM) experts think that the etiologies of chronic atrophic gastritis are mainly related to improper diet, emotional disorders, overexertion, infection by exogenous toxins or pathogens, and weak constitution. The disease is located in the stomach and its onset relates mostly to the spleen, stomach, or liver (gallbladder) organs. The weakness of spleen and stomach, and disturbance in ascending and descending movements are the root causes of the disease, while toxic heat invasion and stagnated heat in the liver and stomach are the manifestations. This affects the inner organs after Qi and blood stasis for a long-term. Spleen qi and stomach yin defficiency are common patterns in weakness of the spleen and stomach, and qi stagnation and blood stasis usually remain throughout the whole course of the disease. The stomach is considered the origin of the five zang-organs and six fu-viscera and the origin of qi and blood production. Only when the middle energizer's qi is enough, can it produce Qi and blood, nourish the five zang-organs and six fu-viscera, including the spleen and stomach. If the function of spleen and stomach declines, there will be changes in the functions of receiving and transporting, and a lack of promoting generation and transformation, which will lead to an inhibited qi movement, heat resulting from stasis, internal accumulation of dampness-heat, stasis and stagnation of toxins. A blockade will consequently happen in the meridian of the stomach, Qi and blood movements will be blocked, and as a result atrophy of gastric mucosa will occur after it hasn't been fully nourished. Modern TCM doctors think that the pathogenesis of CAG takes weakness of spleen and stomach as the root cause, blood stasis obstructing the collaterals as manifestation, and qi deficiency and blood stasis as reciprocal causation. It features deficiency at the root and excess at the surface, a mix of deficiency and excess.

ii. Western medicine

According to Western medicine, the onset of CAG is related to many factors such as helicobacter pylori (HP) infection, bile reflux, changes in vascular active factors and cytokines, immune factors, and other factors, involving atrophy changes of the gastric mucosa. Common signs are mucosal lining thinning, reduced or absent mucosal glands, in some cases accompanied by intestinal epithelial cells to varying degrees of injury. Some researchers believe that when the coexistence of early atrophic gastritis and polyp occurs, there is increased risk of developing gastric cancer. Hence, populations should be informed and pay more attention to the timely treatment of atrophic gastritis.

III.Key points of diagnosis and differential diagnosis

i. Key points of diagnosis

1. Clinical manifestations

Discomfort of the upper abdomen, abdominal stuffiness and fullness, frequent pain, anorexia and loose stools, anorexia in the late stage, emaciation and lack of strength, anemia, pale tongue with white coating, and string-like pulse and thready pulse.

2. Relevant exams

Gastroscopy and pathological diagnosis are the main diagnostic methods of chronic atrophic gastritis.

(1) Gastroscopy diagnosis: Through gastroscopy, changes in the color of mucous membrane can be seen, showing white grey, grey or yellow grey colors, and the atrophy of mucous membrane may be bounded or diffuse with unclear boundaries. The mucous membrane becomes thinner, mucosal folds become flat or smaller. In the early stage of atrophy, minute vessels can be seen in mucous membrane, whereas in the late stage, great vessels can be seen under the mucous membrane. Following the atrophy of the glandular body, there will be hyperplasia, possibly accompanied by intestinal metaplasia, with tissue roughness, granularity or nodular changes in the appearance of the surface of mucous membrane.

(2) Pathology diagnosis: According to the Sydney System for the classification of gastritis, samples are taken to conduct routine biopsy, and patients who have the following pathogenic manifestations can be diagnosed: ① lymphoid follicle formation; ② atrophy of the mucosal glands, displaying a shrinking of volume of glandular epithelial cells, as well as a decrease in the amount of cells, hyperplasia of the inter-glandular fibrous tissue, interstitial lesions; ③ intrinsic membrane inflammation; ④ thickening of the mucosal muscle layer; ⑤ intestinal metaplasia or pseudopyloric metaplasia.

ii. Differential diagnosis

1. Gastric cancer

Symptoms of chronic gastritis, such as anorexia, epigastric discomfort, anemia and other symptoms of antral gastritis are similar to the symptoms of gastric cancer, so special attention should be paid to proper identification. Gastroscopy and biopsies are helpful for identification in most patients.

2. Peptic ulcer

Also manifests as chronic stomach pain in the upper abdominal region, but the symptoms of peptic ulcer are mainly regular and periodic pain in the upper abdomen. Pain in chronic stomach atrophic gatritis is rarely regular and mainly involves indigestion. Diferential diagnosis is based on x-ray barium fluoroscopy and gastroscopy.

3. Bile duct diseases

Chronic bile duct diseases such as chronic cholecystitis, cholelithiasis, are often accompanied by chronic distention in the right upper abdomen, belching and other poor digestion symptoms, so they can easily be misdiagnosed as chronic gastritis. However, there are no abnormalities in gastrointestinal examination, and it can be confirmed after a cholecystogram and type-B ultrasound scan.

4. Other diseases

Such as hepatitis, liver cancer and pancreatic diseases can also be delayed in diagnosis, mistaken as anorexia or poor digestion, thus comprehensive and detailed examinations can be helpful in preventing misdiagnosis

IV. TCM therapy

i. Syndrome differentiation and treatment

1. Liver qi invading the stomach

Main symptoms: distending pain in stomach, tapping up in chest and hypochondrium, belching and acid regurgitation, dry or bitter taste in mouth, anorexia, difficulty in defecation, red tongue texture, pale and thin or yellow and thin tongue coating, string-like pulse pulse or string-like pulse and rapid pulse. The signs are mostly related to emotional factors as well.

Therapeutic method: to disperse stagnated liver qi for regulating the stomach, to promote qi circulation and relieve flatulence.

Prescriptions: modified Chai Hu Shu Gan San. Sini san, modified Chaihu Liugan San; chaihu, zhiqiao, xiangfu, danggui, baishao, muxiang, foshou, pugongying, danshen, yanhusuo, chuanlianzi.

Modifications: patients who suffer from depression of qi, transforming into fire in the liver or stomach, or liver heat invading the stomach, with symptoms such as epigastric scorching pain, acid regurgitation, heartburn, bitter taste in mouth, gastric upset, vexation and irritability, may have modified Zuojin Pills and Jinlingzi San, or modified Danzhixiaoyao San. Patients who have obvious poor appetite can have Liu Shen Qu, shaogu (chao millet sprouts) and maya (maya); shao shanzha (Scorched shanzha) can be added. For patients who also have symptoms of nausea and vomiting, zhuru, banxia, chenpi can be added.

2. Spleen-stomach dampness-heat

Main symptoms: epigastric fullness, discomfort or scorching pain, noisy belching, bitter taste, without desire to drink, or abdominal distension and loose stools, red tongue, yellow or greasy coating, string-like pulse and rapid pulse or slippery pulse. Treatment: clearing away heat and dampness, invigorating spleen and stomach.

Therapeutic method: to clear heat and resolve dampness, to invigorate spleen and harmonize stomach.

Prescriptions: modified San Ren Tang. baidouren, xingren, yiyiren, houpo, banxia, tongcao, huashi, zhuye, huanglian, yinchen, danshen.

Modifications: patients who also have symptoms of superficial dampness, xiangru, huoxiang can be added for releasing the exterior and resolving dampness. Patients who have symptoms of nausea and vomiting, zhuru and shengjiang can be added for harmonizing the stomach and descending adverse qi. Patients who have obvious an-orexia signs, jineijin, shenqu, maiya can be added for promoting digestion and removing food stagnation. In order to treat this disease, Huang Lian Ping Wei San is also indicated.

3. Spleen-stomach weakness

Main symptoms: Epigastric dull pain pain, being improved by slight pressure, stuffiness and fullness in stomach, aggravated after meals, anorexia, borborygmi and loose stools, sometimes accompanied by tiredness and lack of strength, lack of energy and unwillingness to talk, sore and tired limbs, light red tongue texture, thin and pale or pale tongue coating or with teeth prints, deep and thready pulse.

Therapeutic method: to tonify qi and harmonize the middle, to invigorate the spleen and nourish the stomach.

Prescriptions: Xiang Sha Liu Jun Zi Tang or modified Shen Ling Bai Zhu San. Dangshen, chaobaizhu, yiyiren, fuling, muxiang, sharen, chenpi, banxia, maiya, danggui, baishao, guizhi, pugongying, danshen, huanqi.

Modifications: patients who have symptoms of stomach pain, loose stools, cold limbs, pale tongue coating, tight pulse and severe yang deficiency syndrome should be treated by warming and tonifying the spleen and stomach with Huang Qi Jian Zhong Tang and modified Liang Fu Wan. For patients who have symptoms of post-meal severe distention in the stomach and abdomen, jineijin, laifuzi, foshou cn be added. For patients with clear liquid vomit, chenpi, banxia, fuling should be used; if acid regurgitaion is present, Zuo Jin Wan may be added. For patients with severe spleen deficiency with loose stools, shanyao, lianzirou, shengbiandou can be added for invigorating the spleen and resolving dampness. For patients who have black stools, ganjiangtan, fulongdan, baiji, diyutan can be added. Patients with yang deficiency in the middle energizer may take Lizhong Tang, modified with wumei or baishao.

4. Stomach yin deficiency

Main symptoms: Epigastric dull pain or scorching pain, stomach upset similar to being hungry, thirsty, dry lips, dry stools, red and fissured tongue with little saliva, lack of or no tongue coating or scattered ,exfoliated coating, thready and rapid pulse.

Therapeutic method: to clear heat and promote fluids, to nourish yin and tonify the stomach.

Prescriptions: Sha Shen Mai Dong Tang or modified Yi Wei Tang. Shashen, maidong, shihu, tianhuafen, wumei, baishao, shanzha, gancao, dangshen, shanyao, fuling, pugongying, danshen.

Modifications: patients who also suffer from anadipsia, retching and gum bleeding, which are signs of stomach yin deficiency and internal scorching of deficiency fire can have modified Yu Nyu Jian. Patients who also suffer from pain in the chest, hypochondrium and stomach, dry mouth or bitter taste, string-like pulse and rapid pulse which are symptoms of yin deficiency of liver and stomach, blood dryness and Qi-depression can have a decoction of modified Yi Guan Jian. Patients who also have epigastric stuffiness and qi stagnation should have Qi-circulating herbs and formulas for moistening the middle burner, such as foshou, wumei, houpo, and zhiqiao. Patients who have severe dry stools can have the above prescriptions together with Zeng Ye Tang. For patients who have yin deficiency and excessive heat, sheng shigao zhimu can be added according to the disease condition, to strengthen the function of clearing heat and promoting fluid production. Patients with dampness may have yiyiren, baikouren, yinchen. yiyiren, baikouren and yinchen to clear heat and resolve dampness. Patients who also have blood stasis and qi stagnation may have danshen, danggui and taoren to activate blood and resolve stasis. A modified Yi Guan Jian decoction is also helpful.

5. Blood stasis in the stomach collateral

Main symptoms: chronic epigastric pain, or localized, piercing pain and disliking pressure, or sometimes accompanied by hematemesis, black stools, dark purple or dark red tongue texture or with ecchymosis, deep pulse.

Therapeutic method: activate blood and relieve stasis, dredge collaterals and relieve pain

Prescriptions: Tao Hong Si Wu Tang and modified Shi Xiao San. Taoren, honghua, danggui, chuanxiong, chishao, wulingzhi, sheng puhuang, yanhusuo, danshen, zexie, jiangxiang.

Modifications: For patients who have Qi deficiency, huangqi, dangshen, baizhu and huangjing can be added for tonifying Qi. And for patients with qi stagnation, zhiqiao, qingpi, muxiang and sharen can be added for moving Qi accordingly. For patients who also have hematemesis and black stools, if a patients' blood is bright red, along with red tongue texture and yellow tongue coating as well as string-like pulse, rapid pulse, Xie Xin Tang can be used for clearing heat, cooling blood and stopping bleeding; if a patient's blood is dark red, with withered-yellowish complexion, cool limbs or pale tongue as well as weak pulse, it is due to spleen failing to control blood and Huang Tu Tang can be used to warm the spleen, tonify qi and control blood. For patients who have polyps, danshen, danggui, honghua, sanleng, ezhu, jiuxiangchongcan be added.

6. Intermingled cold and heat

Main symptoms: epigastric pain, preferring warmth and liking pressure, nausea with desire to vomit, belching and acid regurgitation, being thirst and easy to feel hunger, constipation and red urine, pale engorged tongue texture, the color of tongue coating alternating between yellow and white, and string-like pulse, thready and rapid pulse.

Therapeutic method: using pungent herbs for dispersing and bitter herbs for descending, and harmonizing cold and heat.

Prescriptions: modified Ban Xia Xie Xin Tang. Zhibanxia, huangqin,huanglian, dangshen, ganjiang, fuling, foshou, gancao, baizhu.

Modifications: For patients with deficient gastric acidity, wumei and mugua can be added; for patients with anorexia, guya and jineijin can be added. For patients with intestinal metaplasia, cigoupi and paoshanjia should be added for softening hardness and dissipating masses, resolving polyps, and resolving blood stasis and qi stagnation. Or baihuasheshecao, tufuling are added. In the case that chronic atrophic gastritis is caused by a deregulated immune system, large dosages of blood-activating and stasis-resolving herbs should be used.

ii. Specific prescription treatment

1. Liver-stomach disharmony

(1) Shu Wei Tang

Components: 10g of chaihu, yujin, xiangfu, banxia, zhiqiao, sharen each, 15g of baishao, 30g of yimi, 5g of gancao.

Indications: Chronic atrophic gastritis belonging to syndrome of liver-stomach disharmony.

(2) Modified Si Ni San

Components: 10g of chaihu, baishao, sheng zhiqiao, foshou, maya, pugongying for each, 5g of gancao, 3g of huanglian and wuzhuyu for each.

Indications: Chronic atrophic gastritis which belongs to the syndrome of liver-spleen disharmony.

(3) Shu Gan Jian Pi Tang

Components: 10g of chaihu, zhiqiao, baishao, yujin, chenpi and baizhu for each, 15g of taizishen and fuling for each, 6g of gancao.

Indications: Chronic atrophic gastritis which belongs to the syndrome of liver depression and spleen deficiency.

2. Dampness-heat in the spleen and stomach

(1) Yi Qi Huo Xue Yang Wei Tang

Components: 15g of huangqin, dangshen, ezhu and wumei for each, 25g of danshen, pugongying and baihuasheshecao for each, 8g of ganjiang, Sanqi San (take infused) and huanglian for each, 10g of zhishi.

Indications: Chronic atrophic gastritis which belongs to syndrome of qi deficiency and heat stagnation.

(2) Jia Wei Huang Liang Wen Dan Tang

Components: 2g of huanglian, 6g of chenpi, 10g of banxia, 12g of fuling, 3g of gancao, 6g of zhishi and zhuru for each.

Indications: Chronic atrophic gastritis which belongs to phlegm-heat resistance and the disorder of the stomach qi.

(3) Jian Zhong Huo Xue Tang

Components: 30g of baihuasheshecao and danshen for each, 10g of chishao, baishao, huangqin and chaihu for each, 15g of taizishen and baizhu for each, 6g of gancao.

Indications: Chronic atrophic gastritis which belongs to stagnated heat of liver and stomach with blood stasis syndrome.

3. Deficiency of spleen and stomach or with blood stasis

(1) Zhi Wei Mixture

Components: 30g of huangqi, dangshen, long kui and baqi for each, 15g of baizhu, danggui, baishao, fuling, shihu and danshen for each, 9g of gancao, 10g of hongzao.

Indications: Chronic atrophic gastritis which belongs to the syndrome of spleen-stomach weakness.

(2) Wen Run Jian Zhong Tang

Components: 20g of huangqin and danshen, 15g of dangshen, xiancao and baihe each, 12g of ezhu and pugongying, 10g of yinyanghuo, chao baizhu and baishao for each, 5g of wuyao, 6g of zhigancao.

Indications: Chronic atrophic gastritis which belongs to syndrome of heat stagnation, qi deficiency and blood stasis.

(3) Jian Pi Kang Wei Tang

Components: 15g of dangshen, 30g of baizhu, huangqi and danshen for each, 10g of zhiqiao, xiangfu and ezhu, 12g of huanglian and lianqiao each, 6g of gancao.

Indications: Chronic atrophic gastritis which belongs to the syndrome of Qi deficiency and blood stasis.

4. Stomach yin deficiency

(1) Yang Yin Hu Wei Tang

Components: shashen, maidong, xuanshen, shihu, shijie, baishao, gancao, wumei, mugua.

Indications: Chronic atrophic gastritis which belongs to the syndrome of stomach yin deficiency.

(2) Zha Mei Yi Wei Tang

Components: 30g of shashen, 10g of maidong, 10g of shijie, 10g of sheng dihuang, 10g of mugua, 15g of shanzha, 15g of shanyao, 12g of shihu, 12g of wumei, 12g of baishao, 6g of gancao.

Indications: Chronic atrophic gastritis which belongs to the syndrome of spleen yin deficiency and dry-heat in stomach earth.

(3) Prescriptions by Dong Jianhua

Components: 10g of shashen, maidong, shihu, yuanshen, chuan lian zi and xiangfu for each, 12g of tianhuafen and sheng dihuang for each, 5g of wumei, gancao and yanhusuo for each.

Indications: Chronic atrophic gastritis which belongs to syndrome of stomach yin deficiency.

(4) Yin Xu Gan Yu Wei Wei Fang

Components: 12g of baishao, wumei, mugua and taizishen for each, 15g of pugongying and baihuasheshecao for each, 10g of foshou, lumeihua and yiyiren for each, 5g of gancao.

Indications: Chronic atrophic gastritis which belongs to syndrome of yin deficiency and liver depression.

5. Blood stasis in the stomach collaterals

(1) Yi Qi Huo Xue Tang

Components: 30g of huangqi, 20g of danshen and pugongying for each, 15g of dangshen, baizhu, danggui, wulingzhi and yanhusuo for each, 5g of gancao and Sanqi San for each.

Indications: Chronic atrophic gastritis which belongs to syndrome of Qi deficiency and blood stasis.

(2) Jian Pi Huo Xue Tang

Components: 30g of huangqi, 20g of baizhu, dangshen and baishao for each, 15g of danshen, 10g of yanhusuo, ezhu and zhiqiao for each, 6g of Sanqi San and gancao.

Indications: Chronic atrophic gastritis which belongs to the syndrome of Qi deficiency and blood stasis.

6. Intermingled cold and heat

(1) Wei Wei Fang

Components: 15g of huangqi and baishao, 12g of sheng dihuang and wumei, 10g of baizhu, muxiang and shanzha for each, 5g of chuanlian and gancao, 3g of wuzhuyu.

Indications: Chronic atrophic gastritis which belongs to the syndrome of Intermingled heat and cold.

(2) He Zhong Xiao Pi Tang

Components: 12g of dangshen, 10g of banxia, 6g of ganjiang and chuanlian each, 12g of baishao, 5g of gancao, 15g of danshen and pugongying for each.

Indications: Chronic atrophic gastritis and bile reflux gastritis which belong to the syndrome of intermingled heat and cold.

iii. Single ingredient prescriptions and proved prescriptions

1. Simple prescriptions

(1) Goji berries

Components: Lycium Barbarum

Indications: Chronic atrophic gastritis which belongs to the syndrome of yin deficiency of liver-kidney.

Direction: Berries are cleaned and put into different bags after dried and crushed. 20g of the medicine is taken daily and chewed in twice on an empty stomach. 2 months as a course of treatment.

(2) Bian Dou Yin

Components: equal amounts of chao biandou (dolichos lablab), dangshen, shanzha and wumei.

Indications: gastritis, especially for chronic atrophic gastritis.

Direction: take orally with the addition of appropriate white sugar when the biandou is well-cooked.

2. Empirical Prescriptions

(1) Wei Wei Tang

Components: 15g of taizishen , 15g of fuling , 15g of baizhu, 15g of baishao, 20g of tieshuye, 20g of pugongying , 20g of danshen , 9g of chaihu , 9g of ezhu , 9g of zhiqiao, 9g of foshou, 9g of prepared gancao.

Efficacy: to invigorate spleen and soothe the liver, tonify Qi and activate blood circulation, and to clear heat and remove toxin.

Indications: it is mainly used for treating chronic atrophic gastritis, distension or dull pain in upper abdomen, nausea and belching, anorexia, light or dark red tongue texture, thin, pale or greasy tongue coating, and even for emaciation and anemia.

Modifications: for patients who have yin deficiency of the spleen and stomach, 10g of maidong, 10g of shihu, 9g of wumei can be added; for patients who have spleen-kidney yang deficiency, 6g of ganjiang, 3g of wuzhuyu, 15g of buguzhi can be added; for patients who have upwelling of stomach turbidity, nausea and belching, 10g of banxia, 6g of chenpi, 10g of sugeng can be added; patients who have dampness in the stomach and greasy tongue coating, 6g of houpo, 9g of huoxiang can be added; for patients who are infected with HP, 9g of huangqin, 3g of chuanlian can be added; patients who have intestinal gland metaplasia and severe atypic hyperplasia, 20g of pingdimu, 20g of banzhilian can be added.

Direction: Take 1/3 of one dose by decocting each time, 3 times a day.

(2) Yu Zhu Huang Jing Tang

Components: 30g of huangjing , 30g of yuzhu, 30g of shihu, 15g of danggui, 15g of baishao, 15g of chuanxiong, 15g of lvmeihua, 15g of Rose Flower, 15g of wumei, 15g of wuweizi, 6g of zhigancao.

Efficacy: to nourish yin and stomach, and to activate blood circulation for removing obstruction in collaterals.

Indications: it is mainly used for treating chronic atrophic gastritis, dull pain in the upper abdomen hunger and gastric upset, hunger without appetite, dry mouth and throat without desire to drink, dry stools, red or dark purple tongue texture, thin or less tongue coating, string-like pulse and rapidor thread or weak pulse and so on.

Modifications: patients who have Qi deficiency, 15g of huangqi and shanyao for each; patients who also have dampness-heat can add 15g of huangqin, 6g of chuanlianzi, 6g of unprocessed gancao can be added; for patients who have liver depression and Qi stagnation, 10g of chaihu and yujin for each can be added.

Direction: decoction was taken an oral dose and one dose per day.

(3) Yi Gan Fu Pi Fang

Components: chaihu, zhiqiao, baishao, baizhu, chenpi, yiyiren, shanzha, danshen, ezhu, sanqi, huanglian, gancao.

Efficacy: to free repressed liver and support spleen, and to activate blood and relieve stasis.

Indications: it is mainly used for treating chronic atrophic gastritis, swelling in upper stomach, dull pain, or accompanied by nausea, belching, anorexia, loose stools or constipation, and also with lusterless complexion, fatigued spirit and lack of strength and weight loss.

Modifications: for patients who have spleen-stomach weakness, dangshen and fuling can be added; patients who have kidney yang deficiency, roudoukou and fuzi can be added; for patients who have stomach yin insufficiency, shashen and maidong can be added; patients who have downward diffusion of dampness-heat, baitouweng and cheqianzi can be added.

Direction: 1 dose a day, and each dose should be decocted for 3 times, and take the decoction in 2 separated times half an hour before meals.

iv. Chinese patent medicine

1. Wen Wei Shu Capsule

Components: dangshen, baizhu, paofuzi, rougui, shanyao, wumei, sharen, chenpi, buguzhi, shanzha, huangqi, roucongrong and so on.

Efficacy: to strengthen and consolidate body resistance, warm and tonify stomach, active Qi and stop pain, assist yang and warm middle.

Indications: it is mainly used for treating chronic atrophic gastritis, chronic gastritis with the symptoms of epigastric cold pain, inflation, belching, anorexia, fear of cold, lack of strength.

Direction: three times a day, 2-4 pills each time, and take the medicine half an hour before meals.

2. Yang Wei Shu Granules

Components: huangjing (steamed), dangshen, baizhu (chao), shanyao, tusizi, beishashen, xuanshen, wumei, chenpi, shanzha, ganjiang.

Efficacy: to tonify Qi and nourish yin, invigorate spleen and harmonize stomach, activate Qi and remove food stagnation.

Indications: it is mainly used for treating the stomachache caused by deficiency of both Qi and yin of spleen and stomach, and patients who also have symptoms of scorching pain in stomach, stuffiness distension and discomfort, dry mouth and bitter taste in mouth, less eating and emaciation, feverish feeling in palms and soles; and chronic gastritiswith the listed symptoms.

Direction: three times a day, 2-4 pills each time, and take the medicine half an hour before meals.

3. San Jiu Wei Tai

Components: Sanyaku, jiulixiang, baishao, sheng dihuang, muxiang.

Efficacy: to diminish inflammation and relieve pain, and to regulate Qi and invigorate the stomach.

Indications: it is mainly used for treating superficial gastritis, erosive gastritis, chronic atrophic gastritis and other types of chronic gastritis.

Direction: three times a day, 1 bag each time, take the medicine half an hour before meals.

4. Hou Gu Jun Pian

Components: Hericium erinaceus.

Efficacy: to diminish inflammation and relieve pain, to support healthy Qi.

Indications: chronic atrophic gastritis, peptic ulcer, gastric cancer, esophaguscancer and so on.

Direction: three times a day, 2-4 pills each time, and take the medicine half an hour before meals.

5. Qi Zhi Wei Tong Capsule

Components: chaihu, chaoxiangfu, baishao, chaoyanhusuo, zhiqiao, zhigancao.

Efficacy: to soothe liver and regulate Qi, to harmonize stomach and relieve pain.

Indications: it is mainly used for treating liver depression and Qi stagnation, distension and stuffiness in chest, epigastric pain and chronic gastritis patients with the above syndromes.

Direction: three times a day, 1 bag each time, take the medicine half an hour before meals.

6. Wei Su Capsule

Components: zisugeng, xiangfu, chenpi, zhiqiao, binlang, foshou, xiangyuan, zhijineijin.

Efficacy: to regulate Qi and disperse swelling, and to harmonize stomach and relieve pain.

Indications: it is mainly used for treating: epigastric pain due to Qi stagnation with the symptoms such as distending pain in stomach which extend to both rib-sides and is relieved after having belching or flatus. And the above symptoms will be severe when the patients become irritated and emotional. It is also used for treating chest tightness and eating less, difficult defecation, thin and white tongue coating, string-like pulse pulse, and chronic gastritis and peptic ulcer with the listed syndromes

Direction: three times a day, 1 dose half an hour before meals.

v. Acupuncture and moxibustion therapy

1. Spleen-stomach weakness, Qi stagnation and blood stasis

Prescription: BL 20, BL 21, BL 17, CV 12, LR 13, CV 6, PC 6, ST 36, SP 10.

Prescription analysis: comprehensive treatment of BL 20, BL 21 and CV 12 can invigorate spleen and harmonize stomach, warm and tonify Zhongzhou; ST 36 is the lower sea point of the stomach, and can tonify the middle energizer and replenish qi, ascend the clear and descend the turbid, with the function of regulating spleen and stomach. Therefore it is an important acupoint for treating spleen-stomach weakness; treatment of PC 6 can be helpful for curing the pain in chest and stomach; LR 13 is the Front-Mu point in spleen meridian at which Qi of zang viscera meet, and can treat stomach and abdominal distension and other digestive system diseases; BL 17 and SP 10 can both treat blood diseases; treatment of CV 6 have the functions of tonifying primordial qi, regulating Qi and relieving stagnation.

Manipulation: adopt reinforcing method on BL 20, BL 21, BL 17 and LR 13; adopt an eutral supplementation and draining method on CV 6, PC 6and ST 36; adopt reinforcing method and moxibustion on CV 12 and SP 10. Retain needles for 30-40 min, and use warming needle moxibustion or moxibustion with moxa stick for 15-20 min.

2. Liver-stomach disharmony and fire stagnant dryness-heat

Prescription: LR 3, PC 6, CV 12, ST 36.

Prescription analysis: the LR 3 is the source point of liver meridian and can soothe the liver and regulate Qi, harmonize stomach and descend adverse Qi; PC 6 can help treat pain in chest and stomach; CV 12 and ST 36 can both invigorate spleen and support earth to restrain liver-wood.

Modifications: ST44 can be helpful for treating stomach fire exuberance; LR 2 can be helpful for treating liver fire exuberance; ST 25 can be helpful for treating constipation.

Manipulation: adopt neutral reinforcement and reduction method on PC 6, CV 12 and ST 36, and adopt purgative method on other ocupoints. Retain needles for 30 min and manipulate needle once every 10 min.

3. Stomach yin deficiency and blood stasis in the collaterals

Prescription: BL 21, CV 12, PC 6, ST 36, SP 6, SP 10

Prescriptions analysis: BL 21 and CV 12, according to back-shu points and front-mu points combination, have the functions of invigorating spleen, harmonizing stomach, and tonifying the middle energizer; PC 6 can help treat pain in the chest and stomach; ST 36 is the lower sea point of stomach and SP 6 is an acupoint in spleen meridian, so they both together can have the functions of invigorating spleen and nourishing yin; SP 10 has the functions of transporting and transforming spleen blood.

Modifications: if the patients has constipation issues, treatment on ST 25 can be added.

Manipulation: adopt reinforcing method on BL 21, SP 10 and CV 12; adopt neutral reinforcement and reduction method on PC 6, SP 6 and ST 36; adopt reducing method on ST 25. Retain needles for 30~40 min and manipulate needle every 10 min.

4. Spleen deficiency and liver depression, Qi deficiency and inharmonious descending

Prescription: CV 12, PC 6, ST 36, LR 3, SP 4.

Prescription analysis: CV 12 and ST 36 can invigorate spleen and support earth to resist liver wood. PC 6 and SP 4 are two of the eight confluence points, and they can soothe chest oppression and relieve a depressed liver, and treat pain in chest and stomach. LR 3 is the source point of liver meridian, and can soothe the liver and regulate Qi, and harmonize stomach and descend adverse Qi.

Manipulation: all of the acupoints should be applied with neutral reinforcement and reduction method. For patients with deficiency syndrome, 3-5 cones of moxibustion over ginger slices can be added on CV 12. Retain needles for 30min and manipulate them every 10 min.

vi. Recipes for dietary therapy

1. Cow milk porridge

Components: 250g of fresh cow milk, 60g of polished round-grain rice and 20g of white sugar.

Efficacy: tonify deficiency and benefit the five zang-organs.

Indication: suitable for patients who suffer from poor gastric acidity, weak health and constipation.

Direction: the polished round-grain rice is washed clean and then put in the pot. It is added with the required amount of water and put on strong fire for boiling. Next, it is boiled into porridge with slow fire; and then white sugar and milk are put in the pot for boiling.

2. Boiled lean meat with hawthorn

Components: Shanzha and qianshi powder (20g for each), 250g of lean pork meat, ginger and green onions (10g for each), 6g of salt and 20g of vegetable oil.

Efficacy: improve retention of food and increase gastric acid.

Indication: lacking gastric acid.

Direction: the hawthorn and lean meat are cut into slices, the ginger into shreds, and the green onion into segments; the pork is dressed with qianshi powder. And then the vegetable oil is added after the pot is put on strong fire for heating. When the temperature reaches up to about 60°C, the ginger and green onion are added for frying. Next, moderate clean water is put before the hawthorn, for boiling. At last, the lean meat dressed with qianshi powder is put for cooking, added with salt.

3. Yang Rou Nuo Zao Wen Wei Porridge

Components: 200 g of fresh mutton, 10g of huangqi, 100g of sticky rice, 10 Chinese dates and 5g of fresh ginger.

Efficacy: nourish spleen and stomach, and taking it for long time can warm yang, tonify Qi and strengthen spleen.

Indication: patients who suffer from gastric ulcer, gastric neurosis, chronic gastritis with stomach cold, limbs cold and stomachache.

Direction: 200g of fresh mutton (stewed and cut into shreds) is added with 10g of huangqi, 100g of sticky rice, 10 Chinese dates and 5g of fresh ginger for cooking porridge. Moderate salt, monosodium glutamate and ground pepper are added after the porridge is well done.

vii. Others

1. Bag for protecting stomach

Components: 30g of banxia prepared with ginger, 30g of baizhu, 30g of baishao, and 30g of foshou.

Efficacy: to strengthen the spleen and harmonize stomach, and to promote qi to relieve pain.

Indications: it is used for treating all kinds of chronic gastritis accompanied with epigastric fullness and pain and related symptoms.

Method: a small bag is made with a handkerchief. All herbs are put in the bag and then the bag is put in cold water for soaking. Next the bag is taken out after it is put to steam of 10 minutes. One towel is covered on the medicine bag first, preventing from being too hot and injure the skin. The medicine bag can be put at the navel position (VC 8 acupoint) after it is cooled a little. The bag is applied in the navel position twice times, with the patient lying still, half an hour each time. The herbs bag is exchanged one time per day. 3 months constitute one treatment course.

2. Yi Wei San bag for protecting the stomach

Components: baijiezi 4g, sharen 1g, dingxiang 4g, wuzhuyu 4g, baikouren 4g, wuyao 2g, xixin 1g, honghua 4g and bingpian 0.5g.

Efficacy: to warm the stomach and relieve pain, and to activate qi and descend adverse qi.

Indications: epigastric pain with fear of cold.

Method: after dried and pounded, the herbs are filtered with a sieve. 10g are put into a small tissue paper bag and then applied at the CV 8 acupoint and a new one is changed one time per day. 30 days constitute one treatment course.

3. Ear points stimulation

Selected points: sympathetic, shenmen, stomache, spleen, liver and subcortex. Efficacy: to invigorate spleen, supplement qi, and activate blood flow

Indications: treatment of epigastric discomfort related to chronic gastritis

Manipulation: after proper desinfection of one of the ears, wangbuliuxingzi seeds are placed in the points. Seeds are used in alternation between the two ears, changed to the other ear once per week. 10 times constitute one treatment course. It is suggested that the patient should press his ear points 3-5 times per day, and it can be stopped when congestion, heating and swelling of auricle is felt.

4. Abdominal massage

(1) Push and pull: It is the first and common manipulation to make abdominal massage, and the force should be determined according to the status and depth of abdominal mass as well as the thickness of the patient abdominal wall, which is usually 10-30kg. It is important that the patient should not feel too painful during massage (the patient often has tenderness at abdominal mass position during touching).

(2) Total pressing: the doctor uses his hands to press from two sides of the abdomen to the central navel, which plays a good role in treatment of abdominal mass in deep part. However, it is difficult to be mastered and the doctor needs a good physical ability.

(3) Supporting and lifting: The doctor uses one or two hands to move upward in Z-shaped way from below the navel. This manipulation is mainly used for masses in hypogastrium.

(4) Kneading and pressing: The doctor should knead and press a little hard with two hands, taking the navel

as the center. The diameter of pressing anticlockwise should be shorter and the diameter of pressing clockwise should be larger. This manipulation should be used at the end of the treatment.

Above manipulations should be used alternately. One treatment should be conducted in two or three stages.

Indications: various kinds of chronic gastritis with epigastric and abdominal distension.

This set of manipulation is designed according to characteristics of smooth muscles of of the abdomen, and determined by the position, hardness and depth of mass. The position of patient during treatment should be the same as that of during abdominal examination. In addition, the patient should take a deep breath for cooperating with the manipulation, best in abdominal respiration. Only when the manipulation is used during expiration, it is the best. Back massage or stepping massage should be conducted after the abdominal massage, in order to improve the curative effect. One treatment course consists of 15-30 times. Massage should be performed once time every two days or every three days.

V. Empirical Prescriptions of famous physicians and experts

i. Yi Wei Ping Wei Decoction (Zhou Xinyou)

Components: dangshen 20g, chao baizhu 9g, huangqi 20g, chenpi 9g, banxia 9g, xiangfu 9g, sharen 9g, jineijin 9g, chao baishao 20g, ezhu 20g, pugongying 15g and gancao 6g.

Efficacy: to tonify qi and harmonize stomach, remove stasis and relieve pain, and promote tissue regeneration and prevent atrophy

Indications: it is used for treatment of atrophic gastritis, showing epigastric swelling pain, belching, poor appetite, lassitude, and decreased gastric acid in clinic.

Direction: decocting in water for an oral dose, twice a day.

ii. Qing Zhong Xiao Pi Tang (Li Shoushan)

Components: taizishen 15g, maidong 15g, zhibanxia 7.5g, chaihu 6g, baishao 10g, chaozhizi 7.5g, mudanpi 7.5g, qingpi 10g, danshen of 15g, and gancao 6g.

Efficacy: to nourish yin and benefit stomach, and disperse masses

Indications: superficial gastritis, reflux gastritis, atrophic gastritis, etc. with manifestations of distension and blockage in the stomach, scorching pain, not wanting to eat when being hungry, not wanting to drink when being thirsty, vexing heat in chest, palms and soles, anorexia and eating less, dry stools, red tongue with scant liquid, uncoated and smooth tongue coating with cracks, and thin and rapid pulse, etc.

Direction: the medicines are decocted after soaking in cold water for 20 minutes. They are decocted with slow fire for 30 minutes after boiling at the first time, and decocted with slow fire for 20 minutes after boiling for a second time. The two decoctions, with a total volume of 200 ml, are mixed well. One dose should be taken every day, split in the morning and evening. Decoction should be warmed and taken 2 hours before or after the dinner. 3 doses or 6 doses should be taken continuously according to the patient' condition, and then stopped for one day. Herbs are stopped after the disease is stable or cured. Other Chinese and western medicines should be avoided when taking this medicine. For chronic atrophic gastritis, usually 3 months constitute one treatment course.

iii. Wei Wei An (Zhang Jingren)

Components: taizishen 9g, chao baizhu 9g, danshen 9g, chaihu 6g, chishao and baishao (9g for each), zhigancao 3g, xuzhangqing of 15g, baihuasheshecao of 30g, and chao huangqin of 9g.

Efficacy: regulating Qi and activating blood circulation

Indications: chronic atrophic gastritis

Direction: decocted with water, one dose is taken per day. It should be taken separately in the morning and evening.

iv. Wei Wei Ning (Yu Jibai)

Components: banxia 10g, huangqin 10g, huanglian 6g, dangshen 12g, zhigancao 10g, ganjiang 10g, daizheshi 20g, laifuzi 15g, zhishi 10g and baishao 15g.

Efficacy: pungent dispersing and bitter descending, and strengthening the spleen and regulating stomach

Indications: it is used for treatment of chronic atrophic gastritis

Modifications: for the patient who has severe epigastric pain, 10g of muxiang and 12g of baizhi should be added, for activating Qi and relieving stagnation, regulating blood circulation and removing stasis, and relieving spasm and pain. For the patient who has borborygmus, diarrhea and loose stools, ganjiang should be replaced by 10g of chaoganjiang, and jiaoshanzha is added, for warming spleen and stomach to dispel cold, invigorating stomach and checking diarrhea. For the patient who has anorexia and eats less food, 10g of chenpi, 6g of sharen, or 15g of jiaoshanzha and 15g of chaomaya should be added for enlivening spleen and stimulating appetite, promoting digestion and removing food stagnation. For the patient who cannot sleep well at night or has insomnia, 20 g of suanzaoren and 12g of chuanxiong should be added, for nourishing heart and tranquilizing mind. For the patient who has excess of cold, 10g of xixin and 10g of chuanjiao should be added for warming spleen and stomach to dispel cold; for the patient who has excess of heat, 10g of binglang and 20g of pugongying should be added for dispelling stomach-heat; for the patient with yin-deficiency, the ganjiang should be removed, and 10g of shashen, 12g of maidong, 10g of shihu should be added, for nourishing yin and promoting fluid production; for the patient who has serious stasis, the ganjiang should be removed, and 20g of danshen, 15g of fresh shanzha should be added, for activating blood circulation and removing stasis. For the patient who suffers from chronic atrophic gastritis with intestinal metaplasia or atypical hyperplasia, 10g of sanleng, 10g of ezhu, for dispersing stasis and eliminating stagnation, and inhibiting intestinal metaplasia should be added to the prescriptions; furthermore, 30g of huangyaozi, or 30g of banzhilian, 12g of shancigu may be added for its anti-cancer properties.

Note: Professor Yu Jibai emphasized that chronic gastritis is caused mainly because of disorders of the stomach qi. The method of harmonizing stomach and its descending-Qi movement should be considered during the treatment. This disease should be treated slowly and carefully. To obtain a curative effect, the importance is in the "preserving". Following the original idea of Zhang Zhongjing, professor Yu takes Banxia Xiexin Tang decoction as a main prescription, and Xuanfu Daizhe Tang decoction as a secondary prescription, modifying them according to syndrome differentiation. To give a comprehensive view of the whole prescriptions, it includes herbs for resolving cold and heat, pungent herbs for opening and bitter discharging bitter, medicines for tonification and purgation, and can resolve both symptoms and root causes. The prescriptions can mildly regulate cold and heat, harmonize yin and yang, restore ascending and descending functions, and stimulate the qi in the middle energizer.

VI. Typical medical records of famous physicians and experts

i. Medical record of Shan Zhaowei

Mr. Zhou, male, 45 years old.

Preliminary diagnosis: on November 29, 2011. Complain of dull epigastric pain occurred 2 months ago, without any obvious improvement. A gastroscopy was performed on October 24, 2011, showing: 1) chronic gastritis; 2) postoperative APC verrucous gastritis. Pathology: (smaller curvature) mild atrophic gastritis with intestinal metaplasia, mild atypical hyperplasia at glandular epithelium in focal area. HP(-). At present: dull epigastric pain, gastric upset when in empty stomach, peculiar taste in the mouth, dark red tongue with thin and yellow coating, as well as string-like pulse and thready pulse.

Differentiation syndrome: deficiency of spleen and stomach qi.

Therapeutic principle: tonify qi and harmonizing stomach.

Prescription: Modified Er Shen San Cao Tang: taizishen 10g, huangqi 10g, chaobaizhu 10g, chaoyiyiren 15g, xianhecao 15g, baihuasheshecao 15g, danshen 15g, zhigancao of 5g, foshou of 5g. It is comprised of 14 doses. Decoct one formula with water for an oral dose and one dose per day, taken separately in two times.

Second diagnosis: Epigastric dull pain pain sometimes occurred after taking the medicine, and it was more serious after eating, with symptoms of gastric upset, peculiar taste in the mouth, anorexia, dry and bitter taste in mouth, dark red tongue, thin and yellow tongue coating, as well as string-like pulse and thready pulse. The previous prescriptions were modified for treatment. Zhigancao was removed from the previous prescriptions, and chaoguya and chaomaya (15 g for each) should be added, for relieving dyspepsia. It is comprised of 14 doses. Decocted one formula with water for an oral dose and one dose per day, taken separately in two times.

Third diagnosis: Epigastric dull pain pain was relieved after taking the herbs. Still had symptoms of the gastric swelling, occasional gastric upset, peculiar taste in the mouth, some lack of appetite, stomach cold, prefering hot food, thin and yellow tongue coating, as well as string-like pulse and thready pulse. The previous prescriptions should be modified for treatment. The chao guya and chao maya should be removed from the previous prescriptions, and 2g of ganjiang should be added for dispelling cold in stomach. It is comprised of 14 doses. Decocted 1 formula with water for an oral dose and one dose per day, taken separately in two times.

Fourth diagnosis: Epigastric dull pain pain and grastic upset were not so obvious after taking the decoctions, and the peculiar taste in the mouth disappeared, but had higher blood pressure. It is still due to deficiency of spleen and stomach. The previous prescriptions were modified for treatment. Ganjiang was removed from the previous prescriptions, and 15g of gouteng, 10g of tianma should be added for pacifying liver and subduing yang. It is comprised of 14 doses. Decocted one formula with water for an oral dose and one dose per day, taken separately in two times.

Fifth diagnosis: The second gastroscopy examination was taken on March 31, 2012, showing: 1) chronic gastritis; Pathology: (smaller curvature) severe superficial gastritis, hP(-). All symptoms were relieved and the previous prescriptions were used for consolidating the effect. Prescriptions: taizishen 10g, huangqi 10g, 10g of chaobaizhu, 15g of chaoyiyiren, 15g of baihuasheshecao, 5g of foshou, 15g of baihe, and 15g of yejiaoteng. It is comprised of 14 doses. Decocted 1 formula with water for an oral dose and one dose per day.

Note: Ershen Sancao Tang is one of the commonly used prescriptions by Professor Shan Zhaowei, in accordance with the pathogenic characteristics of chronic atrophic gastritis. The pathogenic characteristics are that deficiency of spleen and stomach qi with blood stasis will occur if the patient suffers from this disease for a long time. Taizishen and huangqi in the prescriptions can replenish Qi to invigorate the spleen, and strengthen and consolidate body resistance, taking the Qi-tonifying as the main function. Baizhu and yiyiren can tonify the middle energizer, strengthen stomach, activate spleen and eliminate dampness. Xianhecao is a necessary herb to treat spleen and stomach diseases, which can strengthen stomach and tonify deficiency, clear heat and stop bleeding.In the *Bai Cao Jing (Classic of One Hundred Herbs)*, it is recorded that "it can descend Qi and activate blood circulation, treat numerous diseases as well as dispel distention and fullness"; in the *Ben Cao Gang Mu Shi Yi (Supplement to Compendium of Material Medica)*, it is said that "it can help digestion, dispel abdominal distension, descend qi, treat hematemesis and the symptoms of regurgitation and dysphagia". Baihuasheshecao is used for clearing heat and toxic materials; modern pharmacological research shows that baihuasheshecao can inhibit intestinal metaplasia, and prevent intestinal metaplasia from occurring in atrophic gastritis, otherwise it will develop to tumor, like the old saying "nip in the bud"; baihuasheshecao can also inhibit the proliferation and infiltration of tumour cell, reflecting the idea of "preventing disease from exacerbating". danshen can activate and enrich the blood. In *Fu Ren Min Li Lun* (*Famous Theory about Women*), it is praised that "the functions of the single danshen equal to that of Si Jun Zi Tang". It can not only promote blood circulation to remove obstruction in meridian but also enrich and replenish blood; danshen is matched with huangqi and dangshen, because Qi leads the blood, and if the Qi is replenished, blood will move, so that stasis will be removed; blood is the mother of Qi, and "yang can be produced infinitely with the help of yin", having the effect of tonifying Qi and producing blood, nourishing blood and activating collaterals; foshou can soothe the liver and regulate Qi, harmonize stomach and relieve pain; gancao can soften the middle energizer, combining with coordinating the drug actions of a Prescriptions.

ii. Medical record of Xu Jingfan

Mr. San, male, 60 years old, worker.

Preliminary diagnosis: on December 2, 1992. The patient had epigastric pain for more than 10 years, and he was hospitalized because of defecating black stools. Gastroscopy examination showed: chronic atrophic gastritis accompanied by intestinal metaplasia and superficial duodenitis. Blood HP-antibodies was positive. Also positive for ocult blood in faeces. The patient took dissolved Sanqi San, Baiji San and modified Qinlian Pingwei San after admission, in order to clear dampness-heat, harmonize stomach and stop bleeding. The black stools disappeared, and examination to occult blood in faeces changed to negative. However, epigastric pain was still not removed more than 40 days after admission, with a very black tongue coating like sauce. Symptoms included epigastric dull pain pain, anorexia, being thirsty and wanting to drink, abnormal urination and defecation, red tongue, black and yellow as well as sticky and greasy tongue coating like covering with the moldy sauce, and string-like pulse and rapid pulse.

Syndrome differentiation: deficiency of middle energizer, accompanied by dampness-heat.

Therapeutic principle: clear dampness-heat, regulate Qi and harmonize the middle.

Prescription: dongguazi 30g, pei lan 10g, huanglian 3g, yiyiren 20g, diyu 10g, chenpi 10g, zhibanxia 10g, zhijineijin 10g, foshou 6g, baizhu 10g, shanyao 15g, zhigancao 3g. One dose was taken each day.

Second diagnosis: on December 16, 1992. After taking the decoction, the patient had no obvious epigastric pain and his appetite improved. In addition, the problem in the mouth was resolved, and the sign of black and yellow as well as sticky and greasy tongue coating gradually disappeared. The treatment according to the original prescriptions, with little modifications. The patient took more than 20 doses in total and left the hospital after all symptoms were relieved.

Note: *Shejian Bianzheng* (*Tongue Mirror Pattern Differentiation*) recorded that "if a patient's tongue shows dark reddish brown, as well as yellow and black, it is because heat in zang-fu viscera is accompanied with dyspeptic food". It is indicated that this kind of symptom is mainly because dampness-heat is accumulated for long. In this case, dual deficiency-excess occurred, where deficiency is the root cause and dampness-heat is the manifestation. Dampness-heat accumulates, leading to black, yellow and greasy coating like the sauce on the tongue. Mr. Xu mainly cured the disease through mainly treating manifestations, and he focuses on clearing and harmonizing the middle, and eliminated dampness-heat in middle energizer so as to tonify the spleen, therefore hte curdy coating disappeared naturally. Dongguazi is usually used for clearing lung, eliminating phlegm and expelling pus. Dr. Xu thinks that dongguazi can clear dampness-heat of the stomach and intestines, discharge heat-toxicity of the intestines and other viscera, and stimulate appetite. Therefore, it is often used for the treatment of chronic gastritis with syndrome of damp-heat blocking middle energizer. In addition, dongguazi combined with huanglian and diyu in prescriptions can clear heat, dry dampness and eliminate toxic substances. Pei lan, yiyiren and banxia are taken for resolving turbid dampness. Chenpi and foshou are used for regulating Qi and stomach. Jijneijin, baizhu and shanyao are used for tonifying spleen, nourishing the stomach, preventing bitter cold from damaging the middle.gancao is used for relieving the middle and coordinating the herb actions of the prescriptions.

VII. Prevention and aftercare

i. Prevention

(1) Regular examination should be taken. If necessary, the gastroscopy is recommended.

(2) Go for examination as soon as possible when having symptoms of emaciation, anorexia, black stools or other related symptoms.

(3) Control alcohol consumption, do not smoke, for preventing the damage of nicotine to the gastric mucosa; avoid taking analgesics and anti-inflammatory drugs for long time.

(4) Food should be fresh, nutritious. Be sure to ingest enough protein, vitamins and iron. Take meals on time, without overeating. Do not eat food too cold or hot. Do not use pungent spices or any other strong condiments.

ii. Aftercare

(1) Principles of dietary therapy: developing good dietary and living habit. Chew carefully and swallow slowly when eating, for the fully mixing of food and digestive juice. The diet should be light. Do not overeat at supper and sleep after the food is digested. Otherwise, the discomfort of stomach will be increased. Chewing food thoroughly supports the digestion of food. People whose teeth are loose or fall off should treat them in order to ease the burden of the stomach.

(2) Keep an optimistic mood: the gastrointestinal tract has abundant innervation, total amount of which is next only to that in brain and spine, through which mind and emotions may affect the movement in the digestive tract (including the stomach), or disturbing secretion of digestive glands, that may aggravate the gastritis.

(3) Strenghen physical exercise to have a regular lifestyle.

(4) Give up smoking and alcohol: everybody knows that long-term and high alcohol consumption can damage stomach, but people always ignore the damage of smoking. However, multiple chemical components of tobacco can damage the gastric mucosa, even lead to cancer.

VIII. Conclusion

In short, it has obvious advantages to use TCM for treating CAG, which can eliminate or improve clinical symptoms, promote the recovery of gastric mucosa atrophic lesion, block progression of disease and reduce recurrence without obvious toxic and side effects. However, at present there are still some disadvantages in TCM treatment: it lacks unified criterion of differential classification, and medicines are prescribed mainly based on personal experience; there is no unified reference basis for therapeutic effect evaluation; in clinical practice, the disease is always diagnosed through syndrome differentiation and treatment, with fewer reports of individual cases and experience summary samples; follow-up visits are not enough after diagnosis and treatment. Therefore, we should strengthen the pharmacological research of traditional Chinese medical Prescriptions to formulate unified and normative criterion of differential classification of CAG, providing a more exact theoretical basis for TCM therapy of CAG.

(MENG Jingyan)

References

[1] Chen J, Li SY, and Xu H. Research progress of chronic atrophic gastritis [J].Chinese Journal of Gerontology,2013(14):3540-3542.

[2] Wang SQ, Wang YH, Wang F. Syndrome differentiation and treatment in Chinese medicine of chronic atrophic gastritis [J].China Pharmaceuticals, 2015(12):125-127.

[3] Yang WW, Zhou XH. Research progress of TCM therapy of chronic atrophic gastritis[J]. Modernization of Traditional ChineseMedicine and Material Medica-World Science and Technology, 2014, 16 (10):2166-2169.

[4] Gao DW, Liu XW, Chen WJ. Diagnosis and combined treatment of TCM and WM of chronic atrophic gastritis [J]. Journal of Clinical and Experimental Medicine, 2012(10):748-749.

[5] Shen KJ. TCM therapy of common gastrointestinal disorders [M]. Hefei: Anhui Science & Technology Publishing House, 2006.

[6] Li JZ, Zhou L, Liu LG, et al. Clinical observation of 36 cases of chronic atrophic gastritis treated by acupuncture [J]. Acupuncture Research, 2002, 27 (4):280-285.

[7] Zhang D. Prescriptions of distinguished veteran doctors of TCM that are effect through multiple attempts [M]. Beijing: People's Military Medical Press, 2009.

[8] Chen GS, Li JT, Deng Y, et al. Diagnosis and treatment of empirical Prescriptions of professor Yu Jibai [J]. Traditional Chinese Medicinal Research, 2007, 20 (7):50-53.

[9] Gu C, Shan ZW. Empirical medical record that Shan Zhaowei use Ershen Sancao Decoction to treat chronic atrophic gastritis [J]. Journal of Changchun University of Traditional Chinese Medicine, 2013, 29 (2):222-223.

[10] Xu Q. 2 medical records of stomach disease from Xu Jingfan [J].Journal of Traditional Chinese Medicine, 1993, 34 (12):722.

肾病综合征　Nephrotic Syndrome

I. Overview

Nephrotic Syndrome (NS for short) is caused by various etiological factors, and its clinical manifestation shows 4 main features: massive proteinuria; hypoproteinemia; hyperlipidaemia (HLP); different levels of edema. Hypoproteinemia mainly presents decreased plasma-albumin, often less than 30g/L; HLP mainly reflects increased cholesterol; for the patients with different levels of edema, the serious ones may have hydrothorax and ascites. NS can be divided into primary and secondary types. The pathological patterns of primary NS include minimal change disease, mesangial proliferative glomerulonephritis, membrano-proliferative glomerulonephritis, membranous nephropathy and focal segmental glomerulosclerosis, etc., which are more common among children and teenagers. Secondary NS can be caused by multiple paths such as immune diseases (e.g. systemic lupus erythematosus and anaphylactoid purpura), diabetes and secondary infection (e.g. bacteria and hepatitis B virus, etc.), circulation system disease and drug poisoning.

There is no the name of disease "nephritic syndrome" in traditional Chinese medicine. It belongs to "edema", "lumbago", "consumptive disease", "turbid urine" according to clinical symptoms.Edema is the early symptom of this disease, which was recorded earliest in *Edema* of *Miraculous Pivot*. The book recorded that "when the edema occurs in the early time, puffiness of eyelid will happen as you just wake up. Venous engorgement of neck exists, sometimes with cough. It is cold in pudendal thigh, with swollen shin of feet and big abdomen, and then the edema has been formed. When the abdomen is pressed with hands, the symptom is that when the hands rise up, the abdomen is like holding full of water."

II. Etiology and pathogenesis

NS is a common kidney disease but with a lack of epidemiology data. Researcher seldom directly made the statistics of morbidity of NS, but morbidities of various primary diseases which show NS in clinical manifestation were often analyzed further. Llach reported that annual morbidity of adult NS was 3/100,000. Most of NS were caused by primary glomerulopathy. However, there was no reliable data to show how much percentage the primary and secondary took respectively in NS. It can be referenced that primary accounts for 60% of glomerulopathy.

The disease spectrum of NS has a significant difference among regions. Most of researches showed that for the adult NS, the focal segmental glomerulosclerosis is the most common, followed by membranous nephropathy and minimal change nephropathy. Kitiyakara et al. reported that membranous nephropathy and focal segmental glomerulosclerosis account for 1/3 of NS respectively, minimal change nephropathy and IgA nephropathy account for about 1/4 respectively, and Membranoproliferative GNwas seldom seen. There is a great difference in research data of the East Asia. For example, Japan reported that IgA nephropathyaccounts for above 1/3, and focal segmental glomerulosclerosis only accounts for 10%. One research from Beijing showed that according to the percentage in primary NS, the diseases in sequence from high to low is: membranous nephropathy (29.5%), minimal change nephropathy (25.3%), IgA nephropathy (20.0%), mesangial proliferative glomerulonephritis (12.7%), focal segmental glomerulosclerosis (6.0%), membrano-proliferative glomerulonephritis (1.5%), etc. From 1993 to 2010, Shi Suhua et al. had collected 36,379 cases of medical records about needling biopsy of kidney from the Pathology Department of FUZHOU GENERAL HOSPITAL OF NANJING MILITARY COMMAND, which includes the specimens about needling biopsy of kidney posted by near 200 hospitals in China. Ratio of males and females who suffer from kidney disease was similar, but male ratio was a little higher (51.0%). The kidney disease was more seen among the people with the age between 18 years and 37 years. As regards the pathological type, glomerulopathy had the highest morbidity (96.2%), therein the primary glomerulopathy accounts for more (72.5%). Lupus nephritis (41.8%) was the most common pathological type of the secondary glomerulopathy. For the patients who have NS reflected by the primary glomerulopathy, their most common pathological type wasmesangial proliferative glomerulonephritis. These differences might be related to race, environment, renal biopsy indicator and other factors.

Chinese medicine consideres that the NS is caused by deficiency of natural endowment, or damage of vital Qi due to acquired excessive fatigue, or disorder of Qi and blood, yin-yang in zang-fu viscera led by not being treated in time and therapeutic error, especially when there is deficiency of spleen and kidney: spleen deficiency can make nutrient substance and Qi-blood lose the origin of generation and transformation. At the same time with deficiency kidney leakingJing it can also cause losses of essential Qi of body, thus causing hypoproteinemia; the kidney cannot store essence due to kidney deficiency, so that the kidney Qi cannot be secured and essential qi leaks, pouring down to bladder to cause massive proteinuria. Uncontrolled water-dampness transportation and transformation caused by spleen deficiency, disturbance of qi transformation caused by kidney deficiency, both lead todampness accumulated in the body, which is reflected in the skin, i.e. edema; deficiency of both spleen and kidney can damage the liver to cause the deficiency of liver yin, further causing ascendant hyperactivity of liver yang. In development process of the disease, the irregular Qi-blood and yin-yang caused by the dysfunction of liver, spleen and kidney is the root cause of this disease, and water-dampness, dampness-heat and stagnation of blood stasis are the manifestations of this disease, finally showing the complex pathological process of deficiency mixed with excess. The disease condition is aggravated due to deficiency of vital Qi, being infected with exogenous pathogenic factors, forming the vicious circle. The more deficient vital Qi is, the more excess pathogenic Qi will be. Damp turbidity and all pathogenic Qi become more serious, finally the disease will last for long time and be difficult to cure.

III. Key points of diagnosis and differential diagnosis

i. Key points of diagnosis

NS is divided into primary and secondary diseases according to the disease causes. If the disease is deemed to be secondary disease, the causes shall be sought actively. Only the secondary nephritic syndromes, such as henoch-schonlein purpura nephritis, diabetic nephropathy, hepatitis B-related nephritis, lupus nephritis and amyloidosis of the kidney, are excluded, the disease can be diagnosed as the primary nephritic syndrome. Diagnostic criteria are as follows: ① Massive proteinuria: urine protein ≥ 3.5g/d is the main diagnostic basis of NS. ② Hypoalbuminemia: level of serum albumin is at 30g/L or below. ③ Edema: obvious among most patients; the serious patients may have thoracic, celiac and pericardial effusion. ④ Hyperlipidaemia: all kinds of lipoproteins in plasma are increased.

① and ② are the necessary conditions to diagnose NS, and ③ and ④ are the secondary conditions. Clinically, only two necessary conditions are met, the NS can be identified. In fact, "massive proteinuria" is the characteristic manifestation and initiative factor of NS, and latter three items are the results caused by it. Therefore, some scholars considered that it is more correct to use the "nephrotic-range proteinuria" to describe NS. There have been many different standards about the amount of massive proteinuria. At present, it is generally considered that if the urine protein amount of an adult is ≥ $3.5g/(1.73m^2 \cdot d)$ or 3.5g/d, it shall be deemed to be massive proteinuria; for children, it shall be calculated according to the body weight, i.e. urine protein ≥50mg/(kg·d). Besides, the ratio of urine protein to creatinine in the urine expelled at any time shall be taken as standard, if it is ≥ 2mg/mg(0.25mg/mmol), it will be massive proteinuria.

ii. Differential diagnosis

1. Chronic glomerulonephritis

The disease can be seen among the people with any age, concentrated on the young and middle-aged people. The main clinical manifestations include proteinuria, hematuresis, edema, hypertension, and different levels of kidney function decrease. The urine protein is always 1-3g/d. It is not difficult to confirm the diagnosis with the help of laboratory examinations.

2. Systemic lupus erythematosus nephritis

Morbidity of female is higher than that of male, mostly seen among females aged 20-40 years. Main clinical features: ① most patients have fevers; ② multiple joint pain; ③ rash; ④ infiltrated blood system, etc. Serum anti nuclear antibodies, anti-ds-DNA, anti-SM antibody show positive and the level of serum complement is decreased. The lesion shows diversity, in addition to mesangial proliferation under renal biopsy microscope.

3. Chronic pyelonephritis

The patients with this disease always have the recurrent urinary system infection history, probably with lumbago and low-grade fever. There often are leukocytes in urinary sediment. If it shows positive through urinary bacteriologic examination, this disease can be identified.

4. Diabetic nephropathy

Male patients are more than female patients and this disease is mostly seen among patients with more than 10 years of diabetes. In early period, expelled microalbuminuria is increased, later gradually developing to massive proteinuria. The diabetes and diabetic retinopathy are helpful for differential diagnosis.

5. Nephritis of Schonlein-Henoch purpura

In addition to hematuresis, proteinuria, edema, hypertension and other nephritis features, purpura, arthralgia, stomachache, alimentary tract hemorrhage etc. are also accompanied. If there is no typical purpura, it is easy to be misdiagnosed as primary NS. Antinuclear antibodies show negative. Through renal biopsy, the common pathologic change is diffuse mesangial cell proliferation. With respect to the immunopathogenesis, the main sediment is IgA and C3, so it is easy to identify.

IV. TCM therapy

As to the treatment of edema, *Plain Questions* of *Tangye and Laoli Discussionin* pointed out: "Opening pores of sweat duct and cleaning the bladder can eliminate the stagnated pathogen". *On Pulse, Symptom Complex and Treatment of Edema in Synopsis of the Golden Chamber* recorded that: "For the patient with edema, if the edema occurs below waist, the urination shall be induced, and if the edema occurs above waist, it can be cured through sweating". According to *Edema* of *Danxi's Experiential Therapy*, the therapeutic methods can be selected based on the different etiologies and pathogeneses of yin edema and yang edema. The yin edema belongs to interior, deficiency and cold syndrome, so reinforcing vital Qi shall be taken as main therapy, to warm the kidneys and tonify the spleen; because yang edema belongs to exterior, excess and heat syndrome, eliminating pathogen shall be taken as main therapy, such as sweating, inducing urination and purgation; generally, it is considered that at the beginning of the disease, the main pathogenesis is the exogenous pathogenic factors. Sweating, inducing urination, purgation and dispersing stasis can be performed for eliminating pathogen, according to the different symptoms. In addition to tonifying spleen and warming kidneys as adjuvant therapy, its roots caused and symptoms can be achieved by this treatment.However, in the late stage of the disease, vital Qi of the patients become weak gradually, so the treatment shall be changed to reinforce vital Qi and consolidate the body resistance. Warming kidney and tonifying spleen shall be focused on, and the method of reinforcing vital Qito eliminate pathogen can be used depending on the actual situations of exterior excess syndrome.

i. Syndrome differentiation and treatment

In *Inner Canon of Yellow Emperor*, edema is called "edema", "kidney-wind edema", "wind edema" and "edema swelling" etc. In *Synopsis of the Golden Chamber*, edema is divided into "wind edema", "skin edema", "typical edema", "stony edema", provided with therapy and prescription. On this basis, the practitioners of later generations developed a set of improved syndrome differentiation and treatment system to treat edema with TCM. Hereby,

1. Serious wind edema

Main symptoms: firstly the eyelid and facial edema is seen, and then edemarapidly spreads to the whole body, showing sore and heavy limbs, difficult urination, with wind cold syndromes: aversion to wind cold, nasal obstruction, cough, thin and white fur, and floating and tight pulse; as well as wind heat syndromes: red, swollen and sore throat, red tongue and yellow fur, and floating and rapid pulse.

Therapeutic method: expel wind and remove cold, clear damp and promote diuresis; or expel wind and clear heat, clear damp and promote diuresis.

Prescription: ① For the patient who mainly shows wind cold syndrome, modified Ma Xing Wu Pi Yin shall be adopted. Raw Ephedra, Apricot Seed, Indian Bread Exodermis, Dried Tangerine Peel, Areca Peel, White

Mulberry Root-Bark, Plantain Herb and Ginger Peel. ② For the patient who mainly shows wind heat syndrome, the modifiedYue Bi Tang and Ma Huang Lian Qiao Chi Xiao Dou Decoction shall be adopted. Raw Ephedra, Gypsum, Weeping Forsythia Capsule, Lalang Grass Rhizome, Baical Skullcap Root, Rice Bean, Fresh Reed Rhizome, Heartleaf Houttuynia Herb and Platycodon Root.

Modification: if the exterior pathogen disappears, the Ephedra, Apricot Seed or Gypsum shall be removed; for the patient who still has protein or red blood cell in urinethrough urinalysis, Tripterygium Wilfordii tablet shall be added. 20 mg is taken for each time, with 3 times per day.

2. Retention of dampness-heat

Main symptoms: edema over the whole body, lustrous and moisturizing skin color, thoracoabdominal distress, vexation heat and thirst, dry stool, scanty dark urine or skin with sore, ulcer and furuncle, red tongue, yellow and sticky fur, and rapid and slippery pulse.

Therapeutic method: separate and dispel dampness-heat.

Prescription: modified Shu Zao Yin Zi. Pokeberry Root, Oriental Waterplantain Rhizome, Rice Bean, Zanthoxylum Seed, Areca Seed, Areca Peel, Indian Bread Exodermis, Raw Rhubarb, Atractylodes Rhizome, Officinal Magnolia Bark and Incised Notopterygium Rhizome and Root.

Modification: if the patient still has serious condition, showing constipation and dampness-heat stagnation after taking the medicine, modified Ji Jiao Li Huang Wan and Ba Huang Wan, double the Rhubarb, added with Fourstamen Stephania Root and Pepperweed Seed. In addition, the Unprocessed Fructus Crotonis can be ground into fine powder and put into capsule for swallowing. For the patient with sore, ulcer, heat and swollen skin, Honeysuckle Flower, Weeping Forsythia Capsule or Dandelion, Tokyo Violet Herb and so on can be added for clearing heat and removing toxin.

3. Stasis of kidney and collaterals

Main symptoms: puffy face and swollen limbs for long time, scaly skin, or red-streaked furuncle, petechia and ecchymosis, or lumbago and red urine, pale or red tongue, petechia on the margin of tongue, purple and static muscles and tendons under the tongue, thin, yellow and sticky tongue, as well as thin and uneven pulse.

Therapeutic method: tonify kidney and break stasis.

Prescription: modified Tao Hong Si Wu Tang. Peach Seed, Safflower, Chinese Angelica, Sichuan Lovage Rhizome, Red Peony Root, Motherwort Herb, Leech and Hirsute Shiny Bugleweed Herb.

Modification: for the patient who has the serious obstruction of blood vessel, amount of the above prescription shall be increased, adding dormant insect and centipede; for the patient who also has kidney Qi deficiency, Tangshen, Milkvetch Root and Epimedium Herb shall be added; for the patient with liver-kidney yin deficiency, Rehmannia and Turtle Carapace shall be added; for the patient with spleen-kidney yang deficiency, White Atractylodes Rhizome and Aconite shall be added; for the patient with pathogenic heat, Honeysuckle Flower and Tokyo Violet Herb; for the patient with obvious hematuresis, Cattail PollenandSanqi shall be added.

4. Kidney Qi deficiency

Main symptoms: face edema in the morning, acrotarsium edema in the evening or no obvious edema, but soreness of waist, heavy body and fatigue appear, even fatigue appears during walking, sitting cannot last for long time, with pale and red tongue, thin fur as well as deep and thin pulse.

Therapeutic method: tonify kidney Qi.

Prescription: modified Ji Sheng Shen Qi Wan. Prepared Common Monkshood Daughter Root, Cassia Twig, Prepared Rehmannia Root, Asiatic Cornelian Cherry Fruit, Common Yam Rhizome, Indian Bread, Oriental Waterplantain Rhizome, Tree Peony Root Bark, Epimedium Herb, Medicinal Cyathula Root, Plantain Seed and Milkvetch Root.

5. Spleen-kidney yang deficiency

Main symptoms: white complexion, feeling cold in the normal circumstance; edema appears on the whole body and finger will be buried when it is pressed; the serious patient may have hydrothorax and ascite, chest distress and jerky breath, scanty dark urine, thin sloppy stool, pale tongue, fat body, as well as deep and thin pulse.

Therapeutic method: warm spleen and kidney, and activate yang and promote diuresis.

Prescription: modified Zhen Wu Tang and Shi Pi Yin. Prepared Common Monkshood Daughter Root, Cassia Twig, White Atractylodes Rhizome, Debark Peony Root, Dried Ginger, Red Chuling, Indian Bread, Oriental Waterplantain Rhizome, Areca Seed and Calabash Shell.

Modification: if the patient shows aversion to cold without sweat, fever headache, cough and congestion, wind cold so on too, Dried Ginger and White Atractylodes Rhizome shall be removed and Ephedra and Manchurian Wildginger shall be added. For the severe patient who shows yang deficiency and serious edema, and cannot lie on the back with shortness of breath, JiJiaoLiHuang Pill shall be taken for expelling water by purgation, further tonifying yang Qi.

6. Liver-kidney yin deficiency

Main symptoms: not serious edema, dry mouth, dry and sore throat, dizziness, quick temper, sore waist and red urine, night sweat, dysphoria with smothery sensation, red tongue, as well as thin ,wiry and rapid pulse.

Therapeutic method: tonify liver and kidney, and resolve water-dampness

Prescription: modified Er Zhi Wan and Qi Ju Di Huang Wan. Glossy Privet Fruit, Eclipta Prostrata, Adhesive Rehmannia Dried Root, Chrysanthemum Flower, Barbary Wolfberry Fruit, Tree Peony Root Bark, Oriental Waterplantain Rhizome, Indian Bread, Common Yam Rhizome and Motherwort Herb.

Modification: for the patient with more serious edema, the prescription can be added with Plantain Herb, Chinese Lobelia Herb, Barbated Skullcup Herb; for the patient who has red urine without end, it can be added with Raw India Madder Rootand Raw Garden Burnet Root.

7. Debilitation of vital Qi, and accumulated turbid toxins

Main symptoms: sallow complexion, eyelid edema, fatigue, low voice, thoraco-abdominal stuffy sensation, vomiting, anorexia, urine-like smell in the mouth, short and less urine, more nocturnal enuresis, even mental confusion, tic, skin itch, black stool, pale tongue, greasy or bean curd fur, thin or slippery pulse, weakness after being pressed.

Therapeutic method: warm spleen and tonify kidney, and activate yang and descend turbidity.

Prescription: modified Wen Pi Tang is used for oral administration. Ginseng, Processed Prepared Common Monkshood Daughter Root, Salvia Root, Medicinal Evodia Fruit, Golden Thread, Silkworm Feces, Serissa Serissoide, Yushu Dan, Processed Rhubarb, Rhizoma Pinelliae Preparatum. The enema prescription is used for coloclysis. Raw Rhubarb, Fresh Oyster Shell, Prepared Common Monkshood Daughter Root, Garden Burnet Root.

Modification: for the patient who always vomits, Cablin Patchouli Herb and Perilla leaf shall be added; for the patient with black stool, Santi or Yunnan Baiyao shall be added; for the patient with mental confusion, Turmeric Root Tuber and Grassleaf Sweetflag Rhizome shall be added; for the tiqueur, the prescription shall be added with Oyster Shell, Turtle Carapace and Tortoise Carapace and Plastron; in the case that serious edema, damp turbidity attacking heart cause sleeplessness due to breathlessness, Pepperweed Seed shall be added and amount of Rhubarb shall be increased; for the patient with loose stool, processed Rhubarb shall be used. Generally, volume of enema prescription is between 150 and 200ml, with the temperature of about 37℃ -40℃. Retention enema of high position shall be adopted. The breech position need to rise and the anal tube is pulled out slowly after clysis. It is suggested that the patient shall rest with lying for half an hour (as long as possible).

ii. Specific prescription treatment

Dai Luqing considered that because Zhen Wu Tang has the functions of benefiting Qi, warming yang, inducing urine, tonifying spleen and benefiting kidney, it can improve microcirculation of kidneys, correct hypercoagulable state in the body and reduce lesion of glomerular capillary, so as to decrease internal pressure of glomerulus, reducing the leakage of proteinuria. 90 patients with this disease were divided into two groups by Hao Kaihua. 45 patients constituted the treatment group, given the conventional therapy and SupplementedZhenWu Decoction. The control group consisted of 45 patients, only given convention therapy, for the clinical curative effect observation. Results: Cure rate of treatment group is 40.00%, with total effective rate of 87.67%; cure rate of control group is 24.44%, with total effective rate of 66.67% ($P < 0.05$).

Xia Jianhua divided 100 patients with NS into two groups randomly. The treatment group was treated with Supplemented Xiao Chai Hu Tang (Chinese Thorowax Root, Baical Skullcap Root, Rhizoma Pinelliae Preparatum, Tangshen, Fried White Atractylodes Rhizome, Indian Bread, Chuling, Hedyotis, Processed Leech, Unprocessed Milkvetch Root , Lalang Grass Rhizome, Radix Glycyrrhizae Preparata, India Madder Root and Motherwort Herb). The control group was treated with hormone and dipyridamole. The results showed: in the treatment group, 24-hour urine protein quantitation was decreased significantly, plasma-albumin was increased, and total cholesterol was reduced (($P < 0.01$). It indicated that Xiaochaihu Decoction can eliminate the proteinuria of the patient and reduce his blood fat.

From the studies, it is found that the ancient prescriptions, such as Shi Zao Tang or Kong Xian Dan, Xue Fu Zhu Yu Tang, Chai Ling Tang, Chai Ling Tang with Tao Hong Si Wu Tang, also have the functions of removing proteinuria and edema, increasing plasma proteins and improving hyperlipemia, achieving good effect for treatment of this disease.

iii. Chinese patent medicine

1. Shen Yan Kang Fu Pian

Shen Yan Kang Fu Pian mainly comprised by American Ginseng, Ginseng, Rehmannia root, Eucommia Bark, Common Yam Rhizome, Hedyotis, black soybean, Glabrous Greenbrier Rhizome, Motherwort Herb, Salvia Root, Zexie, Lalang Grass Rhizome, Platycodon Root, with the effect of notifying kidney and spleen. It is mainly used for treatment of chronic glomerulonephritis. The patient who belongs to deficiency of both Qi and yin, deficiency of spleen and kidney, with toxic heat syndrome shows symptoms of mental weakness, soreness and weakness of waist and knees, facial edema, bloated legs, dizziness and tinnitus, proteinuria, Hematuria syndrome, etc. Main pharmacological effects include: ① repairing the damaged glomerular podocytes, and reducing protein loss; ② reducing high blood pressure, anti-inflammatory, diuresis, swelling, and improving kidney function; ③ antagonism of side effects of glucocorticoid. In the period of edema of Nephrotic Syndrome, it belongs to syndrome of spleen-kidney deficiency, and the treatment should be performed in the way of reinforcement and elimination in combination: inducing diuresis to reduce edema on the basis of warming kidney and strengthening spleen. Yin Shitao et al. discovered that Shenyan Kangfu Tablet combined with hormone can treat primary nephrotic syndrome, not only the total effective rate in experiment group was more effective than that in control group, but also indexes of urine protein quantitation of 24 h, serum creatinine, serum albumin, total cholesterol1 and triglycerides and so on were all improved. The results indicated that Shenyan Kangfu Tablet played a role in avoiding loss of urinary protein, correcting hypoalbuminemia and lipid-decreasing.

2. Okra Capsules

Okra Capsules are extracted from flowers of Abelmoschus Manihot, and mainly used to clear heat, promote dieresis, resolve toxin and disperse swelling. They are often used in dampness- heat syndrome of chronic nephritis, and the clinical manifestations of which are: swelling, lumbago, proteinuria, bloody urine, yellowish fur, etc. Research of modern pharmacology indicated that Okra Capsules have functions of anti - inflammation of the glomeruli immune response, clearing circulatory system of immune complexes, anti-platelet aggregation, reducing urine albumin, protecting renal function,etc. Experiments on animals indicated Okra Capsules could effectively clean oxygen radical, decrease urine albumin and increase levels of serum protein. Sun Yi et al. discovered that Okra Capsules together with Tripterygium Wilfordii Tablets could be used to treat primary nephrotic syndrome: both of them could reduce proteinuria, delay further failure of renal function, adjust immunity at the same time and reduce side effects of hormones.

3. Jin Shui Bao Capsule and Bai Ling Capsule

Jin Shui Bao and Bai Ling Capsules are Chinese patent medicine made of Chinese Caterpillar Fungus powder fermented through modern technology. Chinese Caterpillar Fungus, a kind of Sphaeria sinensis of Claviceps fungus, is rich in amino acids, polysaccharides, organic acids, a variety of trace elements, sterol and many other chemistry elements and it also has effects of protecting liver and kidney function, anti-inflammatory, adjusting immunity and so on. Hao Li et al. discovered Chinese Caterpillar Fungus together with Tripterygium Wilfordii could be used to reduce proteinuria and side effects of Tripterygium Wilfordii through experiments results of effects of Chinese Caterpillar Fungus together with Tripterygium Glycosides on podocytes of rats with diabetic kidney disease.

4. Tripterygium Wilfordii Tablets

Tripterygium Wilfordii a plant, belongs to Celastaraceae, Tripterygium, and its roots, stems, flowers are all toxic. Root xylem is the medicinal part after two layers of peelare removed,which is one of the most reliable Chinese patent medicines used for immunosuppression at present. Its mechanism action in kidney disease treatments mainly contains: ① anti-inflammatory, immunosuppression; ② protection and repair of damaged podocyte; ③ protection of renal tubular epithelium; ④ inhibition of proliferation of mesangial cells. Presently, research reports about Tripterygium Wilfordii treatment on primary nephrotic syndrome were all small and from single center study and most of them were used together with glucocorticoid (referred to as hormones) with reported effectiveness of 73.1%-96.9%. Many researchers suggested curative effect of Tripterygium Wilfordii should be related to pathological pattern. If pathological patterns wereminimal change nephropathy and mesangial proliferative glomerulonephritis, the curative effect wolud be better, with effective rate above 90%; the medicine's curative effect would be affected if lesion was worse, especially tubulointerstitium was heavily damaged. Previously, routine dose of Tripterygium Wilfordii was 1mg/(kg·d), based on the consideration of the toxicity of it. Researches in recent years verified double dose [2mg/(kg·d)], was better as inductive treatment. A variety researches of the Nanjing Military Region General Hospital verified that double doses of Tripterygium Wilfordii had obvious curative effect on nephrotic syndrome. Its overall response rate achieved 83.3% on the 4th week. For the cases in which hormone therapy was invalid, double doses of Tripterygium Wilfordiiare effective all the same. The best treatment period of double doses of Tripterygium Wilfordiiwas 8-12 weeks. In order to avoid recurrence, during the process of reducing medicine dosage, the dosage should be reduced gradually like hormones, namely reduced to 1.5 mg/(kg·d) at first and then reduce to 1 mg/(kg·d) and maintain it a month later. Patients with nephrotic syndrome were all in good tolerance of double doses of Tripterygium Wilfordii treatment, and the adverse effects rates were not markedly increased.

iv. Others

1. Moxibustion therapy

The therapy is also called "moxa-moxibustion", a treatment method of fumigating body acupoints directly or indirectly by lit moxa with effects of raising yang and lifting prolapsed zang-fu organs and activating yang qi. Its clinical practice forms contain moxibustion with moxa sticks, moxibustion with moxa cones, warming acupuncture and thermal box moxibustion, etc. Zhang Weishi et al. adopted warming acupuncture method together with Chinese materia medica to cure nephrotic syndrome and aimed acupuncture points mainly included CV4, CV6 and CV9. He treated 51 patients, among whom 31 patients'symptoms were relived totally, 8 patients' symptoms were relived basically, partial relief for 9 patients and ineffective for 3 patients, with an effectiveness of 94%. Zhuang Kesheng adopted ginger moxibustion with moxa cones and aimed acupuncture points mainly included CV4, CV3, CV6 CV9 and ST 36 to treat nephrotic syndrome purpuric nephritis for 4 weeks' courses of treatment. The results showed that urinary protein, serum albumin, serum cholesterol and urinary red blood cell count were all improved.

2. Acupoint application method

Attaching drugs to body acupoints to produce therapeutic action by stimulating acupuncture point, is a combined therapy that integrates meridian, acupuncture point and medicine as a whole. Zhang Zhenzhong adopted self-made Shenkang Application Agent (Clove, Milkvetch Root, Cassia Bark, Crystalline Lens, Rhubarb, Gansui Root, Pangolin Scales and Dried Body of Ground Beetle) modulated with ginger sauce and garlic, and applied on BL 23, KI 1, CV 8.c. Results showed that: the effect of experimental group was better than that of control group. This therapy could improve clinical symptoms, reduce proteinuria, relief the side effect of hormone and lower the recurrence rate. The herbal plaster (Gansui Root, Euphorbia pekinensis, Lilac Daphne Flower Bud, Processed Prepared Common Monkshood Daughter Root, Fennel, Plantain Seed andBomeol) was used by Wang Jun to cure primaryNS. Aimed acupuncture points mainly includedCV 8, BL 23, CV9, ST28, BL 22, BL 39 and SP 9. The result showed that in experimental group, the therapy could relieve the edema, increase urine volume, decrease urine protein, of which curative effect was better than that of the basic treatment only using western medicine.

3. Acupoint injection therapy

It is also called "hydro-acupuncture". Chinese and western medicines are injected to the specific acupuncture points for the treatment of the disease, which can improve immunity of the organism and prevent disease. Cao Yang applied acupoint injection therapy combined with prednisone in treatment of NS, with the aimed acupuncture points of BL 23 and ST 36, and injecting medicine of Heartleaf Houttuynia Herb injection. Therein, 1.5 ml was injected in BL 23 and 2 ml was injected in ST 36, with the course of treatment of two months. It was found that total effective rate of experimental group was 96.4% and that of control group was 63.2%. There was statistical difference ($P < 0.05$) in two groups. It was concluded that acupoint injection medicine with prednisone couldeffectively improve immunity of the patient. Yin Baoqi injected Milkvetch Root injection in BL 23 and ST 36 for the adjuvant therapy of primary NS. The result showed: 24-hour urinary protein quantity, plasma-albumin, serum cholesterol were respectively better than that before treatment, with significant difference, through follow-up visit of 2 months.

4. TCM clyster

It means intestinal infusion with TCM liquid or mixed with powder, to achieve treatment by using absorption function of rectal mucosa. Zhao Wei adopted TCM mixture retention enema(Components: Unprocessed Milkvetch Root, stir-frying White Atractylodes Rhizome, Common Yam Rhizome, Baical Skullcap Root, Salvia Root, Gordon Euryale Seed, Dried Tangerine Peel, Cherokee Rose Fruit, Smoked Plum, Liquorice Root. They were prepared to 250ml of decoctum and taken two times per day) to cure primary NS of children. The total effective rate of experimental group was 93.33%, and that of control group was 80.00%. There was significant difference ($P < 0.01$) before and after the treatment, showing a good clinical effect. TCM retention enema (Components: 30g of Milkvetch Root, 15g of Common Yam Rhizome, 20g of Tangshen, 15g of Indian Bread, 15g of Sichuan Lovage Rhizome, 20g of Motherwort Herb, 15g of Songaria Cynomorium Herb, 15g of Hirsute Shiny Bugleweed Herb, 15g of Gordon Euryale Seed, 10g of Divaricate Saposhnikovia Root, 30g of Lalang Grass Rhizome, 15g of Amur Cork-Tree. They were made into 200-300ml of enema liquid) was adopted by Huang Lingli to treatrefractory NS of children. Enema volume: for the patient aged below 3 years, 50-80ml/time; for the patient aged over 3 years, 80-120ml/time. The results showed: compared with the group only using western medicine, the symptom, blood fat and urine protein quantitation were all improved, with significant statistical difference (P<0.05). The author applied Shen Xi Chun Enema Liquid (Unprocessed Milkvetch Root of 30g, Raw Oyster Shell of 30g, Safflower of 15g, Rhubarb of 15g, Dandelion of 30g, Viola of 30g) in the treatment of patient with NS and renal failure. The patient was advised to control the temperature of Shenxichun Enema Liquid between 37℃ and 40℃, with 250ml per time; patient shall lie on right side, with left led bended. Enema tube was slightly put in the anus for about 15cm deep, opening nearly 1/3 of water shut-off valve. Speed should be adjusted depending on condition of each person. If patient has desire to defecate, the speed can be slowed, or the water valve was closed first, enema was continued after desire to defecate was relieved 30 seconds to 1 minute later. The patient shall lie on the back after completion of enema. Left abdomen should be pressed about 3-5 minutes, for ensuring full absorption of medicine in the body. This therapy could effectively improve proteinuria of patient and decrease index of creatinine.

V. Empirical prescription of famous physicians and experts

Treatment based on syndrome differentiation is the process to know and treat the disease in TCM, and the thinking and practice process to analyze data, symptoms and signs of relevant diseases with TCM theory, and to determine syndromes and identify the therapeutic principles and methods so as to put into practice through analysis and synthesis. Now, experience of famous physicians and experts is introduced below.

i. Removing edema based on "circulation" (Zhang Qi)

Professor Zhang Qi thinks that the transportation and transformation of urine are related to all the zang-organs in his treatment of refractory NS edema, and that the edema forms because "Sanjiao stagnates, and the meridians and collaterals are blocked." When treating edema, Professor Zhang emphasizes "circulation", thinking that qi transformation of lung, spleen, kidney, Sanjiao is the first step to treat edema. He classifies the therapies into the following categories: ① Reliving lung for diuresis: it is created by Zhu Danxi, which means "taking ascending as descending". Professor Zhang thinks that refractory NS edema patients take hormone and immunosuppressor over and over again in a long time, which leads to the insufficiency of yang qi in Taiyin and Shaoyin, thus wind edema forms as "it cannot get inside zang-fu organs, nor can it get outside of the skin; it lingers in the sweat pore and under the skin, and then becomes swelling and aching of the instep." In clinic, Supplemented Jia Wei Yue Bi Tang relieving edema is often used (15g of Ephedra, 50g of Gypsum, 15g of Fresh Ginger, 3g Red Dates, 7g of Licorice,10g of Bitter Apricot Seed,10g of Atractylodes, 50g of Watermelon Peel, 50g of Red Beans, 25g of Plantain Seed) for ventilating lungs and stomach, and excreting water. ② Water and heat method to clear the Sanjiao: this method aims at curing the syndrome of water and heat binding together because of diffusive dampness-heat in Sanjiao. It can be used in the treatment of chronic nephritis, NS syndrome. Symptoms include anasarca, abdominal distention, difficult urination, yellow and large quantities of urine, constipation, dry mouth and thirsty, thick and greasy tongue fur, deep and slippery pulse, or quick pulse. Prescription includes Shu Zao Yin Zi. Components: 20g of Areca Seed, 15g of Areca Peel, 15gof Poria Peel, 15g of Seed of Peppertree Pricklyash, 15g of Pokeberry Root, 50g of Red Beans, 15g of Largeleaf Gentian Root, Incised Notopterygium Rhizome and Root of 15g, Akebia Stem of 15g, Ginger Skin of 15g, 15g of Plantain Seed, 20g of Grass of Common KnotGrass, 30g of Seaweed, 20g of Pharbitis Seed. ③ Clearing heat and draining dampness method to replenish qi and nourish yin: this method is used to treat deficiency of both qi and yin and linger dampness and heat. The symptomsshowed fatigue limbs, shortage of qi and declination to speak, mouth parched and tongue scorched, loss of appetite and anorexia, vexing heat in chest, palms and soles, slight edema or no edema, red-tipped tongue, slightly greasy tongue, thread and rapid or slippery pulse. Prescription includes Qin Xin Lian Zi Yin. Components: 15g of Nelumbo nucifera Gaerth, 20g of Tangshen, 15g of Chinese Wolf berry Root-bark, 15g ofIndian Bread, 15g of Bupleurum, 15g of Dwarf Lilyturf Tuber, 15g of Plantain Seed, 30g of Baical Skullcap Root, 30g of Unprocessed Milkvetch Root, 30g of Hedyotis, 30g of Motherwort Herb,10g of Liquorice Root. ④ Tonifying the kidney essence method: this method is aimed at the pathogeneses of insecurity of kidney qi and leaked essential qi. The symptomsshowed sore and weak of waist and knees, dizziness and tinnitus, spermatorrhea and seminal leakage, fat tongue body, pink tongue, deep or weak pulse.Prescription includes modified Ba Wei Shen Qi Wan. Components: 7g of Prepared Common Monkshood Daughter Root, 7g of Cassia Bark, 20g of Prepared Rehmannia Root, 15g of Asiatic Cornelian Cherry Fruit, 20g of Common Yam Rhizome, 20g of Indian Bread, 15g of Tree Peony Root Bark, 15g of Oriental Waterplantain Rhizome, 20g of Dodder Seed, 20g of Barbary Wolfberry Fruit, 15g of Mantis Egg-Case, 20g of Cherokee Rose Fruit.

ii. Treating Children with NS in accordance with clinical stages (Li Shaochuan)

Children's NS is distributed into three stages clinically.

(1) First stage: symptoms showsdeficiency in root, and spleen's failure in transformation, wind pathogen attacking the exterior, stuffy lung qi, dampness impregnation and inundation of adversity. It is always treated with modified Yue Bi Jia Zhu Tang, Yin Qiao Si Ling Tang (Yin Qiao San combined with Si Ling Tang), Xing Su San, Shu Feng Tong Qi Tang. Common components: Ephedra, Apricot Seed, Perilla Stem Leaves, White Atractylodes Rhizome, Indian Bread, Common Anemarrhena Rhizome, Oriental Waterplantain Rhizome, Honeysuckle Flower, Weeping Forsythia Capsule, etc.

(2) Chronic stage: 1) The treatment of syndromeofdampnessstagnancy duetospleendeficiency centers on notifying spleen and clearing dampness, coordinated with promoting the circulation of qi and its prescription is modified Wei Ling Tang. Common components: Perilla Stem, Indian Bread, Officinal Magnolia Bark, Oriental Waterplantain Rhizome, Ophiopogon, Dried Tangerine Peel, Heterophylly Falsestarwort Root, Medicated Leaven, etc. 2) The treatment of syndrome of heat transformed from stagnated dampness centers on eliminating dampness with aromatics, clearing heat and dampness. Sweet Dew Detoxication Pill is chosen for clearing heat without obstructing dampness, draining dampness without impairing yin. The dampness and heat are both treated coordinating with smoothing the movement of qi. Common components: Cablin Patchouli Herb, Weeping Forsythia Capsule, Roud Cardamon Seed, Officinal Magnolia Bark, Indian Bread, Oriental Waterplantain Rhizome, Perilla Stem, Talc, Common Anemarrhena Rhizome, Amur Cork-Tree, etc. 3) The treatment of syndrome of yin deficiency and effulgent fire centers on notifying the liver and kidney, coordinated with strengthening spleen and regulating the stomach. Prescription includes Yu Nyu Jian, Zhen Gan Xi Feng Tang, Zhi Bai Di Huang Tang, modified Three Prescriptions and Stomach Calming Decoction. Common components: Prepared Rehmannia Root, Asiatic Cornelian Cherry Fruit, Common Anemarrhena Rhizome, Amur Cork-Tree, Dwarf Lilyturf Tuber, Common Yam Rhizome, Atractylodes Rhizome, Indian Bread, Officinal Magnolia Bark, Perilla Stem, Oriental Waterplantain Rhizome, Malaytea Scurfpea Fruit, Unprocessed Rehmannia Root, etc.

(3) Remission period: Characteristics of this periodare that the edema abates, proteinuria turns negative, increased diet, pale complexion, lazy and declination to speak, sweat automatically and easily get infected with disease, pale red tongue and white fur, rapid pulse. Deficiency of lung-qi and spleen-qi is a common syndrome in the later stage of nephropathy, and the key point in this period is to easily get infected and recurrence. Cold or diarrhea of the sick children can all cause the recurrence of the disease. The main treatment of the remission period is strengthening the spleen and smoothing qi with Shen Ling Bai Zhu San, Tian Bao Cai Wei Tang, and Fei Er Wan. Common components: Heterophylly Falsestarwort Root, Indian Bread, White Atractylodes Rhizome, Common Yam Rhizome, Kudzuvine Root, Incised Notopterygium Rhizome and Root, Doubleteeth Pubescent Angelica Root, Chinese Thorowax Root, Dried Tangerine Peel, Officinal Magnolia Bark, Common Anemarrhena

Rhizome, etc. Professor Li attaches much importance to strengthening spleen and clearing dampness in the treatment of nephropathy, combining strengthening spleen and draining dampness with nourishing yin and for moistening dryness to avoid dryness and diuresis to damage yin.

iii. Removing edema by differentiating syndrome and diagnosis

(1) Spleen-kidney yang deficiency syndrome: Its treatment focuses on warming yang and excreting water. Its prescription includes Zhen Wu Tang and Wu Ling San, Ji Sheng Shen Qi Wan, and Shen Shui San (experienced prescription). Components: 12g of Prepared Common Monkshood Daughter Root, 12g of White Atractylodes Rhizome, 30g of Indian Bread, 10g of Fresh Ginger, 15g of Oriental Waterplantain Rhizome, 10g of Cassia Bark, 10g of Chuling of 15g, 10g of Fenugreek, Common Curculigo Rhizome.

(2) Syndrome of dampness stagnancy due to spleen deficiency: its treatment centers on replenishing qi and strengthening spleen, drying the dampness and excreting water. Its prescription includes Fang Ji Fu Ling Tang, Shen Ling Bai Zhu San, Wei Ling Tang. Components: 15g of Stephania, 10g of Cassia Twig, 30g of unprocessed Milkvetch Root, 30g of Indian Bread, 12g of Tangshen, 12g of White Atractylodes Rhizome, 15g of Coix Seed, 10g of Hyacinth Bean, 15g of Common Yam Rhizome, 6g of Liquorice Root.

(3) Syndrome of wind pathogen attacking the lungs: its treatment is dispersing wind, ventilating lungs and excreting water. Its prescription includes Yue Bi Jia Zhu Tang and Wu Hu Yin, Ma Huang Lian Qiao Chi Xiao Dou Tang. Components: 10g of Ephedra, 30g of Gypsum, 10g of Liquorice Root, 3 pieces Fresh Ginger, 4 Chinese Date, 12g of White Atractylodes Rhizome, 10g of White Mulberry Root-Bark, 30g of Poria peel, 15g of Dried Tangerine Peel, 10g of Areca Peel.

(4) Syndrome of qi stagnation and water retention: its treatment is replenishing qi and excreting water. Its prescription includes modified Da Ju Pi Tang and Mu Xiang Liu Qi Yin. 10g of Tangerine Peel, 12g of Talc, 15g of Red poria, 15g of Chuling, 15g of Oriental Waterplantain Rhizome, 5g of Cassia Bark, 2 pieces Fresh Ginger, 6g of Common Aucklandia Root, 10g of Areca Seed, 12g of Combined Spicebush Root, 10g of Chinese Clematis Root, 6g of Common Floweringqince Fruit.

(5) Syndrome of blood stasis and water resistance: its treatment is activating blood, resolving stasis and excreting water. Its prescription includes modified Dang Gui Shao Yao San. 12g of Chinese Angelica, 15g of Red Peony Root, 10g of Sichuan Lovage Rhizome, 15g of Indian Bread, 12g of White Atractylodes Rhizome, 15g of Oriental Waterplantain Rhizome, 30g of Salvia Root, 10g of Peach Seed, 10gof Safflower, 30g of Motherwort Herb, 15g of Plantain Seed.

(6) Syndrome of dampness and heat stagnation: its treatment is clearing heat and expelling dampness to disperse the stagnation. Its prescription includes Bi Xie Fen Qing Yin, Wu Wei Xiao Du Yin, with modified Zhu Ling Tang for those patients who have deficiency yin and carry dampness. 15g of Rhizoma Dioscoreae, 10g of Grassleaf Sweetflag Rhizome, 10g of White Atractylodes Rhizome, 15g of Salvia Root, 6g of Lotus Plumule, 15g of Indian Bread, 10g of Amur Cork-Tree, 10g of Plantain Seed, 30g of Honeysuckle Flower, 10g of Weeping Forsythia Capsule, 10g of Dandelion, 10g of Tokyo Violet Herb.

iv. Differentiation treatment based on clinical menifestation (Zhao Yuyong)

Zhao Yuyong thinks that the characteristics of the clinical manifestations should be noted, and NS should be treated by distinguishing its characteristics and studying its symptoms combined with theory of traditional Chinese medicine.

(1) Yin edema is usually treated by strengthening spleen and replenishing qi, abating edema and excreting water. It is usually treated with modified Wu Pi Yin and Wu Ling San: Indian Bread of 15g, Chulingof 10g, White Atractylodes Rhizome of 10g, Oriental Waterplantain Rhizome of 10g, Areca Peel of 10g, Cassia Twig of 6g, White Mulberry Root-Bark of 10g, Dried Tangerine Peel of 6g, Motherwort Herb of 20g, Lalang Grass

Rhizome of 20g. The symptomsof yang edema may appear if the patient is again attacked by wind pathogen. To treat patients with wind-cold, modified Ma Xing Wu Pi Yin are used: Ephedra of 6g, Apricot Seed of 9g, Poria Peel of 15g, Dried Tangerine Peel of 6g, Areca Peel of 9g, White Mulberry Root-Bark of 12g, Fresh Ginger Peel of 3g, Plantain Seed of 15g. For patient whose exterior pathogen disappears, he/she can be treated by the above prescription except Ephedra and Apricot Seed, added with Corn Stigma of 30g, and Lalang Grass Rhizome of 30g. To treat patients with wind-heat, Yue Bi Tang and modified Ma Huang Lian Qiao Chi Xiao Dou Tang used: Ephedra of 6g, Gypsum of 30g, Weeping Forsythia Capsule of 9g, Baical Skullcap Root of 12g, Rice Bean of 30g, Heartleaf Houttuynia Herb of 15g, Platycodon Root of 3g, Lalang Grass Rhizome of 15g, Reed Rhizome of 30g.

(2) Protein malnutrition is the manifestation of syndrome ofspleen and kidney deficiency. It is usually treated with Liu Jun Zi Tang, etc. which can strengthen spleen and smooth qi. In addition, Milkvetch Root has better curative effect in treating protein malnutrition, whose dose of common usage is 10 to 40g. Milkvetch Root can replenish qi, consolidate exterior, excrete water and abate edema, which is a commonly used medicine in treating nephropathy. More unprocessed Milkvetch Root should be used, coordinated with qi-regulating and blood-activating medicine for the treatment.

(3) For those patients with renal collateral stasis and obstruction, Professor Zhao adopts replenishing kidney and dredging collateral method and blood-activating and stasis-resolving method with modified Tao Hong Si Wu Tang: Chinese Angelica of 12g, Unprocessed Rehmannia Root of 15g, Red Peony Root of 12g, Peach Seed of 9g, Safflower of 9g, Sichuan Lovage Rhizome of 9g, Motherwort Herb of 12g, Epimedium Herb of 12g, Salvia Root of12g, Fried Pangolin Scale of 6g, adding Leech of 3g for those with serious blood-stasis. For patients with refractory proteinuria but without blood stasis symptom, worm medicine can be added, such as Black-Tail Snake, Earthworm, Stiff Silkworm, Cicada Slough, Scorpion, Centipede, etc. which has the function of decreasing albuminuria. For some patients, medicines such as Tripterygium wilfordi, Orientvine Vine can also be added, which has the function of adjusting immunity. When Tripterygium wilfordi is put into use, firstly, its peel should be removed; secondly, it should be fried for a long time to decrease its poisonous effects.

VI. Typical medical records of famous physicians and experts

i. Medical record of Zou Yunxiang ——depression and stagnation of Qi and blood as well as phlegm-dampness

Mr. Sun, male, 16 years old, preliminary diagnosis on June 26, 1972.

He came to see a doctor because of edema in February, 1972, who was checked out urine protein (+++), pyocyte (+), erythrocyte 1-3, and was found granular casts and hyaline cast. He was checked out cholesterol 23.34mmol/L, plasma albumin 27g/L and globulin 24g/L, so he was diagnosed as "Nephrotic Syndrome" and he was in hospital to accept treatment in April 20. He was given a treatment of hormone for 2 months. Because of the obvious side effects of hormone, he was discharged in June 20 and went to Mr. Zou's hospital to accept the traditional Chinese medicine's therapy on June 26.

He had distending pain of waist, headache, alopecia and copious sweat. Besides, he was fat and he had edema in whole body. His UV became decreased and he had wiry pulse and greasy tongue fur. Urinalysis: protein was mainly dominant by (+++) and the pyocyte, epithelial cells, erythrocyte and granular casts was in the minority.

Syndrome differentiation: depression and stagnation of Qi and blood as well as phlegm-dampness.

Therapeutic method: dredging and dispersing.

Prescription: 6g Atractylodes Rhizome, 12g Raw Coix Seed, 9g Indian Bread, 6g Prepared Pinellia Tuber, 6g Dried Tangerine Peell, 15g Silktree Albizia Bark, 15g Glutinous Rice Rhizome, 6g Dipsacus Asperoides, 9g

Safflower, 9g Puncturevine Caltrop Fruit, and 12g Yue Ju Wan. It is taken by decoction with 2 does per day.

If one breathes hard, the prescription needs to be added with Heterophylly Falsestarwort Root, Milkvetch Root, Codonopsis pilosula and Chinese Date; if one has anemia, the prescription needs to be added with Chinese Angelica, Debark Peony Root, Barbary Wolfberry Fruit, Magnetite and Whole Deer Pill; if one had dry mouth, the prescription needs to be added with Snakegourd Root, Dendrobium, Adenophora Stricta, Figwort Root and dried Radix Rehmanniae; if one has poor appetite and loose stools, the prescription needs to be added with Fried Common Yam Rhizome and Gordon Euryale Seed; if one has the obvious pain of waist, the prescription needs to be added with Mahonia Leaf; urinalysis: when the erythrocyte is (++), the prescription needs to be added with Lalang Grass Rhizome, Amber, Yerba-Detajo Herb and Glossy Privet Fruit.

The modified prescription had been used for treating the patient for 3 months. His edema was alleviated and the urine volume was about 1000ml per day. Urinalysis: protein (+) – (++). After the 5-month therapy, the urinary protein was in the microscale. Until the autumn in 1973, the patient had no subjective symptoms, the edema disappeared and the spirit recovered. The protein in urinalysis was extremely little. The urine specific gravity was 1.012. The blood pressure was 110/68 mmHg. Disease relapse didn't occur until the summer in 1977 through follow-up.

Note: According to the theory of ascending, descending, exiting and entering in *Inner Canon of Huangdi*, Mr. Zou pointed out that "the disruption of ascending, descending, exiting and entering makes vital activity and Qi configuration die out and disappear." In *Discussion on Principles of Five Normalities* of *Plain Questions* the writer said "There exist all ascending, descending, exiting and entering. It is valuable to keep them, otherwise we will have diseases." In addition, in this book, the writer also said "the four factors can be divided into 2 groups, including ascending and descending, and exiting and entering. The four factors can be classified into a word Qi, which every disease all originated from." In *Danxi's Experiential Therapy*, the writer said "the coordination of Qi and blood can make disease get away and the depression can make us have all kinds of diseases." Depression can cause Qi stagnation so as tomake the function of ascending, descending, exiting and entering ineffective. When ascending, descending, exiting and entering don't work, the clearness becomes turbid and the body has obstruction. Moreover, the surface loses protection and the interior doesn't operate so that they don't work. Cushing syndrome caused by hormone shows dysfunction of ascending, descending, exiting and entering. It can hurt Qi tier at first and after a long time, it also hurts blood tier. Besides, the symbol turns from subtle Qi and blood to dampness turbidity and phlegm and blood stasis. And it is formed by the obstruction of viscera, collateral and muscular striae. In *Discussion and Events of Six Pathogenic Factors* of *Plain Questions,* the writer said "liver Qi depression needs transforming into fire; fire stagnation needs removing; earth stagnation needs eliminating; lung Qi needs expelling and dispersing; fluid stagnation needs regulating." According to the theory of *Inner Canon of Huangdi*, Mr. Zou creates a method of negotiating Qi depression and purging turbid from the therapy of nephrotic syndrome and drug-induced Cushing syndrome. He uses the prescription of Atractylodes Rhizome, Coix Seed, Nutgrass Galingale Rhizome, Turmeric Root Tuber, Silktree Albizia Bark, Pinellia Tuber, Dried Tangerine Peel, Chinese Angelica, Safflower, Sichuan Lovage Rhizome, Peach Seed, medicated leaven, Indian Bread and Reed Rhizome to negotiate Qi and blood and purge dampness turbidity and phlegm and blood stasis. The method and prescription makes the disfunction of ascending, descending, exiting and entering recover and has a satisfactory effect.

ii. Medical record of Zhu Chenyu ——insufficiency of both the spleen and kidneys, internal stagnation of fluid-dampness.

Mr. Yang, male, 18 years old.

Preliminary diagnosis: on April 5,1978. Chief complaint: the patient had edema for more than 2 years. He had lots of proteinuria with edema 2 years ago and then he was diagnosed as Nephrotic Syndrome. During this time, he took hormone to treat without best efficiency, so he came to see a doctor. The patient took prednisone about 400mg/d orally, and PRO was (3+-4+) by examination at that time, and ration of PRO in 24 hours was more than 3g.

Present symptoms: His double lambs were obviously bloated and sunken after pressing. He has plenty of urine volume. The patient was fat but weak. After the cold, he was easy to have sore throat, soreness of the waist and the knees, and the general fatigue. He had swollen tongue, red tip of tongue, tongue with teeth prints and deep and thin pulse.

Syndrome differentiation: insufficiency of both the spleen and kidney, internal stagnation of fluid-dampness.

Therapeutic method: strengthen the spleen and kidney, induce diuresis and alleviate edema.

Prescription: modified Liu Wei Di Huang Tang and Fang Ji Huang Qi Tang. There are 10g of Unprocessed Rehmannia Root, 10g of Prepared Rehmannia Root, 10g ofChinese Magnoliavine Fruit, 10g of Common Yam Rhizome, 10g of Tree Peony Root Bark, 25g ofIndian Bread, 10g of Oriental Waterplantain Rhizome, 30g of Milkvetch Root, 10g of Fourstamen Stephania Root, 10g of Rhizoma Atractylodis Macrocephalae, 5g of Radix Glycyrrhizae Preparata, 15g of black lotus seed, 15g of Hanliancao, 30g of Plantain Herb, and 30g of Hedyotis. It is taken by decoction with 2 doses per day.

After taking more than 30 doses of the modified prescription, the patient felt his physical strength increased and number of having a cold decreased, and his edema was alleviated. The ration of PRO was in range of 2.3 – 3.2g through 24-hours test. Maintained prescriptionwasadded by 15g Dodder Seed. After continuing to take 45 doses of the prescriptions, the patient's edema was alleviated and his physical strength was basically recovered, and the patient was tested PRO (-). The ration of taking prednisone orally was reduced to 30mg/d and the number of taking medicines was totally more than 90 doses. After treating for 3 months, the patient's edema had faded and the ration of 24-hours PRO was little. His ration of taking prednisone orally was reduced to 20mg/d and was maintained. Therefore the original prescription was slightly to make pills. The pills were assigned, sustained and reduced.

Note: When predecessors discussed about edema, they would always mention lungs, spleen and kidneys. Just like Zhang Yueyun said that "edema and other symptoms are the diseases related to lungs, spleen and kidneys. The nature of water pertains to beginning of yin, so edema is controlled by spleen. Water is transformed from Qi, so it appears in lungs; water is suppressed byearth, so it is controlled by the spleen."It is known that controlling the water and reinforcing deficiency are two rules to treat the edema. The course of this medical record had lasted for 2 years. The swell was serious and healthy atmosphere is weak, so it was difficult to treat. If using the method to eliminate the water, t would have been effective in a short term but it could not bea good way to recover the vital Qi.

iii. Medical record of Zhang Qi ——retention of dampness-heat

In May 1989, Mr. Zou, male, 35 years old, was diagnosed as Nephrotic Syndrome. He suffered from high fullness (ascites), nausea and vomiting. In addition, he didn't want to eat and he was parched. There were little urine (about 200-300 milliliters in 24 hours), flushed face, yellow greasy fur and sunken pulse. PRO (++++),urea nitrogen of 13.9mmol/L, creatinine of 176.8 μmol/L. He often used traditional Chinese medicine, western medicine and diuretics, but they were inefficient. Therefore he came to ask for the medical consultation.

Syndrome differentiation: syndrome of damp-heat in spleen and stomach, internal accumulation of damp-heat, mixture of the clear and the turbid, and the adverse kidneys.

Therapeutic method: invigorate spleen and eliminate dampness, distribute clear heat with bitter cold.

Prescription: 15g of Coptis chinensis Franch, 15g of YunQin, 15g of pinellia ternate, 15gof Villons Amomum Fruit, 15g of magnolia obavata, 15g of Immature Orange Fruit, 15g of Dried Tangerine Peel, 15g of anemarrhenae, 15g of Oriental Waterplantain Rhizome, 15g of Turmeric, 15g of Indian Bread, 15g of Chuling, 10g of atractylodes macrocephala koidz, 15g of Tangshen, 10g of Liquorice Root. It is taken decocted with water.

The patient took 5 doses of the medicine and as a result, his abdominal distension was reduced; his urine volume increased; and the medicines relieved edema obviously. The prescription was varied and the patient even took it about more than 30 doses. The appetite of the patient increased and hissymptoms disappeared. Tongue coating was changed and the pulse became slow. PRO (+), 6.35mmol/L urea nitrogen. After the continuing treatment, PRO turned to be negative totally.

Note: Professor Zhang Qi thinks that damp-heat in spleen and stomach, internal accumulation of damp-heatand the adverse kidneys are the etiology of this disease. This prescription was called as ZhongmanfenxiaoPill. LiDongyuan used it to treat damp-heat and flatulence. In this prescription,Coptis chinensisandBaikal Skullcap have function of clearing heat and disintegrating masses with bitter cold. Dried Ginger and Villons Amomum Fruit can warm up stomach, invigorate spleen and eliminate dampness. Turmeric and Fructus Aurantiiand Mangnolia Officinalis promote Qi and relieve fullness. Anemarrhenae nourishes kidney yin. Indian Breadeliminates dampness with bland medicinal. Tangshen,atractylodes macrocephala koidz,Dried Tangerine Peel,Liquorice Root invigorate spleen and reinforce stomach. The therapy of diminishing and nourishing and the use of cold and heat simultaneously make the damp-heat distribute, the lucidity ascend and the turbidity descend, so the edema is eliminated.

iv. Medical record of Yu Chunquan —— deficiency of both the spleen and kidneys

Mr. Wang, male, 66 years old. He was firstly diagnosed on January 21, 2015.

He came to see a doctor because of the edema of double lower limbs. The patient said he had experienced the edema of double lower limbs1 month ago, so he was diagnosed in nephrology outpatientof a Grade 3A hospital in Tianjin. Examination: the ration of PRO in 24h: 5.80g/24h, albumin 32.0g/L, TC: 5.65mmol/L. He was diagnosed as Nephrotic Syndrome. The therapeutic efficacy was not good, thus he came to the Chinese medical department for help. At the time of diagnosis, the patient showed the edema of double lower limbs and higher blood pressure in normal times (up to 160/100mmHg), lumbago, poor appetite, lacking in strength, stable sleep, more foam in urine, less stool (it occured every two days and was drier), pale purple tongue texture, less tongue fur as well as wiry and slippery pulse.

Syndrome differentiation: deficiency of both the spleen and kidney.

Therapeutic method: invigorate spleen, replenish kidney, activate blood and promote the diuresis.

Prescription: 30g of Unprocessed Milkvetch Root, 15g of Indian Bread, 15g of Chuling, 15g ofOriental Waterplantain Rhizome, 15g of White Atractylodes Rhizome, 15g of Cassia Twig, 15g of Chinese Angelica, 15g of Fourstamen Stephania Root, 10g of Prepared Rehmannia Root, 10g of Asiatic Cornelian Cherry Fruit, 10g of Common Yam Rhizome, 10g of Earthworm, 8g of Stiff Silkworm, 8g of Black-Tail Snake, 30g of ustulated malt, 15g ofSpine Date Seed, and 15g ofTuber Fleeceflower Stem. It is taken by decoction with 2 doses per day.

The prescription was varied and he was treated continuously for 3 months. As a result, PRO returned to normal and the edema didn't appear on his double lower limbs. The patient shouldtake hypotensor (Norvasc) in daily life and he was suggested to regulate life style.

Note: The writer uses Wu Ling San with Fang Ji Huang Qi Tang to warm up yang and resolve Qi, and excrete damp and promote water. Milkvetch Root is added into the ration of 30g, which is testified by the modern science that it has the effect of inducing dieresis.Tonifying Qi, fades humidity and eliminates edema. He also uses Chinese Angelica, Earthworm, Black-Tail Snake and Stiff Silkworm. Black-Tail Snake dispels wind and dredges collaterals; Earthworm and Stiff Silkworm resolves stasis and dredges collaterals; Chinese Angelica nourishes blood, activate blood and resolves stasis. Nephrotic Syndromes conforms to the etiology of the long-course cases and kidney collateral stasis. Using pungent and salty salt medicines, such as Black-Tail Snake, Earthworm, Stiff Silkworm and other gondii and ant things, can reach into collaterals toremove obstruction in them. Lots of clinical practice proves that adding the drugs of activating blood and resolving stasis into the therapy of CGD can control the formation of immunocomplex and prevent from and postpone nephrosclerosis.

VII. Prevention and aftercare

Among patients with NS, infection occurs in most of them. In patients with NS and infection, infection sites mainly include respiratory tract, urinary system, peritoneum, skin soft tissue, etc. Water-sodium retention easily occurs in lung tissue space and pleural cavity of patient, providing condition for growth of bacteria. It is easy for pathogenic bacteria to enter the body through respiratory tract because it is connected to the outside world. Combined infection of patients with NS mostly occurs in the respiratory tract. Therefore, the author paid more attention to the thought of TCM, i.e. "A better physician shall not focus on treatment of the disease that has already happened (with obvious symptom), but shall pay attention to the preventive treatment of disease."Patientswere advised to strengthen self-care, especially prevent respiratory disease, and to avoid cold, greasy and spicy food, seafood and red meat in the daily time. Some studies indicated that high protein diet can increase hypertransfusion and high filtration of glomerulus, so as to cause kidney hypertrophy, increase workload of nephron and damage the kidney structure; degree of high filtration can be relieved by taking low-protein diet which can slow down the falling rate of glomerular filtration rate at the same timeso that delay the deterioration of kidney function. As to the selection of proteins, red meat (pork, beef and mutton) has greater effect on hemodynamics of kidney than that of white meat (chicken and fish meat). In the therapeutic measures of preventing patient with chronic renal disease from renal function failure, low-protein diet was considered as one of effective measures in recent years.

(YU Chunquan)

References

[1] Ye RG, Chen YS, Fang JA, et al. Panel discussion summary about diagnosis and treatment of kidney disease[J]. Chinese Journal of Integrated Traditional and Western Nephrology, 2003, 4(6):355-357.

[2] Llach F. Thromboembolic complications in the nephrotic syndrome. Coagulation abnormalities, renal vein thrombosis and other conditions[J]. Postgrad Med, 1984, 76(6): 111-114, 116-118, 121-123.

[3] Nachman PH, Jennette JC, Falk RJ. Primary Glomerular Disease. In: Brenner BM eds. Brenner and Rector's The Kidney[M]. 8th ed. Philadelphia: WB Saunders, 2007: 987-1066.

[4] Kitiyakara C, Kopp JB, Eggers P. Trends in the epidemiology of focal segmental glomerulosclerosis[J]. Semin Nephrol, 2003, 23: 172-182.

[5] Research Group on Progressive Chronic Renal Disease. Nation-wide and long term survey of glomerulone-phritis in Japan as observed in 1850 biopsied cases[J]. Nephron, 1999, 82: 205-213.

[6] Zhou FD, Zhao MH, Zou WZ, et al. The changing spectrum of primary glomerular disease within 15 years: a survey of 3331 patients in a single Chinese centre[J]. Nephrol Dial Transplant, 2009, 24: 870-876.

[7] Shi SH. 36,379 cases of glomerulopathy type and epidemiological analysis in China[D]. Fuzhou: Fujian Medical University, 2012.

[8] Orth SR, Ritz E. The nephrotic syndrome[J]. N Engl J Med, 1998, 338: 1202-1211.

[9]   Eddy AA, Symons JM. Nephrotic syndrome in childhood[J]. Lancet, 2003, 362: 629-639.

[10] Dai LQ. 12 cases with NS are treated with modified ZhenWu Decoction[J]. Journal of Gannan Medical University, 2005, 25(6):834.

[11] Hao KH, Zhang YK. 90 cases with NS are treated with ZhenWu Decoction[J]. Guangming Journal of Chinese Medicine, 2015, 30(6):1231-1232.

[12] Xia JH. 60 cases with primary NS are treated with Supplemented Xiao Chai Hu Decoction[J]. Shandong Journal of Traditional Chinese Medicine, 2010, 29(3):159-160.

[13] Jiang EX. Experience to control saliva, induce diuresis and reduce edema with Ten Jujubes Decoction, as to NS[J]. Henan Traditional Chinese Medicine, 1981, 1(6):32-33.

[14] Tian WJ, Zou J. Mechanism study summary of Blood House Stasis-Expelling Decoction treating NS[J]. Practical Clinical Journal of Integrated Traditional Chinese and Western Medicine, 2005,5(5):90-91.

[15] Kosuke Fujita, Chen YP. Progress of Japan's Chinese medicine treating NS of children[J].Chinese Journal of Integrated Traditional and Western Nephrology, 2008, 9(1):81-82.

[16] Xu DL, Liu CX. Research on Chailing Decoction complicated with Tao Hong Si Wu Tang treating NS with hyperlipidemia[J]. Modern Journal of Integrated Traditional Chinese and Western Medicine, 2004, 13(6):722-723.

[17] Xie H, Huang ZY, Liu Y, et al. Functional mechanism and curative effect observation of Shenyan Kangfu tablet treating glomerulonephritis[J]. Journal of Henan University of Chinese Medicine, 2005, 20(5):22-23.

[18] Yin ST and Peng YP. Clinical observation of Shenyan Kangfu tablet combined with Candesartan treating primary NS[J]. Beijing University of Chinese Medicine, 2012, 31(7):539-541.

[19] Yin LF, Liu L, Gong YX, et al. Research on protective effect of Abelmoschus manihot for kidney tubules damage of NS model rat[J]. Journal of Capital Medical University, 2000, 21(3):209-211.

[20] Sun Y, Fu B. Clinical observation of okra capsule combined with Tripterygium Wilfordii Tablet treating primary NS[J]. Jilin Journal of Traditional Chinese Medicine, 2012, 32(6):596-597.

[21] Hao L, Pan MS, Zheng Y, et al. Experiment research on influence of Chinese Caterpillar Fungus and Tripterygium Wilfordii on sertoli cell of DN rat[J]. Chinese Journal of Integrated Traditional and Western Medicine, 2012, 32(2):261-265.

[22] Lu YQ. 26 cases with primary NS are treated with Tripterygium Wilfordii and Prednisone[J]. China's Naturopathy, 2004, 12(12):46.

[23] Zhai XS. Curative effect analysis of Tripterygium Wilfordii and Prednisone treating 32 cases with NS[J]. Journal of Modern Medicine,2004, 20(21):2246-2247.

[24] Zhu XL. Clinical research of double doses of Tripterygium Wilfordii and Prednisone treating primary NS[J]. Zhejiang Medical Journal, 2007, 9(2):764-765.

[25] Chen Y, Huang JP, Ding J, et al. Evaluation for different programs of Root Leaf or Flower of Common Threewingnut treating primary NS[J]. Chinese Journal of Medicine, 2006, 41(2):41-44.

[26] Li XW. Application of TCM Root Leaf or Flower of Common Threewingnut in treatment of chronic renal

disease[J]. Chinese Journal of Nephrology, Dialysis & Transplantation, 2003, 12(3):251-252.

[27] Hu WX, Tang Z, Yao XD, et al. Short-term curative effect of double doses of Tripterygium Wilfordii treating primary NS[J]. Chinese Journal of Nephrology, Dialysis & Transplantation, 1997, 6(3):210-213.

[28] Rong S, Hu WX, Liu ZH, et al. New therapy of mesangial proliferative nephritis[J]. Chinese Journal of Nephrology, Dialysis & Transplantation, 1998, 7(5):409-413.

[29] Liu ZH, Li SJ, Wu Y, et al. Prospective control study of Tripterygium Wilfordii combined with small dose of hormone treating idiopathic membranous nephropathy [J]. Chinese Journal of Nephrology, Dialysis & Transplantation, 2009, 18(4):303-309.

[30] Li LS, Liu ZH. Chinese Nephrology [M]. Beijing: People's Military Medical Press, 2008.

[31] Zhang WS. Clinical observation of needle warming moxibustion treating 50 cases with NS [J]. China Foreign Medical Treatment, 2009, 28(30):96.

[32] Zhuang KS, Li LC, Li YC, et al. Adjuvant therapy of NS type anaphylactic purpura nephritis with Peiyuan moxibustion therapy [J]. Journal of Emergency in Traditional Chinese Medicine, 2015, 23(10):1803-1805.

[33] Zhang ZZ, Yue J, Li JG, et al. 40 cases with primary NS is treated with Shenkang Application Agent [J]. Journal of External Therapy of Traditional Chinese Medicine, 2000, 9(2):12.

[34] Wang J, Wang HY. Clinical observation of primary NS edema being treated with TCM point application therapy [J]. Shanxi Journal of Traditional Chinese Medicine, 2015, 31(2):30-31.

[35] Cao Y, Zhang YM. Clinical curative effect observation of six points injection and prednisone treating NS as well as influence on immunity [J]. Chinese Acupuncture & Moxibustion, 2015, 25(12):857-859.

[36] Yin BQ, Song PJ. Observation of curative effect of injection at ST 36 and BL 23 treating adult primary NS [J]. Journal of New Chinese Medicine, 2013, 45(1):109-111.

[37] Zhao W, Chen CH. Clinical application of TCM mixture retention enema treating primary NS of children[J]. Chinese Medicine Guides, 2010, 7(12):118-119.

[38] Huang LL. TCM retention enema is used for treatment and nursing of refractory NS of children[J].Hubei Journal of Traditional Chinese Medicine, 2014, 36(10):8-9.

[39] Gao YX, Zhang PQ, Zhang Q, et al. Experience of Professor Zhang Qi treating refractory NS edema through concept of "circulation"[J]. Chinese Journal of Integrated Traditional and Western Nephrology, 2014, 15(8):663-664.

[40] Ma R. Remove nephropathy through tonifying spleen and eliminating dampness——academic idea of Professor Li Shaochuan treating children NS[J]. Tianjin Traditional Chinese Medicine, 2002, 19(3):7-9.

[41] Huang WZ. Experience of combination of TCM and WM treating NS[J]. Journal of Tianjin University of Traditional Chinese Medicine, 2006, 25(3):142-145.

[42] Soeiro EM, Koch VH, Fujimura MD, et al.Influence of nephrotic state on the infectious profile in childhood idiopathic nephrotic syndrotne[J]. Rev Hosp Clin Fac Med Sao Paulo, 2004, 59(5):273-278.

[43] Zhang JJ, Chi ZS. Influence of taking protein on diabetic nephropathy[J]. Foreign Medical Sciences (Section of Endocrinology), 1998, 18(4):26-29.

[44] Teplan V, Schuck O, Votruba M, et al. Metabolic effects of keto acid--amino acid supplementation in patients with chronic renal insufficiency receiving a low-protein diet and recombinant human erythropoietin—a randomized controlled trial[J]. Wien Klin Wochenschr, 2001, 113(17-18): 661-669.

I. Overview

Diabetes is a kind of systemic and metabolic disease characterized by high blood sugar. The reasons of the high blood sugar are insufficiency or deficiency of insulin secretion of pancreas or its physiological malfunction or the combination of both. The long-term high blood sugar caused by diabetes may result in chronic damage and dysfunction of multiple tissues of body, especially the eyes, kidneys, heart, blood vessels and nerve, thus causing various complications.

This disease is equal to consumptive thirst disease called in traditional Chinese medicine, but actually, the clinical range of the consumptive thirst disease is larger than diabetes, for example, the "diabetes insipidus" in modern medicine also can be treated based on syndrome differentiation according to "consumptive thirst", but clinical morbidity of "diabetes insipidus" is much lower than the "diabetes". "Consumptive" means consumption, emaciation and weakness; "thirst" means that patients feel thirsty and drink more water. Basic clinical characteristics of consumptive thirst, as a disease name in traditional Chinese medicine, are polydipsia, polyuria, polyphagia, weariness and emaciation.

In traditional Chinese medicine, it is considered that the basic pathological change of consumptive thirst disease is yin deficiency with internal heat, which mainly involves three viscera: lungs, stomach and kidneys. Pathological changes that are mainly related to lungs are called "upper consumptive thirst" and the thirst and polydipsia are the more significant symptoms; pathological changes that are mainly related to the stomach are called "middle consumptive thirst", and polyphagia and easy hunger are the more significant symptoms; Pathological changes that are mainly related to the kidneys are called "lower consumptive thirst", and polyuria, reproductive system dysfunction and stool abnormity are the more significant symptoms; therefore, "consumptive thirst" is also known as "three types of consumptive thirst".

II. Etiology and pathogenesis

i. Chinese medicine

In traditional Chinese medicine, it is considered that the etiology and pathogenesis of consumptive thirst basically include the several aspects below:

1. Improper diet

Overeating, particularly eating too much fatty, heavy taste, greasy, spicy and fried food which can produce internal heat.

2. Immoderation of labor and rest

More sitting and less movement, lack of activity and sedentariness are easy to result in impairment of the spleen, thus causing obstructed Qi-blood circulation, stagnant Qi function and heat-transmission with the passing of time.

3. Emotional disorder

Thinking too much with heart and brain or anxiety and impatience because one's wants and hopes fail to materialize can result in impairment of yin-blood and yin deficiency, which produce internal heat.

4. Excessive debauchery

It is easy to cause consumptive thirst disease if one has excessive drinking and frequent sexual life, because alcoholic strength is dampness-heat, which can consume fluid and nutrient-blood; while alcohol consumption is easy to cause hyper-eroticism of people, which results in impairment of kidney essence; both can cause deficiency of essence, blood and fluid, thus producing internal heat.

5. Innate factors

This disease has genetic predisposition; if any one of parents, grandparents, or other relatives of last generation is suffering from this disease, the relatives of son generation will have relatively high incidence.

ii. Western medicine

Its basic pathologic changes are damaged pancreas islet of pancreas, deficiency of insulin secretion and insulin dysfunction, which result in higher blood sugar; while the reasons include lifestyle, family heredity, infection and other factors.

III. Key points of diagnosis and differential diagnosis

i. Key points of diagnosis

1. Chinese medicine

(1) The patients show dry mouth, thirst, polydipsia, polyphagia, easy hunger, increased urine volume,

weakness, easy fatigability or emaciation in clinic.

(2) They have four kinds of lifestyles given in the etiology and pathogenesis above and family heredity history.

2. Western medicine

Doctors can make a definite diagnosis when the fasting blood glucose is greater than or equal to 7.0 mmol/L, and/or 2-hour postprandial blood glucose is greater than or equal to 11.1 mmol/L.

(1) Type I diabetes: Onset age of this disease is younger and the age of most patients is less than 30; this disease usually occurs suddenly; patients show obvious polydipsia, polyuria, polyphagia and emaciation and have high blood glucose level; ketoacidosis is the initial symptom of many patients, who have low serum insulin and C peptide level; ICA、 IAA or GAD antibody may show positive. The curative effect of single oral medicine is poor; therefore, insulin is needed for therapy generally.

(2) Type II diabetes: This disease is common in middle aged and elderly people; morbidity of obese group is high, and the disease can be accompanied with hypertension, dyslipidemia, arteriosclerosis and other diseases. Onset of this disease is slow or insidious; patients show unconspicuous symptoms in early stage or only show mild weakness and thirst; for patients whose blood sugar increases is not obviousl, sugar tolerance test is needed to be conducted for definite diagnosis. Serum insulin level is normal or increased in early stage and low at late stage.

ii. Differential diagnosis

(1) Common heat syndrome, such as gastrointestinal heat syndrome and hepatobiliary heat syndrome, may also include dry mouth, thirst, polydipsia and other symptoms; however, these patients show normal urine volume or oliguria and show less weakness and fatigability; special attention shall be paid to the identification of this disease and consumptive thirst disease.

(2) The blood sugar may increase in the cases of hyperthyroidism, chronic renal insufficiency, and liver cirrhosis, as well as under stress states such as trauma; special attention shall be paid to the identification.

IV. TCM therapy

i. Syndrome differentiation and treatment

As described above, in traditional Chinese medicine, it is considered that basic pathological change of consumptive thirst disease is yin deficiency causing internal heat, which mainly involves three viscera: lungs, stomach and kidneys. From specific circumstances of clinical patients, the "upper consumptive thirst" whose lesions are mainly in the lungs is mostly associated with the dysfunction of heart at the same time; "the middle consumptive thirst" whose lesions are mainly in the stomach is mostly associated with the dysfunction of spleen at the same time; "the lower consumptive thirst" whose lesions are mainly in the kidneys is mostly associated with the dysfunction of liver at the same time. Therefore, in traditional Chinese medicine, it is considered that consumptive thirst disease is associated with the dysfunction of multiple viscus in upper, middle and lower jiao, and it is a kind of systemic disease; this disease shows different syndrome types because main pathological changes and clinical manifestation of different patients may be different.

1. Deficiency of lung yin and hyperactivity of heart fire

Main symptoms: dry mouth, thirst, continuous thirst even after drinking water, easy impatience, potential insomnia, dry tongue fur with less fluid, red tip of the tongue or total red tongue and rapid, floating or thready pulse.

Therapeutic methods: to nourish yin, clear heat; generate fluid and quench thirst.

Prescription: Modified Yu Quan San. Snakegourd Root, Unprocessed Rehmannia Root, Dwarf Lilyturf Tuber, Common Anemarrhena Rhizome, Kudzuvine Root, Platycodon Root, Lophatherum Herb, Unprocessed Liquorice Root and Chinese Magnoliavine Fruit.

Prescription analysis: in the prescription, Snakegourd Root, Common Anemarrhena Rhizome, Platycodon Root and Kudzuvine Root clear and purge lung heat and generate fluid production to quench thirst; Unprocessed Rehmannia Root, Dwarf Lilyturf Tuber and Chinese Magnoliavine Fruit nourish yin and generate fluid; Platycodon Root and Lophatherum Herb clear and purge upper jiao and heart-lung heat. The function of nourishing yin and clearing heat and promoting fluid production to quench thirst can be achieved by comprehensive compatibility of medicines.

2. Deficiency of both Qi and yin of heart and lung

Main symptoms: dry mouth, thirst, continuous thirst after drinking water, fatigue, lassitude of the spirit, dry tongue with less fluid and thin and rapid or feeble rapid pulse.

Therapeutic methods: to nourish yin, eplenish Qi; generate fluid and quench thirst.

Prescription: Modified Sha Shen Mai Men Dong Tang. The Root of Straight Ladybell, Dwarf Lilyturf Tuber, Fragrant Solomonseal Rhizome, Mulberry Leaf, Snakegourd Root, Hyacinth Bean, Unprocessed Milkvetch Root, Chinese Wolf berry Root-bark, Unprocessed Liquorice Root and Kudzuvine Root.

Prescription analysis: in the prescription, The Root of Straight Ladybell, Dwarf Lilyturf Tuber, Fragrant Solomonseal Rhizome and Unprocessed Milkvetch Root nourish yin, replenish Qi and promote fluid; Mulberry Leaf, Snakegourd Root, Chinese Wolf berry Root-bark and Kudzuvine Root clear heat, purge fire and promote fluid. Hyacinth Bean and Unprocessed Liquorice Root invigorate spleen, resolve dampness and replenish Qi. The function of nourishing yin and replenishing Qi and promoting fluid production to quench thirst can be achieved by comprehensive compatibility of medicines.

3. Lung-stomach fluid consumption and hyperactivity of fire due to yin deficiency

Main symptoms: dry mouth, thirst, easy hunger and polyphagia, excessive appetite, constipation or viscous stool, red tongue texture, scanty tongue fur or dry and yellow tongue fur and thin and rapid or feeble rapid pulse.

Therapeutic methods: to nourish yin, clear heat, benefit stomach and promote fluid.

Prescription: Modified Yu Nyu Jian. Unprocessed Rehmannia Root, Dwarf Lilyturf Tuber, Common Anemarrhena Rhizome, Gypsum, Golden Thread, Figwortflower Picrorhiza Rhizome, Snakegourd Root, Indian Bread, Kudzuvine Root and Reed Rhizome.

Prescription analysis: in the prescription, Unprocessed Rehmannia Root and Dwarf Lilyturf Tuber nourish yin and clear heat; Gypsum, Common Anemarrhena Rhizome, Golden Thread, Figwortflower Picrorhiza Rhizome, Snakegourd Root and Kudzuvine Root clear heat and purge fire and generate fluid to quench thirst; Indian Bread and Reed Rhizome invigorate spleen and resolve dampness and cause diuresis and purge heat.

4. Deficiency of both Qi and yin in spleen-stomach

Main symptoms: dry mouth, thirst, easy hunger and polyphagia, hunger without appetite, sallow and lusterless complexion, lassitude of the spirit and lack of strength, constipation or loose stool, and thin and rapid or feeble rapid or deep or thin pulse.

Therapeutic method: to invigorate spleen, tonify Qi, nourish yin and generate fluid.

Prescription: modified Shen Ling Bai Zhu San. Ginseng, White Indian Bread, Common Yam Rhizome, Hyacinth Bean, Crystalline Lens, Kudzuvine Root, Platycodon Root, Sacred Lotus Seed and Coix Seed.

Prescription analysis: in the prescription, Ginseng, Common Yam Rhizome, Crystalline Lens and Sacred Lotus Seed invigorate spleen, tonify Qi and nourish yin; Indian Bread, White Atractylodes Rhizome, Hyacinth Bean and Coix Seed invigorate spleen, tonify Qi and resolve dampness; Kudzuvine Root and Platycodon Root produce fluid and quench thirst.

5. Dampness-heat in spleen-stomach

Main symptoms: dry mouth, thirst, polyphagia and easy hunger, or hunger without appetite, bound or viscous stool, red tongue texture, yellow or white greasy tongue fur, soggy rapid or deep rapid or deep wiry pulse.

Therapeutic method: to invigorate spleen and regulate stomach, eliminate dampness and clear heat.

Prescription: modified Ping Wei San and Lian Pu Yin. Atractylodes Rhizome, Dried Tangerine Peel, Officinal Magnolia Bark, Villons Amomum Fruit, Fortune Eupatorium Herb, Golden Thread, Milkvetch Root, Caulis Perillae, Talc and Reed Rhizome.

Prescription: in the prescription, Atractylodes Rhizome, Dried Tangerine Peel, Officinal Magnolia Bark, Villons Amomum Fruit, Fortune Eupatorium Herb and Caulis Perillae invigorate spleen, regulate stomach and eliminate dampness; Milkvetch Root and Golden Thread clear dampness-heat in middle jiao; Talc and Reed Rhizome promote diuresis, purge heat, produce fluid and quench thirst.

6. Liver-kidney yin deficiency

Main symptoms: dry mouth, thirst, soreness and weakness of waist and knees, impatience and irritability, fatigue and weakness, dizziness and tinnitus, constipation, yellow urine or night sweat, insomnia, red tongue texture, scanty tongue fur and thin and rapid or feeble rapid pulse.

Therapeutic method: to nourish liver and kidneys, clear heat and nourish yin.

Prescription: modified Zeng Ye Tang and Liu Wei Di Huang Wan. There are Unprocessed Rehmannia Root, Figwort Root, Dwarf Lilyturf Tuber, Cornus Officinalis, Chinese Magnoliavine Fruit, Chrysanthemum Flower, Chinese Wolfberry Root-bark, Common Yam Rhizome, Indian Bread, Tree Peony Root Bark, Oriental Waterplantain Rhizome and Radix Achyranthis Bidentatae.

Prescription analysis: in the prescription, Unprocessed Rehmannia Root, Figwort Root and Dwarf Lilyturf Tuber nourish yin, produce fluid and clear heat; Cornus Officinalis, Chinese Magnoliavine Fruit and Radix Achyranthis Bidentatae nourish yin essence in liver and kidneys; Common Yam Rhizome, Indian Bread and Oriental Waterplantain Rhizome invigorate spleen and resolve dampness; Chrysanthemum Flower, Tree Peony Root Bark and Chinese Wolf berry Root-bark clear deficient fire in liver and kidneys. The goals of nourishing yin essence in liver and kidneys and clear deficient fire can be achieved by combination of all herbs.

7. Kidney essence deficiency

Main symptoms: dry mouth, thirst, soreness and weakness of waist and knees, dizziness, tinnitus, deafness, blurred vision, lassitude of the spirit and lack of strength, memory deterioration, polyuria, cloudy urine, constipation or loose stool, dry tongue and less fluid, and deep and thin or thin and rapid pulse.

Therapeutic method: to tonify kidneys, benefit Qi and supplement essence.

Prescription: modified Liu Wei Di Huang Wan. Unprocessed Rehmannia Root, Cornus Officinalis, Chinese Magnoliavine Fruit, Dodder Seed, Barbary Wolfberry Fruit, Common Yam Rhizome, Radix Achyranthis Bidentatae, Chinese Taxillus Herb, Unprocessed Milkvetch Root, White Atractylodes Rhizome, Indian Bread and Oriental Waterplantain Rhizome.

Prescription analysis: in the prescription, Unprocessed Rehmannia Root, Cornus Officinalis, Chinese Magnoliavine Fruit, Dodder Seed, Barbary Wolfberry Fruit, Radix Achyranthis Bidentatae and Chinese Taxillus Herb nourish yin essence in liver and kidneys; Milkvetch Root, White Atractylodes Rhizome and Common Yam Rhizome benefit Qi and invigorate spleen, as well as replenish spleen and kidneys; Indian Bread and Oriental Waterplantain Rhizome resolve dampness and promote diuresis. All these make entire prescription present tonification rather than clearing.

8. Deficiency of both yin and yang in liver, spleen and kidney

Main symptoms: dry mouth, thirst, soreness and weakness of waist and knees, dizziness, tinnitus, deafness, blurred vision, memory deterioration, lassitude of the spirit and lack of strength, extremity end numbness, blackish complexion, frequent micturition with polyuria, impotence in men, menstrual disorder in women, loose stool, pale and dry tongue with less fluid, peeling or scanty tongue fur and deep and thin pulse.

Therapeutic method: tonify liver and kidneys, invigorate spleen-stomach and reinforce yang Qi.

Prescription: modified Ba Wei Shen Qi Wan and Si Jun Zi Tang. Unprocessed Rehmannia Root, Cornus Officinalis, Chinese Magnoliavine Fruit, Dodder Seed, Barbary Wolfberry Fruit, Common Yam Rhizome, Radix Achyranthis Bidentatae, Unprocessed Milkvetch Root, Tangshen, White Atractylodes Rhizome, Prepared Common Monkshood Daughter Root, Cinnamon Twig, Epimedium Herb, Indian Bread and Oriental Waterplantain Rhizome.

Prescription analysis: in the prescription, Unprocessed Rehmannia Root, Cornus Officinalis, Chinese Magnoliavine Fruit, Dodder Seed, Barbary Wolfberry Fruit and Radix Achyranthis Bidentatae nourish liver and kidneys; Tangshen, Milkvetch Root, Common Yam Rhizome and White Atractylodes Rhizome invigorate spleen-stomach and replenish Qi; Common Monkshood Daughter Root, Cinnamon Twig and Epimedium Herb reinforce yang Qi in spleen and kidneys; Indian Bread and Oriental Waterplantain Rhizome resolve dampness and promote diuresis, which achieves tonification rather than clearing.

ii. Specific prescription treatment

Hezhitang Xiao Ke Wan Ling Fang mainly treats consumptive thirst disease.

15g of White Atractylodes Rhizome, 15g of Atractylodes Rhizome, 15g of Kudzuvine Root, 15g of Snakegourd Root, 30g of Silkworm Cocoon, 30g of Frosted Mulberry Leaf of, 20g of Dried Corn Stigma, Unprocessed 15g of Milkvetch Root, 15g of Chicken's Gizzard-Skin and 10g of Orange Fruitare decocted in water for oral dose; one dose is taken every day and is divided by two parts and taken while warming.

iii. Single ingredient prescription and proved prescription

30-50g of Potentilla Discolor Bunge is brewed with boiling water and drunk substituting for tea, which has efficacy on mild diabetes.

iv. Chinese patent medicine

(1) Jin Gui Shen Qi Wan: deficiency syndrome of both kidney yin and kidney yang, of consumptive thirst disease.

(2) Liu Wei Di Huang Wan: kidney-yin deficiency syndrome of consumptive thirst disease.

(3) Shen Ling Bai Zhu Wan: spleen Qi deficiency combining with dampness Qi of consumptive thirst disease.

(4) Bu Zhong Yi Qi Wan: syndrome of middle Qi deficiency with exogenous disease of consumptive thirst disease.

(5) Jin Qi Jiang Tang Pian: syndrome of Qi-deficiency combining with hot breath of consumptive thirst disease.

(6) Xiao Ke Wan: syndrome of deficiency of both Qi and yin combining with hot breath of consumptive thirst disease.

v. Acupuncture and moxibustion therapy

Generally, acupuncture therapy is not recommended for consumptive thirst disease, because skin injury caused by acupuncture may result in local infection of needle eye, which is difficult to heal after infection; in particular, acupuncture treatment is not suitable for patients with systemic malnutrition and relatively serious syndrome. ST 36, BL 23, BL 17 and other acupuncture points can be chosen for moxibustion therapy, which needs to be insisted in the long term for being beneficial.

vi. Massage therapy

Selection of acupuncture points for massage and massotherapies may refer to the thinking of foregoing diagnosis and prescription; it starts from three types of diabetes; acupuncture points of lung meridian and heart meridian in upper jiao are selected; acupuncture points of spleen-stomach meridian in middle jiao are selected; acupuncture points of liver meridian, kidney meridian and bladder meridian in lower jiao are selected. Common acupuncture points include BL 43, BL 13, BL 15, BL 17, BL 18, LU 2, GV 4, ST 36, SP 6, KI 2, KI 1, etc. The manipulation is given priority to relatively soft health care manipulation and can be made from light to heavy gradually. Moderate acid swelling or sore feeling on local parts of acupuncture points is taken as proper manipulation. Point pressure method or rotary type point pressure method is chosen. The time shall not be less than 15 minutes each time; generally, 30 to 60 minutes may be appropriate. Massage time shall avoid full and empty stomach time.

VI. Typical medical record of famous physicians and experts

i. Medical record of Ding Ganren —— lung-stomach fluid consumption, yin deficiency with yang hyperactivity and deficiency of liver and kidney

Through feeling the pulse, Yin's left three-position pulses are found to possess wiry and rapid pulses and three-position pulses possess slippery and rapid pulses. Meanwhile, KI 3 is found thin and weak and anterior tibial pulse has soft and and rapid pulses. The clinical manifestations include swift digestion with rapid hungering, emaciated body, poor nutrition absorption, lack of energy, cardiac apex movement, spontaneous sweating and night sweat as well as reheat sweating, fear of cold after sweating and light-headedness. All these symptoms are caused by yin-fluid consumption and failing to nourish wood and excessive liver yang. In such a case, the heart spirit becomes restless and the deficient yang forces fluids to discharge, thereby causing profuse sweating; stomach yin is consumed, thereby leading to swift digestion. As for the symptoms of reheat sweating and fear of cold after sweating, they are related to nutrient qi deficiency failing to protect the interior and defensive-qi deficiency failing to well protect the exterior. In the case that the pulses remain rapid, the symptom develops into consumptive-thirst disease. Under such circumstance, it is recommended to nourish lung yin to suppress liver-wood, clean stomach yin to relieve heart spirit. In such a way, yin becomes at peace and yang becomes compact and water rises and fire reduces. Only in this way can the spirit be normal and the body is in good condition.

Syndrome differentiation: lung-stomach fluid consumption, yin deficiency with yang hyperactivity and deficiency of liver and kidney.

Therapeutic method: nourish yin and subdue yang; clear heat and generate fluid.

Prescription: 12g of Dried Rhizome of Rehmannia, 9g of Indianbread with Pine, 9g of Flatstem Milkuetch, 6g of Tendrilleaf Fritillary Bulb, 12g of Fructus Tritici Levis, 6g of Unprocessed Debark Peony Root, 12g of Oyster Shell, 9g of Prepared Glossy Privet Fruit, 9g of Snakegourd Root, 9g of Fragrant Solomonseal Rhizome, 9g of Flowery Bone Fossil of Big Mammals, Chinese 6g of Caterpillar Fungus, 3g of Chinese Magnoliavine Fruit.

Note: Main pathogenesis of this record includes insufficiency of yin-fluid of lung, stomach, liver and kidney, yin deficiency with yang hyperactivity and non-interaction between heart and kidney. The disease belongs to a relatively typical consumptive thirst disease with dysfunction of multiple viscera. Herbal prescription gives consideration to five zang-organs and all organs, which has demeanor of great master pharmacy.

VII. Prevention and aftercare

i. Prevention

(1) The formation of consumptive thirst disease has more close relationship with lifestyle, especially for people with family history of this disease, whose juvenile years and even childhood shall be paid attention to.

(2) One shall form good and healthy lifestyle, try to eat less sweet food, eat less fried staple food and dishes and reasonably control the intake of the fat, especially the animal fat.

(3) The physical exercise or physical labor shall be arranged scientifically and reasonably, consistently to the best, according to the different age groups. For example, people at the age of less than 50 years old and people in better health status and physical strength may insist on exercise training of moderate intensity, not less than 3 times per week. People at the age of more than 50 years old and people in poorer health status and weaker physical strength may insist on exercise training of less than moderate intensity, not less than 5 times per week.

(4) Office workers, especially white-collar workers, must alternate work with rest, avoid sedentariness and avoid sitting before computer to work for more than one hour.

(5) One shall maintain peaceful mentality and shall be cheerful and optimistic, avoiding excessively severe emotional stimulation, such as great rejoicing and great pity in the aspect of emotion.

ii. Aftercare

(1) The patients, who have been found suffering from the disease, must control diet first, eat less sweet food and drink less carbonated beverages; they shall drink alcoholic drinks according to their own actual situation of body, as appropriate, but the general rule is that it is advisable to drink less. They shall control high fat diet, particularly animal fat diet. Patients shall eat some roughage appropriately and cannot only eat white rice and flour; they also shall eat more bean products and vegetables properly.

(2) The patients shall stick to regular exercise and they can determine the exercise intensity, exercising ways and the duration of each exercise according to their own actual situations, as appropriate; however, no matter what kind of exercise they will choose, they shall do it consistently; exercise intensity and time are appropriate when they sweat slightly; they shall replenish water after exercise.

(3) Daily life of patients shall be regular; they shall sleep, get up and dine on relatively regular time, otherwise it is easier for blood glucose to fluctuate. Patients shall keep optimistic mentality and stable emotion and avoid excessively intense mental stimulation to the greatest extent.

(4) Patients with fasting blood sugar of more than 9mmol/L must use medicine as specified.

(SUN Zhongtang)

头痛　Headache

I. Overview

Headache is a disease that mainly shows pain in the head, and a subjective symptom mostly seen in clinic, which can not only be caused by multiple diseases, but shown by itself. Headache is often seen in various kinds of acute and chronic diseases. All diseases, of which the main symptom is headache, caused by exogenous six excesses and internal injury, are called headache. The disease is called migraine when the ache occurs at one side; the ache is called parietal headache when it occurs at the top of head; the ache is called forehead headache when it is occurring at forehead; the ache is called post-dural puncture headache when it occurs at afterbrain; the disease is called recurrent headache when it lasts for long time without curing; it is called real headache if the head is very painful, and hands and feet are cold to the joints. This disease is described with the terms of the "recurrent headache", "headache", "migraine", "headache due to qi moving on inverse" and so on in traditional Chinese medicine.

According to western medicine, there are various causes of headache. Neuralgia, intracranial infection, encephalic space occupying lesion, cerebrovascular disease, head and face disease outside the cranium, as well as systemic diseases (acute infection, intoxication, etc.) can cause headache. Not all diseases of headache can be treated by the therapy of this article. It is generally considered that hypertension, intracranial tumours, prosopalgia, migraine and psychoneurosis in western medicine can be treated by syndrome referring to this section, if they mainly show headache. In clinic therapy, nerve headache is taken as the main symptom, including tension headache, functional headache and vascular neuralgia headache, etc.

II. Etiology and pathogenesis

i. Chinese medicine

The earliest record of headache was in *Inner Canon of Huangdi*, which is called "Naofeng" and "Shoufeng". Headache is recorded 35 times in *Plain Questions* and 18 times in *Spiritual Pivot*. From etiology and pathogenesis, it is considered that attack of exogenous pathogens is the main cause of headache, diseases in five zang viscera as well as six meridians are all related to headache. In addition, positions are different among different ages, namely "For the older patient, the treatment shall be given in zang-organ; for the younger patient, in meridians; for the patient in the prime of life, in fu-organ". *Classic of Difficulties* put forward headache due to qi moving on inverse and true headache, the former belongs to qi syncope syndrome and the latter belongs to phlegm syncope with the serious disease condition. In *Treatise on Cold Damage*, etiology and pathogenesis, therapy and prescription of headache were recorded systematically, with 14 places of record distributing in four diseases of Taiyang, Yangming, Shaoyang, Jueyin. Headache is divided into headache caused by internal injury and exogenous headache by *Dongyuan Shishu*. *Danxi's Experiential Therapy* recorded that "headache is mainly caused by phlegm, and the serious headache is due to exuberant fire". *Formulary of Universal Relief. Appendix of Headache* recorded: "if a person shows deficiency in both qi and blood, and wind pathogen infects the yang meridians, involving in the head, headache will occur". "If unendurable ache appears in Tianmen acupoint, upwards spreading to the brain, the patient will die quickly", Wang Kentang of Ming Dynasty said.

Head is the confluence of original spirit of people, known as "house of bright essence", "confluence of all yang-channels" and "place of brain marrow". Seven orifices are connected inside and outside, meridians are connected to the viscera, so qi-blood body fluids in five zang- and six fu-organs are all related to the head and gathered to it. *Classified Patterns Syndromes with Clear-Cut Treatments* said: "Head is the top, gathered with all yang-energy. If the head is invaded by six qi, essences are impeded inside, and depression is accumulated in facial orifices, clear yang will not move and the headache will occur." The body is invaded by pathogens of six excesses, affecting seven orifices, blocking meridians; qi depression transforms into fire due to anger and sorrow, wind-yang disturb upside; improper diet damages spleen and causes dampness-gathering, and then phlegm-dampness is converged upward. The head loses normal function because of insufficiency of qi and blood caused by aeipathia and overstrain; an inadequate natural endowment and excessive indulgence in sexual activity lead to essence and marrow deficiency; traumatic injury cause static blood obstructing brain collateral; all conditions above can cause headache.

1. Etiology

It is generally believed that there are various pathogenesis of headache, mainly including external contraction and internal injury. External contraction includes wind-heat, wind-cold, and wind-dampness. Internal injury includes hyperactivity of liver-yang, deficiency of the kidney essence, spleen-stomach weakness, phlegm dampness stagnation and blood stasis obstructing the collaterals.

(1) Exogenous headache: Six climatic exopathogens are caught mostly because of careless life style and sitting and lying against the wind. They invade upward to the top, so clear yang qi is obstructed, and qi and blood stagnates, which obstructs pulse and collaterals, resulting in headache. However, wind is the first cause of many diseases, "if a patient is damaged by wind, the top is affected firstly", therefore, headache caused by Six climatic exopathogens are still subject to wind pathogen and attacks mostly with seasonal epidemic. Cold, heat and dampness pathogens are mostly accompanied.

① Exogenous wind cold invasion: Wind cold mostly occurs in winter when the weather is cold, daily life is inappropriate, causing body deficiency and qi depletion, and insecurity of defensive qi. Cold-pathogen invade and fetter exterior, defensive yang was obstructed. Cold-pathogen invading into the channel and blood vessel stagnation obstruct vessel and collateral, so as to cause interior blood stasis, resulting in headache. As said in *Plain Questions ·Treatise on Listing Pain*: "When cold qi enter channel, the blood will be blocked with astringency. If cold qi is outside of the vessel, it will lead to blood deficiency; if it is inside of vessel, qi will be blocked, causing sudden pain."

② Wind heat invasion: The air temperature suddenly becomes warm, with daily life in an inappropriate way, or the living room is poorly ventilated with stifling heat qi, in addition hair orifice is rare, so the warm-heat pathogen attacks making mutual contention of wind and heat, catharsis of muscular striae is not smooth, thus the fire tends to flame upward, seven orifices are disturbed, at the last qi and blood disorder, causing headache.

③ Wind-dampness invasion: Living in humid place for a long time, wading in the rain, sweating out into water, careless living in the year of wet with rain, or pathogenic dampness maceration. Dampness is yin pathogen, obstructing and damaging yang qi, blocking qi movement, of which nature is dense, sticky and greasy. If dampness pathogen blocks seven orifices, and clear yang fails to ascend, headache will occur. As said in *Plain Questions. Treatise on Generating Qi and Access to the Heaven:* "Due to dampness, the head is like being wrapped." It means that if there is dampness in the head, it feels heavy pain, causing coma, as if the head is wrapped with a towel, and feels tightened during delving in.

(2) Headache caused by internal injury: "The brain is the sea of brain marrow", which means that the head mainly depends on the essence of liver and kidney (essence is mainly stored in kidney which governs bone and generates marrow, and liver and kidney are from same source) and moistening of essence of water and grain transported and transformed by spleen and stomach, hence, the occurrence of headache caused by internal injury is usually related to liver, spleen and kidney.

① Hyperactivity of liver-yang: Liver prefers to free activity and hate depression, easily ascending and stirring, hence called "liver being firm-characterized zang organ". Catharsis of liver qi is mainly related to ascending and descending as well as regulating of qi movement of human body. Only under the normal condition of catharsis of liver qi, can people harmonize qi and blood with ease of mind and not damaged by disease. On the contrary, if the patient is overwhelmed by abnormal emotion, depression and anger will damage the liver, so the liver cannot remain mild and the liver qi will depresse, qi depression will transform into fire. As said in *Case Records as a Guide to Clinical Practice · Depression*: "Depression will result in qi stagnation, and qi stagnation for a long time will transform into fire." Fire tends to flame upward, fire pathogen upward disturbs seven orifices, causing headache. If qi depression transforms into fire for a long time, body fluids will be damaged to make liver yin insufficient and liver fail to be moistened. Kidney fluid is insufficient, which is mostly because sexual strain damages to essence. Water failing to nourish wood results in liver and kidney yin depletion, exuberance of liver yang, and causes damages to liver yin, lower damages to kidney fluid to make liver and kidney yin fluid more insufficient, forming a "vicious circle". "Liver is viscus of wind and wood", fire and wind stirring up each other, fire channeling with qi and upward disturbing the top cause headache.

② Kidney essence deficiency: Kidney essence is deficient mostly due to insufficient natural endowment or excessive sexual strain. As said in *Plain questions · Theories on Inverse Adjustment*: "if kidneys do not generate, marrow cannot be filled". As said in *Spiritual Pivot ·Theories on Sea*: "the brain is the sea of brain marrow". Generation of marrow is from kidneys; kidneys govern bone and generate marrow. Marrow upward connects to the brain; hence, brain marrow depends on continuous generation and transformation of kidney essence. If kidney essence is deficient for a long time, emptiness of brain marrow will cause headache. If kidney yin is damaged for a long time, yin damaging yang (mutual rooting of yin and yang) or body deficiency with long illness will cause kidney yang weakness, clear yang without expansion, resulting in headache.

③ Spleen-stomach weakness: Spleen-stomach is the acquired foundation, and origin of producing qi and blood. In the whole body, four limbs and skeleton, five zang- and six fu-organs depend on the moistening of qi and blood. Hunger-satiety overstrain or body deficiency after the illness and delivery, spleen-stomach weakness, insufficient transformation origin of qi and blood result in nutrient-blood deficiency, which cannot transform nutrient into brain marrow, causing headache.

④ Phlegm-dampness obstruction: It is mainly caused by spleen-stomach weakness, generation and transformation phlegm-turbidity, preference for drinking and fat food, spleen deficiency failing to transport and transform water dampness to produce phlegm. Phlegm-turbidity upward disturbs seven orifices, blocks clear yang and clear yang failing to ascend result in headache.

⑤ Blood-stasis obstructing collateral: Traumatic injury and chronic diseases transforming to collaterals will cause qi stagnation and blood stasis. "Qi being commander of blood and blood being mother of qi" Qi flow promotes blood circulation, qi stagnation makes blood coagulation, and qi deficiency occurs due to a long illness. Qi does not command blood, blood flow will be blocked. Or traumatic injury in head, blood stasis and qi stagnation, blood stasis block brain collaterals, and stagnation leads to pain, headache will appear accordingly.

2. Pathogenesis

Pathogenesis of headache refers to stagnation leading to pain, failure to moistening leading to pain, and disharmony leading to pain. Occurrence of pain is mostly related with disturbance of meridians. Obstruction of pathogen excess and disorder of qi and blood happen, and then pulse passage fails to conduce circulation; due to spleen-stomach weakness, nourishing lacking origin, qi and blood fail to be moistened; or imbalance of yin and yang, yin damage and yang hyperactivity, qi-movement disturbance, upward disturbing to brain, and failure of vessel collateral, all can result in occurrence of headache syndromes.

(1) Stagnation leading to pain: It was said in *Key to Diagnosis and Treatment*: "Pain is caused by obstruction and there is no pain under unobstruction." Unobstruction is one of important reasons for occurrence of pain. Pathogenesis lies in pathogen excess, phlegm-turbidity, qi stagnation, blood stasis, food accumulation and other pathological factors. Obstruction of brain collateral will cause headache. Pathogen of wind-cold stagnates qi and blood and obstructs vessel collateral; or pathogen of wind-heat upward disturbs seven orifices, resulting in disordered qi and blood; or pathogen of wind-dampness confuses seven orifices, resulting in clear yang failing to ascend; improper diet and internal producing phlegm-dampness blocks clear yang; qi and blood obstruction, collateral vessels stasis and obstruction; mental disharmony, constraining of liver qi, qi depression transforming into fire, upward disturbance of seven orifices; long illness invading into collateral and obstructing brain collateral; all conditions above can trigger headache.

(2) Failure to moisten leading to pain: As said in *Plain Questions ·Treatise on Listing Pain*: "Pulse is astringent, causing blood deficiency and then being headache." As said in *Golden Mirror of Medicine*: "Syndrome of injury is caused by blood deficiency". Pathogenesis of failure to moistening leading to pain lies in essence deficiency, qi deficiency and blood deficiency. Insufficiency of natural endowment, kidney essence cannot upward supplement to the brain; or yin impairment affecting yang, declination of kidney yang, clear yang failing to ascend, loss of nourishment of brain house; overfatigue and improper diet damage to spleen-stomach, causing insufficient qi and blood transforming to origin, and loss of nourishment of brain; or consumption for a long illness, both qi and blood deficiency, loss of nourishment of brain orifice; all conditions above can trigger headache.

(3) Disharmony leading to pain: If qi and blood are smooth, all diseases will not generate. Voice of discontent and rebellion will appear when meeting with unsatisfied things. Harmony refers to the state of relative equilibrium of yin-yang. If this balanced state is damaged, disease will appear accordingly. Except stagnation and failure to moisten for occurrence of headache, disharmony leading to pain also exists. Pathogenesis of disharmony leading to pain lies in qi counterflow and yang hyperactivity. Imbalance of yin and yang, liver, kidney and yin deficiency, exuberant fire damage to yin, ascendant hyperactivity of liver yang, upward disturbance of seven orifices; mental disharmony, qi and blood counterflow, upward disturbance of qi counterflow, all can trigger headache.

ii. Western medicine

Headache is a comprehensive disease that is caused by many disease causes, and many causes can result in headache. After Pain peripheral receptors of head and neck is irritated by abnormal nervous impulse, headache will often be triggered. Headache can be generally divided into 4 categories: headache caused by intracranial lesions, such as wind stroke, cerebral arteriosclerosis, and hypertensive encephalopathy; headache caused by extracranial head and neck lesions, such as migraine and cluster headache; headache caused by head and neck skin muscle skull lesion, such as scalp acute infection, tension headache, etc.; headache caused by five sense organs and oral lesions, such as glaucoma and nasosinusitis. There are many common causes as following.

1. Vascular headache

It is mainly caused by expansion or rupture hemorrhage of intracranial and extracranial artery. For example, headache caused by migraine and subarachnoid hemorrhage is often related to vascular factors.

2. Traction headache

It is mostly caused by traction or displacement of intracranial pain sense sensitive tissue. When the edema occurs in the intracranial, edema part squeezes and presses the meningeal tissue, thus causing headache.

3. Meningeal irritation headache

It is mainly caused by inflammation of intracranial and extracranial sense sensitive tissue. When inflammatory exudation occurs in the intracranial, exudative inflammatory substances has a certain irritation to meningeal nerve and blood vessel, thus triggering headache.

4. Tension or muscle contraction headache

It is mainly caused by intracranial and extracranial muscle contraction, which results from mental factors. There are no lesions in the head of patients, but obvious mental symptoms exist.

5. Neural inflammatory headache

It is mainly caused by direct damage or inflammation of cranial nerve and cervical nerve which result in the sense of pain. Intracranial pain sense is sensitive to the conduction of the fifth pairs, the ninth pairs and the tenth pairs of cranial nerve as well as the second to third pairs of cervical nerve. When inflammation occurs in the above nerves, feeling of headache will often appear.

6. Referred headache

It is mainly caused by pain spreading of five sense organs lesions. Headache may result from facial trigeminal nerve and cervical nerve stimulated, at this time, there is no lesions in the intracranial.

7. Hereditary headache

It is mostly caused by hereditary factors. The patient has an obvious family history of genetic disease.

III. Key points of diagnosis and differential diagnosis

i. Key points of diagnosis

The pathogenesis of headache is complex. Onset method, attack frequency, attach time, duration, headache part, nature, pain degree, whether there is premonitory symptom, and specific inducing factor, and factors of headache aggravating and relieving in collection of disease history shall be asked during collecting history. There are various accompanying symptoms of headache, and key points of diagnosis shall be headache part, nature, and disease course and tongue and pulse condition.

1. Chinese medicine

(1) Disease location differentiation by headache part: The head is confluence of all yang channels, three yang channels are along the head, and Jueyin channel upward meets the top. Headache can be judged through channels. Taiyang headache: it mostly occurs in back of the head and lower connects to back of neck. Yangming headache: it mostly occurs in forehead and supraorbitalnidge. Shaoyang headache: it mostly occurs in both side of the head and connects to ear. Jueyin headache: it mostly occurs in parietal part or connects to eye connector. Shaoyin headache: it occurs in the brain or involves in the teeth.

(2) Nature of disease differentiation by nature of the headache: Patients with pulling pain suffer from the headache caused by muscles and tendons obstruction. Patients with throbbing pain suffer from the headache caused by liver yang or blood heat. Patients with burning pain suffer from the headache caused by wind-heat or fire-heart or yin deficiency. Patients with distending pain suffer from the headache caused by qi stagnation or hyperactivity of liver-yang and up-flaming liver fire. Patients with heavy pain suffer from the headache caused by wind-dampness. Patients with dull pain suffer from the headache caused by deficiency of qi and blood. Patients with empty pain suffer from the headache caused by kidney essence depletion. Patients with faint pain suffer from the headache caused by body deficiency and dampness obstruction. Patients with stabbing pain (pain like bore spine, fixation of pain point) suffer from the headache caused by stasis blood.

(3) Division of exogenous pathogenic factors and internal injury through disease course: Headache as new disease is mostly caused by exogenous pathogenic factors and most pain conditions are severe, such as manifesting pulling pain, throbbing pain, burning pain, distending pain, heavy pain and endless pain. Headache for long illness is mainly caused by internal injury, and most pain conditions are mild, such as manifesting dull pain, empty pain, and faint pain, long pain conditions, which will be severe in fatigue and sometimes attack or stop.

(4) Clear diagnosis with tongue picture and pulse condition: Patients with thin and white tongue fur suffer from wind-cold headache; patients with thin and yellow tongue fur suffer from wind-heat headache; patients with white and greasy tongue fur suffer from wind-dampness or phlegm-turbidity headache; patients with red tongue and yellow fur suffer from ascendant hyperactivity of liver yang headache; patients with red tongue and less fur suffer from yin-blood deficiency headache; patients with thin tongue and less fur suffer from kidney deficiency headache; patients with purple tongue body or ecchymosis and petechia suffer from stasis blood headache.

Patients with floating and tense pulse suffer from wind-cold headache; patients with floating and rapid pulse suffer from wind-heat headache; patients with soggy pulse suffer from wind-dampness headache; patients with slippery pulse suffer from phlegm-turbidity headache; patients with wiry pulse suffer from ascendant hyperactivity of liver yang headache; patients with thin rapid pulse suffer from yin deficiency headache; patients with deep and faint pulse suffer from kidney deficiency headache; patients with thread and uneven pulse suffer from stasis blood headache.

2. Western medicine

Patients with sudden headache, accompanying with sweating, nausea, vomiting and headache relief after vomiting, suffer from migraine; patients with headache, accompanying with severe nausea, vomiting, nuchal rigidity, increased intracranial pressure and meningeal irritation sign, suffer from brain tumor, cerebrospinal meningitis, subarachnoid hemorrhage and cerebral hemorrhage; patients with headache, accompanying with obvious dizziness manifests posterior fossa lesions; if mental symptoms appear in headache, especially euphoria, hallucination and abnormal laughing and weeping, it is frontal lobe tumor or viral encephalitis; symptoms of dysfunction of autonomic nerve appear in headache, such as cold sweat, flushed or pale face, fluctuation of blood pressure, nausea, vomiting, lacking in strength, palpitation, and diarrhea, which is vascular headache.

Headache that occurs in head top is mostly functional or nervous headache; headache that occurs in occipital part maybe is subarachnoid hemorrhage, cerebrospinal meningitis, hypertension headache, cervicogenic headache, posterior cranial fossa tumors and great occipital neuralgia; headache that occurs in eyes or eye socket is mostly intracranial hypertension headache, glaucoma, cluster headache, Carbon monoxide poisoning headache and prosopalgia; hemicranias that occurs in lateral head is mostly vascular migraine, otogenic migraine and odontogenic migraine; patients with the whole headache may be with brain tumor, tension headache, intracranial hypertension headache and infectious headache.

ii. Differential diagnosis

When headache is diagnosed, the identification of relevant illness should be paid attention to. There are common diseases of WM that require identification:

1. Tension headache

The prolonged mental stress, anxiety and fatigue, etc. cause head and neck tense, vessel contractile, tissue ischemic, metabolism abnormal and algogenic substance release. These cause tension headache. Headache happens in bilateral frontal, occiput and tempus and the ache show the lasting dull pain, tension and stress. It sometimes shows less pain and sometimes more pain gets worse and the pain never relives. These are the characteristics of headache. In addition, the headache is accompanied with neurosis and other symptoms. Antidepressants and ataractic can relieve headache, but ergotamine is not effective.

2. Intracranial hypertension

Headache is the main and the only early symptom of intracranial hypertension. The headache shows lasting dull pain with nausea and emesis. With the deterioration of the illness, the headache becomes fierce. The headache is obvious in the morning, or one may wake up because of the fierce headache in the evening. Any factors that can cause intracranial hypertension, such as cough, sneeze and stool exerting can make headache fiercer. It can be identified according to medical history, brain CT, DSA and MRI in clinical.

3. Hypertension headache

Severe hypertension is generally accompanied with the headache of occipitalia and frontal part. When the head is down and one holds breath, the headache will be fiercer. There is a direct relationship between headache and hypertension. Controlling hypertension can relieve headache. The migraine is episodic ache and throbbing ache of one side. It can be identified by monitoring the blood pressure.

4. Headache epilepsy

Headache epilepsy is a sort of paroxysm, which doesn't have the signal symptom. The headache epilepsy is fierce with the disturbance of consciousness. The headache is more seen in temples and frontal part. The lasting time is of various lengths and the attack can be ceased by itself. At paroxysm, there is paroxysmal high amplitude in electroencephalogram: the rhythm is 4 – 7 times a second, or it is spike, sharp wave, SSW, etc. It always happens in two sides synchronously. The gap phase is usually normal.

5. Neurosis headache

Neurosis patients always have headache, whose cardinal symptoms are that threshold of ache toleration decreases and the muscle is intense. This is the non-paroxysmal ache and there aren't any premonitory signs. This headache is always accompanied with insomnia, attention deficit disorder, hypomnesia, dizziness and irritation, etc., the appearance and intensify of which are always related to mental conditions of patients.

6. Temporal arteritis

The main symptom is headache that is located in tempus, the peripheral part of eyes, frontal part and occipitalia. This is a kind of fierce throbbing and persistent pain. In addition, it has burning sensation that other vascular headaches don't have. The patient may have ache when he is chewing and this can be regarded as first symptoms. Visual obstacle is a common symptom and there is a possibility of losing part or total vision. Because the retinal arteries in about 1/3 of temporal arteritis cases of illness are invaded, formation of MCAT in the center of retina and ischemic neuritis can be seen through the examination of fundus oculi. Fever, tiredness and discomfort, anorexia, pain of muscle, limb fatigue, anxiety, depression and ESR are the constitutional symptoms. Biopsy can define the diagnosis. The therapy of hormone has evident effects.

7. Trigeminal neuralgia

There is no premonitory stage of trigeminal neuralgia. The pain is fulgurating paroxysmal, electrical symptom or fire iron pain, some of which are limited in three distribution areas of trigeminus. Pain can last from some seconds to a few minutes. Trigeminal neuralgia can be induced by stimulating skin triggering points. Medicinal phenytoin sodium has effects.

IV. TCM therapy

i. Syndrome differentiation and treatment

Syndrome differentiation and treatment should concentrate on dredging, reinforcement and balance according to pathogenesis. In general, excess appears in the early stage of illness, and the treatment shall eliminate pathogen and focus on dredging. However, different therapeutic methods shall be taken according to different disease causes. For example, wind-cold headache shall be treated by dispersing wind and dissipating cold; wind-heat headache shall be treated by dispersing wind and clearing heat; wind-damp headache shall be treated by expelling wind and eliminating dampness. As for deficiency due to long illness, the original qi shall be consolidated, and tonifying deficiency is dominant. However, for the deficiency complicated by excess, such as blood stasis and turbid phlegm, weighing the primary and the secondary. Both dredging and reinforcement are going to be carried out. The liver-yang headache has both deficiency and excess; pacifying liver and subduing yang shall be for the excess. The patients with deficiency in origin and excess in superficiality shall nourish the liver and kidney yin so as to pacify liver. "Patients with temporary diseases shall pay attention to pathogenic qi, while patients on long-term shall consolidate the original qi" said in *Jing-Yue Complete Works* is exactly this meaning. Due to various complex clinical manifestations of headache, the treatments shall be carried out in the light of different clinical manifestations and different stages. In the period of acute attack, the emphasis lies in dredging; dispersing wind, reducing fire (subduing yang), resolving phlegm and removing blood stasis are main therapeutic methods. In the remission stage, the emphasis lies in reinforcement; invigorating spleen, nourishing liver and tonifying kidney are the therapeutic methods, avoiding recurrence. The patients with slow onset and long-term pain can simply receive the comprehensive treatment of Chinese medicine. However, the patients with severe headache are attacked suddenly, and the pain is acute and unbearable; they shall receive combined treatment of traditional Chinese medicine and western medicine. After the remission of the disease, they can recuperate their bodies with Chinese medicine to consolidate the efficacy.

1. Exogenous headache

(1) Exogenous wind-cold

Main symptoms: occasional attack of headache, accompanied back pain, aversion to wind and cold. The headache becomes more severe when wind attacks. Patients like wrapping head. The symptoms are relieved when it is warmer. No thirst. Pale red tongue, thin and white tongue fur and floating pulse.

Therapeutic method: dispersing wind and dissipating cold.

Prescription: Chuan Xiong Cha Tiao San. Sichuan Lovage Rhizome, Incised Notopterygi um Rhizome and Root, Dahurian Angelica Root, Manchurian Wildginger, Peppermint, Fineleaf Schizonepeta Herb, Divaricate Saposhnikovia Root, Liquorice Root and Debark Peony Root.

Modification: In the case of severe headache, no sweating, being more severe when feeling cold and obvious cold manifestations, Radix Aconitilateralis Preparata and Ephedra can be added. If the patients also cough and have white and dilute phlegm, Apricot Seed, Hogfennel Root and Perilla Leaf can be added on the basis of the above prescription to enhance the function of ventilating lung and relieving cough.

Prescription analysis: In the prescription Sichuan Lovage Rhizome treats headache of Shaoyang and Jueyin meridian, Incised Notopterygium Rhizome and Root treats headache of greater yang meridian, Dahurian Angelica Root treats headache of yang brightness meridian, Debark Peony Root relieves acute spasm and stops pain, and they are the base of the prescription. Manchurian Wildginger, Peppermint, Fineleaf Schizonepeta Herb and Divaricate Saposhnikovia Root give off and ascend pesticide effect, disperse the upper wind pathogen, and assist the base in dispersing wind and relieving pain; they are all adjuvant drugs. Liquorice Root coordinates the drug actions of a prescription; it can prevent the warm and dryness of drugs, ascend and disperse, making ascending combined with dispersing; it works as assistant and guide. In the prescription Sichuan Lovage Rhizome can run the qi in the blood, remove the wind in the blood, act on the head and eyes, and is the main drug for treating headache clinically. Various drugs are used together to disperse wind pathogen and to relieve headache. The original prescription was the main prescription for external wind headache. This prescription can also be used for refractory headache to dispel wind, dredge collaterals and relieve pain. Studies have shown that Chuanxiong Chatiao Powder can promote blood circulation, enhance the blood supply to the brain, improve the microcirculation, alleviate head and neck muscle fatigue, and treat nervous headache.

(2) Exogenous wind-heat

Main symptoms: fullness and pain of head, feeling like cleaving head, fever, aversion to wind, red face and eyes, thirst, constipation, yellow urine, red tongue, thin and yellow tongue fur, floating and rapid pulse.

Therapeutic method: disperse wind and clear heat.

Prescription: modified Xiong Zhi Shi Gao Tang. Sichuan Lovage Rhizome, Dahurian Angelica Root, Mulberry Leaf, Chrysanthemum Flower, Gypsum, Tree Peony Root Bark, Red Peony Root, Peppermint, Baical Skullcap Root, Cape Jasmine Fruit, Weeping Forsythia Capsule, Platycodon Root, Manchurian Wildginger and Liquorice Root.

Modification: if there are high fever, thirst, dry nose, red tongue, vexation, less fluid and other syndromes of heat damaging to fluid, Kudzuvine Root can be added to release flesh, and Raw Gypsum, Common Anemarrhena Rhizome and Snakegourd Root are added to clear heat and promote fluid production. If the patients cough with phlegm, have thick and yellow phlegm, feel thirsty and painful in throat, Tendrilleaf Fritillary Bulb, Snakegourd Fruit and the Fourleaf Ladybell Root are added to resolve phlegm and promote fluid production.

Prescription analysis: in the prescription Sichuan Lovage Rhizome, Dahurian Angelica Root, Chrysanthemum Flower and Gypsum disperse wind, clear heat and expel pathogen through exterior; they are sovereign. Tree Peony Root Bark and Red Peony Root can cool and activate blood; Peppermint disperses wind pathogen; Baical Skullcap Root, Cape Jasmine Fruit and Weeping Forsythia Capsule can clear heat and expel pathogen through exterior, and the exterior syndromes are self-relieved. Reed Rhizome ascends lucidity and promotes fluid production to nourish yin. Liquorice Root cooperates to remove wind-heat pathogen without damaging yin and healthy qi. Platycodon Root disperses lung qi; the ascending and descending of qi movement is matched, avoiding the wind pathogen hurting people. Manchurian Wildginger can relieve pain. All are combined to disperse wind, expel pathogen through exterior, dredge collaterals and relieve pain.

(3) Exogenous wind-dampness

Main symptoms: headache as wrapped, heavy sensation in the limbs and body, anorexia and chest tightness, sloppy diarrhea, different urination, pale red tongue, white and greasy tongue fur, soggy pulse.

Therapeutic method: disperse wind and remove dampness.

Prescription: modified Qiang Huo Sheng Shi Tang. Incised Notopterygium Rhizome and Root, Doubleteeth Pubescent Angelica Root, Divaricate Saposhnikovia Root, Chinese Lovage, Sichuan Lovage Rhizome, Shrub Chastetree Fruit, Debark Peony Root, Radix Achyranthis Bidentatae, Manchurian Wildginger and Liquorice Root.

Modification: If the patients are accompanied by vomiting, Rhizoma Pinelliae and stir-baked Pinellia Tuber and Bamboo Shavings with ginger juice are added to descend adverse qi and arrest vomiting. In the case of irritancy, anorexia, bitterness and stickiness in the mouth, yellow urine, yellow and greasy tongue fur, soggy and rapid pulse, which are caused by dampness-stagnation fever, Baical Skullcap Root, Golden Thread, Amur Cork-Tree and Pinellia Tuber can be added to clear heat. In the case of chest tightness, abdominal distension, heavy limbs, loss of appetite, sloppy diarrhea, Atractylodes Rhizome, Officinal Magnolia Bark, Dried Tangerine Peel and Orange Fruit etc. can be added to remove dampness and harmonize the middle jiao.

Prescription analysis: In the prescription, Incised Notopterygium Rhizome and Root, Doubleteeth Pubescent Angelica Root, Divaricate Saposhnikovia Root, Chinese Lovage can expel wind and eliminate dampness, dissipate cold and relieve pain. They dissipate the exterior wind-cold and expel exterior pathogenic dampness. Sichuan Lovage Rhizome can activate blood and move qi, expel wind and relieve pain. Debark Peony Root can relieve acute spasm and pain. Radix Achyranthis Bidentatae can activate blood and relieve pain. Shrub Chastetree Fruit expels wind, relieves pain and clears the head and eyes. Manchurian Wildginger can relieve pain, and the efficacy is more significant when it is matched with Incised Notopterygium Rhizome and Root, Doubleteeth Pubescent Angelica Root and Divaricate Saposhnikovia Root; since wind can eliminate dampness, the wind medicine shall be used more. Liquorice Root is added to coordinate the drug actions and harmonize the middle jiao. The functions of releasing exterior, dissipating cold, eliminating dampness and relieving pain are served, and then headache is cured.

2. Headache caused by internal injury

(1) Headache caused by liver depression

Main symptoms: Headache affected by emotions, or related to women's menstruation, headache on one side, or pain extending to superciliary ridge. Mostly distending pain, repeated pain, chest oppression, sighing many times, emotional depression or irritability, or accompanied hypochondriac pain. Pale red tongue, dark color, thin tongue fur, stringy pulse.

Therapeutic method: soothe liver and relieve depression.

Prescription: modified Xiao Yao San. Chinese Thorowax Root, Nutgrass Galingale Rhizome, Chinese Angelica, Debark Peony Root, White Atractylodes Rhizome, Indian Bread, Liquorice Root, roasting Ginger, Peppermint, Manchurian Wildginger, Radix Achyranthis Bidentatae and Sichuan Lovage Rhizome.

Modification: if the headache is caused by invasion of wind-cold pathogen, Dahurian Angelica Root, Manchurian Wildginger and Chinese Lovage are added to expel wind and dissipate cold. If the headache is caused by wind-heat pathogen, Kudzuvine Root, Dahurian Angelica Root and Chrysanthemum Flower are added to disperse wind and clear heat. Tree Peony Root Bark, Cape Jasmine Fruit, Chrysanthemum Flower and Baical Skullcap Root are added to clear liver and purge fire for the patients with liver depression transforming into fire, dry mouth with bitter taste, and bloodshot eyes. Tall Gastrodia Tuber and Gambir Plant Nod are added to pacify liver and extinguish wind for patients with dizziness. Pinellia Tuber and Bamboo Shavings are added to harmonize the middle and arrest vomiting for the patients with nausea and vomiting.

Prescription analysis: In the prescription, Chinese Thorowax Root can soothe liver and relieve depression; Chinese Angelica and Debark Peony Root tonify blood, nourish and soften liver; White Atractylodes Rhizome and Indian Bread bank up earth to suppress wood, invigorate spleen and remove dampness, entitling transportation and transformation; Liquorice Root replenishes qi , harmonizes the middle and relieves the urgency of liver; Fresh Ginger harmonizes the middle and regulates qi ; Peppermint enhances dispersion of free activity. Nutgrass Galingale Rhizome can regulate qi movement; Radix Achyranthis Bidentatae and Sichuan Lovage Rhizome move qi and activate blood; Manchurian Wildginger relieves pain. All these drugs are used together to sooth liver and relieve depression, invigorate spleen and harmonize stomach, regulate qi and relieve pain.

(2) Up-flaming of liver fire

Main symptoms: splitting headache, flushed face and red eyes, vexation and irascibility, dry and bitter mouth, insomnia, yellow urine and constipation, red tongue and yellow tongue fur and wiry, rapid and forceful pulse.

Therapeutic method: clear liver and discharge fire.

Prescription: modified Long Dan Xie Gan Tang. There are Chinese Gentian, Baical Skullcap Root, Cape Jasmine Fruit, Chinese Angelica, Unprocessed Rehmannia Root, Bupleurum, Plantain Seed, Oriental Waterplantain Rhizome, Akebia and Unprocessed Liquorice Root.

Modification: for dizziness, dizzy vision and tinnitus, Chrysanthemum Flower, Tall Gastrodia Tuber and Magnetite (decocted first) are added to pacify liver and subdue yang; with regard to patients with obvious vexing heat and dry and bitter mouth, Tree Peony Root Bark and Golden Thread are added to clear heat and discharge fire; as to those with nausea and vomiting of yellow water, Bamboo Shavings, Golden Thread and Perilla Leaf are added to clear heart and harmonize stomach; in terms of bound stool, Raw Rhubarb (later addition) is added to relax bowels and discharge heat.

Prescription analysis: in the prescription, Chinese Gentian discharges excessive heat of liver and gallbladder, and clears dampness-heat in lower energizer; Baical Skullcap Root and Cape Jasmine Fruit clear heat and discharge fire; Oriental Waterplantain Rhizome, Akebia and Plantain Seed clear heat and eliminate dampness; Chinese Angelica and Unprocessed Rehmannia Root nourish blood and liver; Bupleurum regulates of qi movement of liver and gallbladder, and makes various medicines entry liver and gallbladder; Unprocessed Liquorice Root discharges fire, detoxicates, and coordinate various medicines. Various medicines are combined to achieve efficacies of soothing liver and relieving depression, clearing liver and discharging fire. With general observation, there is tonification in discharge and nourishment in promotion in entire prescription to reduce fire, clear heat, and circulate in meridians, and then all kinds of symptoms can be correspondingly cured.

(3) Ascendant hyperactivity of liver yang

Main symptoms: vertigo for headache, vexation and irascibility, restless sleep, flushed face and red eyes, bitter mouth, red tongue and yellow tongue fur, wiry and rapid pulse

Therapeutic method: pacify liver and subdue yang.

Prescription: modified Tian Ma Gou Teng Yin. There are Tall Gastrodia Tuber, Gambir Plant Nod, Abalone Shell, Baical Skullcap Root, Cape Jasmine Fruit, Radix Achyranthis Bidentatae, Eucommia Bark, Chinese Taxillus Twing, Tuber Fleeceflower Stem, Indianbread with Pine, Manchurian Wildginger, Red Peony Root and Motherwort Herb.

Modification: in the case that the headache is severe and lingering, with the symptoms of lower back pain and sore legs, red tongue and thin pulse that belong to the syndrome of liver disease into kidneys. For deficiency of water and excess of fire, Unprocessed Rehmannia Root, Fleeceflower Root, Glossy Privet Fruit, Yerbadetajo Herb, Barbary Wolfberry Fruit and Dendrobium and the like are added. If headache is severe, flushed face and red eyes, bitter mouth and hypochondriac pain, constipation and oliguria with reddish urine and yellow tongue fur and wiry and rapid pulse occur, liver fire at hyperactivity side is focus. It is suitable to clear liver and discharge fire. Chinese Gentian and Common Selfheal Fruit-Spike can be added to previous prescription.

Prescription analysis: in the prescription, Tall Gastrodia Tuber is sweet, netural and moistened with micro cold nature. When its efficacy reaches liver meridians, the effects are extinguishing of wind, arrest of convulsion, pacification of liver, suppression of yang, dispelling of wind, dredging of collaterals and relieving pain; Gambir Plant Nod and Abalone Shell both have efficacies of pacifying liver and extinguishing wind; Cape Jasmine Fruit and Baical Skullcap Root clear heat and discharge fire to make heat in liver meridian not to cause hyperactivity; Motherwort Herb activates blood and promotes dieresis; Radix Achyranthis Bidentatae induces downward flow of blood, and it tonifies liver and kidneys with Eucommia Bark and Chinese Taxillus Herb; Tuber Fleeceflower Stem and Indianbread with Pine calm nerves and stabilize the mind. Various medicines are combined to clear liver fire and dispel wind, dredge brain collaterals and make pain automatically relieve.

(4) Upward overflowing of phlegm-turbidity

Main symptoms: headache and daze, full and oppressed chest and gastral cavity, phlegm and retching and nausea, heavy limbs and tired body, indigestion, enlarged tongue with teeth marks, white and greasy tongue fur and deep wiry or deep slippery pulse.

Therapeutic method: resolve phlegm and descend adverse qi.

Prescription: modified Ban Xia Bai Zhu Tian Ma Tang. There are Pinellia Tuber, White Atractylodes Rhizome, Tall Gastrodia Tuber, Dried Tangerine Peel, Indian Bread, Sichuan Lovage Rhizome, Dahurian Angelica Root, Atractylodes Rhizome, Puncturevine Caltrop Fruit, Stiff Silkworm, Debark Peony Root and Radix Achyranthis Bidentatae.

Modification: for patients with severe headache, Shrub Chastetree Fruit and Sichuan Lovage Rhizome can be added. In the case that patients also suffer from qi-deficiency, and lassitude and lack of strength and sallow complexion, Milkvetch Root and Ginseng and the like are added to tonify qi and invigorate spleen. In the case of bitter mouth, worry, oppression in chest and abdominal distension, thirst without desire to drink, reddish urine, yellow and greasy tongue fur and soggy rapid pulse occur, these are caused by stagnation phlegm-dampness and transformation to heat. Baical Skullcap Root, Bamboo Shavings and Immature Orange Fruit and others can be added to clear heat and resolve phlegm. Tall Gastrodia Tuber and Puncturevine Caltrop Fruit pacify liver and extinguish wind, and they are important medicines of treating headache and dizziness; Stiff Silkworm resolves phlegm and extinguishes wind; Sichuan Lovage Rhizome and Dahurian Angelica Root dispel wind and relieve pain. As to patients with fullness, hardness and oppression of chest and gastral cavity, indigestion, retching and nausea, Officinal Magnolia Bark, Cablin Patchouli Herb and Fortune Eupatorium Herb are added to resolve dampness, relieve the chest and descend adverse qi. If qi-deficiency also occurs, Tangshen and Milkvetch Root are added to tonify qi and invigorate spleen. In the case of severe vomiting, Inula Flower (decocted with pack) and Hematitum are added to descend adverse qi and control vomiting. With regard to patients who suffer from stagnation phlegm-dampness and transformation to heat, bitter mouth and yellow and greasy tongue fur, Sichuan Lovage Rhizome and Atractylodes Rhizome are removed, and Baical Skullcap Root, Rhizoma Coptidis from Sichuan of China and Tabasheer are added to clear heat and resolve phlegm.

Prescription analysis: In the prescription, Pinellia Tuber, Tall Gastrodia Tuber, Debark Peony Root and Radix Achyranthis Bidentatae are primarily applied to dispel wind and resolve dampness. Activation of blood and movement of qi and relief of pain are advantages. Modern medical studies show that volatile oily alkaloids substance contained in Pinellia Tuber can restrain central nervous system, and Tall Gastrodia Tuber has wide analgesic effect; White Atractylodes Rhizome and Indian Bread have good efficacies of invigorating spleen, draining dampness and resolving phlegm; Atractylodes Rhizome eliminates dampness, invigorates spleen and dispels wind. Sichuan Lovage Rhizome and Dahurian Angelica Root move qi, dispel wind, dredge collaterals and relive pain. Puncturevine Caltrop Fruit descends qi and activates blood. Dried Tangerine Peel smoothes qi and resolves phlegm, and Stiff Silkworm dispels wind, arrests convulsion, resolves phlegm and dispels mass. Combination of various medicines can resolve phlegm, descend turbidity, smooth qi and relieve pain.

(5) Headache caused by blood-stasis

Main symptoms: Prolonged unhealed headache with fixed and stabbing pain, patient with trauma history on the head, dark complexion, dark purple lip color, purple tongue or tongue with ecchymoses and petechiae, thin and white tongue fur, deep and thin pulse or thin and uneven pulse.

Therapeutic method: Activate blood and resolve stasis.

Prescription: Modified Tong Qiao Huo Xue Tang. Sichuan Lovage Rhizome, Dahurian Angelica Root, Manchurian Wildginger, Debark Peony Root, Liquorice Root, Chinese Thorowax Root, Incised Notopterygium Rhizome and Root, Scorpion, Chinese Lovage, White Mustard Seed, Baical Skullcap Root, Medicinal Cyathula Root, Nutgrass Galingale Rhizome.

Modification: Scorpion, Centipede, Dahurian Angelica Root, Nidus vespae are added for patients with worse headache to relieve spasm and pain; for patients with manifestations of chills, Cassia Twig and Manchurian Wildginger are added to warm channels, to dissipate coldness and to relieve pains; for patients with insomnia and amnesia, Grassleaf Sweetflag Rhizome, Milkwort Root, Tuber Fleeceflower Stem are added to tranquil and sedate the mind; for patients with long blood-stasis and blood deficiency, Prepared Rehmannia Root, Suberect Spatholobus Stem are added to activate and nourish the blood; qi deficiency can be cured by adding Milkvetch Root which can replenish qi and activate blood.

Prescription analysis: In prescription, Dahurian Angelica Root, Chinese Thorowax Root, Chinese Lovage are adopted to dispel wind pathogens, which are the important medicines to cure headache; Sichuan Lovage Rhizome, Medicinal Cyathula Root can activate blood and resolve stasis, promote the circulation of qi and relieve pain; Manchurian Wildginger can dispel cold and relieve pain; Debark Peony Root and Liquorice Root can relieve spasm and pain; Scorpion and White Mustard Seed can dredge collaterals and relieve pain. Prolonged headache can cause stagnated qi and accumulated heat. Therefore, Nutgrass Galingale Rhizome is added to regulate qi and Baical Skullcap Root is added to clear heat.

(6) Qi and blood deficiency

Main symptoms: Continual headache which occurs intermittently, and becomes worse after laboring, lassitude with tired body, tastelessness in mouth, pale complexion, pale tongue with white tongue fur, deep, thin and weak pulse

Therapeutic method: Tonify qi and blood.

Prescription: Modified Bu Zhong Yi Qi Tang. Chinese Angelica, Prepared Rehmannia Root, Debark Peony Root, Medicinal Cyathula Root, Sichuan Lovage Rhizome, Tangshen, White Atractylodes Rhizome, Milkvetch Root, Puncturevine Caltrop Fruit, Manchurian Wildginger, Dahurian Angelica Root, Pinellia Tuber, Largetrifoliolious Bugbane Rhizome, Unprepared Liquorice Root, Ass Hide Glue(melted).

Modification: Fleeceflower Root is added to nourish blood for patients with serious blood deficiency; Stir-fried Date Seed and Chinese Arborvitae Kernel are added to nourish heart and tranquilize mind for patients with palpitation and insomnia; dry eyes can be treated by adding Barbary Wolfberry Fruit and Glossy Privet Fruit which can nourish liver and improve vision. The syndrome can be caused by wind-cold attack, Biond Magnolia Flower and Divaricate Saposhnikovia Root and Chinese Lovage can be added to dissipate cold with pungent warm for patients with anemophobia and who like to wrap the head; Severe headache can be treated by adding Common Monkshood Mother Root and Manchurian Wildginger which can warm channels and dredge collaterals, thus to enhance the effects of dispelling wind and relieving pain.

Prescription analysis: Milkvetch Root which can tonify qi with sweet and warm effects as well as uplift qi should be put into an important position. It is supplemented with Tangshen, White Atractylodes Rhizome, Radix Liquorice Root which can invigorate spleen and replenish qi for the effects of tonifying the middle and replenishing qi; Largetrifoliolious Bugbane Rhizome can promote the rise and dispersion of yang qi in the middle energizer; the function of Sichuan Lovage Rhizome, Dahurian Angelica Root, and Puncturevine Caltrop Fruit to stop headache is obvious; Prepared Rehmannia Root and Debark Peony Root can nourish yin and blood, and Ass Hide Glue and Tangshen can tonify blood and generate blood, thus yin is saved from the harm of warmness and dryness; Pinellia Tuber can descend qi and calm stomach as well as prevent too much uplifting and dispersion. All the medicines are used together to achieve the effects of replenishing qi and nourishing blood, ascending lucidity and descending turbidity, as well as dispelling wind and relieving pain.

ii. Specific prescription treatment

1. Zhen Qing Mian An Tang

Components: 30g of Unprocessed Bone Fossil of Big Mammals, 30g of Unprocessed Oyster Shell, 30g of Nacre, 30g of Stir-Fried Spine Date Seed, 20g of Fourleaf Ladybell Roo, 25g of Debark Peony Root, 15g of Milkwort Root, 15g of Chinese Angelica, 15g of White Atractylodes Rhizome, 10g of Cape Jasmine Fruit, 10g of Grassleaf Sweetflag Rhizome, 10g of Chinese Magnoliavine Frui, 10g of Chinese Thorowax Root, 5g of Manchurian Wildginger, 15g of Sichuan Lovage Rhizome, 25g of Medicinal Cyathula Root.

Indications: headache with syndrome of liver depression, stagnated qi, static blood.

293

2. Xiong Shen Wu Bai Tang

Components: Unprocessed Debark Peony Root of 20g, Salvia Root of 20g, Debark Peony Root of 15g, Dahurian Angelica Root of 5g, Stiff Silkworm of 10g, Feverfew of 10g, White Mustard Seed of 6g.

Indications: Migraine with syndrome of phlegm and blood stasis obstructing the collateral and disturbing upward seven orifices.

3. Self-prescribed prescription for headache

Components: Sichuan Lovage Rhizome of 15g, Chinese Thorowax Root 6g, Manchurian Wildginger of 3g, Dahurian Angelica Root of 6g, Stiff Silkworm of 9g, Liquorice Root of 6g, Tall Gastrodia Tuber of 15g, 2 Centipedes, Debark Peony Root of 25g, Chinese Angelica of 15g.

Indications: Headache with syndrome of qi deficiency and blood stasis, attacked by wind pathogens.

4. Self-prescribed prescription for migraine

Components: Sichuan Lovage Rhizome of 30g, Chinese Thorowax Root of 10g, Biond Magnolia Flower of 10g, Scorpion of 10g, Chinese Angelica of 10g, White Mustard Seed of 15g, Dahurian Angelica Root of 15g, Debark Peony Root of 15g, Chinese Lovage of 15g, Baical Skullcap Root of 15g, Nutgrass Galingale Rhizome of 15g, 2 centipede, Manchurian Wildginger of 3g, Liquorice Root of 3g.

Indications: Migraine.

5. Xiong Ge Tang

Components: Sichuan Lovage Rhizome of 9g, Kudzuvine Root of 15g, Debark Peony Root of 10g, Chinese Angelica of 10g, Chinese Thorowax Root of 10g, Turmeric Root Tuber of 10g, White Mustard Seed of 10g, Chinese Lovage of 8g, Medicinal Cyathula Root of 10g, Liquorice Root of 6g.

Indications: Headache with syndrome of stagnated qi and blood.

6. Xiong Gui Er Ge Tang

Components: Sichuan Lovage Rhizome of 15~50g, Cassia Twig of 10g, Common Selfheal Fruit-Spike of 15~50g, Pinellia Tuber of 10~15g, Manchurian Wildginger of 6~15g (decocted later), Rhizoma Corydalis of 15g, Great Burdock Achene of 10g, Peppermint of 5g.

Indications: Headache with syndrome of brain collateral attacked by wind-heat.

7. Xiong Ju Tang

Components: Chrysanthemum Flower of 60g, Sichuan Lovage Rhizome of 30g, Kudzuvine Root of 30g, Medicinal Cyathula Root of 30g, Silktree Albizia Bark of 30g, Tuber Fleeceflower Stem of 30g, Stir-fried Date Seed of 30g, Divaricate Saposhnikovia Root of 15g, Dahurian Angelica Root of 15g, White Mustard Seed of 15g, Cicada Slough of 10g, Liquorice Root of 6g.

Indications: Headache with syndrome of brain collateral is attacked by wind pathogens.

8. Xiong Ma Zhi Tong Tang

Components: Sichuan Lovage Rhizome of 10g, Chinese Angelica of 10g, Tall Gastrodia Tuber of 6g, Debark Peony Root of 15g, Unprocessed Rehmannia Root of 10g, Chinese Thorowax Root of 10g, Common Aucklandia Root of 6g, Dried Tangerine Peel of 10g, Chrysanthemum Flower of 10g, Salvia Root of 10g, Liquorice Root of 6g.

Indications: Headache with syndrome of blood stasis turning heat.

9. Xiong Niu Hu Po Tang

Components: Sichuan Lovage Rhizome of 20~30g, Medicinal Cyathula Root of 30~45g, Amber of 5~10g (dissolved), Shrub Chastetree Fruit of 10~15g, Stiff Silkworm of 5~10g, Unprocessed Abalone Shell of 20~50g (decocted first).

Indications: Headache with syndrome of obstructed phlegm and blood stasis.

10. Xiong Qi Shao Zhi Tang

Components: Sichuan Lovage Rhizome of 15g, Dahurian Angelica Root of 12g, Sanqi of 6g, Debark Peony Root of 30g, Chrysanthemum Flower of 10g, Shrub Chastetree Fruit of 10g, Unprocessed Rehmannia Root of 20g, Stiff Silkworm of 6g, Earthworm of 10g, Liquorice Root of 6g.

Indications: Headache with syndrome of obstructed phlegm and blood stasis.

iii. Single ingredient prescription and proved prescription

(1) 12g of Mulberry Leaf, 12g of Chrysanthemum Flower, 12g of Sichuan Lovage Rhizome, 12g of Climbing Nightshade, 6g of Zanthoxylum Bungeanum, 30g of Gypsum, 3g of Manchurian Wildginger, all of these are decocted. Migraine can be cured with one dose a day.

(2) Abalone Shell of 30g, Chrysanthemum morifolium of 9g, Puncturevine Caltrop Fruit of 9g, Sichuan Lovage Rhizome of 9g, Gambir Plant Nod of 15g are decocted. Migraine can be cured after consecutive 3~5 doses, with one dose a day.

(3) 21g Unprocessed Common Monkshood Mother Root and 15g Jackinthepulpit Tuber are ground together. Take 3g of the ground medicine by dissolving it in plain boiled water one time a day, and the migraine can be cured.

(4) 90g Common Selfheal Fruit-Spike, 60g Nutgrass Galingale Rhizome, and 120g Liquorice Root are ground. Take 4.5g the ground medicine by dissolving it in plain boiled water, and the pain on the forehead and the supraorbital ridge can be cured.

(5) 6~10g Chrysanthemum Flower and 10g Cassia Seed are dissolved in boiled water which is taken as tea, and the headache caused by ascendant hyperactivity of liver yang can be cured.

(6) 1ground Goat Horn, 10g Tall Gastrodia Tuber, 9g Sichuan Lovage Rhizome are decocted together and taken, and the headache can be cured.

(7) 4~5 Rose Flowers, 9~12g Broad Bean Flowers are mixed with boiled water. Take it as tea and drink it frequently, and headache caused by liver wind can be cured.

(8) 3g Nutgrass Galingale Rhizome, 3g Sichuan Lovage Rhizome, and 3g tea leaves are roughly ground and dissolved in boiled water. Take it as tea and drink it frequently, and chronic headache caused by stagnated qi can be cured.

iv. Chinese patent medicine

(1) Qi Ye Shen An Tablets: 50~100mg each time; three times a day or 100mg before sleep. it is applicable to curing headache caused by worries and liver qi depression due to depression and fidgeting.

(2) Xiao Chai Hu Infusion Granule: 1 package each time, twice a day. it is applicable to headache caused by liver depression and qi stagnation which are usually onset in menstrual period.

(3) Tai Ji Tong Tian Liquid: 1 piece each time, three times a day, and 15 days constitute a course of treatment; It is applicable to headache caused by qi and blood deficiency, blood stasis and qi stagnation or headache with wind-cold.

(4) Zheng Tian Pills: 1 package each time, 3 times a day, and 15 days constitute a course of treatment; it is applicable to headache caused by qi and blood deficiency together with stasis.

(5) Quan Tian Ma Capsules: 2~3 grains each time, three times a day, and 15 days are a course of treatment; It is applicable to headache caused by ascendant hyperactivity of liver yang, and liver and kidney deficiency.

(6) Liu Wei Di Huang Wan: 6~8g each time, three times each day; It is applicable to headache caused by liver-kidney yin deficiency.

(7) Qi Ju Di Huang Wan: 6~8g a time, three times a day; it is applicable to headache caused by liver-kidney yin deficiency.

(8) Jin Gui Shen Qi Wan: 6~8g each time, three times a day; It is applicable to headache caused by kidney yang deficiency.

(9) Zheng Nao Ling: 5 pieces each time, three times a day, and 15 days are a course of treatment; it is applicable to headache caused by collaterals obstructed by static blood.

(10) Dang Gui Su Pian: 100mg each time, three times a day, and one month constitutes a course of treatment; It is applicable to headache caused by collaterals obstructed by stasis blood.

(11) Qing Kai Ling Injection: 60ml injection is added to 500 ml of glucose injection intravenous drip of 5%, one time a day, 10 days are a course of treatment; It is applicable to headache caused by hyperactivity of liver yang, up-flaming of liver fire, or headache with wind-heat.

(12) Dang Gui Su Injectable Powder: 100mg of the powder is added to 500 ml of glucose injection intravenous drip of 5%, one time a day, 10-15 days are a course of treatment; It is applicable to headache caused by qi and blood deficiency, and static blood and obstructed collateral.

(13) Ligustrazine Hydrochloride Injection: 120-160mg injection is added to 500 ml of glucose injection intravenous drip of 5%, one time a day, ten days are a course of treatment; It is applicable to headache caused by static blood and obstructed collateral

(14) Puerarin Injection: 400mg is added to 5% 500 ml of glucose injection intravenous drip, one time a day, 10-15 days are a course of treatment; it is applicable to headache caused by wind-fire invading upward, wind phlegm invading upward, static blood and obstructed collateral.

v. Acupuncture and moxibustion treatment

1. Selection of acupuncture and moxibustion therapy

Filiform needle therapy has positive effect on most kinds of headache. However, to improve the therapeutic effects and shorten the treatment course, appropriate acupuncture and moxibustion method should be selected according to the sickness of the patient. For example, for patients infected with wind-cold, filiform needle coordinated with warm needling or moxibustion can enhance the effect of dispersing wind and dispersing wind and dissipating cold; For patients with qi deficiency and whose clear yang fails to ascend, filiform needle coordinated with moxibustion on GV 20 and ST 36 to uplift yang qi; For unhealed headache after long-term treatment with no heat manifestation, filiform needle coordinated with moxibustion or warm needling can warm and dredge channels and collaterals to enhance the effect.

2. Commonly used basic acupoints

LR 3, LI 4, GB 20, GV 20, EX-H N 5, EX-HN 3, ST8, LI 11.

GV 20 is on the head, 5 cun straight above the middle of anterior hair line and at the middle point of the connecting lines of two ear apexes. It has the function of extinguishing wind, refreshing mind, raising yang to stop collapse, which is the key point to cure headache. GB 20 is parallel to GV 16, which is between sternocleidomastoid muscle and cucullaris. It is effective in dispersing wind, dredging collateral, making people calm, relieving pain and tranquilizing the mind. It also has hypnotic effect. LR 3 is located in the crater in front of the joint part of the first and second metatarsus on the dorsum of foot. It can pacify liver, extinguish wind, and invigorate spleen and resolving dampness, which is the key point of tranquilizing mind and relieving pain. LI 4 is located parallel to the middle point of the second metacarpus between the first and second metacarpus. It, together with LR 3, is called Siguan points, which is the key point of tranquilizing and calming mind as well as relieving pain. EX-HN 5 is located in the crater one horizontal finger distance from the middle of the brow top and outer corner of the eye. It can clear heat and disperse wind, relieve headache and dispel dysphoria. LI 11 is located in the middle point of the connecting line between LU 5 and Lateral Epicondyle at the outboard end of cubital crease.

It can disperse wind, clear heat, dredge collateral, relieve pain, tranquilize and calm the mind. EX-HN 3 is located in the middle of the eyebrows, which is effective in tranquilizing and calming mind, dredging collaterals and dispersing wind. ST8 is located 0.5 cun above the temple hairline, which is effective in extinguishing wind and calming mind, relieving pain and improving vision.

3. Point selection by syndrome differentiation

(1) Exogenous headache

① Wind-cold headache: BL 12, B L 60, TE 5 are added; or moxibustion therapy is added.

Prescription analysis: acupuncture and moxibustion on BL 12, B L 60 can soothe and regulate greater yang channel qi, disperse wind-cold, dissolve exterior depression; acupuncture and moxibustion on TE 5 can dredge channels and collaterals; All the points together can realize the effect of dispersing wind, dissipating cold and relieving pain.

② Wind-heat headache: LU 7, SI 3 and GV 14 are added.

Prescription analysis: LU 7 can dredge lung qi; SI 3 and GV 14 can discharge heat and release exterior.

③ Wind-dampness headache: CV 12, ST 36, SP 9, ST40 and SP 6 are added.

Prescription analysis: SP 6 is the front-mu point of the stomach channel and fu organ; ST40 is the luo-connecting point of stomach channel; ST 36 is the sea point of stomach channel. Paired with SP 6, it can invigorate middle energizer to transport and transform water and dampness, as well as help SP 9 expel wind and eliminate dampness, make the invading upward turbid pathogen move downward, thus the headache can be cured naturally.

(2) Headache caused by internal injury

① Headache caused by liver depression: LR 2, CV 17, BL 18 are added.

Prescription analysis: LR 2 is the spring point of liver channel, and BL 18 is the transport point of liver channel; the two points combined can soothe liver and relieve depression; CV 17 is the qi-assembling point, which can regulate qi movements over the body.

② Up-flaming of liver fire: GV 14, GB 21 and LR 2 are added.

Prescription analysis: GV 14 and GB 21 can disperse wind and clear heat. Coordinated with LR 2, they can succeed in clearing and purging liver flame.

③ Hyperactivity of liver yang: LR 4, GB 38, SP 6, KI 3, GB 34 are added.

LR 4, GB 38 are the jing-river points of liver and gallbladder channel.

Prescription analysis: They are also paired points of clearing liver and gallbladder, coordinated with KI 3 on kidney channel of foot lesser yin and GB 34 on kidney channel of foot lesser yin, and are the points with special effects in curing headache caused by hyperactivity of liver yang.

④ Upward overflowing of phlegm-turbidity: SP 9, CV 12, ST40, GV 23 are added.

Prescription analysis: ST40 is the connecting point of the stomach, SP 9 is the sea point of the spleen channel, and V 12 is the front-mu point of the stomach channel; the three points have the effects of invigorating Zhongzhou and resolving phlegm-turbidity; GV 23 and GV 20 can refresh mind and brain, and it is also effective in curing partial headache and muddled head.

⑤ Headache caused by static blood: SP 10, SP 8 and SP 6 are added.

Prescription analysis: SP 8 paired with SP 6 can move qi and activate blood; the two can dredge and regulate collaterals and channels coordinated with SP 8.

⑥ Qi and blood deficiency: CV 6, CV 4, BL 20, SP 6, ST 36 are added.

Prescription: CV 6, CV 4 are all the key points of tonifying qi. BL 20 and ST 36 can strengthen spleen and replenish qi; SP 6 can replenish qi and tonify blood.

⑦ Liver-kidney yin deficiency: BL 23, GV4, ST 36, KI 3, GB 12, BL 10 are added.

Prescription Analysis: GB 12 and BL 10 can replenish marrow and tonify brain, BL 23, GV 4, and KI 3 can tonify kidney and supplement essence, CV 4 is the key point of tonifying qi. These points together can cure the headache caused by kidney yin deficiency.

vi. Manipulation

1. Massage therapy

Massage not only has positive effect on curing headache, including chronic headache, angioneurotic headache, neurotic headache, but also has efficacy in relieving pain rapidly. The manipulations should be done following thesixteen steps:

(1) Massage EX-H N 5: massage EX-H N 5 for 100 times with middle finger or index finger. EX-H N 5 is located in the crater about one horizontal finger distance from behind the part between the brow tip and the outer corner of the eye. Massage of the point can clear heat and dispel dysphoria.

(2) Massage BL 2: massage BL 2 for 100 times with middle finger or index finger. The point is located in the crater of the brow and the supraorbital incisures place. Massaging this point can clear heat and improve vision, activate collaterals and disperse wind.

(3) Push the Kangong: part-push 36 times from brow head to brow tip with two fingers to opposite directions. Such massage can refresh the mind and improve vision.

(4) Massage the EX-HN 3: Massage EX-HN 3 for 100 times with middle finger or index finger. EX-HN 3 is located in the middle of two brows. Such massage has the effect of calming and soothing nerves as well as activating collaterals and dispersing wind.

(5) Massage life gate: Push from between the eyes to GV 23 using the ribbed surface of the two fingers alternatively for 36 times. Such massage can refresh and tranquil the mind, improve vision and calm the heart.

(6) Uplift BL7: Massage EX-H N 5 for several times with two hands and then uplift it rapidly upward to BL7 for 3 times (4 cun straight above the middle of the anterior hairline, 1.5 cun beside).This method can activate collateral and relieve stuffy orifices, clear heat and disperse wind.

(7) Massage ST8: Massage ST8 for 100 times with middle finger and index finger. ST8 is located 0.5 cun above the temple hairline.

(8) Comb with five parted fingers: Comb from anterior hairline to posterior hairline for 66 times with five parted fingers of the two hands. Such massage can dredge collaterals and channels, disperse wind, relieve pain, tranquilize mind and tonify the brain.

(9) Click on the head: Hit the head slightly with the ends of the two fingers alternatively with the fingers slightly bent like quincunx for 100 times. It has the function of tranquil mind, tonify the brain, promote the flow of qi and blood.

(10) Knock the head: Knock the head with small fingers for 100 times, with hands held together and five fingers slightly bent. Such massage can eliminate fatigue and dredge collaterals and channels.

(11) Twist gallbladder channel: Twist the running courses of the gallbladder (lateral head above two ears) on two ears with other four fingers of two hands except thumbs for 100 times. Such massage can dredge collaterals and channels, move qi and activate blood.

(12) Massage GB 20: Massage GB 20 for 100 times with fingers. GB 20 is located in the crater in the hairline behind the neck (in the crater between Sternocleidomastoid muscle and cucullaris). Massage of the point can improve vision, open orifices, tranquilize and calm mind.

(13) Grasp the neck: Grasp the neck along the running courses of bladder channel on the neck from top to bottom for 6 times. Such massage can make people calm, relieve pain, open orifice and refresh mind.

(14) Grasp G21: Grasp G21 for three times. G21 is located on the middle point of the connecting line between GV 14(under the seventh spinous process of cervical vertebra) and acromial end. It can regulate qi and blood over the body and invigorate yang qi.

(15) Rub the neck: Rub the neck with hypothenar until there are some heat on the neck.

(16) Konck the back and shoulder: Knock back and shoulder with slightly bent fingers hands.

2. Modification of massage by differentiation of syndromes

For patients with partial headache, massage of GB8 can be added (straight above the ear tip and 1.5 cun into the hair line). For patients with partial pain on the forehead, 100 times massage of GV 23 (1 cun straight above the part right in the middle of the hairline) and 100 times massage of GB 14(straight above the pupil and 1 cun distance from above the eyebrow) are added. For patients with severe headache, he can massage GB 20 for 10 times with bent fingers, which has immediate effect. For patients with side stitches and bitter taste, massage of SP 9 is added; Patients with restless sleep can also massage the PC 6. For patients with sore waist and loss of kidney essence, massage of KI 3 is added. Massage of EX-B7(in the waist, in the crater 3.5 cun distance from beside the fourth spinous process of lumbar vertebra) is added. For patients with spermatorrhea and leukorrhea problems, massage of CV 4 is added. For patient with palpitation, they can also massage HT7 and PC7. Massage of CV 12 is added for patients with anorexia and massage of CV 17 is added for patients with chest tightness. For patients with nausea and vomiting syndromes, massage of PC 6 is added.

3. Self-massage

(1) Exogenous headache: Massage EX-H N 5 for 100 times, left and right side of LI 11 for 100 times respectively, left and right side of LI 4 for 100 times respectively, BL 10(with 1.3 cun distance from GV 15), GB 20 for 50 times, and left and right G21 for 10 times respectively.

(2) Liver yang headache: Massage GV 20 and EX-H N 5 100 times respectively. Rub the gallbladder channels separately, knead LI 15, LI 11, and LR 3 100 times respectively. Rub KI 1 until there is some heat.

4. Massage contraindication

(1) Patients with headache and ejecting vomiting;

(2) Patients with headache and stiff neck;

(3) Patients with headache and hypertensive crisis;

(4) Patients with headache and hemorrhagic diathesis;

(5) Patients with headache and muddled feeling.

vii. Others

1. Ear acupuncture

AT (3), AT (1), brain and HT7 are selected. CowHerb Seed Pressing or auricular point needle-embedding method can be applied. For stubborn headache, doctors can prick vein in posterior surface of ear to bleed.

2. Picking and cupping

GV 14 and back-shu points are pricked, bled and cupped to treat exogenous headache.

3. Point injection

GB 20 is injected with 1% procaine hydrochloride or vitamin B12 injection, and 0.5-1.0ml for each side. It is carried out every day or once every other day. The method applies to treating stubborn headache.

V. Empirical prescriptions of famous physicians and experts

i. Modified Tian Ma Gou Teng Yin (Dong Guoli)

1. Treat headache with syndrome of liver depression

Components: Tall Gastrodia Tuber, Gambir Plant Nod, Concha Haliotidis and Tuber Fleeceflower Stem are selected in the first prescription, and Scorpion, Centipede, Bombyx Batryticatus, Shrub Chastetree Fruit, Dahurian Angelica Root, Chrysanthemum Flower, Bupleurum, Sichuan Lovage Rhizome, Pinellia Tuber, Divaricate Saposhnikovia Root, Manchurian Wildginger, Liquorice Root and the like are added.

Efficacy: the prescription is used for headache caused by liver depression with vertigo for headache, vexation and irascibility, restless sleep, nausea and desire to vomit, bitter mouth and red tongue, wiry and forceful pulse, elevated blood pressure, and so on. It shall be decocted in water for oral dose.

Prescription analysis: Tall Gastrodia Tuber is used to pacify liver and subdue wind, and treat headache and vertigo; Gambir Plant Nod can clear heat, pacify liver and subdue wind, thus treat elevated blood pressure; Concha Haliotidis can calm the liver and suppress yang, and treat headache; Tuber Fleeceflower Stem can nourish heart and calm the nerves, and dispel wind and active meridians to treat debilitated spirit and insomnia. Efficacies of these herbs all can enter liver, so they are first selected. However, there is a concern that the efficacy can't reach the top disease location, so Scorpion, Centipede, Bombyx Batryticatus whose efficacies can enter liver are added to subdue wind, relieve spasm, resolve mass, dredge collaterals and relieve pain. Chrysanthemum Flower clears upper part to treat head wind, Shrub Chastetree Fruit enters liver to clear heat manifestations in head and eyes, Dahurian Angelica Root eliminates blood stasis and stops pain, Bupleurum soothes liver and relieves stagnation, Manchurian Wildginger promotes orifices and stops pain, and Sichuan Lovage Rhizome eliminates blood stasis, activates blood and promotes qi, which makes qi present circulating without pain, and qi moves without blood stasis, choroids in upper parts circulate, and blockage disappear. Both headache and elevated blood pressure can be cured. More than ten cases of patients with "headache caused by liver depression" ever were treated with the foregoing prescription, and all treatment obtained satisfactory efficacy. In terms of the prescription, Chinese Lovage can be added to treat partial headache; Giant Typhonium Rhizome, Arisaema and Pinellia Tuber and the like are added to dispel wind, resolve mass, resolve phlegm, relieve spasm and relieve pain; Divaricate Saposhnikovia Root, Fineleaf Schizonepeta Herb and Incised Notopterygium Rhizome and Root and others are added to dispel wind and eliminate blood stasis. To sum up, the medicines that can reach the head shall not be neglected, and there is no limitation in selection of diagnosis and treatment.

2. Treat nerve-racking headache

Components: In the prescription, some herbs like Gambir Plant Nod, Concha Haliotidis, Giant Typhonium Rhizome, Divaricate Saposhnikovia Root, Fineleaf Schizonepeta Herb and Incised Notopterygium Rhizome and Root are decreased from prescription I, and Fleeceflower Root, Date Seed and Milkwort Root are added.

Efficacy: With regard to nerve-racking headache, headache and dizziness (worse after laboring), nausea, loose of appetite, lassitude and lack of strength, absent mind, hypomnesia, insomnia and dreaminess, thin and weak pulse, etc. The prescription is decocted in water for oral dose.

Prescription analysis: In the prescription, Fleeceflower Root neutrally nourishes liver and kidneys to treat debilitated spirit, Date Seed nourishes heart and calms nerves to treat dreaminess, Milkwort Root clams mind and nerves, dispel phlegm and open orifices. Tonification is used, but is not focused on; calm of nerves is applied, but is not emphasized; relief stagnation and opening orifices shall be taken as urgent tasks, thus orifices can be opened, and movements are flexible, then insomnia, amnesia, headache and vertigo can be eliminated.

ii. Xiong Gui San (Li Shoushan)

Indication: headache.

Components: Chinese Angelica Root of 10-30g, Sichuan Lovage Rhizome of 15-50g, Manchurian Wildginger of 3-9g and Centipedes in range of 1-3 (the effect is better in the case of taking after grinding into fine powder and mixing it with water).

Direction: Decoction with water. The powder is taken 3 times a day for the patients with serious headache.

Efficacy: This prescription has effects clinically. If there were patients who were injected with pethidine, but headache was not relieved, they could be cured with the prescription. There are two reasons in the prescription why it can obtain efficacy: first is few but fine herbs with strong pertinence. In the prescription, main herb of Sichuan Lovage Rhizome is warm with slight taste, but the smell is strong, which can be better in dredging, travelling up to head and eyes, and down to SP 10. qi moves and blood activates, so barrier of static blood can be broken down; Chinese Angelica nourishes and activates blood, induces menstruation and relieves blood, which assists efficacy of relieving pain in Sichuan Lovage Rhizome, and inhibits the shortcoming of excessive travel. Though Manchurian Wildginger and Centipede are assistant medicines, they can't be omitted in the prescription, because the two are first medicines to destroy obstructions, as well as top grade drugs of relieving pain and astringent. Second, large quantity, special herbs and proper selection. Common people suppose that since Sichuan Lovage Rhizome is warm with fragrance drifting, it couldn't be excessively used. Actually, it is not the case. Chronic and stubborn diseases and ailment disease are like fortresses of enemy camps, insufficient explosives are an ineffective solution. Minimum dosage applied by Li starts from 15 g, and increases subsequently. To patients with severe headache, more than 50 g Sichuan Lovage Rhizome was often applied. There were no shortcomings of yin damage and fragrance drifting in practices. Surely, this is involved with soft and moist natures of Angelica and prevention of side effects. This reflects beauty of combination of sovereign, minister and assistant medicines. Additionally, the saying of "no more than one Qian of Manchurian Wildginger (Qian= 3.72 g)"is discredited. Li used Manchurian Wildginger to relieve pain, and the dose varied from 3 g to 9 g, then there were no adverse reactions. Centipedes are poisonous, and all people are in fear of them. Whereas, they can be used to treat static blood and headache, which really have efficacies of dispelling wind, calming spasm, searching wind, promoting orifices, eliminating blood stasis and reliving pain. 3 Centipedes are applied in one dose without toxic reactions. As a result, effects of large application are like drum beat with drumsticks.

iii. Modified Liu Wei Xin Zhi Liang Fang (Zheng Sunmou)

Indication: internal injury and migraine with sydrome of ascendant hyperactivity of liver yang.

Components: 2.5g Manchurian Wildginger, 3g Dahurian Angelica Root, 18 g Prepared Rehmannia Root, 6g Tree Peony Root Bark, 15g Common Yam Rhizome, 9 g Indian Bread, 9 g Asiatic Cornelian Cherry Fruit, 9 g Alisma, 9 g Radix Achyranthis Bidentatae, 24 g Nacre (decocted first) or 18g Magnetite (decocted first).

Application: Decoct Nacre or Magnetite first for 15 min, throw them to various herbs and decoct, take 750ml water, and decoct them to 500 ml. Patients take one dose of decoction two times in two days. In terms of patients who suffer from pain for a long time, 3 g Sichuan Lovage Rhizome is added; for the patients with dizziness, a Sunflower is added; Arnebia Root for constipation during menstruation.

Efficacy: The prescription applies to headache resulting from liver-kidney yin deficiency or ascendant hyperactivity of liver yang, and patients with yang deficiency and exogenous headache shall avoid taking it.

Prescription analysis: This prescription derives from ancient prescriptions. Zhou Shenzhai in Ming Dynasty ever prescribed Liu Wei Di Huang Tang modified with Dahurian Angelica Root and Manchurian Wildginger to treat one female with "Yegeng". This is the meaning that disease occurred in upper part, and treatment is begun from lower parts, which offers deep enlightenment. Since it is thought that headache belongs to syndrome of lower excess and upper deficiency with liver and kidney yin deficiency. Blood in essence can't face toward top; yin deficiency leads to internal heat, floating fire flames up, which disturb mind, then various pains are produced. Following the meaning of Zhou Shenzhai treating "Yegeng", Liu Wei Di Huang Tang is taken to nourish kidney yin to consolidate root. As wind medicines can reach top, Manchurian Wildginger and Dahurian Angelica Root are added. The light and rising taste is applied to dispel pain and promote efficacy. Then, various medicines are made to travel to top. Nacre is added to calm again, which makes the efficacy flow downward with Radix Achyranthis Bidentatae to let qi in liver and kidneys be recovered, and exerts efficacies of nourishing water and covering fire. Genuine yin is abundant, marrow sea is full, and when there is the relative equilibrium of yin-yang, then headache is naturally eliminated.

iv. Gou Xie San (Zhu Liangchun)

Indication: migraine.

Components: Scorpion, Tall Gastrodia Tuber, Human Placenta, Earthworm, Sichuan Lovage Rhizome and other herbs. These herbs are grinded into find powder, and held with capsules for convenience of taking.

Efficacy: patients shall take 4g each time. The powder shall be taken for 2-3 times each day in onset, and once in other occasions for consecutive 2 weeks, thus the efficacy can be consolidated. As to patients with significant yin deficiency, dry mouth, red tongue and wiry and rapid pulse, 6g Chuanshihu and 6g Dwarf Lilyturf Tuber are made teas to take powder, which is able to nourish yin and generate fluid.

Prescription analysis: Scorpion is good at quenching wind and relieving pain, which has efficacies of opening blood stasis and dredging collaterals; Tall Gastrodia Tuber not only quenches wind and relieves convulsion, but also is better in treating recurrent headache, so Zhang Yuansu said that it "has efficacies of treating wind deficiency, vertigo and headache" as well as "dredging blood vessels"; Earthworm clears heat, pacifies liver, activates blood and dredges collaterals. In *Compendium of Materia Medica*, it is used to treat recurrent headache; Sichuan Lovage Rhizome activates blood and stops pain. Wang Haogu praised it for efficacies of "searching liver qi, nourish liver blood, moistening liver dryness, and supplementing wind deficiency"; "there is more deficiency in long-term pain", so Human Placenta of nourishing qi and blood and tonfying liver and kidneys is prescribed. Such integration and supplement and complement each other achieve a good efficacy.

VI. Typical medical record of famous physicians and experts

i. Medical record of Shi Jinmo —— headache caused by blood deficiency

Ms. Fu, female, 22.

Preliminary diagnosis: The patient had been ill for more than a year. In the beginning, overstrained nerves, painful and full head (in particular, the feeling was serious in occiput), short breath, impatience and irascibility, defecation once in several days, malaise, menstrual irregularities with small quantity and light color, pale complexion, thin and white tongue fur and deep and soft pulse.

Syndrome differentiation: Menstrual irregularities and small quantity and light color belong to blood deficiency with weak and consumption of real blood and loss of main auxiliary substance in heart. Therefore, there were palpitation and short breath, and blood failed to nourish liver, and then patients suffered from impatience and irascibility, painful and full head and defecation once in several days. These don't belong to heat accumulation, but manifestations of desiccated intestines without embellishment and qi deficiency.

Therapeutic methods: Nourish blood, promote heart, soothe liver and activate meridians.

Prescription: 10g Concha Mauritiae (decocted first), 10g Fluorite (decocted first), 5g Chinese Thorowax Root Red Thorowax Root, 15g Hemp Seed, 10g Yellow Chrysanthemum, 10g Chinese Arborvitae Kernel, 5g Stir-fried Sichuan Lovage Rhizome with Yellow Rice Wine, 6g Unprocessed and 6g Prepared Rehmannia Root, 5g Villons Amomum Fruit, 1.5g Manchurian Wildginger, 5g Chinese Thorowax Root Red Thorowax Root, 10g Debark Peony Root, 5g Shrub Chastetree Fruit, 6g Deer-Horn Glue (melted and taken with other herbs), 10g Radix Astragali Preparata , 10g Chinese Angelica with Vegetable Oil, 15g Puncturevine Caltrop Fruit, 10g Fleeceflower Root, 10g Stir-fried Milkwort Root and 3g Prepared Radix Glycyrrhizae.

Second diagnosis: 3 doses of medicines were taken, and full and painful head relived, and spirit was better. When she thought more, dysphoria and irascibility, palpitation and short breath happened. There was defecation, but stool was obstructed. Milkvetch Root was removed from the previous prescription, and 6g Blackend Swallowwort Root was added.

Third diagnosis: in the last year, the patient received diagnosis for consecutive twice. The medicine had effect on the patient. She returned to Beijing after a year due to business trips. Now, she still had symptoms of painful and full head, urgent temperament, boredom of noisiness, love of solitude, hate of loud voices and sounds, inhibited defecation and anorexia.

Prescription: 10g Concha Mauritiae (decocted first), 10g Fluorite (decocted first), 10g Indianbread with Pine (mixed with cinnabar), 6g Dwarf Lilyturf Tuber with Cinnabar, 10g Hemp Seed, 10g Unprocessed Bone Fossil of Big Mammals (decocted first), 10g Unprocessed Oyster Shell (decocted first), 5g Officinal Magnolia Flower, 5g Rose Flower, 3g Prepared Radixglycyrrhizae, 5g Inula Flower, 10g Haematitum, 5g Chinese Rose Flower (later addition) and 5g Seville Orange Flower (later addition).

Fourth diagnosis: the patient took 5 doses of medicines according to previous prescription, and the effect showed was not obvious except for improved appetite. The rest of symptoms were as usual, and sleep was not good, and she could only sleep for 4-5 h every night.

Prescription: 6g Magnetic Bead Pill, 12g Husked Sorghum, 5g Chinese Thorowax Root Red Thorowax Root, 10g Debark Peony Root, 10g Chinese Angelica with Vegetable Oil, 5g Stir-fried Sichuan Lovage Rhizome with Yellow Rice Wine, 10g Unprocessed Bone Fossil of Big Mammals (decocted first), 10g Unprocessed Oyster Shell (decocted first), 5g Villons Amomum Fruit, 6g Unprocessed and 6g Prepared Rehmannia Root, 1.5g Manchurian Wildginger, 6g Inula Flower, 10g Haematitum, 18g Snakegourd Fruit, 10g Longstamen Onion Bulb, 3g Prepared Radix Glycyrrhizae, 5g Stir-fried Green Tangerine Peel with Strong fire, 5g Orange Peel and 12g Hemp Seed.

Fifth diagnosis: with 6 doses of prescription, sleep improved, mind was calm without serious dysphoria, stool was unobstructed, and appetite increased, but only headache wasn't eliminated.

Prescription: 5g Tangerine Peel, 5g Tangerine Pith, 12g Puncturevine Caltrop Fruit, 5g Stir-fried Sichuan Lovage Rhizome with Yellow Rice Wine, 10g Yellow Chrysanthemum, 6g Folium Mori, 10g Poria Cocos, 10g Indianbread with Pine, 3g Dahurian Angelica Root, 6g Stir-fried Milkwort Root, 10g Unprocessed Bone Fossil of Big Mammals (decocted first) and 10g Unprocessed Oyster Shell (decocted first).

Sixth diagnosis: with 8 doses, headache was relieved. Because she went on business trip for more than 1 month, and failed to receive treatment, then headache happened to her as before, stool was obstructed, and limbs felt acid and numb.

Prescription: 10 g Concha Mauritiae, 10g Fluorite, 12g Unprocessed Bone Fossil of Big Mammals (decocted first) , 12g Unprocessed Oyster Shell (decocted first), 6g Folium Mori, 3g Stir-fried Milkwort Root, 6g Rhubarb , 5g Stir-fried Sichuan Lovage Rhizome with Yellow Rice Wine, 10g Indian bread with Pine (mixed with cinnabar), 10g Dwarf Lilyturf Tuber, 10g Chinese Angelica with Vegetable Oil, 18g Chinese Taxillus Herb, 15g Hemp Seed, 10g Flatstem Milkvetch Seed and 10g Puncturevine Caltrop Fruit.

Seventh diagnosis: with consecutive 10 doses, symptoms had been relieved, and all were nearly normal except headache and palpitation in overwork.

Prescription: twice of dose of prescription in the sixth diagnosis were added, and 30g Chinese Arborvitae

Kernel, 30g Spine Date Seed were added. They were ground into fine powder, and processed into pills with honey. Each pill weighs 10g, and the patient took 1 pill in the morning and evening with plain boiled water.

Note: the case belongs to headache due to blood deficiency. The disease resulted from overstrained nerves, potential consumption of yin-blood, blood flow failure and nutrient loss in brain, then headache and amnesia occurred. The disease was involved with heart and liver, so there were manifestations of palpitation and dysphoria. The effects of nourishing blood, promoting heart, soothing liver and activating collaterals were supposed to be obvious. The patient received treatment for twice, and took medicines of less than 10 doses, then stopped the medicines to go on business trip for 1 year. Since treatment couldn't be sustained, and she felt tired in trip. The condition could only deteriorate. She returned to Beijing and received treatment, and took 19 doses of medicines, then went on business trip again. In such twists and turns, good effects still could be achieved, it is because that syndrome differentiation was correct, and proper methods were adopted in prescriptions. Patients with anemia and dry stool mostly belong to moistureless intestines with weak movement, not heat manifestation excess syndrome. If blood is sufficient, and qi circulates, then stool is moistened, and there is no need to take medicines for discharging.

ii. Medical record of Zhang Qi ——headache with syndrome of stasis blood

Mr. Li, male, 43.

Preliminary diagnosis: on November 1, 1998. The patient suffered from headache for 10 years, and effects of treatment in many hospitals were insignificant. The disease was diagnosed as angioneurotic headache. The condition was deteriorated in recent year, and usually occurred on the right side. He suffered from poor sleep, fat body, confused dreaminess, tinnitus and amnesia, vexation, dark purple tongue, greasy tongue fur and deep pulse.

Syndrome differentiation: The syndrome belongs to long-term disease invading collaterals, choroid blockage, blood stasis, qi stagnation and phlegm coagulation.

Therapeutic methods: Activate blood, disperse blood stasis, move qi and clear up phlegm.

Prescription: Modified Xue Fu Zhu Yu Tang and San Pian San.

There are 20g Chinese Angelica, 20g Red Peony Root, 20g Unprocessed Rehmannia Root, 20g Peach Seed, 25g Sichuan Lovage Rhizome, 25g Common Selfheal Fruit-Spike, 15g Safflower, 15g Bupleurum, 15g Orange Fruit, 15g White Mustard Seed, 15g Nutgrass Galingale Rhizome and 15g Dahurian Angelica Root.

Second diagnosis: on November 15, 1998. The patient took 7 doses of prescription and headache was significantly relieved. He only suffered from slight headache and discomfort. The prescription wasn't changed.

Third diagnosis: on November 22, 1998. With 6 doses the symptoms eliminated again. However, cross pain constantly appeared, with purple tongue and deep pulse. The patient still had symptoms of bad sleep and vexation. The medicines of dispelling wind, calming nerves and nourishing heart were added to previous prescription.

Prescription: 30g Unprocessed Rehmannia Root, 20g Chinese Angelica, 20g Peach Seed, 20g Red Peony Root, 20g Bupleurum, 20g Sichuan Lovage Rhizome, 20g Chrysanthemum Flower, 20g Spine Date Seed, 15g Safflower, 15g White Mustard Seed, 15g Milkwort Root, 25g Common Selfheal Fruit-Spike and 15g Chinese Dwarf Cherry Seed.

Fourth diagnosis: on December 16, 1998. With 16 doses prescription There was no headache with good sleep. The mild diarrhea occurred. Chinese Dwarf Cherry Seed was removed from the previous prescription, and 15g White Atractylodes Rhizome was added. The patient should take 7 doses of prescription, and headache and other symptoms didn't recur with follow-up after 1 year.

Note: The case belongs to headache due to stasis blood. Long-term headache, dark purple tongue or tongue with ecchymosis and deep or deep and unsmooth pulse belong to blood stasis, and the patient has fat body and greasy tongue fur, so the syndrome belongs to blood stasis with phlegm-dampness inside. Xue Fu Zhu Yu Tang and San Pian Tang are modified to achieve efficacy. In the prescription, Sichuan Lovage Rhizome can flow up to head and eyes, and it is better in divergency and dredging of collaterals. The herb is an important medicine for treating headache; White Mustard Seed eliminates dampness and resolves phlegm, and it is an important medicine for treating phlegm. Combination of two herbs in San Pian Tang is a medicament of treating phlegm and blood stasis. Sanpian Decoction was from prescription in Volume II of *Syndrome differentiation Record*. It was said in formulary that "syndrome of migraine is mostly because that liver wind invades upward, disease lasts for a long time, pathogenic factors enter brain collaterals, and meridians are blocked, then it is hard to avoid qi stagnation and phlegm coagulation. Seldom, these are triggered by cold and summer heat or anger-in. Onset is normal". Beauty of the prescription lies in large application of Sichuan Lovage Rhizome with Dahurian Angelica Root to make it travel to heads and qi motion, White Mustard Seed to resolve phlegm, Bupleurum into meridian of Lesser Yang to make it reach the affected area to exert effects of dredging meridians. Common Selfheal Fruit-Spike clears liver and scatters collaterals. For patients with phlegm blood stasis and heat transformation, effects of pacifying liver and clearing heat can be obtained with the herb. Chrysanthemum Flower removes heat for treating head and ocular diseases, and it is a good match for medicines of activating blood and resolving blood stasis. As a result, convergent effect is quick. Modern pharmacological studies show that Sichuan Lovage Rhizome contains alkaloids and tetramethylpyrazine, which can obviously dilate blood vessels, relieve vasospasm, and increase blood flow, thus make blood in brain circulate normally.

iii. Medical record of Lu Xiaozuo ——ascendant hyperactivity of liver yang

Mz. Chen, female, 51, bank clerk.

Preliminary diagnosis: on March 31, 2011. The patient suffered from headache and dizziness for one year, and the two deteriorated for half a year. The patient stated that one year ago, she got angry and felt tired because of work, then began to suffer from high blood pressure, fullness and pain in head and dizziness. Then, blood pressure was 155/85mmHg. She had no hypertension disease history before, and blood pressure was about 110/70mmHg at usual time. Later, the symptom was relieved after patients taking antihypertensive drugs with western medicine treatment. Half a year ago, since she was unpleasant, blood pressure was elevated again, and systolic pressure was up to 155mmHg. Fullness and pain in head, dizziness, headache in right side, flushed face and red eyes and hot face occurred. These symptoms hadn't been relieved with Chinese and western medicines. The disease was diagnosed as cerebral ischemia in western medicine. The patient had appetite, and could sleep with more than 20 years' constipation, and pee without thirst and desire for drinks. Legs were painful and full, and soles were painful. Tongue was red, with sharp thorn-like thing, tongue fur was thin and yellow, and pulse was deep and wiry.

Syndrome differentiation: Liver depression transforming into heat, ascendant hyperactivity of liver yang, upward disturbance of orifices by liver wind.

Therapeutic method: Tonify qi, nourish blood, soothe and pacify liver, quench wind, relieve pain, move qi and relax bowels.

Prescription:

(1) Take orally: 25g Debark Peony Root, 20g Cochinchinese Asparagus Root, 15g Figwort Root, 15g Gui Ban (decocted first), 30g Haematitum, 30g Unprocessed Bone Fossil of Big Mammals, 30g Unprocessed Oyster Shell, 20ggerminated Barley, 30g Radix Achyranthis Bidentatae, 10g Unprocessed Liquorice Root, 10g Bupleurum, 10g Dahurian Angelica Root, 15g Tall Gastrodia Tuber, 30ggambir Plant Nod, 10g Rhubarb, 15g Salvia Root, 10g Villons Amomum Fruit and30g Milkvetch Root. There were 7 doses. The medicines should be decocted in water for oral use, and1 dose should be taken daily in the morning and evening.

(2) 2 doses of external application prescription for pacifying liver and calm nerves should be used to soak foot to pacify liver, subdue yang and extinguish wind.

(3) Acupuncture and moxibustion should be conducted for 1 course to reinforce healthy qi, calm nerves and smooth Ren.

(4) Ear acupuncture should be leveled, and nutrient-defense should be regulated to dredge collaterals, calm nerves and relieve pain.

Second diagnosis: on April 7, 2011. The patient stated that fullness and pain in head and dizziness were obviously relieved, and she could defecate and have appetite. Seldom, abdominal distension after meal was seen. Recently, she had insomnia, dreaminess, light and shallow sleep, somnolence and lack of strength in the daytime, red tongue, thin and yellow tongue fur and deep and wiry pulse.

Prescription:

(1) In the first prescription, 15g White Atractylodes Rhizome, 30g Magnetite and 30g Caulis Polygoni Multiflori are added to invigorate spleen, harmonize the middle and tranquilize mind. There were 7 doses, and the medicines shall be decocted in water for oral dose. One dose was taken daily in the morning and evening.

(2) Acupuncture and moxibustion was conducted for 1 course. Original scheme of diagnosis and treatment was kept in other aspects.

Third diagnosis: on April 14, 2011. The patient stated that headache obviously relieved. Now, distending pain in right side of head, dizziness (serious or deterioration in lowering head), nausea and vomiting, short of breath and lack of strength, heavy legs also occurred. The left foot sole was still painful. After meal, distending pain in lateral thorax, stomach and gastral cavity appeared. She had proper appetite and normal urine and stool. However, she still had poor sleep, dreaminess, red tongue and thin and yellow tongue fur, tip with spines and deep and wiry pulse. Blood pressure was 100/70mmHg.

Prescription: Rhubarb and Sandalwood were removed from the prescription in the second diagnosis, and 60g Milkvetch Root rather than 20g Kudzuvine Root was added to tonify qi, reinforce healthy qi, relieve restlessness and calm nerves. There were 7 doses, and the medicines were decocted in water for oral dose. One dose was taken daily in the morning and evening. Original scheme of diagnosis and treatment was kept in other aspects.

Fourth diagnosis: on April 21, 2011. The patient stated that various symptoms were relieved, and seldom had short breath and love of quietness. However, dreaminess, proper appetite, distending pain in hypochondrium, belching, slight relief of pain in soles, dry stool, yellow urine, dark red tongue (especially tip), thin and yellow tongue fur and blood pressure was 100/80mmHg.

Prescription: 10g Rhubarb, 10g Sandalwood, 15g Rhizoma Corydalis, 15g Turmeric Root Tuber and 15g Nutgrassgalingale Rhizome are added on basis of the prescription in the third diagnosis. There are 7 doses, and the medicines shall be decocted in water for oral dose. One dose is taken daily in the morning and evening. Original scheme of diagnosis and treatment is kept in other aspects.

Fifth diagnosis: on April 28, 2011. After acupuncture and medical treatment, the patient felt well, headache and dizziness didn't occur, and qi movement was smooth with good mood. To consolidate efficacy, acupuncture and moxibustion should be conducted for 1 course to observe changes. The patient was asked to eat more fresh fruits and vegetables , avoid fatty and spicy food, and keep clam.

With follow-up after two months, the patients had recovered.

Note: The patient was depressed and angry. Emotion dissatisfaction, liver failing to act freely, qi depression and predominant yang, stirring wind and disturbed orifices belong to pain for meridian obstruction. Due to old age, qi and blood were deficient, and orifices failed to be moistened, which is called malnutrition. Therefore, headache, dizziness, elevated blood pressure, flushed face and red eyes and hot face occurred. qi movement stagnated, and couldn't disperse, pass-down was abnormal, residue accumulates inside, stool was bound, qi stagnates in blood vessels, and qi and blood couldn't moisten lower limbs, so distending pain in legs and pain in soles were seen. The patient was treated by Chinese medicines. Chinese Thorowax Root and Debark Peony Root were applied to regulate and smoothen liver meridians, Gui Ban, Unprocessed Bone Fossil of Big Mammals, Unprocessed Oyster Shell, Haematitum, Tall Gastrodia Tuber and Gambir Plant Nod pacify liver, subdue yang and tranquilize mind. Cochinchinese Asparagus Root, Milkvetch Root and Radix Achyranthis Bidentatae nourish liver and kidneys, and Rhubarb and Villons Amomum Fruit move qi, make diarrhea and loose bowels. External application prescription for pacifying liver and calm nerves is decocted with water to wash externally to pacify liver, subdue yang. By combination of acupuncture and moxibustion therapy and ear acupuncture treatment, it can reinforce healthy, regulate and smoothen meridians, relieve symptoms, make multi-adjustment and enhance efficacy.

VII. Prevention and aftercare

(1) Effects of climate shall be paid attention to. In weather variations, people shall avoid wind cold and keep warm, not be exposed to sun and rain to prevent from nducing disease.

(2) Regular sleep, combination of exertion and rest, eye adjustment and maintenance of quiet environment shall be noticed.

(3) People shall positively quit smoking, keep indoor air ventilation and avoid contacting allergen, etc.

(4) Some medicines that can induce headache shall not be taken to avoid inducing disease, such as contraceptive, nitroglycerin, histamine, reserpine, hydralazine and estrogen.

(5) In the case of exogenous headache, patients shall adopt light diet, and not the medicines for tonifying deficiency. It is suitable for them to eat food with effects of dispelling wind and pathogenic factors, e.g. onions, gingers, lobster sauces, Cablin Patchouli Herb, celery and Chrysanthemum Flower. For patients with wind-heat and headache, they shall eat foods with effect of clearing heat, for instance, green beans, cabbages, carrots, celeries, lotus rhizomes, Lily Bulb and pears. With regard to patients who have headache caused by internal injury, headache and deficiency syndrome, tonifying deficiency is the priority, they shall eat foods that can nourish liver and kidneys, nourish blood and tonify qi, for example, jujubes, black soybeans, litchis, arillus longan, chicken, beef and turtle meat. Excess syndrome of headache by internal injury is treated by eliminating pathogenic factors. In terms of patients with phlegm-dampness and blood stasis, it is suitable to select foods with effects of invigorating spleen, removing dampness or activating blood and resolving blood stasis, such as Common Yam Rhizome, Coix Seed, oranges, haws and brown sugar.

(6) If patients suffer from headache, hams, dry cheese and the like should be prohibited. They shall select less milk, chocolate, cheese, alcoholic drinks, coffee, tea , etc.

(LU Xiaozuo)

References

[1] Shi YG, Shan SJ. Essence of clinical syndromes from contemporary famous physicians: headache and vertigo [M]. Beijing: Publishing House of Ancient Chinese Medical Book, 1992.

[2] Shan SJ, Chen ZH. Golden mirror of clinical syndrome from ancient and modern famous physicians: headache and vertigo [M]. Beijing: China Press of Traditional Chinese Medicine, 1999.

[3] Song ZQ. Mixture of syndrome treatment from contemporary famous physicians [M]. Shijiazhuang: Hebei Science & Technology Press, 1990.

[4] Lyu JS. Interpretation of medical record of Shi Jinmo [M]. Beijing: People's Military Medical Press, 2009. 248-251

[5] Zhang PQ. Memoir of clinical experience from Traditional Chinese medicine master: Traditional Chinese medicine master of Zhang Qi [M]. Beijing: China Medical Science Press, 2011.

[6] Hu GQ, Liu HY. Treatment of form and spirit and application of needles and medicines: collection of

experience from Lu Xiaozuo [M]. Beijing: China Press of Traditional Chinese Medicine, 2012.

[7] Wu FC, Kan XL. Medication and prescription rules of common diseases [M]. Beijing: People's Military Medical Press, 2015.

[8] Fang YZ, Deng TT, Li KG, et al. Practical Traditional Chinese Internal Medicine [M], Shanghai: Shanghai Press of Science and Technology, 1985.

[9] Lyu JS. Interpretation of medical record of Shi Jinmo [M]. Beijing: People's Military Medical Pres, 2009.

类风湿关节炎　　Rheumatoid
Arthritis

I. Overview

Rheumatoid arthritis (RA), "rheumatoid" for short, is a kind of chronic systemic autoimmune disease with a focus in joint synovitis. Joint lesions are symmetric and multiple, and frequent and repeated attacks happen. It mostly happens in facet joints of the hand and foot. In the early stage or acute activity period, the joints that suffer from the disease mostly show redness, swelling, fever and pain as well as motion disorders. In the advanced stage, joint worm erosion, ankylosis or deformity of joints appear, as well as skeletal muscle atrophy. In the whole course of the disease, fever, anemia, weight loss, vasculitis and subcutaneous nodules and other lesions can also be present. Furthermore, the disease also involves some organs like the heart, lungs, kidneys, nerve and eyes. The disease is a common and frequently occurring disease, and RA morbidity in China affects 0.32%-0.36% of the population. At present, there are still no particularly effective treatment methods. Disease age onset is mostly between 25 and 55 years old, and morbidity is 3~5 times higher in females than males. Optimal treatment period for RA is between 3 months and 6 months after the disease attack. Irreversible damage of joints generally happen within 2 years after the disease onset. Mostly, the disease doesn't affect people's life, but a few patients may suffer from severe disability, which makes capacity for work in patients partially or completely lost. It has also pointed by researchers that the disease can shorten lifespan of patients for 5-10 years.

In Chinese medicine, RA belongs to the scope of "Bi syndrome".

Clinically, syndrome differentiation and treatment is conducted according to "bone bi syndrome" and "persistent bi-syndrome". Rich experience on the treatment of Bi syndromes has been gathered in Chinese Medicine. Etiology, pathogenesis, syndrome classification and sequelae and prognosis of Bi syndromes were systematically discussed in the *Huangdi Neijing* (*Internal Canon of the Yellow Emperor*) early, where "wind, cold and dampness are mixed and combined into arthralgia" was noted etiologies. The name of "Lijie Disease" was first recorded in the *Zhong Feng Li Jie Bing of Jin Gui Yao Lue* (*Synopsis of the Golden Chamber · Apoplexy and Lijie Disease*) by Zhang Zhongjing in the Han Dynasty. The main clinical characteristics are moving arthralgia, failure to flex joints, dragging-like pain, frail body with swelling joints, especially in the legs, with swelling, painful feet. They are similar to the symptoms of rheumatic arthritis in the advanced stage. WutouTang decoction, GuizhiBaishaoZhi-muTang decoction and the like, recorded in the classic book are still common effective prescriptions in modern clinical practice. In the *Synopsis of the Golden Chamber* the disease name "wind-dampness" was first suggested, saying: "if patients feel painful all over the body, and the pain is severe in the late afternoon, then the disease is called wind-dampness".

Opinions of medical practitioners of past ages evolved, and they realized further causes of Bi syndrome. For example, a discussion on causes of Bi by Li Yongcui in the Qing dynasty in Supplement to Diagnosis and Treatment says: "due to attack from three conditions of Qi movement and deficiency of original Qi and fluid, Qi can't be freely dispelled, and it flows to meridians, then forming Bi for a long time"; it is further pointed in the book that "dampness and hot phlegm fire, stagnated Qi and blood stasis flow through meridians and limbs, and numbness and Bi can appear". In the discussion of etiology and pathogenesis of Bi syndrome, Wang Wenqi in the same dynasty also said in Zazheng Huixinlu that: "liver and kidneys are disease locations, sinews fails to receive nourishment, and deficient fire flows in meridians" and "medical practitioners mostly treat exogenous pathogenic factors, then the disease trend increases, yin liquids are gradually depleted. It is a disaster of worsening deficiency beyond description". Many medical practitioners developed a thought regarding the research of Bi syndrome. In recent decades, prevention and treatment of RA drew extensive interest in the field of medicine. The disease is prevented and treated by the combination of Chinese and Western medicine in China, and remarkable results were achieved in syndrome differentiation and treatment, specific prescription for certain illness, research and applications of single medicines.

II. Etiology and pathogenesis

i. Chinese medicine

1. Etiology

Rheumatoid arthritis is different from the general Bi syndrome in terms of clinical manifestations, treatment and prognosis, so it is called "obstinate bi-syndrome" or "bone bi". In etiology and pathogenesis, a relationship with deficient healthy Qi in body is stressed in addition to invasion of exogenous pathogenic factors. Deficient healthy Qi refers to instability of defensive qi, deficient blood, deficient Qi and blood, liver-kidney depletion and so on. Invasion of exogenous pathogenic factors include pathogenic factors of wind, cold, dampness and heat. In the process of the development of the pathology, phlegm and blood stasis may be intermingled. They can also combine with exogenous pathogenic factors that block meridians, going deep into bone joints, then causing an obstinate illness.

2. Pathogenesis

The basic pathogenesis is mainly characterized by pathogenic factors attacking a weak body and staying in the meridians, which block Qi and Blood and cause intermingled phlegm and blood stasis settling in bone joints.

Also, most patients suffer from poor constitution, which leads to insufficient yingqi and weiqi, and Qi and blood, as well as poor tissue function in the zangfu meridians. Or, yingqi and weiqi, as well as Qi and blood are injured by excessive overstrain, so that yang Qi become deficient, weiqi is unstable, and pathogenic toxins stay in the meridians, joints and muscles; or, excess sexual activity consumes kidney Qi, thus resulting in weak liver and kidney as well as fragile sinews and bones. The invasion of pathogenic factors of wind, cold, dampness and heat affect Qi and blood, and block joints. The movement of Qi, blood and fluids is unsmooth, which may generate phlegm and blood stasis, as well as intermingled phlegm and blood stasis just like flour mixed with oil. The retention in joints develops obstinate bi-syndrome.

As shown in the diagram:

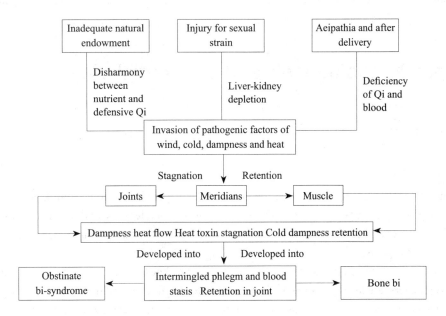

ii. Western medicine

1. Etiology

The etiology of RA disease hasn't been completely defined yet. However, studies in recent years showed that it is associated with factors such as autoimmune disorders, inherited disorders, infections and endocrine disorders.

(1) Immune system factors: many researches support an onset related to immunity. For example, there is large amount of lymphocytes and plasma cells infiltration in the affected bones, and there are immune complexes formed by degenerated IgG and rheumatoid factor (RF). The higher the rate in serum of RF in RA positive patients, the more severe the condition will be.

(2) Genetic factors: results from family pedigree surveys show that direct descendants of patients suffering from RA are more likely to suffer from the disease. It is known that the human leukocyte antigen (HLA) is an important genetic gene, and HLA-DW4 in 70% of patients is positive.

(3) Infection factors: it is believed that streptococcus, diphthemid bacillus, mycoplasma, Epstein-Barr virus and the like are rheumatoid elementary bodies. Although researchers have generated rheumatoid arthritis on animals by means of an infection, this it hasn't been confirmed clinically.

(4) Endocrine disorders: mostly seen in female. Lower morbidity in women who take oral contraceptive drugs, but higher RA morbidity in obese patients and onset peak in menopause tells us that the disease has a relation to endocrine factors.

(5) Others: coldness, dampness, fatigue, malnutrition, trauma, psychoaffective issues and other factors are

incentives to the onset of disease.

2. Pathological mechanism

Pathological changes in rheumatoid arthritis happen to the joint synovium first, then involving the tissues around cartilages and joints. The majority of patients suffer from vasculitis, and the systemic connective tissues may be involved. In the early stage, the disease manifests as acute or subacute joint synovitis, and synovial hyperplasia and hypertrophy appear, then granulation forms and further develop abnormal layer of fibrovascular tissue in blood vessels. Because the fibrovascular tissue contains hydrolase, it can promote the destruction of articular cartilage, the collagen in the tendon of the subchondral bone ligament is eroded, resulting in the destruction of articular cartilage, bone and articular capsule, and joint surfaces are fused with each other to form a fibrous or osseous joint. Muscle and skin near the joints gradually atrophy, and decalcification and osteoporosis happen to bone.

III. Key points of diagnosis and differential diagnosis

i. Diagnostic bases

1. Clinical manifestations

Three kinds of onset form of rheumatoid are generally considered, i.e. hidden onset, acute onset and intermediate onset (happening between the first and second). Clinically, hidden onset is the most prevalent, which can account for 60~70%. General clinical manifestations are sorted into systematic symptoms, articular symptoms and extra-articular manifestations.

(1) Systematic symptoms: Patients often manifest fatigue, weakness, anorexia, weight loss, muscular atrophy, numb limbs, cold fingers, anemia, etc. Some patients may suffer from fever and related symptoms.

(2) Articular symptoms: Symmetric painful swelling of joints, characterized by ankylosis in the morning is the most prevalent. Swelling, pain, restricted movements and other symptoms are local manifestations.

① Morning stiffness: joint morning stiffness refers to ankylosis and inflexible movement of patients after waking up in the morning. In severe cases, catalepsy can happen to the whole body. After patients get out of bed, stiffness may be relieved or disappear with movement or warmth. It is a characteristic symptom of the disease and one of the important diagnostic bases. The duration and degree of morning stiffness can be considered indexes for evaluating disease progression and changes.

② Pain: it is the most prominent symptom of the disease, and a clinical manifestation in all patients' active stages of the disease. The degree of pain is related to individual tolerance, is affected by emotion, climate, environment, and so on. Its characteristic is aggravation with movement and relief after movement. Clinical pain can be divided into tenderness, motion pain (pain when involved joint moves) and spontaneous pain (pain in a resting position, even awakening patients from their sleep). Obvious tenderness and spontaneous pain shows that the disease it is in an acute inflammatory stage, or disease is progressing fast and it's quite severe.

③ Swelling: as a sign of inflammation, swelling is also a quite prominent symptom of the disease. Swelling presents as a homogeneous swelling near the joints, and it is always symmetric. Local swelling presents normal complexion, rather than a redness. But localized redness can also be seen, as well as a heat sensation when the site is touched, and the skin is purplish in color.

④ Movement disorders: it is also a common sign. In the early stage, as inflammatory pain and tissue swelling may cause movement disorder, if edema-related pain is relieved, the joint can be recovered. When the disease is in an advanced stage, muscular atrophy, adhesions and fibrous tissue hyperplasia of bones and joints, as well as bone fusion and malformation may happen, and joint function can't be recovered.

⑤ Joint deformity or stiffness: it is the worst result of joint change in advanced period of the disease. Joint stability, muscular atrophy near the joint and destruction of ligament and joints make joint present one kind of special deformity, e.g. characteristic swan-neck deformity, buttonhole deformity and the like.

(3) Extra-articular manifestations: As the disease belongs to systemic disease, its lesion is not only limited to joints, but involves with other tissues and organs. Common complications are as the following.

① Rheumatoid nodules: among about 20%-25% of patients, subcutaneous nodules occur in the bulky parts of joints and parts that are easily pressed or worn-out. Small nodules are like mung beans, big ones like broad beans, in low number. The appearance of nodules tells us that the disease is in continuous change.

② Rheumatoid vasculitis: inflammation and depositions in blood vessels resulting from immune complexes depositing in vessel walls is clinically called as rheumatoid vasculitis, and also called malignant rheumatoid arthritis. There are two kinds, clinically: one is peripheral vasculitis, and it manifests in the fingers and toes, and nail beds, as ecchymosis. The other is systematic vasculitis, involving multiple organs and viscera. There may be fever, leukocytosis, limb necrosis, various visceral damages and so on. The prognosis is generally poor.

③ Heart damage: heart damage can be seen in the pericardium, myocardium and cardiac valves, and it may cause pericarditis, myocarditis and valve regurgitation. However, heart damage in most patients is mild, and there are no clinical symptoms. Positive rate in autopsy and ultrasonic wave examination is higher, and obvious symptoms are primarily seen in high activity of rheumatoid arthritis.

④ Lung damage: lung damage is manifested as chronic interstitial pneumonia and rheumatoid pleuritis. Main manifestations are fever, cough, expectoration, dyspnea, chest pain, lung rale and other symptoms for a long time with unknown causes. Antibiotic treatment has no effect, but the efficacy of hormonal treatment is significant.

⑤ Eye damage: the symptoms are episcleral inflammation, scleritis, iritis, iridocyclitis, conjunctivitis, uveitis, and so on. There is no efficacy with general therapy and antibiotics, and adrenal corticosteroids has obvious and rapid efficacy.

2. Diagnosis standards

Currently, the diagnosis criteria of rheumatoid arthritis from the American Rheumatism Association (ARA) revised in 1987 is still adopted in RA diagnosis. The disease can be diagnosed as rheumatoid arthritis, if 4 or more in 7 items are present: ① morning stiffness for at least 1 h (≥ 6 weeks) ② 3 or more swollen joints (≥ 6 weeks) ③ swollen joints between proximal fingers on joints of hand or metacarpophalangeal joints (≥ 6 weeks) ④ symmetric swollen joints ⑤ X ray change of finger joints ⑥ subcutaneous rheumatoid nodule ⑦ positive rheumatoid factor. New RA classification criteria were established by the American College of Rheumatology (ACR) and the European League Against Rheumatism (EULAR) in 2009, in which early diagnosis is more emphasized, but they were generally less applied in clinical practice. In the criteria, four parts, including involvement situation, serum antibody examination results, synovitis duration and acute phase reactions are scored, and RA can be confirmed in the case that the total score is over 6 points. Morning stiffness, subcutaneous nodules, symmetric arthritis and X-ray examination were cancelled.

Classification criteria of rheumatoid arthritis from American Rheumatism Association/ European League Against Rheumatism in 2009.

Scores according to the following criteria

A. Involved joints

1 big joint (0)

2~ 10 big joints (1)

1~ 3 facet joints (with or without big joints) (2)

4~ 10 facet joints (with or without big joints) (3)

Over 10 joints (at least of one facet joint) (5)

B: serology (the result on 1 item is required at least)

Negative rheumatoid factor and anti-citrullinated protein antibody (0)

One of rheumatoid factor and anti-citrullinated protein presents low titer and positive (2) at least

One of rheumatoid factor and anti-citrullinated protein presents high titer and positive (3) at least

C: reactant in acute period (the result on 1 item is required at least)

C: normal reactive protein and erythrocyte sedimentation rate (0)

C abnormal reactive protein or erythrocyte sedimentation rate (1)

D: duration of symptoms

< 6 weeks (0)

6 weeks (1)

The case that 6 points or more are obtained is classified as rheumatoid arthritis.

ii. Differential diagnosis

There are various manifestation patterns in rheumatoid arthritis. In particular, shortage of specific symptoms and signs in early period is similar to many other rheumatic diseases. Therefore, it can be quite difficult to make an early diagnosis, and the disease needs to be distinguished from various joint diseases, such as rheumatic arthritis and gout. See the table below for details.

Rheumatoid Arthritis Differentiation Table

Disease name	Differential diagnosis	
	Differentiation basis	Clinical manifestations and laboratory examinations
Rheumatoid arthritis		(1) Young women are the main patients (2) Symmetric swelling and pain of facet joints (3) Positive rheumatoid factor by examination (4) Typical rheumatoid change in X ray
Ankylosing spondylitis		(1) It mostly happens to male youth (2) It mainly invades sacroiliac joint and spine (3) Positive HLA-B27 (4) Spine can present bamboo joint-like change
Proliferative arthritis	(1) Occult or acute onset (2) Swelling and pain in joints of four limbs or spinal joints (3) Joint motion disorder of different degrees	(1) It mostly happens to the patients aged above 40 (2) Main symptom is involvement of weight-bearing joint (3) Affected joint is often asymmetric (4) Labial hyperplasia can be seen in joint margin by X ray.
Gout		(1) Onset age is above 40. (2) More than 95% are male patients. (3) Mainly show redness, swelling, heat and pain of the first metatarsophalangeal joint. (4) Hyperuricemia
Rheumatic fever		(1) It mostly happens to adolescents. (2) The onset is often acute. (3) Swelling and pain of big joints of four limbs (4) Positive anti-streptolysin "O" in serum (5) No positive change in X ray examination

IV. TCM therapy

Until now, there is still no targeted specific therapy for rheumatoid arthritis, but a certain effect can be obtained in the majority of patients in the case of integrated treatment of Chinese medicine and western medicine. Treatment objectives lie in controlling inflammation in joints and other tissues, alleviating pain and relieving symptoms as early as possible. Meanwhile, maintenance of joint functions and prevention of joint deformity should be carried out as possible.

i. Treatment principles

1. Eliminating pathogenic factors, activation of collaterals and relieving spasms and pain.

"Bi" is a disease that can be mild or severe. In any case, it it presents itself with severe syndromes. Consequently, doctors should be proficient at grasping main symptoms and distinguishing levels in treatment. For patients with wind invasion, wind should be primarily dispelled. When patients recover, they should stop taking the originally prescribed medicines, rather than taking more to prevent that medicines to exples wind and dampness damage yin, dry blood and consume Qi; with regard to patients with cold domination, herbs to reinforce yang should be also taken, along with wind-dispelling herbs, so as to make their yang Qi sufficient, support healthy Qi, so as to activate blood, dispell cold, remove stagnation, and unobstruct Bi, so that patients may finally recover; in terms of patients with predominant dampness, medicines for invigorating spleen and replenishing Qi need to be taken as well, while taking herbs for draining dampness and resolve the turbid, so as to make their spleen vigorous enough to dominate dampness and supply sufficient Qi, treating persistent numbness; as to patients with predominant heat, clearing of stagnated heat is the focus. Medicines for activating blood and dredging collaterals should be also taken. However, damaged yang and dampness stagnation due to bitter and cold should be prevented; for patients whose disease lasts for a long time and enters collateral meridians, doctors should follow "blood should be treated first to treat wind, and when blood moves, then wind will be automatically extinguished", and prescribe the medicines for enforcing healthy Qi.

2. Reinforcement of liver and kidneys, resolution of phlegm and expelling of blood stasis

If a Bi syndrome isn't cured for a long time, it easily consumes Qi and blood, affects the meridians, and zang-fu organs will be damaged. Hence, medicines for replenishing Qi, activating blood, nourishing liver and kidneys, reinforcing healthy Qi and eliminating pathogenic factors are often prescribed while eliminating pathogenic factors and dredging collaterals, thus obtaining better efficacy. When Bi lasts for a long time, "wet condensation develops into phlegm, and blood stagnation develops into blood stasis", phlegm and blood stasis combine, and circulation in the meridians is blocked. Therefore, the method of expelling blood stasis and resolving phlegm should be given full attention, and doctors should properly adopt warm herbs. Phlegm and blood stasis enter bone joints and can't be eliminated without warm drugs to expell wind and dredge collaterals.

ii. Syndrome differentiation

1. Dampness-cold Bi

Main symptoms: pain in joints of limbs (facet joints are the main parts), morning stiffness, inhibited bending and stretching of joints (this is mild during the day and severe at night), severe disease in the case of cold, relieved pain in the case of heat with fear of cold and cold limbs, white complexion and pale lips, pale tongue texture, white and greasy white tongue fur, or having tooth marks, and deep and thin or soggy and moderate pulse.

Therapeutic method: to warm meridians and dissipate cold, and to remove dampness and dredge collaterals.

Prescription: modified Wu Tou Tang. It includes wutou, zhifuzi, rougui, xixin, baishao, mugua, huangqi, wu-jiapi, lulutong, shenggangcao.

Prescription analysis: mahuang in the prescription induces perspiration and removes obstructions, and zhifuzi removes cold and stops pain; baishao and gancao relieve spasms and relaxes muscles; huangqi replenishes Qi and stabilizes weiqi, and plays a supporting role in warming the meridians and stopping pain, along with ma-huang and fuzi, and can also prevent an excessive diffusion of mahuang; white honey is sweet and slow, which reduces the toxicity of fuzi. The combination of the various herbs can resolve the pathogenic factors of cold and dampness by stimulating slight diaphoresis, so that they are removed, and pain is stopped.

Modifications: for the patients with swelling, 15~30g of unprocessed yiyiren and 10~15g of fuling are add-ed; with regard to patients who suffer from muscular atrophy, 10~15g of shudihuang and 10~15g of dangshen are added.

2. Dampness-heat Bi

Main symptoms: redness, swelling, fixed pain in joints or muscles, heaviness feeling, heat or burning sensa-tion once they are touched, no desire to drink even in thirst, with feelings of stuffed chest and esophagus, sallow complexion, constipation, anuria, yellow urine, red tongue, white and greasy tongue fur or yellow and greasy tongue fur and soggy and rapid or slippery and rapid pulse.

Therapeutic method: to clear heat and remove dampness, dredge channel blockages and collaterals.

Prescription: Er Miao San and Fang Ji Huang Qi Tang with additional herbs. The formulas contain huangqi, huangbai, cangzhu and baizhu, weilingxian, chuanbixie, shengyimi, fuling, sangzhi, dilong, qinjiao and fangji.

Prescription analysis: huangqi replenishes Qi, eliminates dampness, promotes diuresis, dispels pathogenic factors and strengthens the surface. It is a chief herb. It will dispel dampness and support the spleen, along with the bitter warm nature of cangzhu, a minister herb; fangji and bixie with their acrid and pungent flavours, expel wind and remove dampness, promote diuresis and reduce swelling. Baizhu and fuling nourish the spleen and re-move dampness, namely they assist huangqi in replenishing Qi and strengthening the surface. Also, it facilitates the function of fangji in terms of dispelling dampness and promoting diuresis. Hence, their belong to the category of assistant herbs. Dilong and cangzhu dispel wind and remove dampness, drain collaterals, remove obstructions and stop pain; sangzhi eases joints.

Modifications: with regard to patients with dampness-heat syndrome with predominant heat, 30g of huzhang and 30g of tufuling; if a patient also suffers from chest distension and tightness, nausea and vomiting, 15g of huoxianggeng, 15g of Rhizoma Pinelliae and 10g Radix Scutellariae are added.

3. Heat-toxin Bi

Main symptoms: severe pain in the joints and muscles that cannot stand touching, localized redness in the joints, possibly accompanied with movement restriction or fever , thirst and irritability, dry throat with a bitter taste, dry stools, dark urine, red or purple tongue color, yellow tongue fur and reduced saliva, and large and bounding or slippery and raid pulse.

Therapeutic method: to clear heat-toxicity , and activate blood and remove blood stasis.

Prescription: modified Xi Jiao Di Huang Tang. Xijiao or Niujiao, sheng dihuang, chishao, baishao mudanpi, tufuling , dilong, jinhua, yinteng, baihuasheshecao, gancao and dahuang.

Prescription analysis: xijiao clears heat and cools blood, and it is a chief herb. Dihuang, a minister herb, assists xijiao in clearing heat and cooling blood; chishao and mudanpi are bitter and slightly cold, and are used as assistant herbs to clear heat, cool and activate blood, dispersing blood stasis; compatible characteristics are simul-taneous nourishment of blood, activation and cooling, which clear heat and stabilize the blood without concerns of consuming and stirring it.

Modifications: in case that toxemic symptoms in patients are insignificant with excessive heat in lung and stomach, xijiao can be removed, 30g of shigao and 15g of zhizi are added; with regard to patients who suffer from serious thirst and dry throat, 15g of yuzhu and 15g shashen are added; for patients who suffer from constipation as well as fluids depletion, 15g of quangualou and 15g of baiziren are added.

4. Phlegm and blood stasis Bi

Main symptoms: asymmetric pain in joints and muscles, mostly a sharp kind of pain, even joint deformity, restricted bending and stretching movements, swollen joints, slightly hard, local skin color is purple dark, purple tongue or ecchymosis, white greasy tongue coating and deep and uneven pulse manifestation.

Therapeutic method: to activate blood, remove blood stasis, resolve phlegm and dredge collaterals.

Prescription: modified Yang He Tang and Tao Hong Si Wu Tang. Dihuang , lujiao, jiangtan, rougui, mahuang, baijiezi, taoren, honghua, danggui, chishao, baishao, shenggancao and duhuo.

Prescription analysis: in the prescription, as a chief herb, shudihuang is largely centered in nourishing the blood; lujiao generates fluids, supplements the bone marrow, nourishes blood and warms yang, and it is the minister herb; jiangtan breaks yin and harmonizes yang, while rougui warms meridians and dredges collaterals, Baijiezi removes phlegm and eliminates stagnation, mahuang regulates blood vessels, and dredges muscle and opens the pores. Taoren, honghua, chishao, baishao, and danggui nourish and activate blood, and they all are assistant herbs; shenggancao clears heat and detoxifies and it works as a guiding herb. The combination of the various herbs may remove blood stasis, dissolve phlegm-dampness and dredge the collateral meridians.

Modifications: in the case of serious swelling, 15g of zaoci and 10g of zhechong; for patients with serious pain in the upper limbs, 15g of jianghuang and 10g of guizhi are added; for patients who suffer from serious pain in the lower limbs, 15g of niuxi and 15g of xuanmugua.

5. Qi and blood deficiency

Main symptoms: chronic joint pain, occasional soreness, spasms in the joints regions or muscle spasms, and yellowish and lusterless complexion, short breath and lack of strength, spontaneous sweating and palpitations, muscular atrophy, lack of appetite and loose stools, pale tongue and weak or fine pulse.

Therapeutic method: to replenish Qi, activate blood, dredge collaterals and stop pain.

Prescription: Fangji Huanqi Tang and modified Siwu Tang decoctions. It includes huangqi, shudihuang , chaocangzhu, fangji, danggui , jixueteng, chuanxiong , chishao, baishao, weilingxian,xixiancao, xixin and gancao.

Prescription analysis: huangqi replenishes Qi, eliminates dampness, promotes diuresis, dispels pathogenic factors and strengthens superficies. Shudihuang largely replenishes nutrient blood. The two are sovereign medicines. Cangzhu assists huangqi in strengthening spleen and replenishing Qi, and danggui, jixueteng, baishao and chishao nourish and activate blood, which aupport the effect of shudihuang. They are minister herbs. Fangji and weilingxian can dispel wind, remove dampness and dredge collaterals; xixiancao assists fangji in the effect of removing dampness to ease joints; gancao is a guiding herb that regulates the various medicines.

Modifications: for patients with loose stools, roudoukou of 10g and 30g shengyiyiren; with regard to the patients with obvious Qi deficiency, 15g dangshen is added.

6. Dual deficiency of liver and kidney

Main symptoms: joint swelling, pain (mild during the day and severe at night), joint stiffness, restricted movement, soreness and weakness of waist and knees and heel pain, and bright pale complexion, dizziness and tinnitus, fear of cold and cold limbs, spontaneous sweating, clear abundant urine, nocturia, deep, thin and weak pulse, pale tongue texture and thin and white tongue fur.

Therapeutic method: to nourish liver and kidneys, dispel cold and remove dampness.

Prescription: modified Du Huo Ji Sheng Tang. Rensheng, fuling, fangfeng, duhuo, qinjiao, fangji , xixin , danggui , shudihuang , baishao, sangjisheng, niuxi, duzhong, gouqizi, huangqi, chaobaizhu, and gancao.

Prescription analysis: in the prescription, niuxi, duzhong and shudihuang nourish and reinforce liver and kidneys and strengthen the muscles and bones, duhuo and sangjisheng dispel wind, remove dampness, nourish blood, harmonize ying, activate collaterals and dredge Bi, and they are the main herbs; shudihuang and baishao nourish and activate blood; renshen, fuling and gancao reinforce Qi and replenish spleen, which generates strong Qi and blood, and facilitates dispelling of wind-dampness. They all are minister herbs; xixin is used to treat wind Bi. Qinjiao is used to remove wind cold and dampness from the whole body. The prescription reinforces healthy Qi and eliminates pathogens with the combination of herbs to treat the manifestations and root causes of the disease.

Modifications: with regard to patients with serious cold manifestation, 10g of ganjiang and 15g lujiaopian are added; in terms of the patients with deficient spleen and dampness prevailing, 30g of yiyiren and 15g of mugua are added.

iii. Specific prescription treatment

1. Hua Yu Tong Bi Tang (Bi Zheng Zhi Yan)

Prescription: 18g of danggui , 30g of danshen, 21g of jixueteng , 9g of zhiruxiang, 9g of moyao, 12g of yuanhusuo, 12g of xiangfu, 30g of tougucao. guizhi, chuanwu, zhicaowu and xixin should be added to the prescription for the patients whose constitution slants cold; for patients whose constitution slants hot add baijiangcao and mudanpi; huangqi for the patients with Qi-deficiency; chuanshanjia, wushaoshe, dilong, wugong, chuanxie and processed zhimaqianzi for patients with long-time blockage and swelling deformation of joints.

Indications: blood stasis Bi syndrome; chronic, localized deformation; fixed pain that feels like needles or a knife piercing; obvious pain under pressure; localized dark purple skin color; chronic, obstinate bi-syndrome; swelling deformation of joints; scaly skin; dark purple tongue with ecchymosis and wiry and uneven pulse.

2. Xuan Bi Tang (Wen Bing Tiao Bian)

Prescription: 15g of fangji ,15g of xingren, 15g of huashi,9g of lianqiao, 9g of shanzhi, 15g of yiyiren, 9g of banxia (stir-fried with vinegar) and 9g of wancansha. Eight cups of water are prepared and boiled, the resulting decoction divided into three parts and be taken for three times with warm water; 6g of jianghuang and 9g of haitongpi should be added when patients suffer from severely pain.

Indications: heat bi syndrome; shivering and excessive feeling of heat; frequent joint pain; sallow complexion; grey tongue.

3. Chu Shi Yi Tong Tang (Lei Zheng Zhi Cai)

Prescription: 3g of cangzhu, baizhu, fuling , qianghuo, zexie and chenpi, each; 1.5g of gancao; three scoops of ginger and bamboo juice, each. It should be decocted in water for oral dose.

Indications: dampness syndromes, heavy body, aching and localized pain, worst in cloudy days.

iv. Single ingredient prescriptions and proved prescriptions

(1) 15g of qingfengteng and 10g of hanfangji, decocted in water for oral administration.

(2) 10g of wujiapi and 30g of yinhuateng, decocted in water for oral administration. It should be taken twice a day, for heat Bi syndrome pain.

(3) 24~30 g of xuzhangqing and 200g of lean pork and two liang of old wine (one liang = 37.2 g) are decocted in water for oral administration. It should be taken for twice per day.

(4) 120g of shengdihuang is decocted in water, to be taken as a daily beverage.

(5) Shi Bi Fang: 1g of mahuang, 5g of xiqipi, 10g of xigualou, 10g of shenjincao, 2g of fuzi, 5g of baishao, 5g of zhigancao, 5g of baizhu, 5g of qiannianjiao, decocted in water for oral administration. Indications: damp bi syndrome, with pain in the feet and walking with difficulty.

(6) 30g of songjie and 30g of ruxiang are fried with slow fire until scorched, 3 to 6 g which could be im-

mersed in hot papaya wine and taken accordingly. Apply to patients whose legs twitch, with muscular spasms and pain.

(7) 4 fen (1 fen = 0.375 g) of chuanxie every morning. Apply to bi syndrome with spasms, pain and numbness of limbs.

v. Chinese patent medicine

(1) Lei Gong Teng Duo Gan Pian: 2 tablets each time, 2~3 times a day after meals.

(2) Kun Ming Shan Hai Tang Pian: 2 tablets each time, 3 times a day after meals.

(3) Zheng Qing Feng Tong Ning Pian: 50 ~ 100mg each time, 2~3 times a day, orally; injection: 50~100mg each time, 1~2 times a day, intramuscular injection, course of treatment for 3 ~ 12 months.

(4) Wan Bi Granule: 2 bags each time, 3 times a day. It has the functions of nourishing liver and kidney, strengthening the sinews and bones, dispelling wind and dissipating cold and removing dampness and dredging collaterals.

vi. Acupuncture and moxibustion therapy

As an adjuvant therapy, acupuncture can regulate the function of synovial cells, and inhibit immune factors related to synovial secretion inflammatory markers.

Common points selection: GV 14, GB 20, GV 16 and BL 10 are selected on the neck joints; LI 15 and TE 14 are selected on the shoulder joints; LI 11, PC 3 and ST 36 are selected on elbow joints; TE 4, TE 5, LI 5 and SI 4 are selected on wrist joints; EX-LE 10, EX-UE 9 and LI 4 are selected on finger joints; GV 14, GV 12, GV 3 and GV 2 are selected on spinal joints; GB 30 and B L 54 are selected on hip joints EX-LE 5, GB 34, GB 33, ST 34 and ST 35 are selected on knee joints; and BL 60, GB 40, KI 6 and ST 41 are selected on ankle joints. Ashipoints are selected to suport the above recommendations.

For excess syndrome, draining methods are given priority; moxibustion or deep needling and needle retaining can be used for patients with strong cold symptomatic features; ginger moxibustion can be used for patients in severe pain; acupuncture and moxibustion can be used simultaneously or warming needle moxibustion, grain-size moxibustion and cupping methods can be used in combination for patients with strong dampness symptoms. For deficiency syndrome, tonifying methods are given priority. Moxibustion or warming needle moxibustion can be used for patients with deficiency-cold. Each therapy should be conducted every day or every two days; 15~20 sessions make one course of treatment. All therapies can effectively improve clinical symptoms, relieving pain and enhancing the quality of life.

vii. Massage therapy

Massage can stimulate the meridian points or specific parts of the human body through different forms of operation methods, which has the functions of regulating yin and yang, draining meridians, activating and harmonizing Qi and blood, lubricating joints, strengthening sinews and bones, dispersing blood stasis, relieving stagnation, decreasing edema and pain, increasing local nutrition, improving blood circulation, preventing muscle atrophy and improving the function of joint mobility.

Common points: BL 25, GB 30, BL 36, BL 40, ST 36, and so on.

There are more than one hundred of manipulations in total, such as pressing manipulation, squeezing and pressing manipulation, one-point manipulation, rubbing manipulation, pushing manipulation, grasping manipulation, scrubbing manipulation, twisting manipulation, finger-nail pressing, kneading manipulation, vibrating manipulation, wiping manipulation, shaking manipulation, rotating manipulation, patting-striking manipulation and pinching manipulation. Among them, one or several kinds can be selected for comprehensive treatment according to specific situations. Course of treatment: once to twice a day, 15-20 min each time until illness state remission.

viii. Others

1. External therapy

(1) Herbal rod method: The prepared medicinal liquid is dipped with specially-made stick; then tapping manipulation will be conducted with the stick on appropriate acupuncture points of human body to relieve muscles and tendons in contracture and dredge meridians in deficiency, thus Qi and blood circulation is improved; patients will stop feeling pain once there is unobstruction.

Herbal tincture preparation: it consists of chuanwu, caowu, sanqi, xixin, ruxiang, moyao, and so on. They are immersed into commercial white wine for seven days and then the filtrate may be used.

Tapping method: a stick with the length of 25-50cm is selected. Its shape and length are different according to the different requirements of the treated body parts.

Tapping point selection: point selection is conducted according to different affected joints of patients. The principles of point selection: pain indicates the points and areas to treat; a combination of local points, meridian points and points near the joints and sinews insertions are selected. Common acupuncture points include LI 15, TE 14, LI 16, SI 12, LI 14 and SI9; LI 11, LI 12, TE 10, LI 10, HT3 and SI 7 in the elbows; SI 4, LI 5, TE 4, HT 7, SI 6, LU 9 and TE 5 in the wrist; GB 30, GB 29 and BL 36 in the hips; each phalangeal joint is selected for fingers; ST 35, GB 34, EX-LE 5, EX-LE 2, KI 6, KI 10, BL 39, Binzhong and Binyuan in the knees are selected; GB 40, ST 41, B L 60 and Genping of ankle are selected; BL 23 and ST 36 are selected for patients in pain; ST40 and GV 14 are selected for patients with fever; LI 11, B23, and ashipoints are selected for patients in severe pain.

Tapping manipulation: hard and quick tapping should be given to patients with excess syndrome, the tap frequency being about 200 times/min; soft tap and slow tap should be given to deficiency syndrome patients, the tap frequency is about 90 times/min.

(2) Fumigation and washing therapy: These are treatment methods whereby herb decoctions are administered through the skin of the affected body parts by fumigation or washings while the preparations are still hot. It acts on the body through the skin by means of penetration and the heating power of traditional Chinese herbs to soothe acupoints, harmonize meridians, activate Qi and blood, thus achieve treatment goal.

① Hand steaming-washing therapy: Drugs are selected and wrapped with gauze first. A wash basin, towel and sheet should be prepared. The decocted decoction is poured into the wash basin while it is hot. The patients should put their arms on the edge of wash basin first, which then should be covered with the sheet to prevent that hot vapor flows outside. The affected hands will be immersed into the decoction when it is not so hot anymore. The affected hands should be wiped dry with a dry towel after steaming-washing therapy and avoid exposure to wind.

② Foot steaming-washing therapy: Drugs are selected and wrapped with gauze first. A wooden barrel (a high and thin wooden barrel is appropriate), a small wooden stool, sheet and towel should be prepared. The decoction is poured into the wooden barrel while it is hot. The small wooden stool is placed into the barrel; the height of the small wooden stool should be slightly higher than the liquid level of decoction. The patient should sit on the chair and put its feet on the small wooden stool. The edge of the barrel and the legs should be wrapped fully for steaming therapy. The small wooden stool should be taken out when the decoction is not hot for feet. The affected feet are immersed into the decoction for steeping and washing. The liquid level of decoction can reach ankle joint or knee joint according to the type of pathology. The skin should be wiped dry with a towel after steaming-washing therapy and exposure to wind should be prevented.

Prescriptions: 15~30g of tougucao, 10~15g of honghua, 10~20g of wujiapi, 10~15g of baizhi, 10~20g of chuanxiong , 10~20g of haitongpi, 10~20g of jixueteng , 10~20g of chishao, 10~15g of shenjincao, 10~15g of sangzhi and 15~30g of baihuasheshecao.

The prescription above is decocted in water for 30 min. The affected parts should be steamed and washed by the method above. It should be conducted once or twice every day and 20-30min every time.

(3) External application: It is a method whereby the drugs are applied on specific parts of the body surface for the treatment of disease. The methods are as follows: if the used herbs have been dried, they should be grinded into small parts; then, a suitable amount of blending agent (vinegar, wine, etc) should be added to make a herbal paste with for application; if the used herb itself contains juice, it just needs to be smashed into paste directly for use.

Prescription I: 30g of chuanwu, caowu, shengnanxing and xixin, respectively. 90g of paojiang and chishao each, 15g of rougui and baizhi each, and xixin of 12 g are all grinded, and then put into a bottle for application. Appropriate amount of herbs should be taken for use according to the affected areas. The formula is made into a pasty mixture with a little hot white wine and applied on the affected parts with a thickness of 0.5 cm. Then the affected parts should be covered with oiled paper and wrapped and fixed with gauze. Dressing change should be conducted once every day, or twice a day for serious patients. This prescription is suitable for patients under the attack of wind-cold-damapness bi syndrome, but it is should not be used for patients with heat bi syndrome.

Prescription II: shengbanxia 30g, shengzhiziren 60g, 15g of shengdahuang, taoren 15g and honghua 10g. All drugs above are grinded into powder and made into a paste by vinegar, which will be applied on the affected parts. This prescription is suitable for heat bi syndrome with redness, swelling, heat and joint pain.

Prescription III: Leigongteng San Concentrate. Composition: 15g of leigongteng 45g, 15g of chishao, 15g of danshen, 15g of tougucao, 15g of shenjincao, 20g of laoguancao, 15g of huangjiezi, 20g of fangji . Grinded powder is made into a herbal paste with 1/2 wine and 1/2 vinegar respectively, and applied on a plastic cloth with a thickness of 2mm. It should be applied externally on the periphery of the elbow and knee joints and wrapped with bandage, of which the upper and lower end should be tightened to avoid spilling the decoction. It should be applied for 24h every time, every two days. This type of external application has significant healing effect when there is pain with redness, swelling and heat in an active stage of RA.

2. Point injection

Point injection should be conducted with Fufang Danggui Injection or Guning Injection. Ashipoints or meridian points selection can be selected according to the affected parts. Generally, LI 15, LI 11, Bizhong, LI 4, GB 30, ST 36 can be selected as main treatment. Generally, EX-UE 9 in the finger joints is selected for point combination; LI 5 for wrist joints; PC 3 for elbow joints; LI 15 for shoulder joints; GB 31 for hip joints; EX-LE 5 for knee joints; B L 60 for ankle joints; EX-LE 10 for toe joints; HuaTuo Jiaji for the spine. 2~6 points should be injected every time, 2ml into each point, every two days.

3. Rehabilitation therapy

Receiving rehabilitation therapy is beneficial to maintain or restore joint function and relieving pain, reducing swelling, improving dysfunction and preventing and correcting joint deformity. Different methods can be used according to different disease stages, specifically including physiotherapy, physical exercise therapy, massage, daily life movement training, application of rehabilitation equipment, etc.

V. Empirical prescription of famous experts

i. Tong Bi Tang (Lou Duofeng)

Indication: excess pathogen cold syndrome of Bi syndrome.

Components: 18g of danggui, 18g of danshen, 21g of jixueteng, 18g of haifengteng, 21 g of tougucao, 18 g of duhuo, 21 g of xiangfu and 18 g of difeng.

Usage: it should be decocted in water for oral administration; 1 dose a day; it should be taken in the morning and the evening respectively.

Efficacy: dispel wind, dissipate cold, remove dampness, activate blood, nourish blood and dredge collaterals

ii. Chu Zheng Li Wan Tang (Li Zhiming)

Indication: Bi syndrome joint and swelling and pain in yin-deficiency fever.

Component: 30g of qinghao, 20g of digupi, 15g of huangqi, 15g of fangji, 12g of fangfeng, 12 g of qianghuo, 12g of duhuo, 15 g of wushaoshe, 12g of baizhu, 15g of gouteng, 30g of sangjisheng, 15g of difengpi, 12g of dilong, 12g of danggui , 8g of honghua, 15g of yuanshen and 10~15g of leigongteng.

Usage: it should be decocted in water for oral administration; 1 dose/day; it should be taken in the morning and the evening respectively.

Efficacy: nourish yin, clear heat, dispel wind, dredge collaterals and relieve pain.

iii. Bu Shen Qu Han Zhi Wan Tang (Jiao Shude)

Indication: heat bi syndrome with kidney deficieney.

Component: 12~15g of chuanduan, 12~15g of shudihuang , 9~12 g of buguzhi, yinyanghuo, guizhi and chishao, each, 6~12g of zhifuzi, 10g of gusuibu, 9g of duhuo, niuxi, zhimu, each, 6 g of cangzhu, 12g of weilingxian, 6~9g of fangfeng, zhishanjia, 20~30g of shenjincao, 3g of mahuang and 10~15g of songjie.

Usage: it should be decocted in water for oral dose; 1 dose/day; it should be taken in the morning and the evening respectively.

Efficacy: to tonify kidney, clear heat, disperse wind, resolve dampness, activate and dispel stasis, and to strengthen sinews and bones.

VI. Typical medical records from famous experts

i. Medical record of Lou Duofeng — cold-dampness bi syndrome

Ms Zhang, female, 56 years old, housewife. She had painful swelling of joints in the whole body for 36 years, while hand disability lasted for 6 years.

She pumped bellows for several days after childbirth in June 1956. Her finger joints were seriously swollen and painful for ten days, which affected more joints of the whole body when her child was one month old. It was diagnosed as "postpartum bodily pain" by the local county hospital; hormones were given to relieve symptoms temporarily. Both her hands showed finger joint alterations after 10 years, developing into typical gooseneck type of rheumatoid hands after 20 years. At the time of diagnosis, more joints of her whole body were swelling, painful, aching, tired and stiff; among which the limbs and mandibular joint were more serious. She had difficult in opening the mouth and attending to daily life routine. Her limbs felt weak and sensitive to cold. Emotionally, she was pessimistic, tongue color was dark, tongue fur was thin and white, and pulse was thin and uneven.

Syndrome differentiation: blood stasis and coagulation.

Therapeutic method: nourish blood and activate blood, replenish rheumatism and dredge collaterals.

Prescription: 30g of danggui, 30g of danshen, 30g of jixueteng, 12g of chaoshanjia, 12g of guizhi, 20g of duhuo, 30g of qiannianjian, 18g of mugua, 30g of xiangfu, 30g of chuanniuxi, 15g of chenpi and 9g of gancao.

Note: the author thinks that the syndrome of blood stasis and stubborn phlegm coagulation should be treated by methods of eliminating wind and collateral dredging, so as to remove stasis and eliminate phlegm. Simultaneously, healthy Qi should be reinforced and patient constitution should be strengthened, because when healthy

Qi is weak diseases can linger. With a focuses in activating and nourishing blood with danggui, danshen and jixueteng, blood movement and pain relief are achieved with chaoshanjia; duhuo, qiannianjian, mugua, guizhi and chuanniuxi are supporting agents for dispelling wind, eliminating dampness and dispelling cold, which eliminate pathogenic factors, but do not damage healthy Qi. Chenpi and gancao are both assistant and guiding herbs. This prescription activates and nourishes blood, replenishes bi syndrome, dredges collaterals and regulates the body slowly.

ii. Medical record of Lu Zhizheng — dampness-heat bi syndrome

Ms Ma, female, 27 years old. She came to hospital for treatment, because her joints in the whole body were painful and numb for four years, and became more serious for the last two months on October 1982. Four years before, the patient started to suffer from this disease after miscarriage; all her joints were in pain and couldn't be cured for a long time. Blood sedimentation was 46mm/h before she came to the hospital; rheumatoid factors were positive; her disease was diagnosed as primary rheumatoid arthritis. At the time of diagnosis, the joints of her whole body were numb and painful, the neck and waist were stiff and both ankles were seriously painful. It was difficult for her to walk, and she required support with one hand. She had a slim constitution and weak; her breath was feeble and her voice was hoarse. Her hands were too weak to hold things, and the pharynx was dry and mouth felt bitter; she had indigestion and lack of appetite. Her sleep was poor with plenty of dreaming, stools were soft, defecating two or three times every day, urine was scanty and very yellow, lips were deep red, tongue tip was deep red with petechiae, her tongue fur was yellow, thick and dry and her pulse was uneven.

Syndrome differentiation: the patient has congenital deficiency for a long time. Besides, her pulse became feeble due to hemorrhage after miscarriage. Simultaneously, the patient suffered invasion by wind cold and dampness. What's more, these pathogenic factors were lingering in her body and eventually shifted to pathogenic fire, leading to fluid consumption. Suffering from long-term heat stagnation, the patient grew frail day by day and the condition became severe.

Therapeutic method: dredge dampness-heat.

Prescription: Xuan Bi Tang. Composition: 9g of lianqiao, 15g of chixiaodou, 15 g of wancansha (boiled in cloth bag), 9g of fangfeng, 9g of fangji, 15g of chaosangzhi, 9g of chishao, 9g of baishao, 9g of haitongpi, 12 g of shengdihuang, 9g of bixie, 6g of duhuo, 12g of yinchen, 3g of mahuang and 10g of cangzhu; 5 doses.

Note: this patient was weak, and affected by exogenous pathogenic factors. Doctor Lu takes fangji as the main drug to eliminate dampness and heat and govern meridians; bixie and yinchen are beneficial to the functions of resolving dampness and clearing heat of fangji; chixiaodou, wanchansha and haitongpi remove dampness and eliminate turbidity; sangzhi and duhuo dispel wind and dredge collaterals; chishao, baishao and shengdihuang are added for nourishing yin and blood; and lianqiao clears stagnated heat.

VII. Prevention and aftercare

i. Prevention

1. Prevention from cold and damp environment

Cold and dampness are important factors for inducing AR disease. People should avoid sweating while exposed to wind, contacting cold water, sitting and lying on wet places.

2. Prevention and treatment of infections

Infections may also be related to RA onset, as there is a relationship between AR and previous tonsillitis, pharyngolaryngitis, sinusitis and other infectious diseases. So infection may also be related to the incidence of this diseases.

3. Early diagnosis and treatment

Patients with joint pain symptoms should go to hospital to get an early diagnosis and treatment, control disease development, reduce potential for disability and avoid losing capability for work.

ii. Aftercare

1. Psychological aftercare

Clinically, some patients show obvious psychological symptoms before onset, such as depression or excessive sadness. Emotional fluctuations after onset often exacerbate the disease; therefore, physicians must guide patients to better understand this disease, alleviate mental burden, and cooperate with treatment actively.

2. Life care

Both medical workers and family members should give patients a very supportive help and guidance, because AR disease may bring a lot of inconvenience to their lifes. For bed-ridden patients with loss of limb function, the occurrence of bedsores should be prevented. For patients with joint dysfunction who are unable to move freely, special attention should be paid to preventing falls. Diet should be restrained and special attention should be paid to nutrition supplements as well.

3. Functional exercise

Patients should adhere to functional exercise and undergo specific joint function recovery training, by calisthenics, jogging, bicycle riding and so on; in addition, Chinese traditional exercises, such as taijiquan and qigong, can relax muscles and stimulate blood circulation by combining movement and breathing exercises, and promoting the circulation of Qi. This type of traditional exercise can also protect joints, effectively improve joint movement and slow joint deformities. High intensity exercise is advisable if there is no new and obvious discomfort in joints after activity. It can avoid spasticity, prevent muscle atrophy, promote the blood circulation of body, improve local tissue nutrition, boost spirit and keep good physique.

(YING Senlin)

References

[1] Tang JW. Pathology [M]. Version 2. Beijing: Science Press, 2012: 227.

[2] Sun T, Xiong F, Wang CX. Research Progress of the Diagnosis of Rheumatoid Arthritis with Anti Citrullinated Protein Antibodies [J]. Rheumatism and Arthritis, 2014, 5(3):5-7.

[3] Alsalahy MM, Nasser HS, Hashem MM, et al. Effect of tobacco smoking on tissue protein citrullination and disease progression in patients with rheumatoid arthritis[J].Saudi Pharmaceutical Journal, 2010, 18(2): 75-80.

[4] Vossenaar ER,Van Venrooij WJ.Citrullinated proteins: sparks that may ignite the fire in rheumatoid arthritis[J]. Arthritis research and therapy,2004, 6(3):107-111.

[5] Farid SS,Azizi G,Mirshafiey A.Anti-citrullinated protein antibodies and their clinical utility in rheumatoid arthritis[J]. International journal of rheumatic diseases,2013,16（4）: 379-386.

[6] Wang GH. Research Progress for Immune Pathogenesis of Rheumatoid Arthritis [J]. Chinese Journal of Histochemistry and Cytochemistry, 2010, 19(3): 19-22.

[7] Huang J, Huang CB. Diagnostic and Therapeutic Progresses in Rheumatoid Arthritis [J]. Clinical Medication Journal, 2010, 8 (1): 1-5.

[8] Chinese Rheumatology Association. Diagnosis and Treatment Guideline for Rheumatoid Arthritis [J]. Chinese Journal of Rheumatology, 2010, 14 (4): 265- 269.

[9] Lou GF, Lou Y. Diagnosis and treatment of Lou Duofeng for Rheumatism[M]. Beijing: People's Medical Publishing House, 2007.

[10] Lu ZZ. Lu Zhizheng medical circles portfolio[M]. in Li JD. Collection of national TCM masters' medical records. Beijing: People's Medical Publishing House, 2009.

Metrorrhagia and Metrostaxis 崩漏

I. Overview

i. Definition

Metrorrhagia and Metrostaxis refers to sudden profuse bleeding or dripping menses in non-menstrual period, the former is called "metrorrhagia" and the latter is "metrostaxis".

Although metrorrhagia and metrostaxis refer to different bleeding conditions, they often appear alternately with the basically same disease cause and pathogenesis, so they are generally called "metrorrhagia and metrostaxis".

"Metrorrhagia and metrostaxis" means serious imbalance of menstrual cycle, period and volume caused by the disorder of the reproductive axis: kidney-Reproduction-stimulating essence—thoroughfare and conception vessels—womb.

Menstrual cycle disorder, "menses in non-menstrual period"; menstrual volume disorder, the abnormal increase or decrease of menstrual volume, or dripping continuously.

ii. Characteristics

This disease is a common gynecological disease, and also a puzzling, difficult, acute and severe disease.

Puzzle refers that the disease is described in emmeniopathy, but the bleeding does not appear in menstrual period, so it is called "a severely irregular menstruation" by *Jing-Yue Complete Works*. Most of modern physicians consider that "metrorrhagia and metrostaxis" should be studied by classing it as emmeniopathy.

Difficulty means it is difficult to obtain the curative effect, because of the complex pathogenesis, causal correlation, Qi and Blood diseases and involvement in multiple viscera.

Severity means that great loss of Qi and blood can lead to hemorrhagic shock.

iii. The relationship between metrorrhagia and metrostaxis

(1) **Common point:** the bleeding appears both in non-menstrual period.

(2) **Different point:** "metrorrhagia" is more severe as it breaks out urgently with more blood loss, while the "metrostaxis" is milder as it arises slowly with less bleeding amount, and less bleeding amount per unit time

(3) **Mutual transformation:** if "metrostaxis" lasts for long time and never ends, it will get more and more serious——then leads to "metrorrhagia", If "metrorrhagia" lasts for long time, it will cause the Qi and Blood loss——"metrostaxis"; "metrorrhagia is caused by too much metrostaxis, and metrorrhagia can gradually become metrostaxis"

iv. Relationship with Western medicine

As a symptom, metrorrhagia and metrostaxis can appear in the following various diseases :

(1) Diseases of internal secretion: dysfunctional uterine bleeding, often found in puberty and menopause.

(2) Diseases related to gestation, such as threatened abortion, incomplete abortion and drug abortion.

(3) Diseases related to inflammation, such as colpitis, cervicitis, uterus body inflammation, intimitis and pelvic inflammation

(4) Tumour, such as myoma of uterus, ovary tumor and cervical cancer

(5) Traumatic diseases related to trauma

(6) Systemic diseases, such as thrombopenia and cirrhosis

Among all kinds of diseases above, only dysfunctional uterine bleeding can be recognized as metrorrhagia and metrostaxis. It includes two types: ① Anovulatory type: the symptoms of this type of bleeding include period disorder, bleeding amount going up and down, or menelipsis in short time, and excessive blood loss. ② Ovulatory type: luteal hypoplasia due to advanced menstruation; withered corpus luteum due to menostaxis.

II. Etiology and pathogenesis

i. Chinese medicine

The main pathogenesis of this disease is that thoroughfare and conception channels cannot restrict the menstrual blood because of their unconsolidation, so that the uterus storing and discharging get abnormal. The common clinical symptoms are as follows:

1. Spleen deficiency

The spleen qi is damaged because of spleen deficiency, overstrain and anxiety, as well as improper diet. Because of spleen deficiency, or the blood cannot be controlled, or even collapse. Also, because of the unconsolidation of thoroughfare and conception channels, the menstrual blood cannot be restricted, which causes metrorrhagia and metrostaxis. Just as shown in *Fuke Yuchi*, "Anxiety damages spleen and makes it lose the control for the blood, causing the abnormal blood circulation".

2. Kidney deficiency

(1) Kidney qi deficiency: It involves the following circumstances: kidney qi is congenitally deficient;or

maidens' kidney qi and sex-stimulating essence is not abundant; or kidney qi is damaged due to too many sexual activities or having too many babies; kidney is affected by chronic diseases and serious diseases ; it can also happen to women who reaches 49 and have weak kidney qi. Kidney qi deficiency causes the dysfunction in essence storage and pattern of insecurity of thoroughfare and conception channel. Due to kidney qi deficiency menstruation can't be restricted, and the storage and excretion of uterus are abnormal, thus causing the metrorrhagia and metrostaxis.

(2) Kidney yang deficiency: body usually suffers from yang deficiency and the decline of vital gate fire. Or As yin deficiency involves yang and yang failed to control yin because of metrorrhagia and metrostaxis for a long time, and dysfunction in essence storage and unsolidation of thoroughfare and conception channels occur, so that the menstruation cannot be controlled,and the metrorrhagia and metrostaxis are caused.

(3) Kidney yin deficiency: It happens because the patient usually suffers from kidney yin deficiency, or has too many sexual activities or babies, which consumes kidney-yin. Yin deficiency makes it unable to defense blood, and the deficient fire leads to bleeding, so that the storing and excretion of uterus cannot be controlled, and the metrorrhagia and metrostaxis are caused.

3. Blood heat

Blood heat caused by yang exuberance or internal heat due to yin deficiency usually occurs; or seven emotions cause internal injuries and depressed liver qi transforms into heat; or pathogenic factor of damp-heat is hidden in the body. The heat injures thoroughfare and conception channels and causes frenetic movement of the blood, causing the metrorrhagia and metrostaxis.

4. Blood stasis

Blood stasis can be caused by the internal damages and qi stagnation caused by the seven emotions; or heat consuming, cold congelation, deficiency and stagnation; or sexual activities cause blood stasis. When there is menstrual blood or blood after giving birth; or the abnormal flow of blood due to long-term metrorrhagia and metrostaxis, blood stasis appeared. Blood stasis blocks thoroughfare and conception channels and uterus, and blood fails to circulate in channels, which causes metrorrhagia and metrostaxis.

In conclusion, the metrorrhagia and metrostaxis is a kind of disease, summed up in pathology of deficiency, heat and stagnation. Because zang-fu organs reinforce each other and there is close correlation among zang-fu organs, Qi and blood and meridians, as well as the course of the disease is long, the metrorrhagia and metrostaxis always involve qi, blood and many organs, which makes it difficult to tell the causal connection.

No matter in which organ the disease occurs, "it will transfer among the four zang-fu organs and finally come to spleen and kidney". As the "injury of five zang viscera must affect the kidney in the end", the kidney catches a disease. Kidney is divided into kidney Qi, kidney yin and kidney yang. If yin pulse is feeble and yang pulse is strong, metrorrhagia occurs. The disease is mainly caused by kidney water and yin deficiency, so heart and liver cannot get nourished, and the patient shall avoid heart-fire hyperactivity; otherwise, the disease may develop to the metrorrhagia and metrostaxis due to diseases in the heart, liver and kidney. When it lasts for long, there is the loss of blood and the consumption of qi, and blood out of channe develops into stagnation. The pathogenesis of deficiency of both Qi and yin with stagnation exists to the different extent.

For metrorrhagia and metrostaxis, its root lies in the kidney, and it is located in thoroughfare and conception channels. It causes the change of qi and blood, with the syndromes of uncontrolled storage and excretion of uterus.

ii. Western medicine

1. Anovulatory dysfunctional uterine bleeding

Factors inside and outside the body: spiritual hypertension, fear, depression and extreme changes of the environment and climate; systemic disease, malnutrition, anemia and metabolic disorders; all factors above can affect the mutual regulation functions of hypothalamus-hypophysis-ovarian axis through cerebral cortex and central nervous system, finally causing the dysfunctional uterine bleeding.

Anovulatory dysfunctional uterine bleeding often happens to women in adolescence and perimenopause, but with completely different pathogenesis.

Adolescence: the regulating function of hypothalamus and hypophyseal is not mature.There is not a regular periodic regulation between hypothalamus, hypophyseal and ovary. Although some follicles grow in this period, when they grow to a certain extent, they will have degeneration without ovulation, forming the atretic follicle.

Perimenopause: because of hypo-ovaria,, the ovarian follicles are almost used up, and the remained follicles have a weak reactivity for gonadotropin of hypophysis and the secretion of estrogen declines sharply with weaker negative feedback for the hypophysis, and gonadotropin level rises, so the non-ovulation dysfunctional uterine bleeding occurs.

Anovulatory dysfunctional uterine bleeding is an estrogen withdrawal or break-through bleeding which is caused by single estrogen stimulation without the antagonism of progestogen and   endometrial hyper-plasia with no restraint

2. Estrogen withdrawal bleeding:

Under the long-term stimulation of single estrogen, the simple hyperplasia, complex hyperplasia and so on happens in endometrium. If there is a group of atretic follicles, estrogen level may decrease suddenly, so that the bleeding occurs because the endometrium loses its support and exfoliates

Estrogen break-through bleeding can be divided into two types: ① If low level estrogen is maintained at the threshold level, intermittent small amount bleeding may occur. The slow endometrium restoration can prolong the bleeding. ② If high level estrogen is maintained at effective concentration, the long time of amenorrhea will occur. Endometrium is thickened and loosened because there is no progestaational hormomne to participate in, so as to cause the spontaneous, acute breakthrough bleeding, with large amount of blood. Because the endometrium blood channel is lack of coiling and the segmental contraction and relaxation do not happen, the endometrium cannot fall off synchronously. Therefore, when one part is restored, the other part will fall off with bleeding, so as to cause the large amount of bleeding for long time which cannot be stopped by itself. The fibrinolysin in the blood is activated because of the damage of tissue for many times, As a result, more fibrin is dissolved, which causes more bleeding..

III. Key points of diagnosis and differential diagnosis

i. Key points of diagnosis

1. Medical history

(1) Age: it is closely related to the occurrence of metrorrhagia and metrostaxis

(2) Menstrual history: whether there is abnormity in cycle, menstrual period and blood volume; whether there is history of metrorrhagia and metrostaxis.

(3) History of contraception: whether the contraceptive or other hormones are taken orally; whether the patient accepted the intrauterine device and tubal ligation, etc.

(4) Whether there is medical bleeding disease history.

2. Clinical manifestation

Irregular menstrual periods; menstrual period exceeding more than half month or even lasting for several months; or sudden profuse discharge or dripping menses after amenorrhea for several months; the different levels of anemia often exist.

3. Examination

(1) Gynecologic examination: There should be no organic pathologic changes; if the cervical polyp and uterus myoma are found, they shall be treated according to this disease theory.

(2) Auxiliary examination: Excluding the genital neoplasms uterus myoma, endometrial cancer and ovarian tumor); inflammations (endometritis, myometritis, cervical polyp, endometrial polyp and pelvic inflammation); the colporrhagia caused by systemic diseases (such as aplastic anemia, thrombocytopenia).

ultrasound, MRI, hysteroscopy, diagnostic curettage or examination of basal body temperature and so on is selected according to the patient's condition.

ii. Differential diagnosis

1. Distinguishing from menstrual disorder

	Cycle	Menstrual period	Menstrual volume
Advanced menstruation	Yes, it is shortened	Normal	Normal, or more or less
Hypermenorrhea	Normal	Normal	More, like metrorrhagia
Menostaxis	Normal	Prolonged, like metrostaxis	More or less
Irregular menstrual period	Early or late	Normal	Normal
Metrorrhagia and metrostaxia	Serious disorders occur at the same time.		

2. Intermenstrual bleeding

Metrorrhagia and metrostaxis as well as intermenstrual bleeding all occur in non-menstrual period, but the intermenstrual bleeding regularly happens between the two adjacent menstruation, and lasts only 2-3 days. The bleeding stops naturally within 7 days. However, metrorrhagia and metrostaxis shows serious disorder of cycle, menstrual period and menstrual volume, and the bleeding cannot stop naturally.

3. Red vaginal discharge

The identification of red vaginal discharge and metrostaxis depends on enquiry of medical history and the examination. The red vaginal discharge figures the blood streak in leucorrhea but it is normal for menstruation.

4. Bleeding during giving birth to a child

To distinguish it from hemorrhagic disorders in early pregnancy such as vaginal bleeding during pregnancy, threatened abortion, ectopic gestation, diagnosis can be clarified by asking medical history, taking pregnancy tests and B ultrasound examination.. To distinguish it from postpartum lochiorrhea, the disease history should be equired. If the disease occurs after giving birth to a child, it can be identified as lochiorrhea.

5. Genital tumor bleeding

The clinical feature of genital tumor bleeding is colporrhagia like metrorrhagia and merostaxis, which can be clarified through gynecologic examination, B ultrasound, MRI examination or diagnostic curettage.

6. Reproductive system inflammations

The inflammations include cervical polyp, endometrial polyps, endometritis, pelvic inflammation.It has many clinical manifestations, such as dripping menses, and can be identified through gynecologic examination, diagnostic curettage or hysteroscopy.

7. Bleeding due to trauma on the vulva

Injuries caused by trip, sexual intercourse in violent way,which can be identified through asking disease history and gynecologic examination.

8. Medical blood disease

Medical blood diseases such as aplastic anemia and thrombocytopenia can cause a large amount of bleeding by the primary medical blood disease during the vaginal bleeding, or even cause sudden profuse discharge or dripping menses. It is not difficult to be identified through blood analysis, examination of blood coagulation factor or analysis of bone marrow cell.

IV. TCM therapy

i. Principle of differentiation syndrome and treatment

1. Differentiation syndrome

(1) Differentiating deficiency and excess: deficiency: spleen deficiency, kidney deficiency; excess: blood heat, blood stasis.

(2) Differentiating whether it is in bleeding period or after hemostasis: in bleeding period: it is often a syndrome of manifestation ora syndrome of intermingled deficiency and excess; after hemostasis: it is often a root cause syndrome or deficiency syndrome.

During bleeding period, first it is necessary to distinguish whether the syndrome is cold, heat, deficiency or excess: heat syndrome - sudden profuse discharge in non-menstrual period, large amount in short time, subsequently dripping continuously with fresh red or dark red menses; deficiency syndrome-sudden profuse discharge or dripping menses, in light color and thick quality; blood stasis-menses in non-menstrual period, which can be metrorrhagia or amenorrhea with irregular bleeding period and amount, and blood color is dark purple, together with blood clots and abdominal pain; cold syndrome–continuous menses metrorrhagia, or metrorrhagia and metrostaxis for a long time, with thin menses of light color..

2. Treatment

According to the principle of "treatment of manifestations for acute disease and root cause for chronic disease", the treatment of metrorrhagia and metrostaxis should involve three methods, including stopping bleeding, clarifying source and recovery.

(1) Stopping bleeding: also called hemostasis, it is used for urgent haemorrhage, in case that the patient is collapsed.

(2) Clarifying source: it means to identify the root cause and treat it.. It is an important stage of treating metrorrhagia and metrostaxis. It is used for treatment based on syndrome differentiation after the bleeding has been controlled. Be careful not to use warm or cold formulas or astringing formulas without asking the cause, thus deteriorating conditions of patients.

(3) Recovery: it means to consolidate origin and rehabilitation, which is an important phase of consolidating metrorrhagia and metrostaxis treatment. It is used for recuperating after the bleeding is stopped. Different therapys are chosen based on different age stages to adjust menstrual cycle or promote ovulation. In this period, the treatment is a therapy for tonifying kidney, assisting spleen and soothing the liver, three regulating bodily functions are adjusted and each has emphasis.

Three methods for treating metrorrhagia and metrostaxis are different, but cannot be separated completely and must be applied flexibly in clinical syndrome. To stop bleeding, the source must be must be clarified, and clarifying the source shall consolidate origin, and causes need to be found for redintegration. Three methods are premises for each other and reinforce each other. Each of them has emphasis, but the spirit of differentiating syndromes for causes runs through each method.

ii. Dialectical therapy

1. Bleeding period

(1) Spleen deficiency

Main Symptoms: sudden profuse discharge of menses in non-menstrual period or dripping menses without stopping, thin menses with light color, pale complexion, mental fatigue and short breath, empty sagging in the lower abdomen, lack of warmth in the limbs, puffy face and swollen limbs, loss of appetite and loose stool, pale and enlarged tongue texture, dental mark on the side, white tongue fur and weak sunken pulse.

Therapeutic method: Tonify Qi and control blood, secure thoroughfare and stop metrorrhagia.

Prescription: Gu Ben Zhi Beng Tang or Gu Chong Tang.

Gu Ben Zhi Beng Tang Ginseng: Milkvetch Root, White Atractylodes Rhizome, Prepared Rehmannia Root, Chinese Angelica and Black ginger.

Prescription analysis: In this prescription, Ginseng and Milkvetch Root greatly tonify original qi, raise Yang and consolidate origin; White Atractylodes Rhizome is the source of tonifying spleen as well as governing blood to circulate in channels; Radix Rehmanniae nourishes Yin and blood, "stopping metrorrhagia and metrostaxis while nourishing Yin". Black ginger guides blood normal circulation in channels and is suitable for reinforcing fire, warming yang and astringing; Milkvetch Root and Chinese Angelica means "Angelica Blood-Tonifying Decoction"; Prepared Rehmannia Root and Chinese Angelica as yin and yang replenish and promote blood circulation. The prescription replenishes blood and invigorates qi, so that blood can be controlled as blood is strengthened and origin is consolidated, and the sufficiency of qi leads to the enrichment of blood, while the growth of yin and yang promotes each other mutually. In this way, thoroughfare channel is consolidated and metrorrhagia stops naturally.

Fu Qingzhu's Obstetrics and Gynecology said: "the prescription is so extraordinary that it focuses not on stopping bleeding but on enriching blood. What is more, it can invigorate qi and supplement fire. If dark appears in front of eyes, and patient faints because of metrorrhagia, her blood is almost all lost and there is only a little qi left to keep her alive. If blood gets enriched but qi doesn't get invigorated, the tangible blood cannot be generated quickly enough while the intangible qi must be completely lost. That is why qi must be invigorated first in this case. However, it is not easy for blood to be generated when only qi gets invigorated. Enriching blood without supplementing fire leads to blood stagnation, as blood cannot get promoted by qi. Furthermore, as black ginger introduces blood to circulate normally in channels, it can be used for strengthening middle and astringing. Therefore, it can be used together with herbal medicines for enriching blood and invigorating qi."

Modification: when blood cannot get promoted because of qi deficiency, it is easy to form blood stasis. Sanqi pseudo-ginseng, Motherwort Herb or Sudden Smile Powder are often added to remove blood stasis and stop bleeding.

Gu Chong Tang: White Atractylodes Rhizome, Milkvetch Root, calcined Bone Fossil of Big Mammals, calcined oyster, Asiatic Cornelian Cherry Fruit, Debark Peony Root, Cuttlebone, Roots of Madder, Carbonized Windmill-Palm Petiole and Chinese Gall.

Prescription analysis: In this prescription, Milkvetch Root and White Atractylodes Rhizome can strengthen spleen and benefti Qito control blood; calcined Bone Fossil of Big Mammals, calcined oyster and Cuttlebone secure thoroughfare and conception channels; Asiatic Cornelian Cherry Fruit and Debark Peony Root can tonify kidney and nourish blood, collect acid and stop bleeding; Carbonized Windmill-Palm Petiole and Chinese Gall astringe blood and stop bleeding; Roots of Madder disperses blood stasis and stops bleeding, blood stops without stasis. In the whole prescription, all the medicines can invigorate spleen, benefit Qi, secure thoroughfare and stop bleeding.

If sudden streams down, which makes the patient unconscious with cold limbs, sweat and barely palpable pulse, it should be diagnosed as an urgent syndrome called the exhaustion of qi resulting from hemorrhea. The treatment for this urgent syndrome involves benefiting qi, reviving yang and relieving abiotrophy. When necessary, blood volume is supplemented quickly through transfusion and blood transfusion to avoid shock.

(2) Kidney deficiency

① Kidney Qi deficiency

Main symptoms: irregular menstrual period, more bleeding amount or dripping from metrorrhagia to metrostaxis or from metrostaxis to metrorrhagia, thin menstrual blood with light red or dark, darkish complexion, dark eye socket, empty sagging in the lower abdomen, limp and painful spinal column, light dark tongue, moistening white tongue fur and weak sunken pulse for adolescent girls or women before and after menopause.

Therapeutic method: to nourish kidney and benefit Qi, secure thoroughfare and stop bleeding.

Prescription: modified Cong Rong Tu Si Zi Wan. adding Tangshen, Milkvetch Root ,Ass Hide Glue, Prepared Rehmannia Root, Desertliving Cistanche, Palm leaf Raspberry Fruit, Chinese Angelica, Barbary Wolfberry Fruit, Chinese Taxillus Herb, Dodder Seed and Argy Wormwood Leaf.

Prescription analysis: In this prescription, Desertliving Cistanche and Palm leaf Raspberry Fruit can warm and tonify kidney Qi; Dodder Seed can tonify yang and benefit yin as well as supplement yin and yang; Prepared Rehmannia Root can nourish kidney and tonify yin to make kidney Qi abundant with solid storing to stop metrorrhagia; Milkvetch Root and Tangshen can tonify Qi and control blood; Ass Hide Glue and Argy Wormwood Leaf can enrich blood, consolidate Chong and control blood; Barbary Wolfberry Fruit and Chinese Taxillus Herb can nourish liver and kidney; Chinese Angelica enriches and activates blood, while guiding blood to circulate normally in channels; in the whole prescription, all the medicines work together to tonify kidney, benefit qi, secure thoroughfare and stop blood.. Chinese Angelica can be removed if it is thought to be too strong.

② Kidney yang deficiency

Main Symptoms: irregular menstrual period, more bleeding amount or dripping continuously, or sudden profuse discharge after several months of menelipsis, thin menstrual blood with light red color, darkish complexion, cold limbs and fear of coldness, soreness and weakness of waist and knees, clear urine in large amount, frequent urination at night, dark eye socket, light dark tongue, moistening white tongue fur, deep, thread and weak pulse.

Therapeutic method: to warm kidney and benefit Qi, secure thoroughfare and stop bleeding.

Prescription: You Gui Wan. Tangshen, Milkvetch Root, Sanqi. Preparing Aconite, Cinnamon Bark, Prepared Rehmannia Root, Common Yam Rhizome, Pulp of Dogwood Fruit, Barbary Wolfberry Fruit, Dodder Seed, Deer-Horn Glue, Chinese Angelica and Eucommia Bark.

In this prescription, Prepared Rehmannia Root can nourish kidney and blood, replenish essence and benefit marrow, matched with pulp of dogwood fruit and Common Yam Rhizome, the three herbal medicines, which are used in Six-Ingredient Rehmannia Pill for invigoration, are used to generate water.; Prepared Common Monkshood Daughter Root and Cinnamon Bark can warm kidney and tonify yang, benefit life gate, warm yang and stop metrorrhagia and regulate water and fire; Deer-Horn Glue a tonic coming from animal and building up strength, complements life gate, warms governor channel and nourish and consolidates thoroughfare and conception channels; Dodder Seed and Eucommia Bark can warm liver and kidney; Chinese Angelica and Barbary Wolfberry Fruit can nourish blood and liver and benefit thoroughfare and conception channels; Tangshen and Milkvetch Root are added to tonify sQi and control blood; If there are blood stases caused by coldness, Sanqi is added to remove blood stasis and stop bleeding. In the whole prescription, all herbs can warm kidney and benefit Qi, secure thoroughfare and stop bleeding.

③ Kidney yin deficiency

Main Symptoms: irregular menstrual period, less blood amount, dripping several months without stopping, or sudden metrorrhagia after several months of amenorrhea, slightly thick menstrual blood in light red dizziness and tinnitus, soreness and weakness of waist and knees, burning sensation of chest, palms and soles, restless sleep at night, red tongue, less furred tongue or fissured tongue and thready rapid pulse.

Therapeutic method: nourishing kidney and benefiting yin, securing thoroughfare and stopping bleeding.

Prescription: Zuo Gui Wan and Er Zhi Wan or Zi Yin Gu Qi Tang.

Zuo Gui Wan and Er Zhi Wan Prepared Rehmannia Root, Common Yam Rhizome, Barbary Wolfberry Fruit, Pulp of Dogwood Fruit, Dodder Seed, Deer-Horn Glue, Tortoise-Shell Glue, Medicinal Cyathula Root, Glossy Privet Fruit and Eclipta Alba.

Prescription analysis: in this prescription, Prepared Rehmannia Root, pulp of dogwood fruit and Common Yam Rhizome can nourish liver and kidney, which is " the three tonics" in Six-Ingredient Rehmannia Pill; Tortoise-Shell Glue can tonify deficiency of conception channel; Deer-Horn Glue can replensih the weakness of governor channel; Barbary Wolfberry Fruit, Dodder Seed and Two Solstices Pill can nourish liver and kidney and benefit thoroughfare and conception channels; Medicinal Cyathula Root can supplement liver and kidney and also promote blood promotion. The prescription reinforces water, replenishes essence and strengthens thoroughfare, conception and governor channels, so as to make kidney yin sufficient, strengthen extra channels and stop bleeding.

Modification: the heart fire cannot be replenished due to kidney yin deficiency or exuberant fire due to yin deficiency, dysphoria and insomnia, palpitation with severe palpitation, In this case, Pulse-Reinforcing Powder can be added to benefit Qi, nourish yin and calm heart as well as stop bleeding.

Zi Yin Gu Qi Tang. Dodder Seed, Asiatic Cornelian Cherry Fruit, Tangshen, Milkvetch Root, White Atractylodes Rhizome, Zhigancao, Ass Hide Glue, Degelatined Deer-Horn, Fleeceflower Root, Debark Peony Root, Himalayan Teasel Root.

Prescription analysis: in this prescription, Asiatic Cornelian Cherry Fruit can tonify kidney and benefit essence; Fleeceflower Root and Debark Peony Root can enrich and nourish the blood; Ass Hide Glue can nourish yin and tonify blood and stop bleeding; Dodder Seed can tonify yang and replenish yin; Degelatined Deer-Horn can warm kidney and assist yang as well as astringe and stop bleeding; Himalayan Teasel Root can tonify the liver and kidney; Tangshen, Milkvetch Root, White Atractylodes Rhizome and Zhigancao can benfit Qi and control blood.

(3) Blood heat

① Deficiency-heat

Main symptoms: menstrual unspecified period, less amount but dripping continuously or more amount streaming down, fresh red menstrual blood, flushed cheeks, vexing heat, little sleep, dry throat and mouth, stool constipation, red tongue, less tongue fur and thready rapid pulse.

Therapeutic method: Nourishing yin and clearing heat, securing thoroughfare and stopping bleeding

Prescription: Shang Xia Xiang Zi Tang. Ginseng, Radix Adenophorea, Figwort Root, Dwarf Lilyturf Tuber, Fragrant Solomonseal Rhizome, Chinese Magnoliavine Fruit, Prepared Rehmannia Root, Pulp of Dogwood Fruit, Plantain Seed and Radix Achyranthis Bidentatae.

Prescription analysis: in this prescription, Rehmannia Root and pulp of dogwood fruit are used as the principal medicine to nourish kidney and yin; Ginseng and Radix Adenophorea are used as the adjuvant medicines to benefit qi and moisten lung; Figwort Root, Dwarf Lilyturf Tuber and Fragrant Solomonseal Rhizome can increase fluid, nourish water and reduce fire; Plantain Seed can nourish lung, reinforce yin and benefit essence; Radix Achyranthis Bidentatae can nourish liver and kidney; the prescription contains Fluid-Increasing Decoction to nourish water and Sheng Mai San to replenish Qi, nourish yin and stop bleeding, as well as clear heart, eliminate vexation and tranquillize mind. In the whole prescription, nourishing kidney foucused on accompanied with herbs for moistening lung, which moistens both lung-yin and kidney water. Therefore, lung and kidney nourish each other and both the upper and the lower get moistened, so as to make essence and liquid grown, blood generated and fluid returned. All herbs play the role of nourishing yin and clearing heat, securing thoroughfare and stopping bleeding.

② Excess heat syndrome

Main symptoms: irregular menstrual period sudden profuse discharge or dripping menses, thick menstrual blood in dark red, feeling thirsty, hot and restless, constipation drowning yellow, red tongue, yellow tongue fur and slippery and rapid pulse.

Therapeutic method: Clearing heat and cooling blood, securing thoroughfare and stopping bleeding.

Prescription: Qing Re Gu Jing Tang. Baical Skullcap Root, Fructus Gardeniae Praeparatus, Unprocessed Rehmannia Root, Chinese Wolf berry Root-bark, Garden Burnet Root, fresh Lotus Rhizome Node, Ass Hide Glue, Carbonized Petiole of Windmill-Palm, Tortoise Carapace and Plastron, Oyster Shell and Fresh Liquorice Root.

Prescription analysis: in this prescription, Baical Skullcap Root and Gardenia Jasminoides Ellis can clear heat and purge fire; Unprocessed Rehmannia Root, Garden Burnet Root and Lotus Rhizome Node can clear heat and cool blood, secure thoroughfare and stop bleeding; Chinese Wolf berry Root-bark, Tortoise Carapace and Plastron and oyster shell can nourish yin and supress yang; Tortoise Carapace and Plastron can reinforce deficiency of conception channel, disperse blood stasis to promote regeneration; Ass Hide Glue can enrich blood and stop bleeding; Carbonized Petiole of Windmill-Palm can induce astringency and stop bleeding; fresh Liquorice Root coordinate action of other herbs All herbs perform their own functions, involving integrating clearing heat, purging fire, cooling blood, nourishing yin, stasis-dispelling, glue-securing, astringent, calm and suppress, supplementing Ren, securing thoroughfare and many hemostasia in one prescription, which therefore can have the effects of heat-clearing and blood-cooling and thoroughfare-securing and stopping bleeding.

Modification: If there are also symptoms such as dysphoria and irritability, distending pain in chest and hypochondrium, dry mouth with bitter taste and thready rapid pulse, it can be diagnosed as the syndrome of liver depression transforming into heat or exuberant fire in liver. The treatment should focuses on clearing liver, purging heat and stopping bleeding. Bupleurum Liver-Soothing Powder, Common Selfheal Fruit-Spike and Chinese Gentian should be used together with the prescription above to disperse the depressed liver energy and clear the liver heat.. If there are also symptoms such as pain in lesser abdomen or small abdomen, scorching hot and discomfort, yellow greasy furred tongue, it can be diagnosed as the syndrome of dampness-heat blocking thoroughfare and conception channels.. Amur Cork-Tree, Clematoclethra loniceroides, Weeping Forsythia Capsule and Virgate Wormwood Herb should be added in the previous prescription to clear heat and excrete dampness and remove nourishing and slimy of Ass Hide Glue.

(4) Blood stasis

Main symptoms: sudden profuse discharge or dripping menses in non-menstrual period, sometimes more or less amount, occasionally dripping or stopping or sudden metrorrhagia after several months of menelipsis, followed by metrostaxis, dark menses with blood clot, pain or distension of lower abdomen, dark purple tongue or petechia on the edge of tongue and wiry and thready pulse or unsmooth pulse.

Therapeutic method: activating blood and resolving stasis, securing thoroughfare and stopping bleeding.

Prescription: Zhu Yu Zhi Xue Tang or Jiang Jun Zhan Guan Tang.

Zhu Yu Zhi Xue Tang, Unprocessed Rehmannia Root, Rhubarb, Red Peony Root, Tree Peony Root Bark, Chinese Angelica Tail, Orange Fruit, Tortoise Carapace and Plastron and Peach Seed

Prescripttion analysis: the prescription originates from Peach Seed Four Ingredients Decoction and Peach Seed Purgative Decoction with some changes. Unprocessed Rehmannia Root is reused to clear heat and cool blood. When it is fried with wine, it has the effect of stopping in promoting. Chinese Angelica tail, Peach Seed and Red Peony Root can remove stasis and relieve pain; Tree Peony Root Bark can promote blood circulation and purge fire; Rhubarb can cool blood, remove stasis and descend stagnation, and can descend Qi and strength effect of clearing stasis and stagnation with Orange Fruit; Tortoise Carapace and Plastron is to nourish yin and resolve stasis.

Jiang Jun Zhan Guan Tang. Pollen Typhae Preparatae, fried Trogopterus Dung, Carbonized Rhubarb, Rhizoma Zingiberis Preparatae, India Madder Root, Motherwort Herb, Hairyvein Agrimonia Herb, Mantis Egg-

Case and Cuttlebone, Sanqi Powder, Yam Rhizoma, Coix Seed, Amur Cork-Tree, red Poria cocos, Tree Peony Root Bark, Oriental Waterplantain Rhizome, Ricepaperplant Pith and Talc.

Prescription analysis: in this prescription, Pollen Typhae Preparatae, fried Trogopterus Dung can dispel stasis, stop bleeding and fix pain; Carbonized Rhubarb can clear heat and dispel stasis, accompanying with heat or cold and attacking and maintaining. Rhizoma Zingiberis Preparatae has the effect of both promoting blood circulation and astringing; Motherwort Herb can promote blood circulation; Hairyvein Agrimonia Herb and India Madder Root can activate blood, dispel stasis and stop bleeding; Mantis Egg-Case can tonify kidney and control thoroughfare; Cuttlebone and Sanqi Powder is has great effects of removing blood stasis and stopping bleeding. The prescription focuses more on promotion of blood circulation and also astringency, which has the effect of attacking in reinforcement. It always works on the patients who suffer from metrorrhagia and metrostaxis with both deficiency and excess symptoms.

2. After stopping bleeding

(1) Personal medicine: Treatement after stopping bleeding is the key to cure metrorrhagia and metrostaxis. In clinical practice, the treatment needs to be modified according to patients' condition.

For patients in puberty, there are two therapeutic goals: one is to adjust menstrual cycle and establish ovulation function to avoid recurrence; the other is to adjust menstrual cycle, not focusing on ovulation. Because puberty is not the best age for giving birth, organism can gradually sound ovulation function under natural condition.

Patients in child-bearing period: for these patients, metrorrhagia and metrostaxis often lead to infertility, and treatment should focus on the regulation of menstruation and bring reproductive function back to normal.

Patients in menopause: focusing on body deficiency and anemia caused by metrorrhagia and metrostaxis, prevent recurrence and malignant changes.

(2) Differentiation syndrome and treatment: Cold, heat, deficiency and excess can all result in metrorrhagia and metrostaxis. Treatment should be carried out according to the disease cause and pathogenesis to prevent recurrence. Treatment based on syndrome differentiation can be subject to each pattern of syndrome during bleeding period, but hemostatic medicinal in each prescription shall be removed.

(3) TCM artificial periodic therapy: Due to "menses originate from the kidney" and "menstrual blood comes from kidney", the therapeutic principle of emmeniopathy focuses on curing the root cause to adjust menstruation. The redintegration objectives of the patients in puberty and child-bearing period is to adjust kidney - reproduction-stimulating essence - thoroughfare and conception channels - uterus axis to adjust menstrual cycle or establish ovulation function at the same time. TCM artificial periodic therapy is adopted.In accordance with follicular phase, ovulatory period, luteal phase, menstrual period respectively, follicular promotion decoction, ovulation promotion decoction, luteal promotion decoction and menstruation-regulating and blood-activation decoction, which are all designed for invigorating kidney, should be used one after another for more than three menstrual periods, then it is possible to establish or re-establish a normal menstrual period.

(4) Method of tonifying before attacking the pathogens: According to the mechanism of menstruation, the prescription focuses mainly on tonifying kidney. After bleeding has been stopped, nourishing kidney, supplementing essence, nourish blood and regulate menstruation are the most important. Left-Restoring Pill, Guishen Pill or Menses-fixing decoction is often used to supplement for about 3 weeks, On the fourth week, after menstrual blood gradually stored in uterus, it is time to activate blood circulation, remove blood stasis and induce menstruation. Peach Four Ingredients Decoction is selected with adding Nutgrass Galingale Rhizome, Orange Fruit, Motherwort Herb and Medicinal Cyathula Root. It is traditional menstruation-regulating method, which can reach up to the therapeutic objectives of adjusting menstrual cycle or promoting menstrual cycle.

(5) Invigorating spleen and tonifying blood method: it applies to patients with metrorrhagia and metrostaxis in menopause; anemia and weakness caused by metrorrhagia and metrostaxis shall be eliminated as soon as possible; Major Original-Qi Tonifying Decoction or Ginseng Nutrient-Nourishing Decoction can be selected.

(6) Surgical treatment: it applies to intractable metrorrhagia and metrostaxis for long term in child-bearing period and menopause; or patients with cancerational tendency indicated by the pathological examination due to endometrium by diagnostic curettage.

iii. Specific prescription treatment

Modified Gu Chong Tang: 15g of fresh Milkvetch Root, 15g of Tangshen, 30g of fried White Atractylodes Rhizome, 15g of Prepared Rehmannia Root, 15g of Dodder Seed, 10g of Carbonized Cattail Pollen, 10g of Ophicalcite, 10g of Debark Peony Root, 10g of Ass Hide Glue, 10g of Chinese Gall, 10g of Carbonized Windmill-Palm, 15g of calcining Bone Fossil of Big Mammals, 15g of calcining Oyster Shell, 3g of Sanqi Calomel, 10g of Carbonized Hair. Mainly treat metrorrhagia and metrostaxis that are caused by much bleeding amount caused by blood stasis, with blood clot, accompanied by lack of strength of the whole body, breathe hard and unwilling to talk, dim tongue texture with teeth mark, ecchymosis, white tongue fur, thin and weak pulse;.

iv. Single ingredient prescriptions and proved prescription prescription

(1) Single Ginseng Decoction: 10g of Ginseng, take the medicine after being decocted with water
(2) Shen Fu Tang: 10g of Ginseng, 10g of Prepared Aconite, and take the medicine after being decocted with water on strong fire.
(3) Liu Wei Hui Yang Tang: Ginseng, Processed Aconite, Blast-Fried Ginger, Zhigancao, Prepared Rehmannia Root, Angelica.
(4) 3-6g of pseudo-ginseng powder, and take infused with warm boiled water.
(5) Yunnan Baiyao, and take infused with warm boiled water.

v. Chinese patent drug

Gong Xue Ning Capsule: 2 pills a time, 3 time a day, and take infused with warm boiled water.

vi. Acupuncture and moxibustion therapy (stop bleeding)

Moxibustion Baihui acupoint, Ta Tum acupoint (double), Yinbai acupoint (double).

V. Empirical prescription of famous experts

i. Yu Yin Zhi Beng Tang (Han Bailing)

Indication: menstruation ahead of the time, hypermenorrhea, metrorrhagia and metrostaxis, intermenstrual bleeding, vaginal bleeding during pregnancy and threatened abortion caused by yin deficiency of liver and kidney. The patients suffer from Hypermenorrhea, metrorrhagia and metrostaxis and intermenstrual bleeding caused by yin deficiency for a long time or many babies after early marriage, consumption of essence and blood caused by intemperance in sexual life, yin deficiency with internal heat, heat lodging in thoroughfare and conception channels, advanced menstruation caused by forcing the blood to move frenetically.

Clinical manifestation: soreness of the loins, feebleness of the legs and lack of strength, heel pain, dizziness and tinnitus, amnesia, tidal fever and night sweat, feverish feeling in palms and soles, flush of face and zygomatic region, red tongue with little or no tongue fur, and thready and rapid pulse manifestation.

Component: 10-15g of Prepared Rehmannia Root, 15-20g of Asiatic Cornelian Cherry Fruit, 15-20g of Common Yam Rhizome, 15-20g of Dipsacus, 15-20g of Chinese Taxillus Herb, 15-20g of cuttlebone, 20-30g of Oyster Shell, 15-20g of Debark Peony Root, 10-15g of Ass Hide Glue (melting), 10-20g of Tortoise Carapace and Plastron, 20-50g of fried Garden Burnet Root, 5-10g of Liquorice Root.

Prescription analysis: In the prescription, Prepared Rehmannia Root, Asiatic Cornelian Cherry Fruit and Ass Hide Glue are used as the principal medicines, among which the Prepared Rehmannia Root can nourish yin and tonify kidney and is a kind of significant drug for tonifying blood. According to the record in *Pouch of Pearls,* the Prepared Rehmannia Root can "strongly reinforce qi and blood, promote blood circulation and benefit energy."; and *Compendium of Materia Medica* said Prepared Rehmannia Root "fills the bone marrow, regenerate the muscle and promote generation of vital essence and blood. It also can reduce the insufficiency of the five zang-fu organs, promote blood and do good to eyes and years, darken the beard and hair. It can be used to treat men who suffer from the five consumption and the seven damages, and the women who suffer from vaginal bleeding during pregnancy, irregular menstrual period and other diseases related to pregnancy and birth-giving." Asiatic Cornelian Cherry Fruit can enter lower jiao to tonify liver and kidney and consolidate the conception channels for stopping bleeding It can be used to treat metrorrhagia and metrostaxis and hypermenorrhea that are caused by the deficiency of liver and kidney and unconsolidated conception channels. It is said in *New Compilation of Materia Medica* that Asiatic Cornelian Cherry Fruit as "there is no un-partial yin-tonifying medicine and the Asiatic Cornelian Cherry Fruit is the best yin-tonifying medicine for tonify liver and kidney without complicated functions. It is not too hot or cold, or too abundant of yin or yang." It is called the most effective medicine for tonifying yin; the Debark Peony Root can astringe liver yin, nourish blood and liver, so it can be used to treat irregular menstruation and metrorrhagia and leukorrheal caused by the failure to sooth liver. The Ass Hide Glue has the functions of enrich blood and nourish yin and it is a medicinal with affinity to flesh and blood. It can be used to treat many kinds of syndromes of bleeding, especially bleeding syndrome with yin deficiency or blood deficiency. It is said in *Shennong's Classic of Materia Medica* that "(The Ass Hide Glue) is mainly used to treat internal metrorrhagia in chest and abdomen, hematuria and calm fetus". Take Common Yam Rhizome as adjuvant medicine. In *Compendium of Materia Medica,*"tonify kidney Qi and invigorate spleen and kidney." It can also tonify acquired to nourish inborn; *Mescellaneous Records of Famous Physicians* says Himalayan Teasel Root can treat: "the metrorrhagia and internal metrostaxis of incised wound blood of women……"Chinese Taxillus Herb can nourish liver and kidney, nourish blood and consolidate conception channels. The Oyster Shell is a medicinal with affinity to flesh and blood, and it can not only nourish liver and kidney but also can secure essence and stop bleeding In *Penetrating the Mysterious of Materia Medica,* it is said that Tortoise Carapace and Plastron "can strongly promote water and control fire, so it can strengthen the bones and muscles, benefit mind……dispel blood stasis and stop new bleeding." In *Yangxinglun* there is "the prescription of sovereign medicinal can treat women's metrorrhagia". As fried Garden Burnet Root enter blood, and the drug property of Garden Burnet Root is cold and tastes bitter and good at going downwards, it can be used to treat many kinds of blood heat syndromes and bleeding syndromes, especially bleeding in lower energizer. In *Orthodox Interpretation of Materia Medica*, it is said that Garden Burnet Root "tastes slight bitter and sour, and it is cold and good at going downwards ,which is both consumption and astringent. It can be used for treating women's metrorrhagia and metrostaxis and endless menstruation " The drug property of Cuttlebone is salty, sour and slightly damp, and it has the functions of astring and stop bleeding, secure ssence and leukorrhagia, relieve hyperacidity and pain. It can treat many kinds of internal and external bleeding. When treating trauma bleeding, doctors can singly use Cuttlebone levigation powder for external application. It is said in *Shennong Classic of Materia Medica* that it " is mainly for women's red and white metrostaxis of menstruation." *Collected Essentials of Species of Meteria Medica*: "stop sperm sliding and dispel eye nebula." They two are all assistant medicines used to stop bleeding and help the function of stopping bleeding of both principle medicine and minister medicinal; Liquorice Root adjust all drugs asassistant medicine.

Efficacy: nourish yin and tonify kidney, secure thoroughfare and stop bleeding.

Modification: patients who have large amount of bleeding can use more fried Garden Burnet Root together with Carbonized Windmill-Palm to strengthen the effect of stopping bleeding; patients who have haemal strand or clotted blood can use fried Cattail Pollen and Sanqi to activate blood and stop bleeding.

For patients who always suffer from yin deficiency, as Qi and blood pour down in pregnancy to nourish original qi of fetus, vaginal bleeding during pregnancy and fetal irritability, and the like will be caused by deficiency of yin blood, internal heat due to yin deficiency, disturbance of heat to uterine vessels which force blood to move frenetically.. Taking into consideration the circumstances, doctors shall add Barbary Wolfberry Fruit and Glossy Privet Fruit to nourish yin and clear heat; patients who have large amount of bleeding can use Yerba-Detajo Herb and fried Milkvetch Root for cooling and stopping blood; patients who have stasis can add India Madder Root and fried Cattail Pollen to dispel stasis and stop bleeding.

ii. Qin Re Gu Jing Wan (Gu Xiaochi)

Indication: hypermenorrhea, prolonged menstruation, metrorrhagia and metrostaxis , intermenstrual bleeding caused by yin deficiency and blood heat.

Component: 1.2kg of stir-frying with liquid adjuvant tortoise plastron, 6kg of Unprocessed Rehmannia Root, 3.6kg of Tree Peony Root Bark, 3.6kg of Baical Skullcap Root, 3.6kg of Amur Cork-Tree, 4.8kg of Ass Hide Glue Pellets, 6kg of Carbonized Garden Burnet Root, 6kg of Unprocessed Oyster Shell, 6kg of Cortex Ailanthic, 6kg of Eclipta Prostrata. Grind these drugs into powder and refine the juice into pills. Each pill weights 9 grams. Patients shall take the medicine two times a day and one pill for each time.

Prescription analysis: in the prescription, the stir-frying with liquid adjuvant tortoise plastron, Unprocessed Rehmannia Root and Ass Hide Glue Pellets are principle medicine, which can be used to tonify kidney and nourish yin. Besides, tortoise plastron and Ass Hide Glue are both medicinal with affinity to flesh and blood and can tonify true yin and invigorate yin; Carbonized Garden Burnet Root and unprocessed Oyster Shell as minister medicinal can astringe and stop bleeding; Tree Peony Root Bark, Baical Skullcap Root, Baical Skullcap Root and Cortex Ailanthic can clear heat, cool blood and stop bleeding as assistant medicine; Eclipta Prostrata can enter the kidney to nourish yin and stop bleeding as a assistant medicine.

Efficacy: to nourish yin and clear heat, astringe menses and stop bleeding

iii. Zi Yin Gu Qi Tang (Luo Yuankai)

Indication: metrorrhagia and metrostaxis. It can be used for treating functional uterine bleeding.

Component: 12g of Tangshen, 15g of Milkvetch Root, 9g of White Atractylodes Rhizome, 6g of Ass Hide Glue(melting), 9g of Himalayan Teasel Root, 15g of Dodder Seed, 12g of Polygoni Multiflori, 15g of Fructus Corni, 15g of Degelati ned Deer-Horn, 9g of Debark Peony Root, 6g of Zhigancao. Take the medicine after decocting with water. And take 1 bag a day for two times a day.

Prescription analysis: in the prescription, the Tangshen and Milkvetch Root can tonify Qi and blood; the White Atractylodes Rhizome can invigorate spleen and tonify Qi; Polygoni Multiflori, Dodder Seed and Fructus Corni can tonify liver and kidney; the Debark Peony Root can astringe yin and regulate the nutrient; the Himalayan Teasel Root can regulate and promote blood circulation; the Liquorice Root can coordinate the functions of other drugs. The whole prescription mainly concentrates on tonifying Qi. Once Qi is full enough, blood; can be controlled. The prescription also focuses on nourishing yin and blood, As blood is full enough, it can help liver store blood. And if the blood is controlled, the metrorrhagia will be avoided.

Efficacy: nourish yin, tonify Qi and control blood.

Modification: patients who have much bleeding, Carbonized Windmill-Palm, Red Halloysite and Motherwort Herb are added; accompanied by Ginseng, Milkvetch Root and moxa-moxibustion Yin Pai, Ta Tum, san yin chiao, which have the effect of stopping bleeding; after the bleeding stops, Barbary Wolfberry Fruit, Malaytea Scurfpea

Fruit, Morinda Root, Epimedium Herb, Eucommia Bark, and others are added to strengthen the effect of tonifying kidney.

VI. Typical medical records of famous experts

i. Medical records of Liu Fengwu

Ms. Shi, 41 years old.

Preliminary diagnosis: on June 6, 1975. Chief complaint of irregular menstrual cycle, and menstruate period lasting for more than a year.

Current medical history: the menstruation was regular in the past, but the blood amount increases in this year, which is purple with blood clots. The patient had massive hemorrhage last August for more than 10m days and then the menstruation became frequent or even two times in a month and last for more than 10 days in large amount. In January of this year, the patient received uterine curettage because of massive hemorrhage of vagina, and the pathology was diagnosed as "Endometrium Hyperplasia". Two months after the menstruation, bleeding in vagina has lasted for more than 10 days. The patient has been treated by progesterone and the menstruation was endless and in dark-purple color with large amount and small blood clot. In recent two years, the patient became irritable, accompanied by fullness in chest and hypochondrium, anorexia, abdominal distension, soreness and pain in waist, dry stool 1 time in every 2-3 days. The last menstruation was on April 22 and then the menstruation stopped until now for 54 days. Pink tongue and wiry and smooth pulse.

Western medicine diagnosis: functional uterine bleeding.

TCM differentiation: spleen and kidney deficiency, blood heat, liver-yang hyperactivity.

Therapeutic method: strengthen spleen and nourish kidney, cool the blood and soothe the liver.

Prescription: five qian of Common Yam Rhizome, three qian of Sinocrassula Indica, three qian of Dodder Seed, three qian of Himalayan Teasel Root, three qian of Unprocessed Rehmannia Root, three qian of Prepared Rehmannia Root, four qian of Debark Peony Root, one and a half qian of fried Herba Schizonepetae, one and a half qian of Chinese Thorowax Root, three qian of Baical Skullcap Root, three qian of Tree Peony Root Bark and two qian of Motherwort Herb (One qian equals to about 3.72g).

Second diagnosis: on June 26, 1975. Menses occurred after taking 3 doses of the prescription above. The menses lasted 4 days with red blood of medium amount. Because sterna rib has obvious swelling and pain, three qian of Szechwan Chinaberry Fruit was added, and 7 doses were taken continually.

Third diagnosis: on August 1, 1975. Menses occurred for two times in one month (6 days). The patient continued to take 5 doses of the previous prescription.

Fourth diagnosis: on September 27, 1975, she took 23 doses from June 19 to August 1. All her symptoms disappeared, the menstruation came on time and the blood volume decreased. Menses lasted 3-5 days and the normal menses occurred for 3 times. The menstruation came on time for two times again after stopping taking medicine. In addition, it is a little ahead of the time (23 to 25 days). The last menstruation came on September 24.

ii. Medical record of Song Guangji

Ms Chen, 16 years old, student.

Preliminary diagnosis: on August 40, 1979. Symptoms include: kidney Qi deficiency, deficiency both in thoroughfare and conception channels, advanced menstruation, several times of menses in one month, menorrhagia with dark red blood or dripping menses, lusterless complexion, soreness of waist, cold limbs, poor sleep, thin pulse and whitish fur. Prescription focuses on warming the kidney and tonifying Qi, nourishing blood and securing thoroughfare: Rehmannia, fried Common Yam Rhizome, Radix Astragali Preparata, Tuber Fleeceflower Stem, fried Red Halloysite, Carbonized Petiole of Windmill-palm, 12 g for each foregoing Chinese herbal medicine, Barbary Wolfberry Fruit, Dodder Seed, fried Ass Hide Glue, Indianbread with Pine, 9 g for each foregoing Chinese herbal medicine, 6 g of Common Macrocarpium Fruit, and 3 g of charred Folium Artemisiae Argyi. 5 doses were taken.

Secondary diagnosis: on September 6, 1979. Stopped bleeding, the sleep got better, with increased vaginal dis and whitish fur after taking the previous prescription. Prescription invigorating spleen to eliminate dampness and check vaginal discharge: Codonopsis pilosula var. modesta, fried White Atractylodes Rhizome, Radix Astragali Preparata, Cherokee Rose Fruit, Gordon Euryale Seed and Plantain Herb (9g for each Chinese herbal medicine), Lotus Stamen and calcined Oyster Shell (12 g for each), fried Dried Tangerine Peel and Radix Glycyrrhizae Preparata (3 g for each). 5 doses were taken.

Third diagnosis: on September 30, 1979. Cycle became normal, morbid leucorrhoea quantity increased with light yellow color and the patient has dry stool, thin and slow pulse, as well as thin fur. Prescription invigorating spleen to eliminate dampness, clear heat and check vaginal discharge was prepared again: Codonopsis pilosula var. modesta, Plantain Herb, Lotus Stamen, Glossy Privet Fruit, Cockcomb Flower, brown Millet Sprout (9 g for each), Common Yam Rhizome and calcined Oyster Shell (12g for each), Chinese Thorowax Root, phellodendri, fried Dried Tangerine Peel (3 g for each). 5 doses were taken.

Note: In this case, although reproduction-stimulating essence is enough, kidney Qi is deficient, and storage function is lost, which leads to menorrhagia, mild lumbago and cold limbs, as well as deep and thin pulse. Therefore, the prescription warming kidney and benefiting Qi was prepared. The prescription was a modification of Tiaochong decoction. The Rehmannia, Barbary Wolfberry Fruit, Dodder Seed, Common Macrocarpium Fruit were used for nourishing liver and kiney. Milkvetch Root and Ass Hide Glue were used for benefiting Qi and nourishing blood. Indianbread with Pine and Tuber Fleeceflower Stem were used for nourishing the blood and tranquilization. Carbonized Petiole of Windmill-palm, Red Halloysite and charred Folium Artemisiae Argyi were used for warming the kidney and stopping bleeding. Common Yam Rhizome was used for invigorating spleen and nourishing kidney. They together played the role in invigorating the kidney and regulating the thoroughfare channel.

iii. Medical record of Han Bailing

Ms. Lv, 21 years old.

Preliminary diagnosis: on September 28, 2011. in recent 3 years, the menstrual blood kept dripping without stop, always lasting for more than a month Vagina bleeding has lasted for more than one month since August 25. There was not much blood in light red. Other symptoms include: soreness of waist, fatigue, lack of energy and lazy to speak, eating less food, feeling dizzy, poor memory, lusterless complexion, thinner body as well as more body hair and pubes; pale tongue, thin and white fur, as well as deep and thin pulse. Menstruation first came when the patient was 17 years old, with oligomenorrhea. She has taken the western medicine Ethinylestradiol and Cyproterone Acetate Tablets (Diane-35) for more than 2 years. The menstruation was normal when the drug was taken, but the menstruation was still abnormal after stopping the drug.

Auxiliary examination: six items of serum sex hormone: FSH: 4.22mU/ml, LH: 18.35mU/ml, PRL: 11.96ng/ml, E2: 70.16pg/ml, P: 0.51ng/ml, T: 85.37ng/dl. Sugar tolerance, insulin and thyroid function are all normal. The ultrasound shows the uterus is a little small; polycystic ovary, left ovary is 35mm×22mm in size and 13 follicles of 2-4mm can be seen; right ovary is 37mm×24mm in size and 16 follicles of 2-5mm can be seen.

Diagnosis: metrorrhagia and metrostaxis (polycystic ovarian syndrome)

Differential diagnosis: deficiency of both spleen and kidney, caused by deficiency of thoroughfare and conception channels.

Therapeutic method: tonifying kidney and strengthening spleen, secure thoroughfare and stop bleeding.

Prescription: 20 g of Prepared Rehmannia Root, 15 g of Asiatic Cornelian Cherry Fruit, 15 g of calcined Eucommia Bark, 20 g of Himalayan Teasel Root, 20 g of Chinese Taxillus Herb, 20 g of Milkvetch Root, 20g of Tangshen, 15g of Common Yam Rhizome, 15g of Indian Bread, 15g of Debark Peony Root, 10g of Ass Hide Glue, calcined Oyster Shell, 50g of Carbonized garden Burnet Root, and 5 g of Liquorice Root. 7 doses were decocted in water for oral dose. One dose each day, taken in the morning and evening.

Secondary diagnosis: on October 13, 2012. The bleeding stopped after taking the medicine for 3 days. On October 9, vaginal bleeding occurred again as the patient got frightened from the outside world.. The bleeding lasted 5 days till the day of diagnosis, therein the more bleeding amount appeared in 4 days. Hands and feet were cold, with cool in back; light red tongue, thin and white fur, as well as deep and slow pulse.

15 g of calcined Eucommia Bark, 20 g of Himalayan Teasel Root, 20 g of Chinese Taxillus Herb, 20 g of Milkvetch Root, 20g of Tangshen, 15g of Common Yam Rhizome, 15g of Indian Bread, 15g of Debark Peony Root, 10g of Ass Hide Glue, calcined Oyster Shell, 50g of Carbonized garden Burnet Root, 5g of Liquorice Root. 10 doses were decocted in water for oral dose. One dose each day, taken in the morning and evening.

Third diagnosis: on December 12, 2012. The patient didn't feel quite cold in hands and feet, also not cold in the back. The last menstruation occurred on November 18, 2012, lasting for 6 days. Considering that her menstruation was coming, the medicine for tonifying kidney and regulating menstruation was given.

20g of Prepared Rehmannia Root, 15g of Dodder Seed, 15g of Morinda Root, 15g of Red Peony Root, 15g of Motherwort Herb, 10g of Nutgrass Galingale Rhizome, 15g of Chinese Angelica, 15g of Tangshen, 20g of Common Yam Rhizome, 10g of Radix Glycyrrhizae Preparata. 10 doses were taken in the same way as before.

Combining with the menstrual cycle, the patient accepted the treatment with the prescriptions above and their modifications for half a year. In recent 3 months, the menstruation occurred one time every 25-37 days, lasting 5-7 days each time. She gained 3 kg in weightd, and her complexion is similar with the normal person and all the symptoms disappeared. Blood FSH: 3.71mU/ml, LH: 8.92mU/ml and T: 53.31ng/dl. The patient stopped taking decoction, and changed to take Yuyin pill and Guipi pill for consolidating for 1-2 months. She shall avoiding being scared and defatigation, and pay attention to diet. After 3 months later, her menstruation was normal and the constitution was improved significantly when she took the follow-up examination.

Note: polycystic ovarian syndrome is a complex endocrine disorder disease with diversified clinical manifestations. The patient of this case who is relatively thin has later menarche accompanied with waist ache and soreness, fatigue and atony, dizziness and poor memory which are caused by kidney deficiency. As "the menstrual blood is from all kidneys"; the kidney governing reproduction boosts kidney yin and generates kidney-yang. "Without it, yin Qi in thefive zang-fu organ cannot be nourished and yang Qi in thefive zang-fu organ cannot be emitted"; both kidney yin deficiency and kidney yang deficiency will cause blood flowing and metrorrhagia. *Compendium of Medince* says that "menstruation-regulating shall give priority to tonifying kidney". In clinical syndrome inspection, based on "Liver and kidney theory", Han's treats menstrual disorder starting with kidney and supplies for innateness and after birth by taking Bailing yin-nourishing and Metrorrhagia-stopping Decoction and Returning to Spleen Decoction with the method of acquirement nourishing innateness. Tonifying kidney shall be considered first; invigorating spleen and nourishing blood shall be conducted at the same time to ensure the origin of producing Qi and blood. Menstruation will become normal by tonifying spleen and kidney, harmonizing yin and yang as well as regulating yin and yang. if bleeding is stopped only without clarifying the source and recovery, it is difficult to solve emergent problem . Treatment principles of radically reform and treatment of both primary and secondary symptoms must be considered in the process of stop bleeding.

VII. Prevention and aftercare

(1) Metrorrhagia and metrostaxis can be prevented. Special attention shall be paid to menstrual hygiene, and the uterine cavity operation shall be avoided to the greatest extent.Menorrhagia, menostaxis, advanced menstruation and other menstrual diseases with bleeding tendency shall be treated in time so as to avoid that the diseases develop into metrorrhagia and metrostaxis.

(2) Once metrorrhagia and metrostaxis happened, it must be treated as soon as possible according to three methods for stopping bleeding, clarifying the source and redintegration to establish a normal menstrual cycle and prevent recurrence.

(3) For aftercare of metrorrhagia and metrostaxis, initial attention shall be paid to personal hygiene to prevent infection; diet shall be adjusted, nutrition shall be increased and anemia, which results from bleeding, shall be corrected; work and rest shall be moderate; the patient shall have a good mood.

(LUO Meiyu)

References

[1] Zhang YZ. Gynecology of Traditional Chinese Medicine[M]. 2nd ed. Beijing: Chinese Medicine Press, 2007.

[2] Han YH. Han's Medical Department for Women [M]. Beijing: People's Military Medical Press, 2015.

[3] Beijing Traditional Chinese Medicine Hospital, Beijing Chinese Medical School. Experience in Gynecology of Liu Fengwu [M]. Beijing: People's Medical Publishing House, 1977.

[4] Zhejiang Administration of Traditional Chinese Medicine. Famous TCM Clinical Experience Selections of Zhejiang Province [M]. Hangzhou: Zhejiang Science and Technology Press, 1990.

[5] Chen ZL. Characteristic Experience Essence of Famous Doctors [M]. Shanghai: Shanghai College of Traditional Chinese Medicine Press, 1987.

Infertility 不孕症

I. Overview

If the couples live together with normal sexual life, male reproductive function is normal and the female is not pregnant with 1 year of unprotected intercourse, then it is called infertility. Female who has never been pregnant is primary infertility, which is called "complete infertility" in traditional chinese medicine; female who had pregnancy history before is secondary infertility, which is called "Duan Xu" in traditional Chinese medicine. (In 1991, Infertility standard was amended by Obstetrics and Gynecology Committee of Chinese Association of the Integration of Traditional and Western Medicine on the third academic conference). As early as more than two thousand years ago, traditional chinese medicine already had a systematic understanding of the disease. In the ancient books of traditional chinese medicine, disease names of infertility include "Bu Yun" "Wu Zi" "Jue Chan", in addition to "complete infertility" and "Duan Xu". Infertility is related to the couples. Diseased region can be located in reproductive organs and also in zang-fu organs- meridian. In recent years, infertility patients have shown rising tendency year by year, which has become a global medical and social problem influencing development and health of human. Therefore, World Health Organization has declared that infertility, cardiovascular disease and phymatosis are listed as three main diseases that influence human life and health.

II. Etiology and pathogenesis

i. Etiology

Etiology of infertility is complex. Pathogenic factor can appear independently or compositely. The etiology can be divided into the following two categories.

1. Congenital defect

Ancient physicians already had known that infertility was related to both the couples and proposed that etiology of a part of patients was that one of the couples or the couples presented congenital or acquired genital defects. In Jin and Yuan Dynasties, Zhu Zhenheng had pointed out in *Further Discourses on Acquiring Knowledge by Studying Properties of Things · Conception Theory* that true sexual intersex and false sexual intersex exist: "the male cannot be the father, the female cannot be the mother or the person can not only be matched with male but also with female... the category is different. There are two conditions about both sexes. The one is to be wife together with male, and be husband together with female. The other one is to be wife not a husband or male and female both are parents." Such people cannot be pregnant normally due to abnormal genitals. For another example, in Ming Dynasty, Wan Quan had proposed "five types of female sterility" in *Ze Pei Pian* of *Guang Si Ji Yao*: firstly called spiral, referring to external spiral of vaginal orifice spins into human body like a river snail; secondly called grain, vaginal orifice is small like tendon head, and only can be open to drown, but is difficult to make intercourse. The person in such condition is called a female with a hypoplastic vagina; thirdly called tympan, flower head is intense like atresia; fourthly called angle, flower head is sharp like angle; fifthly called pulse, menstruation comes first before fourteen years old, or appears in fifteen or sixteen years old or is irregularities or never appears. Such five organs without tissues of external genitalia cannot coordinate with greater yang, so how to be pregnant?" In Qing Dynasty, Lu Ruoteng had put forward "five types of male sterility" in *Dao Ju Sui Bi*: male has five types of male sterility: earlier-heaven eunuchism, cutting, fistula, timidity and change. For male with the earlier-heaven eunuchism, impotence is just the earlier-heaven eunuchism as said in ancient times; for male with cutting, the male acts as palace attendant after the male genitals is cut; as to male with fistula, automatic seminal emission often occurs due to insecurity due to semen cold; for male with timidity, penis erects weakly and is not excited when meeting the female; male with change, who is both male and female, is called sexual dimorphism. "Five types of female sterility" and "five types of male sterility" respectively indicate five syndromes that both male and female has no ability to have children due to congenital physiological defects, reproductive organs malformations or other lesions.

2. Acquired pathological changes

(1) Exogenous factors: in pathogenic qi of six excesses, wind, cold and dampness directly attack uterus, resulting in dysfunction of uterus. Cold makes blood congealed and stagnated, causing stasis. Dampness blocks qi movement, thus causing hypomenorrhea, unsmooth menstruation even amenorrhea, metrorrhagia and metrostaxis, leucorrhea and other diseases, so that infertility occurs. In Ming Dynasty, Xue Ji had put forward the opinion that "infertility of women is caused by damage to thoroughfare and conception vessels due to pathogenic Qi of six excesses and seven emotions" in *Xue's Medical Record*.

(2) Factor of internal injuries caused by seven emotions: in mental factor, internal causes and seven emotions both can influence conception. In seven emotions, violent rage and worry have the greatest influence on conception. If violent rage damages liver and emotion shows upset, liver will fail to free flow of qi and qi movement is under depression, causing inharmonious qi and blood, so that thoroughfare and conception vessels

cannot complement each other. Therefore, it is difficult to be pregnant. Worry damages spleen. And then if spleen has dysfunction in transportation, phlegm-dampness is generated from interior, qi movement is constrained, and uterine vessels are blocked. It will be difficult to consolidate semen to be pregnant.

(3) Constitution factor: different constitutions are formed due to natural endowment and acquired differences. Different constitutions have different sensitivities to different diseases, and infertility is closely related to some constitution factors. As *Volume Seven* in *The Heart and Essence of Dan Xi's Methods of treatment* said, "the obese cannot be pregnant, because body fat blocks uterus and menstruation fails to come regularly...... the thin cannot be pregnant, owing that there is no blood in the uterus, essential qi cannot be concentrated." The obese people are phlegm-dampness type constitution and exuberance of internal phlegm-dampness blocks uterus, so they cannot be pregnant; the thin is yin deficiency constitution, internal heat is caused by yin deficiency, fire-heat scorches yin, blood depletion and less menses occur, and it is difficult for yin essence to be concentrated, also causing infertility; people with yang deficiency cannot warm uterus due to weak yang qi, which easily causes cold in uterus and lead to infertility.

(4) Others: in the aspect of life, due to female's unrestricted sexual strain, overabundance and over frequency of pregnancy and birth, kidney qi deficiency, consumption of qi and blood, damage to thoroughfare and conception vessels can be caused, and further infertility occurs. Or crapulence gluttony and arbitrarily eating raw or cold food cause damage to spleen-stomach, failure in transportation and transformation, which cause no nourishing in thoroughfare and conception vessels, or result in endogenous phlegm-dampness, obstructing uterine vessels to cause infertility.

ii. Pathogenesis

Pathogenesis of infertility is a chronic process and the pathogenesis is divided into deficiency and excess. Ancient physicians had discussion on the pathogenesis of infertility. The main pathogenesis is dysfunction of thoroughfare and conception vessels, uterus, kidney and liver.

1. Deficiency and damage of zang-fu organs function

(1) Kidney deficiency: kidney is innate foundation, stores essence qi and controls reproduction. ① Insufficiency of kidney Qi: kidney stores essence, and essence transforms into qi. Essence qi in the kidney dominates growth, development and reproduction of human body. Female cannot consolidate semen to be pregnant due to thoroughfare and conception vessels deficiencies caused by kidney qi insufficiency. ② Deficiency debilitation of kidney yang: deficiency debilitation of kidney yang and debilitation of life gate fire cannot warm uterus and consolidate semen to be pregnant. ③ Deficiency debilitation of kidney yin: deficiency of kidney yin will lead to internal heat. Internal heat will disturb thoroughfare and conception vessels, causing difficulty in pregnancy. Therefore, insufficiency of kidney qi, deficiency debilitation of kidney yang and kidney essence deficiency can lead to infertility.

(2) Liver depression: female represents upset emotion, depression or quick temper, violent rage damaging liver, causing dysfunction of free flow of liver qi, so that liver depresses and qi stagnates, qi and blood are in disharmony and thoroughfare and conception vessels cannot complement each other, leading to infertility.

2. Meridian pathopoiesia

As said in Plain Questions: "if governor vessel was ill, the female would be infertility." It has proposed the relation between infertility and meridian. Further Discourses in Acquiring Knowledge by Studying Properties of Things had advocated "too heat ofblood sea. Profound Scholarship in Women's Diseases had cited "female has no child for a long time, because heat is hidden in thoroughfare and conception vessels...... heat in the interior will cause blood depletion" said Zhu Danxi. In the meridians, thoroughfare and conception vessels are especially important. "Thoroughfare vessel is blood sea", "thoroughfare vessel is sea of twelve meridians" and can adjust qi and blood of twelve meridians. "Conception vessel governing uterus and gestation" and damage of thoroughfare and conception vessels inevitably lead to gynecological diseases.

3. Abnormal metabolism of qi and blood

(1) Blood stasis: in Jin Dynasty, as *Women's Diseases* of *A-B Classic of Acupuncture and Moxibustion* of Huang Fumi said: "the female cannot be pregnant and blood cannot be discharged, which is governed by CV 4. " This is the earliest record about blood stasis and infertility. Blood stasis and qi stagnation, irregular menstruation make menses accumulated in the uterus, or cause obstruction of uterine vessels, so it is difficult for semen to be incorporated, causing difficulty in pregnancy.

(2) Phlegm-dampness: this syndrome mostly appears in the obese. Because fat body or arbitrarily eating greasy and surfeit flavor can damage spleen-stomach and fail in transportation and transformation, resulting in endogenous phlegm-dampness, unsmooth qi movement, and obstruction of uterus and pulse. Therefore, female cannot be pregnant.

Kidney deficiency is the root cause in infertility; however, five zang-organs are connected. Liver depression, phlegm-dampness, blood stasis and other factors can affect kidney and liver functions. Several pathogenesis can be mutually transformed with the presence of many etiologies, finally resulting in menstrual irregularities and obstruction of uterine vessels and causing infertility.

III. Key points of diagnosis and differential diagnosis

i. Key points of diagnosis

From the definition of disease, definition of years of infertility is the premise of diagnosis of this disease. If women are not pregnant for 1 year without contraception, it is called infertility. In disease diagnosis, causes for infertility are found out through overall examination of both sexes, which is the diagnostic key to infertility. Examination steps for female mainly include marriageable age, sexual life condition, menstrual history, previous history (for example, whether there is appendectomy, gynecological operation, thyropathy, diabetes and so on), family history, previous reproductive history and male health condition. Whether women with secondary infertility have abortion history, ectopic pregnancy history and infectious history shall be asked. Moreover, in physical examination, the development of secondary sex characteristic, development condition of internal and external genitals, whether there is malformation, masses, inflammation and milk regurgitation of breast shall be noticed.

ii. Key points of differentiation

1. Distinguishing infertility and sterility

Infertility and sterility are different; infertility refers to the inability to conceive; sterility refers to being pregnant but cannot give a birth. Although one was pregnant, ended by early abortion, habitual abortion and abortion. Another implication of sterility means that the male is infertile.

2. Identifying primary infertility and secondary infertility

Infertility is divided into primary infertility and secondary infertility. Primary infertility refers to those who fail to be pregnant with effective sexual life of married couples for more than 12 months of menstrual cycles. Secondary infertility refers to those who cannot be pregnant again with effective sexual life for more than 12 months of menstrual cycles after having one or more previous pregnancies.

3. Identification of infertility and abortion within the first month of pregnancy

Abortion within the first month of pregnancy refers to those who are spontaneous abortion at the beginning of embryo in very early pregnancy period. As said in *Diagnosis and Treatment of Yeshi's on Women's Diseases · Notice on Abortion within the First Month of Pregnancy*: "if a woman had early abortion only within one month and no one knows that she was pregnant and said she was infertile, without knowing she already conception but have a early abortion". It can be considered as biochemical pregnancy of modern medicine. At that moment, there is no obvious pregnant reaction or only delayed menstrual cycle on pregnant women, resulting in misdiagnosis as primary pregnancy due to difficult awareness. In very early pregnancy period, auxiliary examination is conducted through BBT, one step pregnancy test and human chorionic gonadotropin to clear diagnosis.

IV. TCM therapy

i. Syndrome differentiation and treatment

Key points of syndrome differentiation and treatment of infertility lie in distinguishing the condition of zang-fu organs, meridian qi and blood, thoroughfare and conception vessels and uterus. Essentials of therapy is to nurse thoroughfare and conception vessels, warm kidney and uterus, smooth liver and relieve depression, tonify qi and blood, dry dampness and resolve phlegm as well as activate blood and resolve stasis.

1. Deficiency debilitation of kidney yang

Main symptoms: infertility after married for a long time, delayed menstruation, frigidity, cold pain in lower abdomen, dizziness and tinnitus, soreness and weakness of waist and knees, frequent enuresis nocturna, pale tongue and white tongue coating, deep,thready and weak pulse.

Therapeutic method: warm kidney and uterus. With regard to the patients with deficiency debilitation of kidney yang, uterine cold infertility, it is appropriate to warm kidney and uterus, accompanying with herbs tonifying heart fire. Just as said in *Semen of Fu Qingzhu's Obstetrics and Gynecology*: "Tonifying heart is tonifying kidney, and warming kidney is warming heart. Due to heart kidney with sufficient qi, fire of heart kidney will generate automatically, fire of heart kidney generates, and cold of uterus will disperse automatically. If uterus is warm, why not be pregnant?"

Prescription: Wen Bo Yin or You Gui Wan.

Wen Bao Yin. Ginseng, White Atractylodes Rhizome, Morinda Root, Malaytea Scurfpea Fruit, Eucommia Bark, Dodder Seed, Gordon Euryale Seed, Common Yam Rhizome, Cinnamon Bark, Prepared Common Monkshood Daughter Root.

You Gui Wan. Prepared Rehmannia Root, processed Prepared Common Monkshood Daughter Root, Cinnamon Bark, Common Yam Rhizome, Asiatic Cornelian Cherry Fruit, Dodder Seed, Deer-Horn Glue, Barbary Wolfberry Fruit, Chinese Angelica, Eucommia Bark.

2. Liver depression and qi stagnation

Main Symptoms: Infertility after married for a long time, advanced or delayed menstruation, abdominal pain before menstruation, premenstrual distending pain of breasts, dysphoria and irritability, depression, dark red tongue or ecchymosis, wiry and thready pulse.

Therapeutic method: sooth liver and relieve depression.

Relive depression of liver qi, soothe the retention of spleen qi, heart and kidney qi are soothed, therefore, waist and navel are benefited and conception and belt vessels are open. It is not necessary for gate of uterine vessels to be opened, uterine vessels will start automatically.

Prescription: Kai Yu Zhong Yu Tang. Debark Peony Root, Nutgrass Galingale Rhizome, Chinese Angelica, White Atractylodes Rhizome, Tree Peony Root Bark, Indian Bread, Pollen.

3. Static blood obstructing uterus

Main symptoms: Infertility after married for a long time, delayed menstruation, abdominal pain in menstruation, dark menses, blood clot, dark tongue body, thin and white tongue coating, wiry and thready or thready and hesitant pulse.

Therapeutic method: activate blood and resolve stasis.

Wang Qingren makes good use of method of activating blood and resolving stasis to treat many diseases. Infertility is diagnosed and treated, which has a wonderful effect.

Prescription: Shao Fu Zhu Yu Tang. Fennel, Dried Ginger, Yanhusuo, Myrrh, Chinese Angelica, Sichuan Lovage Rhizome, Cinnamomum Cassia Presel, Red Peony Root, Cattail Pollen, Trogopterus Dung.

4. Phlegm-dampness stasis and obstruction

Main symptoms: Infertility after married for a long time, fat body, often delayed menstruation, hypotrichosis, even amenorrhea, more leucorrhea amount, dizziness and palpitation, pale red and enlarged tongue and greasy white tongue coating.

The rapeutic method: dry dampness and resolve phlegm.

Zhu Danxi firstly advocates that "the body is filled with fat, which will obstruct uterus, should be treated by drying dampness and resolving phlegm." As said in *Fu Qingzhu's Obstetrics and Gynecology*: "therapeutic method should be discharge and resolve phlegm. However, if discharging and resolving phlegm are only carried out, qi of spleen and stomach cannot be supplemented immediately. Yang qi is not strong, dampness-phlegm cannot be resolved, as a result, people get ill firstly. It has proposed method of tonifying spleen and resolving phlegm to treat infertility."

Prescription: Cang Fu Dao Tan Tang. Atractylodes Rhizome, Nutgrass Galingale Rhizome, Dried Tangerine Peel, Jackinthepulpit Tuber, Orange Fruit, Pinellia Tuber, Sichuan Lovage Rhizome, Talc, Indian Bread, Medicated Leaven.

ii. Specific prescription treatment

1. Nuan Gong Yun Zi Wan

Component: Chinese Angelica, Debark Peony Root, Sichuan Lovage Rhizome, Prepared Rehmannia Root, Ass Hide Glue, Milkvetch Root, Himalayan Teasel Root, Eucommia Bark, Nutgrass Galingale Rhizome and Argy Wormwood Leaf.

Usage: 8g is taken each time, with 2-3 times every day. It is taken with warm boiled water.

Indications: failing to be pregnant for a long time after marriage, delayed menstruation, less amount and light menses, dark complexion, soreness of waist and weakness of legs, erotic apathy, clear abundant urine, loose stool, pale red tongue body, thin and white tongue coating, deep and thready pulse or deep and slow pulse.

2. Ding Kun Wan

Component: American Ginseng, White Atractylodes Rhizome, Indian Bread, Prepared Rehmannia Root, Chinese Angelica, Debark Peony Root, Sichuan Lovage Rhizome, Milkvetch Root, Ass Hide Glue, Chinese Magnoliavine Fruit, Pilose Antler, Cinnamon Bark, Argy Wormwood Leaf, Eucommia Bark, Himalayan Teasel Root, Finger Citron, Dried Tangerine Peel, Officinal Magnolia Bark, Chinese Thorowax Root, Nutgrass Galingale Rhizome, Yanhusuo, Tree Peony Root Bark, Amber, Tortoise Plastron, Rehmannia Root, Dwarf Lilyturf Tuber, Baical Skullcap Root.

Usage: 1 pill is taken for each time, with 2 times every day. It is taken with warm boiled water.

Indications: it is used for failing to be pregnant for a long time after marriage, delayed menstruation, less amount and light menses, dark complexion, soreness of waist and weakness of legs, erotic apathy, clear abundant urine, loose stool, pale red tongue body, thin and white tongue coating, deep and thready pulse or deep and slow pulse.

3. Fu Ke De Sheng Wan

Component: Motherwort Herb, Debark Peony Root, Chinese Angelica, Incised Notopterygi um Rhizome and Root, Chinese Thorowax Root, Common Aucklandia Root.

Usage: 1 pill is taken for each time and 2 times every day with warm boiled water.

Indications: it is used for failing to be pregnant for a long time after marriage, irregular menstrual cycle, abdominal pain in menstruation, less amount and dark color, blood clot, premenstrual distending pain of breasts, depression, anxiety and irritability, normal or dark red tongue body, thin and white tongue coating, wiry pulse.

4. Shi Er Wen Jing Wan

Component: Medicinal Evodia Fruit, Cinnamon Bark, Chinese Angelica, Sichuan Lovage Rhizome, Ass Hide Glue Pearl, Debark Peony Root, Dwarf Lilyturf Tuber, Tangshen, Fresh Ginger, Pinellia Tuber, Tree Peony Root Bark, Zhigancao.

Usage: 1 pill is taken for each time and 2 times every day with warm yellow rice or millet wine.

Indications: it is used for failing to be pregnant for a long time after marriage, having obvious history of catching a cold, delayed menstruation, less amount and dark color, often feeling cold in lower abdomen, preferring warm and rejecting press, thin and white tongue coating, deep and tight pulse.

5. Er Chen Wan and Yue Ju Wan

Component: Dried Tangerine Peel, Pinellia Tuber, Indian Bread, Liquorice Root, Fresh Ginger, Nutgrass Galingale Rhizome, Sichuan Lovage Rhizome, Medicated Leaven, Cape Jasmine Fruit, Orange Fruit, Areca Seed.

Usage: 12g is taken every time and 2 times daily with warm boiled water or water with ginger and jujube.

Indications: it is used for failing to be pregnant for a long time after marriage, fat body, delayed menstruation, even amenorrhea, more leucorrhea, sticky and thick quality, pale complexion, dizziness and palpitation, chest distress and nausea, white and greasy tongue coating, slippery pulse.

iii. Acupuncture and moxibustion therapy

Acupuncture and moxibustion as one of the clinical commonly used therapies is mostly seen in treating gynecological diseases. Acupuncture and moxibustion not only can adjust menstruation, but can induce ovulation as well. With regard to kidney deficiency, liver depression, blood stasis and other pathogenesis, acupoints of thoroughfare vessel, conception vessel and governor vessel as well as some acupoints of kidney, liver and spleen meridian can be selected to treat commonly. Commonly used acupoints are SP 6, CV 6, LR 3, CV 4, SP 10, ST 29, CV 3, KI 12, BL 20, BL 23, GV4, KI 3, ST 36 and so on, among which SP 6 is the commonly used, and then CV 6, CV 4, EX-CA 1, SP 10, ST 36, BL 23.

iv. Others

1. TCM application

Point application method has point stimulation effect and also plays a role through absorption of herbs on specific part, so as to achieve the therapeutic purpose. Drug application method has direct effect on warming qi and blood, smoothing meridian, can improve local blood circulation and is beneficial to absorption of inflammatory focus, thus playing a role of releasing the conglutination, eliminating lump, activating blood and dispelling stasis. In clinic, 60g of fresh Prepared Common Monkshood Daughter Root, Garden Balsam Stem, Sodium Sulfate, Cinnamon Twig respectively, 120g of Salvia Root, 5g of Wuzhuying, Fennel respectively, 30g of Argy Wormwood Leaf and 20g of Beautiful Sweetgum Fruit are milled into power, and then they are soaked with white wine, blended, bagged, steamed, next put on CV 4. Hot compresses with heat preservation is done for 15-20 minutes, starting from the first day of menstruation, once every night, continuously for 2 weeks, coordinating with oral chinese medicine, which has a preferred effect on treating oviduct obstructive infertility.

2. Enema

Anal tube or catheter is put into anus and drug is injected into rectum and retained for 30-60 minutes after injection, once a day, 10 days as each treatment course, stopping during menstruation. 100ml retention enema is decocted with 15g of Garden Balsam Stem, Chinese Honeylocust Spine, Glabrous Greenbrier Rhizome respectively, 12g of Chinese Clematis Root, 9g of prepared Frankincense, Myrrh, Common Buried Tuber, Lightyellow Sophora Root respectively, coordinating with TCM syndrome differentiation to treat infertility caused by fallopian tube lesion, which has a preferred effect.

V. Empirical prescriptions of famous physicians and experts

i. Ancient famous physicians

1. Wen Jing Tang (Zhang Zhongjing)

Famous prescription of Zhang Zhongjing in Eastern Han Dynasty is "Jingui Wenjing Decoction" also called "Dawenjing Decoction", which is widely used in ancient and modern TCM gynecology and is a multiple functions prescription.

Component: "three liang of Medicinal Evodia Fruit, two liang of Chinese Angelica, two liang of Sichuan Lovage Rhizome, two liang of Peony, two liang of Ginseng, two liang of Cinnamon Twig, two liang of Ass Hide Glue, two liang of Fresh Ginger, two liang of Tree Peony Root Bark, two liang of Liquorice Root, half sheng of Pinellia Tuber, one sheng of Dwarf Lilyturf Tuber. The above twelve herbs are boiled with one dou of water for three sheng and then taken for three times. " (one liang = 37.2 g, one dou = 10 L)

Efficacy: the women who have abdominal cold and no conception for a long time; concurrently treating metrorrhagia bleeding, or hypermenorrhea and amenorrhea.

2. Bu Gong Pill (Bian Que Heart Book)

Component: two liang of Chinese Angelica, two liang of Prepared Rehmannia Root, two liang of Desertliving Cistanche, two liang of Dodder Seed, two liang of Radix Achyranthis Bidentatae, one liang of Cinnamon Bark, one liang of Chinese Eaglewood Wood, one liang of Bibo, one liang of Medicinal Evodia Fruit, one liang of fleshy fruit, five qian of real Dragon's Blood, five qian of Argy Wormwood Leaf are milled into powder, and then vinegar and paste are as pills, just as big as Phoenix Tree Seed. 50 pills are taken with wine or plain soup each time. (one liang = 37.2 g, one qian = 3.72 g)

Efficacy: female with cold uterus for a long time and infertility, menstrual irregularities, causing pain in lower abdomen and waist, emaciation with sallow complexion, weakness of limbs, less eating and fever, more night sweat, red and white leucorrhea.

3. Wu Ji Wan (Zhang Jingyue)

Component: three liang of Ginseng, three liang of Unprocessed Rehmannia Root, three liang of Prepared Rehmannia Root, three liang of Sweet Wormwood Herb Seed, three liang of Nutgrass Galingale Rhizome, three liang of Turtle Carapace, two liang of White Atractylodes Rhizome, two liang of Spine Date Seed Fruit, two liang of Barbary Wolfberry Fruit, two liang of Dwarf Lilyturf Tuber, two liang of Indian Bread, two liang of Chinese Wolf berry Root-bark, two liang of Tree Peony Root Bark, two liang of Debark Peony Root, two and half liang of Chinese Angelica body, one liang of Sichuan Lovage Rhizome, one liang of Liquorice Root. (one liang = 37.2 g)

Usage: the above herbs are prepared for standby; 1 silky black-bone white cock is taken (about 1 kg weight), removing hair, dirty, head, feet and intestines, and the cock is divided into 4 pieces; firstly Turtle Carapace is arranged on bottom of copper pot, and then miscellaneous herbs are put, in order to avoid scorching and rotting. Urine of boys of about several dou are gradually added, afterwards boiled to extreme minced, picked up to dry in the sun, make it into powder. Turtle Carapace and cock bone with original juice are fried to be dry until becoming powder after removed skirt, and refined to be pill with honey and the previous herbs, as big as Phoenix Tree Seed.

Efficacy: mainly curing emaciation and weakness of women, blood deficiency with heat, menstrual irregularities, metrorrhagia and metrostaxis and leucorrhea, steaming bone and women who cannot be pregnant.

4. Yang Jing Zhong Yu Tang (Fu Shan)

Compenent: 30g of Prepared Rehmannia Root, 15g of Chinese Angelica, 15g of Debark Peony Root, 15g of Pulp of Dogwood Fruit.

Efficacy: kidney depletion and blood deficiency, thin body, persistent failure to conceive.

5. Kai Yu Zhong Yu Tang (Fu Shan)

Component: 30g of Debark Peony Root, 9g of Nutgrass Galingale Rhizome, 15g of Chinese Angelica, 15g of White Atractylodes Rhizome, 9g of Tree Peony Root Bark, 9g of Indian Bread, 6g of Snakegourd Root.

Efficacy: Mainly curing female infertility caused by liver qi depression.

6. Cang Fu Dao Tan Wan (Wan Quan)

Component: 60g of Atractylodes Rhizome and Nutgrass Galingale Rhizome respectively, 45g of Dried Tangerine Peel and Indian Bread respectively, 30g of Orange Fruit, Pinellia Tuber, Jackinthepulpit Tuber, zhigancao respectively.

Efficacy: open phlegm and dissipate masses, dispel dampness and resolve depression, move qi and activate blood

7. Shao Fu Zhu Yu Tang (Wang Qingren)

Component: 7 pieces of Fennel, 6g of Dried Ginger, 3g of Yanhusuo, 6g of Myrrh, 9g Chinese Angelica, 6g of Sichuan Lovage Rhizome, 3g of Cinnamomum Cassia Presel, 6g of Red Peony Root, 9g of Cattail Pollen, 6g of Trogopterus Dung.

Efficacy: expel stasis inuterus, regulate menstruation and assist pregnancy.

ii. Modern physicians

1. Famous veteran doctors of TCM — Han Bing

Professor Han Bing, expert of national TCM gynecology, thinks that menstrual irregularity is one of the most important factors causing infertility. Menses is subject to the kidney, and it is important for treating infertility to tonify kidney and adjust menstruation. Whether menstruation is normal or not is related to dysfunction of liver and kidney as well as dysfunction of thoroughfare and conception vessels. Professor Han aims to follow concept of former physicians and sets great store on the role of liver and kidney function on infertility. Tonifying kidney and adjusting thoroughfare is considered as therapeutic method. In clinical practice for many years, herb pair with relative compatibility and unique form is formed, which has specific efficiency, quick effect-orientation, modification according to symptoms, flexible application and significant effect. Now brief description on commonly used herb pairs of Professor Han to treat infertility is as follows:

(1) Dodder Seed and Palm leaf Raspberry Fruit: two herbs are promoted mutually, supplement yin and yang, treat liver and kidney concurrently, nourish thoroughfare and conception vessels, which have a great efficiency on treating infertility caused by insufficiency of liver and kidney and deficiency of essence and blood.

(2) Glossy Privet Fruit and Yerba-Detajo Herb: ancient name is Er Zhi Pill, tonifying kidney and nourishing liver, cooling blood and stopping bleeding, which can be used for infertility caused by prolonged menstruation, intermenstrual bleeding due to liver-kidney yin deficiency in gynecology.

(3) Himalayan Teasel Root and Chinese Taxillus Herb: two herbs are used together and play the role of tonifying liver and kidney and adjusting thoroughfare and conception vessels, which has a remarkable efficiency on infertility resulting from insecurity of thoroughfare and conception vessels and liver-kidney depletion. It is worth learning.

(4) Chinese Eaglewood Wood and Cinnamon Bark: two herbs are compatible to regulate Qi and dredge collaterals, warm kidney and disperse cold and are usually used for treating dysmenorrhea due to cold congealing and, infertility caused by cold uterus , and also suitable for infertility of oviduct obstruction.

(5) Rhizoma Polygonati and processed Fleeceflower Root: two herbs play the role of tonifying kidney-yin and replenishing essence and blood. Sufficient kidney essence and replenished blood sea can promote the growth of ovum to assist pregnancy.

(6) Salvia Root and Suberect Spatholobus Stem: "efficiency of Salvia Root is the same as SiWu Decoction." Salvia Root can activate blood and adjust menstruation without damage to the blood. When it is used with Suberect Spatholobus Stem, it either can activate blood, or tonify blood and is suitable for blood stasis and blood deficiency as well as used to treat blood deficiency and stasis, infertility caused by hypomenorrhea and delayed menstruation because blood sea cannot overflow timely.

(7) Degelatined Deer-Horn and Fluorite: Degelatined Deer-Horn warm and smooth governor vessel. Fluorite leads qi and blood to descend, warms kidney, nourishes liver and warms uterus. Combination of two herbs can tonify kidney and strength yang, consolidate and control thoroughfare and conception vessels, and also warm kidney and nourish liver, adjust menstruation and warm uterus, which is used for female deficiency-cold amenorrhea and infertility due to cold uterus.

Moreover, Professor Han Bing has proposed Futongning according to infertility formed by insufficiency of kidney qi, blood stasis, successive dampness turbidity and abdominal mass. The medicine contains Common Buried Tuber, Zedoray Rhizome, Dragon's Blood, Salvia Root, Pangolin Scales, Chinese Honeylocust Spine, Seaweed, Turtle Carapace, Coix Seed and so on. Common Buried Tuber, Zedoray Rhizome, Dragon's Blood, Salvia Root, Pangolin Scales and Chinese Honeylocust Spine can activate blood and resolve stasis; Seaweed and Turtle Carapace can resolve hard lump; Coix Seed can drain dampness. In the whole prescription, the composition and structure are rigorous and modified with syndrome, showing an obvious efficiency. Professor Han Bing modifies the prescription combined with his many years of clinical experience. Female with kidney deficiency are treated with Desertliving Cistanche, Morinda Root and Degelatined Deer-Horn to tonify kidney and resolve stasis; female with liver depression and qi stagnation is treated by adding considerably Chinese Thorowax Root, combined spicebush Root, Nutgrass Galingale Rhizome and Tangerine Seed to regulate qi and resolve stasis; female with congealing cold and blood stasis is treated by adding Cassia Twig and Manchurian Wildginger to warm meridian and dredge collaterals, resolve stasis and relieve pain; for female carrying with phlegm-dampness, Tendrilleaf Fritillary Bulb, Chinese Honeylocust Spine and Appendiculate Cremastra Pseudobulb or Common Pleione Pseudobulb are adopted to resolve phlegm-dampness and disperse stasis and stagnation.

2. Tianjin Ha Family — Ha Xiaoxian

Ha Xiaoxian, the fourth generation successor of Ha Family medicine ,divided menstrual cycle into four stages, complying with cycles and conforming to yin and yang in the treatment of infertility:

(1) Postmenstrual period : products for nourishing kidney and emolliating liver and tonifying both yin and blood are used to supplement blood sea and replenish thoroughfare and conception vessels. Herbs are: Prepared Rehmannia Root, Pulp of Dogwood Fruit, Barbary Wolfberry Fruit, Ass Hide Glue, Dodder Seed, Debark Peony Root, Dwarf Lilyturf Tuber, Chinese Angelica and so on.

(2) Ovulatory phase: herbs can nourish kidney and dredge collaterals on the basis of nourishing yin and tonifying blood, adding Common Curculigo Rhizome, Epimedium Herb, Fluorite and other herbs to assist yang and transport qi, and adding CowHerb Seed, Beautiful Sweetgum Fruit, Suberect Spatholobus Stem, Diverse Wormwood Herb and other herbs to dredge collaterals and activate blood. It creates prerequisite conditions for conception.

(3) Post-ovulation phase: herbs for warming kidney and replenishing essence, such as Chinese Taxillus Herb, stir-fried Eucommia Bark, Dodder Seed, Himalayan Teasel Root and other herbs, can make yang qi filled, in the case of being pregnant, even can strengthen kidney and calm fetus.

(4) Premenstrual and menstrual period: in the case of not being pregnant in this period, modified xiaoyao Powder is used to make menstruation smooth; in the case of being pregnant, modified shoutai Pill is used to strengthen kidney and calm fetus.

3. Jiangwan Cai Family — Cai Xiaosun

Professor Cai Xiaosun, who is from Cai Family in gynecology, thinks that insufficiency of kidney Qi and thoroughfare and conception vessels depletion are main pathogenesis of infertility. Periodic therapy is adopted in clinic. According to menstrual cycle, pregnancy I and pregnancy II are supposed as basic prescription.

Prescription for pregnancy I: 12g of Indian Bread, 9g of Unprocessed Rehmannia Root and Prepared Rehmannia Root respectively, 9g of Radix Achyranthis Bidentatae, 9g of Beautiful Sweetgum Fruit, 9g of Processed Turtle Piece, 2.5g of Flos Caryophyllata, 12g of Epimedium Herb, 9g of Chinese Photinia Leaf, 12g of Processed Crystalline Lens and 3g of Cassia Twig are used to nourish kidney, dredge collaterals and promote ovulation.

Prescription for pregnancy II: 12g of Indian Bread, 9g of Unprocessed Rehmannia Root and Prepared Rehmannia Root respectively, 9g of Chinese Photinia Leaf, 12g of Fluorite, 9g of Glossy Privet Fruit, 12g of Cibot Rhizome, 12g of Epimedium Herb, 9g of Common Curculigo Rhizome, 9g of Common Fenugreek Seed, 9g of Degelatined Deer-Horn and 9g of Desertliving Cistanche are used to nourish kidney, complement original-qi and invigorate corpus luteum.

After menstruation disappear completely, pregnancy I prescription is taken for 7 doses; and then during ovulatory period ,pregnancy II prescription is taken for 8 doses.the prescription can be adjusted with syndrome in menstruation. Nourishing kidney cycle method is used to promote menstrual rule, in order to be pregnant by seizing the opportunity.

4. Pudong Wang Family — Wang Huiping

Professor Wang Huiping of Wang Family gynecology thinks that insufficiency of liver-kidney is the root of infertility, while qi stagnation, blood stasis and phlegm-dampness are the symptoms. Therapy is given priority to adjusting and tonifying liver and kidney and Dingjing Decoction is modified to soothe Qi of liver and kidney and tonify the essence of liver and kidney. Herbs: 20g of Dodder Seed, 12g of Prepared Rehmannia Root, 12g of Chinese Angelica, 10g of Debark Peony Root, 12g of Chinese Thorowax Root, 15g of Epimedium Herb, 15g of Morinda Root, 12g of pulp of dogwood fruit, 12g of Tree Peony Root Bark and 10g of costus root are basic prescription. Patients with deficiency of Qi and blood are treated to tonify Qi and nourish blood as well as activate blood and dredge channels. Herbs: 12g of Tangshen, 15g of Milkvetch Root, 15g of Chinese Angelica,

12g of Debark Peony Root, 8g of Sichuan Lovage Rhizome, 12g of Salvia Root, 12g of Peach Seed, 15g of Radix Achyranthis Bidentatae and 10g of Costus Root are basic prescription, which make acquired biochemistry active, thoroughfare and conception vessels filled and menstruation occurred on time.

5. Shanghai Famous Physician — Pang Panchi

Famous Professor Pang Panchi of shanghai TCM gynecology has three treasures to treat infertility, i.e.: oviduct opening , ovulation induction and corpus luteum-invigorating.

(1) Oviduct opening: so-called "oviduct opening" is recanalization therapy of oviduct, and Tongguan Decoction is proposed: 9g of Chinese Angelica, 9g of Prepared Rehmannia Root, 9g of Red Peony Root, 9g of Debark Peony Root, 9g of Sichuan Lovage Rhizome, 12g of peach seed, 9g of Saff lower, 9g of Fresh India Madder Root, 12g of cuttlebone, 12g of Processed Nutgrass Galingale Rhizome, 9g of Beautiful Sweetgum Fruit, 9g of Grassleaf Sweetflag Rhizome, 12g of Unprocessed Coix Seed, 9g of Chinese Honeylocust Spine, 15g of Herba Patriniae, 15g of sargentgloryvine stem. It can activate blood, resolve stasis and dredge collaterals. If it is taken for a long time, it will play its efficiency slowly.

(2) Ovulation induction: Ovulatory dysfunction is the common etiology of infertility. Professor Pang thinks that kidney deficiency is main pathogenesis, and should be treated in way of tonifying kidney and harmonizing thoroughfare vessel. Siwu Decoction is used for nourishing and harmonizing blood, adding crystalline lens, Dodder Seed, Eucommia Bark, Desertliving Cistanche and Epimedium Herb to tonify kidney and promote ovulation; Fluorite and Chinese photinia leaf can warm yang and uterus; Motherwort Fruit, Hirsute Shiny Bugleweed Herb Leaf, CowHerb Seed and Radix Achyranthis Bidentatae can activate blood and dredge channels.

(3) Corpus luteum-invigorating: hypofunction of corpus luteum goes against implantation and growth of fertilized ovum, which easily results in infertility or threatened abortion. Professor Pang thinks that the pathogenesis is insufficiency of spleen-kidney, essence and blood depletion, deficient transformation of yin and yang during ovulatory period, even if semen can be consolidated, but it is difficult to be pregnant. Dodder Seed, Desertliving Cistanche , crystalline lens, Hirsute Shiny Bugleweed Herb leaf, Motherwort Fruit are added on the basis of Sage Cure Decoction with appropriate Chinese Angelica, Sichuan Lovage Rhizome, Nutgrass Galingale Rhizome and other herbs to activate blood without damage to fetus.

VI. Typical medical records from famous physicians and experts

i. Medical record of Han Bing — Deficiency of liver and kidney

Mrs. Xu, female, 29 years old.

Preliminary diagnosis: on February 6, 2012. The patient has been married for 3 years, has regular sexual life but is not pregnant without contraception. Menstrual rule was 6-7/28-30 days, with less volume, red color, less blood clot, dysmenorrheal (-), history of pregnancy G1P0(1 time of induced abortion in 2009). LMP: January 22, 2012. Six items of sex hormone (M3): FSH 6.54 mIU/ml, LH 1.57 mIU/ml, E2 23. 00 mIU/ml, PRL 11.43 mIU/ml, P 0.30 mIU/ml, T 0.57 mIU/ml. There is no abnormality after examined by B ultrasound and gynecologic examination. Rortine semen analysis of male is normal. Now: soreness of the waist, sound night sleep, normal urine and stool, slightly dark tongue, thin and white tongue coating and wiry and thready pulse.

Western medicine diagnosis: Secondary infertility.

TCM diagnosis: infertility, syndrome of deficiency of liver and kidney.

Therapeutic method: tonify liver and kidney, regulate thoroughfare and conception vessels, replenish essence and blood.

Prescription: 30g of Dodder Seed, 15g of Palm leaf Raspberry Fruit, 15g of Malaytea Scurfpea Fruit, 10g of Morinda Root, 20g of Dendrobium nobile, 30g crystalline lens, 30g Fleeceflower Root, 30g Salvia Root, 30g Suberect Spatholobus Stem, 10g Chinese Rose Flower, 10g Folium Citri Reticulatae, 15g Degelatined Deer-Horn, 30g Fluorite.

Second diagnosis: on February 20, 2012. Menses came on the previous day, and menstrual volume obviously increased than before, with red color and no blood clot. Lumbago was improved obviously, tongue is red and slightly dark, tongue fur is thin and white and pulse is deep. Considering that patient was in menstrual period, deficiency of liver and kidney and insufficiency of essence and blood in normal times ,was treated with modified SiwuDecoction

Prescription: 20g of Prepared Rehmannia Root, 10g of Chinese Angelica, 10g of Sichuan Lovage Rhizome, 30g of Salvia Root, 20g of Red Peony Root, 10g of Cassia Twig, 6g of Dried Ginger, 30g of Suberect Spatholobus Stem, 20g of Tangerine Seed, 20g of Lychee Seed, 30g of Motherwort Herb, 10g of Chinese Rose Flower, 15g of Degelatined Deer-Horn.

Third diagnosis: on February 27, 2012. LMP: February 19, 2012, menstruation lasted for 6 days and then disappeared completely, with appropriate volume. The color was red, there was no blood clot, tongue was red, tongue coating was thin and white, and pulse was slightly deep. The patient was postmenstural periodyin was generated and yang was grown, and the prescription was subject to nourishing liver, kidney, yin and yang. Herbs are: 30g Dodder Seed, 15g Palm leaf Raspberry Fruit, 10g Morinda Root, 15g Malaytea Scurfpea Fruit, 20g Dendrobium nobile, 30g Fleeceflower Root, 30g crystalline lens, 30g Salvia Root, 30g Suberect Spatholobus Stem, 30g Fluorite, 10g Human Placenta.

The dose of above herbs was modified with syndromes for 6 months. Menstruation of patients was delayed, blood HCG was found to be 123mIU/mL after examination, after 50 days of amenorrhea, examining B ultrasound and showing: Intrauterine early pregnancy, fetal heart and embryo could be seen. We knew that the patient gave birth to a child by way of telephone follow-up and both mother and child were healthy.

Note: the above herbs-prescribing is long-term practical experience summary and essence of Professor Han on treating infertility. Especially application of herb pair has embodied the feature of combination of traditional Chinese medicine with rich connotation, expending ideas of therapeutic medication of clinical infertility. It is worthy of our study and learning.

ii. Medical record of Ha Xiaoxian ——liver depression and kidney deficiency

Mrs. Liu, female, 30 years old.

Preliminary diagnosis: on January 22, 2014. Regular sexual life, not being pregnant for more than 1 year without contraception. Her menophania appeared at the age of 13, menstrual rule was usually 5 - 6/26-28 days, with less volume, black color and less blood clot. Dysmenorrheal was not obvious, history of pregnancy G1P0 (1 time of induced abortion in 2012). LMP: January 12, 2014. Patient complained that pain in lower abdomen was unbearable within several days before and after ovulatory period. Salpingography from other hospital has shown: left oviduct was open and remote adhesion, discharge of right oviduct was unobstructed. Now: soreness of the waist, dull pain in abdomen, dryness of the mouth, frequent micturition, more leucorrhea, red tongue, white and greasy tongue coating, deep and slippery pulse.

Western medicine diagnosis: pelvic inflammation, mild adhesion on remote left oviduct, infertility.

TCM diagnosis: infertility, syndrome of liver depression and kidney deficiency.

Therapeutic method: replenish kidney and nourish yin, sooth liver and dredge collaterals.

Prescription: 30g of Colored Mistletoe Herb, 15g of Eucommia Bark, 15g of Unprocessed Rehmannia Root, Prepared Rehmannia Root respectively, 30g of Mantis Egg-Case, 15g of Diverse Wormwood Herb, 30g of Dwarf Lilyturf Tuber, 15g of Dendrobium nobile, 30g of Coastal Glehnia Root, 15g of Pinellia Tuber, 9g of Golden

References

[1] Tian DH. Textual criticism[M]. Beijing: China Medical Science Press, 1995.

[2] Li JW, Yu YA, Cai JF, et al. Great Dictionary of Traditional Chinese Medicine[M]. 2nd ed. Beijing: People's Medical Publishing House, 2004.

[3] Xue J. Xue's Medical Record [M]. Beijing: China Press of Traditional Chinese Medicine, 1997, the First Edition.

[4] Fu QZ. Fu Qingzhu's Obstetrics and Gynecology [M]. Beijing: People's Medical Publishing House, 2006.

[5] Kou JM, Kou Z. Clinical observation of acupuncture treatment of 50 cases of syndrome of anovulatory infertility [J]. China Journal of Chinese Medicine, 1997, 12 (4): 45-46.

[6] Ban XY, He C. External and internal treatment of 86 cases of oviduct obstructive infertility [J]. Beijing Journal of Traditional Chinese Medicine, 1996, 15 (1): 33-34.

[7] Bei RP. 150 cases of reports about treating infertility caused by oviduct lesion [J]. Journal of Traditional Chinese Medicine, 1992, 33(5): 37-38.

[8] Han YH, Bai L, Yao TT. Exploration and analysis of diagnosis and treatment of infertility from zang-fu organs of Fu Qingzhu [J]. Liaoning Journal of Traditional Chinese Medicine, 2011, 38 (2): 267.

[9] Xu J, Luo LY, Wu TR. Study on relation of clinical application and dose of Two Solstices Pill [J]. Asia-Pacific Traditional Medicine 2011, 7 (1): 132.

[10] Chang N, Han B, Li TX, et al. Clinical and experimental study on treating endometriosis with Futongning [J]. Journal of Traditional Chinese Medicine 1997, 38(8): 488-490.

[11] Ma PZ, Wu YX. Clinical experience of professor Han Bing on treating endometriosis accompanying with infertility [J]. Hunan Guiding Journal of Traditional Chinese Medicine and Pharmacology 1998,4 (7): 13.

[12] Wang GP, Xuan MS. Experience of Ha Xiaoxian on treating infertility. [J]. Journal of Traditional Chinese Medicine, 2014, 55(3): 195-196.

[13] Zhang YN, Huang SY, Hu GH. A brief description on menstruation-regulating and pregnancy-assisting of Shanghai TCM Gynecology School. [J]. Sichuan traditional Chinese medicine, 2012, 30 (6): 33-34.

Recurrent Respiratory Tract Infection

反复呼吸道感染

I. Overview

Recurrent respiratory tract infection is one of common diseases for children. Recurrent respiratory tract infection means that times of upper and lower respiratory infection within one year exceeds normal range in clinic. Upper respiratory infection includes rhinitis, pharyngitis and amygdalitis, whilelower respiratory infection includes bronchitis, capillary bronchitis and pneumonia. This disease occurs throughout the year, easily relapses in fierce change of winter-spring air temperature and has the trend of natural relief in summer. Infection times of people before and after school age are obviously reduced. This disease is mostly seen among 6 months to 6 years old children, among whom 1~3 years old infants can be more susceptible. If recurrent respiratory tract infection cannot be cured for a long time, some diseases can easily occur, such as chronic rhinitis, cough and nephritis as well as rheumatism, which seriously affectsthe growth and development as well as physical and mental health of infants. It is equivalent to"spontaneous perspiration and being susceptible" in ancient medical books of traditional Chinese medicine. They are generally called "easily infected children" or "recurrent respiratory tract infection" (called "recurrent susceptible children" for short).

This disease is prevented with traditional Chinese medicine to highlight syndrome differentiation and treatment as well as combination of internal and external treatment and to emphasize the prevention, which has a certain advantage on improving children's constitution and enhancing ability of disease resistance and thereforedraws more and more attention from people.

II. Etiology and pathogenesis

i. Chinese Medicine

Children recurrent respiratory infection mostly occurs due to deficiency of natural endowment, improper feeding, improper medications, improper nursing, endowment and body heat. Pathogenesis of this disease attributes to both deficiency and excess: deficiency refers to insufficiency of healthy Qi, insecurity of exterior of defense Qi; excess means pathogen heat is hidden in interior and occurs when meeting withexogenous pathogenic factors.

1. Deficiency of natural endowment and weak constitation

Insufficient of natural endowment is caused by the following aspects, for example, parents are weak and sickly or constantly get ill during pregnancy, or premature delivery, multiple births and frail fetal Qi. And the children have loose striae, tender and lovely skin, and they will get ill once being infected due to intolerance of invasion of pathogenic Qi.

2. Damage to spleen and stomach caused by the improper feeding

Artificial feeding, insufficient breast-milk, early weaning, careless milk change, inappropriate space complementary food, food preference, anorexia, malnutrition, insufficient uptake of food essence, spleen-stomach weakness, inability to generation and transformation, lung-spleen qi deficiency, so patients are invaded by exogenous pathogenic factors easilyas a result; or patients arbitrarily eat fresh and cold, fullness and greasy foods which damage spleen-stomach and healthy Qi, therefore easily invaded by exogenous pathogenic factors.

3. Intolerance of cold and heat due to inappropriate nursing

Patient have weak ability for adapting to abrupt change of climate due to the lack of outside activities, insufficient sunlight, soft skin, insecurity of exterior of defensive Qi and then cold occurs. Or parents cannot add or subtract clothes and bedclothes for sick children timely without proper regulating and nursing, therefore, the disease easily occurs or once sick children are infected by others, they will be sick immediately.

4. Damages to healthy Qi owing to improper medication

After being affected by exopathogen, taking too much formulas relieving superficies damages yang Qi to cause defense yang, exterior defense Qideficiency, disharmony between nutrient and defensive Qi so as to result in excessive sweating due to insecurity of nutrient-yin, and easy being infected due to insecurity of defensive yang. Hence, sick children will be easily and repeatedly infected by pathogen.

5. Disease will occur once meeting exogenous pathogenic factors because of bodyheat

In case of preferred to eat fat and greasy, spicy and hot foods, which results in stagnated heat in lung-stomach or accumulated heat in stomach and intestine. Or because of the not cleared residual pathogen after thepyreticosis, orliving in wet land for long time leading to dampness-heat interior accumulation, or exuberant heat of body, pathogen-heat latent retention, once being invaded by exogenous pathogenic factors, the patient will be easily infected again with internal occurrence of retention pathogen, so that this disease occurs.

All in all, the onset of this disease is divided into deficiency and excess: Children have tender zang-fu organs and weak skin and they are easily infected by exogenous pathogenic factors. Deficiency is caused by Qi and yin depletion of lung, spleen, kidney, insufficiency of healthy Qi, insecurity of defense exterior, additionally improper feeding, inappropriate regulating and nursing, and then the disease can occur once invaded by exogenous pathogenic factors. Excess exists in disease in lung and kidney. Sick children prefer eating spicy, fat and greasy food, or residual pathogen of pyreticosis is not cleared, therefore pathogen and heat are retained in lung and stomach or accumulated in stomach and intestines. If invaded by exogenous pathogenic factors, syndrome of external cold and internal heat can be caused easily If recurrent respiratory tract infection cannot be cured for a long time, healthy Qi is damaged seriously, resistance of sick children will decrease continuously; therefore, other diseases occur easily.

ii. Western medicine

The recurrent respiratory tract infection is closely related to physiology characteristic of respiratory system anatomy and immature immunologic function of children themselves. Other, common causes of recurrent upper respiratory tract infection include: trace elements and vitamin deficiency, environmental pollution, passive smoking, chronic upper respiratory tract lesions, such as rhinitis, nasosinusitis, tonsil and adenoidal hypertrophy etc. Basic diseases mostly exist in sick children with recurrent lower respiratory tract infections, especially recurrent pneumonia, including congenital or acquired respiratory anatomic abnormalities, inhalation, congenital heart disease, immunodeficiency disease and primary ciliary dyskinesia.

III. Key points of diagnosis and differential diagnosis

i. Diagnosis

In the light of age, potential reason and different parts, recurrent respiratory tract infection is divided into recurrent upper respiratory infection and recurrent lower respiratory infection, the latter of which is also divided into recurrent tracheobronchitis and recurrent pneumonia.

Table 1 Judgment Condition of Recurrent Respiratory Tract Infection

Age (year)	Recurrent upper respiratory tract infection (time/year)	Recurrent lower respiratory infection (time/year)	
		Recurrent tracheobronchitis	Recurrent pneumonia
0-2	7	3	2
2^+-5	6	2	2
5^+-14	5	2	2

Note: ① The interval between two infections is at least above 7d. ② Ifthe times of upper respiratory infection are not enough, the times of upper and lower respiratory infection can be added together, conversely, it cannot be done. However, if recurrent infection is mainly lower respiratory tract, it should be defined as recurrent lower respiratory infection. ③ It requires 1 year for observation to determine times. ④ Recurrent pneumonia means suffering from pneumonia for twice within 1 year. Pneumonia needs to be confirmed through lung signs and imageology.During the time betweentwo diagnoses of pneumonia, lung signs and imageological changes shall be removed totally.

It shall be noted to search the cause of the disease when it is diagnosed in clinic, for example, improper nursing, the lack of exercises, migration of accommodation, the initial phase of nurseries and kindergartens, environmental pollution, lack of trace elements or inappropriate matching of other nutrient ingredients. For sick children with recurrentpneumonia, in addition to consideration of pathogenic microorganism, it is necessary to carefully search basic lesions of recurrentpneumonia, such as primary immunodeficiency diseases (primary antibody immunodeficiency disease, cellular immunodeficiency disease, combined immunodeficiency disease, complement deficiency disease, dysphagocytosis and other primary immunodeficiency diseases), congenital lung parenchymal abnormalities, pulmonary vascular dysplasia, congenital dysplasia of the airway, congenital heart malformation, primary ciliary dyskinesia, cystic fibrosis, airway obstruction or exterior oppression, bronchiectasia and repeated inhalation. Disease history shall be asked in details clinically and it shall be noted to differentiate the constitution of the sick child. Immunologyexamination, chest X-ray, detection of trace elements and otorhinolaryn gologicexaminations are carried out according to conditions. When necessary, pulmonary function, bronchoscope, lung CT, airway, vascular reconstruction development and other examinations can be selected.

ii. Differential diagnosis

Allergic rhinitis: it is called "anaphylactic rhinitis" or "allergic rhinitis" in western medicine. Main features are sudden and recurrent rhinocnesmus, nasal obstruction, thin nasqal discharge and frequent sneezing, accompanied by eye itching and other eye allergic symptoms. The onset is always related to contacting wormwood, pollen and other foreign matters, which mostly occurs to patients with allergic constitution and anaphylactic rhinitis family history.

IV. TCM therapy

i. Syndrome differentiation and treatment

1. Key points of syndrome differentiation

The diagnosis of this disease is mainly based on eight-principle syndrome differentiation and visceral syndrome differentiation. In clinic, first it should be differentiated whether the disease is due to deficiency r excess then which viscera is involved.

(1) Deficiency and excess differentiation: if sick children are thin or obese and have the syndromes, mainly including hidrosis and shortness of breath, lassitude and lacking in strength, poor appetite and loose stool, lusterless complexion or growth retardation, it can be differentiated as deficiency syndrome. If they usually show excessive heat and prefer eating greasy, sweet and strong taste food, commonly having bad breath, or easily growing boils in mouth and tongue, feverish feeling in palms and soles, dry stool, then the syndrome is due to excess syndrome.

(2) Zang-fu organs differentiation: patients with deficiency of healthy Qi are subject to deficiency and depletion of Qi and yin of lung, spleen and kidney. If patients represent spontaneous perspiration, short of breath, laziness to speak, lower voice, it is lung deficiency; if patients represent yellowish and lusterlesscomplexion, lassitude and lacking in strength, loss of appetite, and abdominal distension and loose stool, it is spleen deficiency; if they represent growth retardation, not strong or even malformation of bones, it is kidney deficiency. Patients with Qi deficiency syndrome show yellowish and lusterlesscomplexion, short of breath, lassitude, faint low voice, slightly tender tongue, teeth-mark on side of tongue and thin and weak pulse; patients with yin deficiency have lower fever and night sweat, feverish feeling in palms and soles, dry mouth and throat, red and dry tongue, and thready rapid pulse.

Patients with excess pathogen mainly show syndrome of accumulated heat in lung and stomach, commonly accompanied with reddish throat, bad breath, or easily growing a boil in mouth and tongue, feverish feeling in palms and soles, abdominal distension, dry stool, thick or yellowish tongue fur, slippery and rapid pulse.

2. Therapeutic principle

This disease is mainly due to deficiency and treated mainly by tonifying. In clinic, it emphasizes on mastering the timing of administration, invigorating spleen and tonifying lung, replenishing Qi and nourishing yin, or warming and tonifying spleen and kidney. In the case of excess syndrome, clearing lung and stomach is the main principle. This therapeutic principle is used in the period of sick patients with recurrent respiratory tract infection that do not show acute respiratory infection symptoms. If respiratory tract infection appears in therapeutic period, corresponding therapies are given combining with the constitution of sick children according to different diseases.

3. Categorization of differentiation and treatment

(1) Lung-spleen Qi deficiency

Main symptoms: recurrent affection by exogenous pathogenic factors, shortness of breath, profuse sweating, lightly colored lips and mouths, yellowish and lusterlesscomplexion, indigestion and loss of appetite, stool irregularities, slightly red tongue body, thin and weak pulse or light fingerprint.

Syndrome differentiation: this syndrome is mostly seen in children with acquired disorders, improper feeding and the lack of milk and being weaned too early, or patients with long term illness and Qi consumption, clinically featured by recurrent affection by exogenous pathogenic factors, shortness of breath, profuse sweating, yellowish and lusterlesscomplexion, poor appetite and stool irregularities.

Therapentic method: to invigorate spleen and space replenish Qi, to tonify lung space and consolidate exterior.

Prescription: Supplemented Yu Ping Feng San. Milkvetch Root, Divaricate Saposhnikovia Root, White Atractylodes Rhizome, Tangshen, Common Yam Rhizome, Oyster Shell, Dried Tangerine Peel, Liquorice Root.

Prescription analysis: Milkvetch Root is sweet and warm, and can tonify spleen and lung in interior and consolidate exterior to stop sweating in exterior. White Atractylodes Rhizome, Tangshen and Common Yam Rhizome can invigorate spleen and replenish Qi, assistingMilkvetch Root to strengthen the efficacy of benefiting Qi and consolidate superficies; Divaricate Saposhnikovia Root slides exterior and disperse wind pathogen, combing with Milkvetch Root and White Atractylodes Rhizome to benefit Qi and eliminate pathogen; Oyster Shell can astring exterior and stop sweating; Dried Tangerine Peel can invigoratie spleen and resolve phlegm; Liquorice Root harmonizes all herbs. The whole prescription plays the role of smoothing while having efficacy of tonifying, and vice versa. .

Modification: for patients with more much sweating, Chinese Magnoliavine Fruit is added; for patients with loss of appetite and anorexia, Chicken's Gizzard-Skin and charred triplet are added; for patients with loose stool, stir-fried Coix Seed and Indian Bread are added; for patients with constipation, Raw Rhubarb and Orange Fruit are added.

(2) Disharmony between ying and wei

Mains ymptoms: regularly affection by exogenous pathogenic factors, recurrently getting cold, being averse to wind and intolerance of cold, commonly sweating much, sweating out without warming, muscular flaccidity, lusterless complexion, lack of warmth in the limbs, lightly red tongue body, thin and white tongue fur, weak pulse or slightly purple fingerprint.

Syndrome differentiation: this syndrome is mostly seen in children with lung space qi deficiency and insufficient defensive yang, or patients with improper therapies for affection by exogenous pathogenic factors, for example, overtaking medicine of relieving exterior and sweating. Excessive sweating damages yang, resulting in the insecurity ofdefensive yang, dispersing of nutrient-yin and the easy invasion of exogenous pathogenic factors. Children with improper feeding, the lack of milk or being weaned too early, or patients with long illness and Qi consumption are clinically featured by aversion to wind, fear of cold, commonly more sweating and sweating out without warming.

Therapeutic method: to reinforce healthy Qi and consolidate exterior, to harmonize nutrient and defensive aspects.

Prescription: Supplemented Huang Qi Gui Zhi Wu Wu Tang. Milkvetch Root, Peony, Cassia Twig, Fresh Ginger, Chinese Date, Unprocessed Bone Fossil of Big Mammals, Unprocessed Oyster Shell.

Prescription analysis: Milkvetch Rootare sweet and warm and can tonifies Qi, and tonifydefense Qi of exterior; Cassia Twig can disperse wind-cold, warm meridians and dredge blockade; Peony can nourish blood and nutrient and dredge blood stasis; Fresh Ginger is pungent and warm and disperses wind and pathogen; Chinese Date is sweet and warm and can nourish blood and benefit Qi; Unprocessed Bone Fossil of Big Mammals and Unprocessed Oyster Shell can consolidate superficies and stop sweating.

Modification: for patients concurrently with cough, Stemona Root, Bitter Apricot SeedandCommon Coltsfoot Flower are added; for patients with fever, Sweet Wormwood Herb and Weeping Forsythia Capsule are added.

(3) Deficiency of both Qi and yin

Main symptoms: recurrent infection by exogenous pathogenic factors, red complexion, feverish feeling in palms and soles, or low heat, night sweat or spontaneous sweating, dry mouth, lassitude and lack of strength, anorexia and lack of appetite, dry stool, red tongue texture, scanty or exfoliative tongue fur, thin and rapid pulse or faint red fingerprints.

Syndrome differentiation: the syndrome is mostly seen in the patients with yin deficiency constitution, or those who often suffered from febrile diseases and damage yin due to being addicted to eating pungent and hot and dry foods. Characteristics are red complexion, dry mouth and dry stool clinically.

Therapeutic method: to nourish yin and moisten lung, to benefit Qi and invigorate spleen.

Prescription: Supplemented Sheng Mai San. Ginseng, Ophiopogon, Chinese Magnoliavine Fruit, White Atractylodes Rhizome, Coastal Glehnia Root and Unprocessed Oyster Shell.

Prescription analysis: Ginseng is sweet and warm, which replenishes original qi, reinforces lung qi and generates fluid. Ophiopogon is sweet and cold, which nourishes yin, clears heat, moistens lung and generates fluid. Combination of Ginseng and Ophiopogon can replenish Qi and nourish yin; Chinese Magnoliavine Fruit is sour and warm, which astringes lung, arrests sweating, generates fluid and quenches thirst; White Atractylodes Rhizome invigorates spleen and reinforces Qi; Coastal Glehnia Root nourishes yin, clears lung, benefits stomach and generates fluid; unprocessed Oyster Shellconsolidates superficies and arrests sweating.

Modification: for the patients with Qi deficiency, Milkvetch Root is added; in the case of poor appetite, VillonsAmomum Fruit and Chicken's Gizzard-Skin are added; with regard to dry stool, Snakegourd Fruit Seed and Chinese Arborvitae Kernel are added; in terms of night sweat and low heat, Chinese Wolf berry Root-bark and Tree Peony Root Bark are added;

(4) Deficiency of both spleen and kidney

Main symptoms: recurring common cold, even cough asthma, white and lusterless complexion, relaxed muscle, profuse sweating and easy sweating, restless sleep, lack of appetite and anorexia, loose stool, retardation in standing, walking, tooth eruption, hair growth and speech, or chicken-breast and humpback, soreness and weakness of waist and knees, cold body and limbs, more nocturia, thin and white tongue fur and rapid and weak pulse.

Syndrome differentiation: the syndrome results from congenital insufficiency and acquired care imbalance. Characteristics are lusterless complexion, relaxed muscle, growth retardation, soreness and weakness of waist and knees and cold body and limbs clinically.

Therapeutic method: to warm and reinforce kidney yang, to invigorate spleen and benefit Qi.

Prescription: Supplemented Jin Gui Shen Qi Wan. Radix Rehmanniae, Indian Bread, Common Yam Rhizome, Asiatic Cornelian Cherry Fruit, Tree Peony Root Bark, Oriental Waterplantain Rhizome, Cassia Twig, Prepared Common Monkshood Daughter Root, Ginseng, Liquorice Root and White Atractylodes Rhizome.

Prescription analysis: Rehmannia Root and Asiatic Cornelian Cherry Fruit nourish and replenish kidney yin and control pure air; Common Yam Rhizome and Indian Breadinvigorate spleen and remove dampness; Oriental Waterplantain Rhizome discharges water pathogenic factors in kidney; Tree Peony Root Bark clears liver-gallbladderministerial fire; Cassia Twig and Prepared Common Monkshood Daughter Root warm and reinforce real fire of vital gate; White Atractylodes Rhizome and Ginseng invigorate spleen and benefit Qi; Liquorice Root harmonizes the property of herbs.

Modification: in terms of the patients with five retardation, Degelatined Deer-Horn, MalayteaScurfpea Fruit and Unprocessed Oyster Shell are added; for the patients with copious sweat, Milkvetch Root and calcined Bone Fossil of Big Mammals are added; with regard to patients with low fever, Turtle Carapace and Chinese Wolf berry Root-bark are added; in the case of patients with yang deficiency, Pilose Antler, Human Placenta and DesertlivingCistanche are added.

(5) Accumulation of heat in lung and stomach

Main symptoms: recurrent infection by exogenous pathogenic factors, reddish throat, fetid breath, more aphtha possibility of the mouth and tongue, copious and stickysweat, restless sleep at night, feverish feeling in palms and soles, dry stool, red tongue texture, thick or yellow tongue fur and slippery and rapid pulse.

Syndrome differentiation: the syndrome mostly happens to the patients who are usually addicted to eating fat and spicy foods or those with internal heat in body. Characteristics are fetid breath, more aphtha possibility of the mouth and tongue and dry stool clinically.

Therapeutic method: to clear lung-stomach.

Prescription: modified Liang Ge San. Herbs commonly used: Weeping Forsythia Capsule, Cape Jasmine Fruit, Baical Skullcap Root, Fermented Soybean, Peppermint, Platycodon Root, Great Burdock Achene, Reed Rhizome, Rhubarb, Sodium Sulphate, Bamboo Leaf, Gypsum and Liquorice Root.

Prescription analysis: Baical Skullcap Root and Cape Jasmine Fruit are bitter and cold with efficacy of drainage, and can clear pathogenic heat in chest and diaphragm; Weeping Forsythia Capsule and Peppermint are cold-pungent and can clear heat and pathogenic heat in heart and chest; Fermented Soybean relieves muscles, makes diaphoresis, removes blood stasis and eliminates vexation; Rhubarb, Sodium Sulphate and Gypsumpurge fire, relax bowels and induce downward movement of pathogenic heat; Bamboo Leaf clears heart, promotes diuresis, and induces heat outward; Liquorice Root clears heat, moistens dryness and harmonizes the property of herbs.

Modification: in the case of aphtha in the mouth and tongue, Cape Jasmine Fruit and Ricepaperplant Pith are added; in terms of patients with fetid breath, Golden Thread and Hawthorn Fruit are added; for the patients with abdominal distention, Orange Fruit and Radish Seed are added;

ii. Chinese patent medicines

(1) Yu Ping Feng Liquid: it is applicable for syndrome of deficiency of lung-spleen qi. Children sub anno old shall take 5 ml a time, 5~10ml for children aged 2~5 years old, and 10ml for people aged above 5. It is taken three times a day orally.

(2) Huai Qi Huang Granules: it is applicable for syndrome of deficiency of both Qi and yin. Children aged between 1 and 3 shall take 5g each time, and 10 g for children in range of 3~ 12 years old. It is taken twice a day orally.

(3) Tong Kang Tablet: it is applicable for patients with syndrome of deficiency of both lung and spleen (spleen qi is deficient). 3-4 tablets are taken a time and 4 times a day. They should be swallowed after chewing up.

(4) Long Mu Zhuang Gu Granules: it is applicable for syndrome of deficiency of both spleen and kidney. Children with age of less than 2 years old shall take 5 g each time, 7g for child in range of 2~7 years old, and 10g for patients with age of greater than 7. It is taken 3 times a day after being mixed with water.

(5) Qing Jiang Pian: it is applicable for syndrome of accumulation of heat in lung-stomach. Children aged 1 shall take 3 tablets orallyand twice a day, and 4 tablets and 3 times a day for children aged 3, and 6 plates and 3 times a day for children aged 6 orally.

ii. Acupuncture and moxibustion therapy

(1) Ear pressing method: CO (14), spleen, large intestine, kidneys, TG (3), CO (16), CO (18), AT (4), HT7, AT (3, 4i) and EX-HN 6 (bloodletting) are selected. Skin in auricle is disinfected with 75%alcohol cotton ball. Take 0.4cm×0.4cm square rubberized fabric, label 1 CowHerb Seed in the middle, and press to auricular point, and slightly press for a moment with hands. 6 days belong to 1 course.

(2) Point injection method: Milkvetch Root Injection is injected on ST 36 in both sides. Routine disinfection is conducted, and injection is carried out after Qi is obtained. Each point is injected with 0.2~0.3ml injection. Injection is performed every 3~4 days, and twice in 1 week. 4 weeks belong to 1 course.

iv. Massage treatment

(1) Therapy of pinding the skin along the spinal column: Clench middle fingers, the third fingers and the little fingers of both hands into half fist, incompletely fold index fingers, unbent thumbs to direct at the first half segment of index finger, then withstand skin of a child, and lift and grasp flesh by moving thumbs and index fingers forward. Move both hands forward since both sides of coccygeal vertebra alternatively to both sides of GV 14. This can be regarded as one time of spine chiropractic. 6 times of chiropractic is repeated each time, and 1 time is conducted daily. Patients shall be treated for 5 days every week, and 4 weeks belong to 1 course.

(2) Four-season chiropractic therapies: Based on chiropractic, BL 18 and BL 13 are also kneaded in spring; in summer, BL 15 and BL 27 shall be added; in fall, BL 13 and BL 25 are added; in winter, BL 23 and BL 28 are added.

(3) Basic prescription of treatment according to syndrome and season differentiation: There are four-season chiropractic and four manipulation of kneading of GB 20 and head and face (opening of "Tian Men", push of Hom Palace, swing of EX-H N 5 and kneading of high bones behind ears).

① Syndrome of deficiency of lung-spleen qi: swing of lung meridian, wipe of BL 13, swing of Neibagua, swing of spleen meridian and kneading of ST 36 are added.

② Syndrome of deficiency of both Qi and yin: kneading of CV 6, swing of lung meridian, swing of spleen meridian, kneading of Erma, removal of Tianheshui and push of Tianzhugu are added.

③ Syndrome of deficiency of both spleen and kidney: swing of spleen meridian, swing of kidney meridian, kneading of SP 6, kneading of KI 1 and push of three passes are added.

④ Syndrome of disharmony between nutrient and defense Qi: swing of lung meridian, swing of spleen meridian, kneading of Shending, kneading of EX-U E 8 and push of three passes are added.

⑤ Syndrome of accumulation of heat in lung-stomach: clearing of lung meridian, clear of stomach meridian, withdrawal of six fu-organs, clockwise rubbing of abdomen and kneading of TE4 in arms are added.

v. External application of Chinese medicine

3 portions of White Mustard Seed, 2 portions of Manchurian Wildginger, 1 portion of Gansui Root, 1 portion of Gleditsiasinensis Lam., 3 portions of Chinese Gall and 0.052g Bomeol are grinded into fine powder. 1~ 2 g of the powder is taken each time, and made into paste with ginger juice, then applied to points. BL 13 in both sides are the main points, and other points like GV 14 and BL 17 are assistant points. Finally, these points are fixed with adhesive tapes. The treatment is Given once in the first 3 days of first dog days, middle dog days and last dog days, as well as Yijiu, Erjiu and Sanjiu, and there are 6 times of treatment in total.

V. Empirical prescriptions of famous physicians and experts

i. Kang Gan Zhi Bao Oral Liquid (Li Shaochun)

Indication: children suffered from recurrent respiratory tract infection due to syndrome of deficiency of lung and spleen qi.

Components: Cablin Patchouli Herb, Officinal MagnoliaBark, Dried Tangerine Peel, Pinellia Tuber,Medicated Leaven, Hyacinth Bean, Chinese Thorowax Root, Hogfennel Root, Platycodon Root, Orange Fruit, Incised Notopterygium Rhizome and Root, Doubleteeth Pubescent Angelica Root, Sichuan Lovage Rhizome, Red Peony Root, Largetrifoliolious Bugbane Rhizomeand Kudzuvine Root.

Usage: 6 ml is taken each time for children under 3 years old, 10ml for those between 3 and 6 years old, and 20ml for those who are older than 6 years old. The oral fluid is taken 3 times a day, and 1 month belongs to one course.

ii. Fang Gan Mixture (Jiang Yuren)

Indication: children with recurrent respiratory tract infection due to nutrient-defense disharmony.

Components: Cassia Twig, Milkvetch Root, Liquorice Root, Debark Peony Root, Dry Ginger and Chinese Date, and so on.

Usage: 10ml is taken each time for children under 3 years old, 15 ml for those from3+to6 years old, and 20ml for those with age of older than 6 years old. It is taken twice a day, and 2 months belong to one course.

iii. Jian Yi Fang (Yu Jian'er)

Indication: children recurrent respiratory tract infection due to lung-spleen qi deficiency syndrome.

Components: Unprocessed Milkvetch Root, Stir-fried White Atractylodes Rhizome, Divaricate Saposhnikovia Root, RhizomaPinelliaePreparatum, Dried Tangerine Peel, Indian Bread, Baical Skullcap Root, Liquorice Root, Earthworm, Plantain Seed and Biond Magnolia Flower.

Usage: 1 formula should be decocted with water and the decoction (100 ml) should be taken both in the morning and in the evening.

iv. Zhuang Er Granules (Wang Xuefeng)

Indication: children suffered from recurrent respiratory tract infection due to syndrome of both Qi and yin deficiency.

Components: Unprocessed Milkvetch Root, Unprocessed Rehmannia Root, HeterophyllyFalsestarwort Root, Salvia Root, Mushroom and Liquorice Root.

Usage: 4 g is taken for twice a day for children with the age of less than 6 years old; 8ga time and twice a day for patients whose age is greater than 6 years old. Consecutive use of 1 month is 1 course.

v. Shen Qi Gu Ben Tang (Han Xinmin)

Indication: children with recurrent respiratory tract infection due to lung-spleen qi deficiency syndrome.

Components: Tangshen, Radix AstragaliPreparata, White Atractylodes Rhizome, Divaricate Saposhnikovia

Root, Common Yam Rhizome, Lily Bulb, Stemona Root, Dried Tangerine Peel and Prepared LiquoriceRoot.

Usage: 1 dose should be taken by patients orally. For children who are 3 to 4 years old, 60 to 100 ml of the decoction should be taken every day., and who are 5 to 14 years old , 100~150mlof the decoction. The decoction is taken for 1 month.

vi. Na Qi San to compress the navel (Wang Lining)

Indication: children with recurrent respiratory tract infection due to lung-spleen qi deficiency syndrome and syndrome of both Qi and yin deficiency.

Components: Medicinal Evodia Fruit, Pepper Fruit, Chinese Gall, Clove, Atractylodes Rhizome, etc.

Usage: CV 8 is selected for application.

vii. Fang Gan Sachet (Han Xinmin)

Indication: children suffered from recurrent respiratory tract infection due to syndrome of lung-spleen qi deficiency.

Components: Atractylodes Rhizome, White Atractylodes Rhizome, GrassleafSweetflag Rhizome, Dahurian Angelica Root, Manchurian Wildginger and Bomeol.

Usage: the sachet is placed in a pocket next to skin in front of chest and beside pillow at night. It is replaced once every 10 days. It is used for consecutive 4 days.

VI. Typical medical records of famous physicians and experts

Medical record from Li Shaochuan——lung-spleen qi deficiency

Wang, male, 3 years and 8 months old.

Preliminary diagnosis: on February 1, 2004. The child usually had yellowish complexion and slim body, poor appetite and dry stool. He had a cold 8 times and pneumonia 2 times within one year. The child is a premature infant, who was easily infected once the weather slightly changed. During the diagnosis, he had symptoms of nasal discharge and cough (severe in the morning and evening), periumbilical abdominal pain sometimes, reddish tongue texture, thin and yellow tongue fur and floating, thin and weak pulse.

Diagnosis: recurrent respiratory tract infection with syndrome of lung-spleen qideficiency.

Syndrome differentiation: dysfunction of spleen in generation and transformation, lung qi failed to dispersion and purification and defense-exterior insecurity.

Therapeutic method: to ease, clear and regulate spleen-stomach.

Prescription: 5g Cablin Patchouli Herb, 3gIncised Notopterygium Rhizome and Root, 3gDoubleteeth Pubescent Angelica Root, 5gChinese Thorowax Root, 6gHogfennel Root, 5gOrange Fruit, 6gPlatycodon Root, 5gPinellia Tuber, 3gSichuan Lovage Rhizome, 5gDried Tangerine Peel, 5gPoria, 5g Magnolia Obavata, 5 g Red Peony Root, 5 g Largetrifoliolious Bugbane Rhizome, 3gPueraria, 5gMedicated Leaven and 3gLiquorice Root. There are 7 doses. 1 dose of decoction is taken by times in 2 days.

Second diagnosis: on February 5, 2005. Cough stopped, appetite increased, abdominal pain lost, dry stool, and thin and weak pulse. 3g Prepared Rhubarb was added to the previous prescription for continuing conditioning.

Third diagnosis: on March 6, 2005. Guardians of the child said that by 2-month conditioning with the previous prescription, the child had big appetite and stronger constitution. He totally took more than 40 doses, and didn't get a cold in nearly 1 year.

Note: the child suffered from lung-spleen qi deficiency, then constitution was weak, and easy to be infected. Critical factors of lung-spleen qi deficiency are spleen deficiency. Insufficient spleen qi, and mother-organ disorder involving its child-organ, then lung-spleen qi deficiency is occured. In treatment, we should not nourish spleen for spleen deficiency, and nourish lung for lung deficiency, but follow overall principle to adjust the transportation and transformation of body vital energy. Both the superficies of Taiyang, pivot of Shaoyang and interior of Yangmingintestines and stomach shall be taken into account. To sum up, it is suitable to invigorate spleen for spleen deficiency, rather than to nourish spleen, and disperse lung for deficient lung, rather than to reinforce lung.

The prescription is a modification of TianbaoCaiweiDecoction in*YoukeTiejing*. In the prescription, Cablin Patchouli Herb, Officinal Magnolia Bark, Dried Tangerine Peel, Pinellia Tuber and Medicated Leaven are fragrant, which dissolveturbidity; Bupleurum, Hogfennel Root, Platycodon Root and Orange Fruit relieve Shaoyang and ventilate lung qi; bitter and warm effects of Incised Notopterygium Rhizome and Root and Doubleteeth Pubescent Angelica Root are used to take care of Shaoyin kidney meridian and resolve exterior of Superficies of Taiyang; Sichuan Lovage Rhizome and Red Peony Root active blood and promote Qi, which are applicable for long illness into blood and obstructed Qi movement; Puerariaand Largetrifoliolious Bugbane Rhizome can rise Qi of Qingyang in spleen-stomach, ascendinglucidity and reducing turbidity, and harmonize nutrient and defense Qi.

VII. Prevention and aftercare

i. Prevention

(1) Keep environmental sanitation, avoid pollution, and keep indoor air circulating, do suitable outdoor activities, be exposed to sun more and inoculate for prevention on time.

(2) During an influenza epidemic, do not go to public places. When family members catch a cold, vinegar can be used to fumigate room;2~5ml vinegar is applied in per cubic meter of space, and 1~twice of water is added to the vinegar, and the mixture is placed in a container, then heated until all vinegar gasifies. Fumigation is carried out once every day, which shall last for 3~5 days.

(3) Avoid contacting with allergic substances.

ii. Aftercare

(1) Balanced and nutrient diet and no food preference.

(2) Avoid wind cold and cold air. Wipe away the sweat timely in the case of sweating much, especially when taking a bath.

(LI Xinmin)

References

[1] Ma R, Han XM. Pediatrics of Chinese medicine [M]. 2th ed. Beijing: People's Medical Publishing House, 2012.

[2] Wang SC, Yu JM. Clinical study on pediatrics of Chinese medicine in Postgraduate Planning Textbook of National higher institutions of Chinese medicine [M]. Beijing: People's Medical Publishing House, 2009.

[3] Zhao SY, Hu YJ, Chen HZ. The clinical definition and therapeutic principle of recurrent respiratory tract infection [J]. Chinese Journal of Pediatrics, 2008, 46(2): 108-110.

[4] Ma R, Li SC. Pediatrics Experience Set [M]. Beijing: People's Medical Publishing House, 2013.

[5] Ma R, Wang PF, Zheng YM, et al. Clinical study of children recurrent respiratory tract infection treated with Fanggan Mixture [J]. Integrated Traditional Chinese and Western Medicine, 1991, 11(10): 592-594.

[6] Zhang ZQ, Yu JE. Several cases of Yu Jianer treating pediatric diseases with syndrome differentiation and treatment [J]. Shanghai Journal of Traditional Chinese Medicine, 2011, 45 (10): 16-17.

[7] Song TD, Li H, Wang XF, et al. Clinical observation of 50 children recurrent respiratory tract infection treated with Zhuang'er Granules[J]. Journal of Traditional Chinese Medicine, 2006, 47(12): 917-919.

[8] Liu CQ, Han XM. Clinical observation of 68 children recurrent respiratory tract infection treated with Ginseng and AstragalusRoot-ConsolidatingDecoction and Fanggan Sachet[J]. Journal of Emergency in Traditional Chinese Medicine, 2013, 22(6): 900-901.

[9] Chen W, Wang LN, Yang Y. Experience on nursing and prevention with Chinese medicine of children recurrent respiratory tract infection from Professor Wang Lining [J].Chinese Pediatrics of Integrated Traditional and Western Medicine, 2010, 2(6): 491-493.